Thomas

Foreplay – Jazz

Mosby's
Q&A
for
NCLEX-RN

Questions,
Answers, &
Rationales

Ms. Lee
274-2898

Robin Robertson

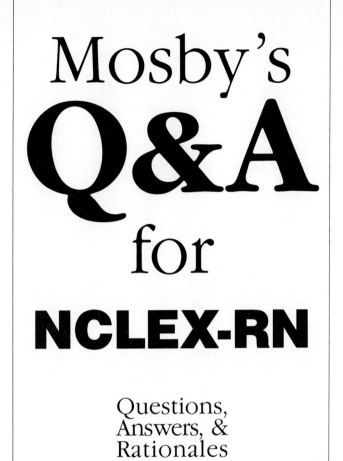

Mosby's Q&A for NCLEX-RN

Questions,
Answers, &
Rationales

Editor

DOLORES F. SAXTON, RN, BS IN ED, MA, EdD

Associate Editors

PHYLLIS K. PELIKAN, RN, AAS, BS, MA
PATRICIA M. NUGENT, RN, AAS, BS, MS, EdM, EdD
SELMA R. NEEDLEMAN, RN, BA, MA

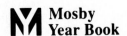

Mosby
Year Book

St. Louis   Baltimore   Boston   Chicago   London   Philadelphia   Sydney   Toronto

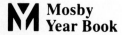

**Mosby
Year Book**

Dedicated to Publishing Excellence

Editor: Nancy L. Coon
Senior developmental editor: Susan R. Epstein
Project manager: John A. Rogers
Production editor: Ann E. Mannle
Designer: Susan E. Lane

Printed in the United States of America

Mosby–Year Book, Inc.
11830 Westline Industrial Drive
St. Louis, MO 63146

Library of Congress Cataloging in Publication Data

Mosby's Q & A for NCLEX-RN: questions, answers, and rationales/
   editor, Dolores F. Saxton; associate editors, Phyllis K. Pelikan,
   Patricia M. Nugent, Selma R. Needleman.
       p.   cm.
   ISBN 0-8016-5211-1
   1. Nursing—Examinations, questions, etc.   I. Saxton, Dolores F.
II. Title: Mosby's Q and A for NCLEX-RN.
   [DNLM: 1. Nursing—examination questions.   WY 18 M89445]
RT55.M65   1990
610.73'076—dc20
DNLM/DLC
for Library of Congress   90-13341
                                                        CIP

C/VH/VH   9   8   7   6   5   4   3   2

CONTRIBUTORS

JUDITH E. BEYER, R.N., B.S.N.E., M.S., Ph.D.
University of Colorado,
Denver, Colorado

AGNES BIEGEL, R.N., B.S., M.S., A.N.P.
University of Northern Colorado,
Greeley, Colorado

JOAN CERNIGLIA-LOWENSEN, R.N., B.S.N., M.S.N.
Union Memorial Hospital,
Baltimore, Maryland

ANNIE SUE CLIFT, R.N., B.S.N., M.R.E., M.N.
University of Tennessee,
Martin, Tennessee

SHERRILYN COFFMAN, R.N., D.N.S.
Florida Atlantic University,
Boca Raton, Florida

GERALDINE C. COLOMBRARO, R.N., B.S.N., M.A.
Consultant, Nursing Education,
Brewster, New York

MARY A. CROSLEY, R.N., B.S., M.S.
Suffolk County Community College,
Brentwood, New York

PENELOPE L. DANIELS, R.N., A.D.N., B.S., B.S.N., M.S.
St. Mary's Hospital School of Nursing,
Huntington, West Virginia

PHYLLIS E. DAWE, R.N., B.S., M.S.
Ona M. Wilcox School of Nursing,
Middlesex Memorial Hospital,
Middletown, Connecticut

GWEN M. DEAN, R.N., B.S.N., M.A.
Prairie State College,
Chicago Heights, Illinois

SUSAN NABHOLZ DENYS, R.N., B.S.N., M.S.N., R.N.C., A.C.C.E.
University of Arkansas,
Little Rock, Arkansas

ELIZABETH FALSETTI DICHIARA, R.N., B.S.N., M.S.Ed., M.S.
Niagara University,
Niagara University, New York

SHIRLEY A. DUFRESNE, R.N., B.S., M.S.
Southeastern Massachusetts University,
North Dartmouth, Massachusetts

CARMEL A. ESPOSITO, R.N., B.S.N., M.S.N.
Ohio Valley Hospital School of Nursing,
Steubenville, Ohio

JANICE COOKE FEIGENBAUM, R.N., B.S., M.S.N.
D'Youville College,
Buffalo, New York

JOANN FESTA, R.N., A.A.S, B.S., M.S., Ph.D.
Nassau Community College,
Garden City, New York

CAROL FLAUGHER, R.N., B.S., M.S.
State University of New York at Buffalo,
Buffalo, New York

MARIE FLICKINGER, R.N., B.S., M.S.
Clark Technical College,
Springfield, Ohio

ROBERT R. GWYDIR, B.S., M.A., Ph.D.
Nassau Community College,
Garden City, New York

RITA M. HAMMER, R.N., B.S., M.A.
Quinnipiac College,
Hamden, Connecticut

LYNDA HARRISON, R.N., B.S.N., M.S.N., Ph.D.
University of Tennessee,
Knoxville, Tennessee

MARY ANN HELLMER, R.N., A.A.S., B.S., M.S., Ph.D.
Nassau Community College,
Garden City, New York

CAROL J. HILL, R.N., M.S.
University of North Dakota,
Grand Forks, North Dakota

ANNETTE H. HUTCHERSON, R.N., B.S.N., M.N., Ed.D.
Mississippi Gulf Coast Junior College,
Gautier, Mississippi

JANET T. IHLENFELD, R.N., B.S.N., M.S.N., Ph.D.
D'Youville College,
Buffalo, New York

FRANCES S. IZZO, R.N., A.A.S., B.S.N., M.S.N.
Nassau Community College,
Garden City, New York

NANCY A. JACKSON, R.N., B.S., M.N.Ed., Ph.D.
West Virginia Wesleyan College,
Buckhannon, West Virginia

GRACE G. JOHNSON, R.N., M.S.N.E.
Houston Baptist University,
Houston, Texas

BERNADETTE KAHLER, R.N., M.N.
Kansas Newman College,
Wichita, Kansas

CHRISTINA ALGIERE KASPRISIN, R.N., M.S.
University of Oklahoma,
Tulsa, Oklahoma

LAURIE GASPARI KAUDEWITZ, R.N., B.S.N., M.S.N.,
   R.N.C.
East Tennessee State University,
Johnson City, Tennessee

CAROLE KENNER, R.N., B.S.N., M.S.N., D.N.S
University of Cincinnati,
Cincinnati, Ohio

DOROTHY L. KOELBL, R.N., B.S., M.S
University of Kentucky;
Henderson Community College,
Henderson, Kentucky

MARY R. KOLBE, R.N., B.S.N., M.S.N.
University of Nebraska,
Lincoln, Nebraska

SHELIA M. KYLE, R.N., A.A.S., B.S.N., M.S., M.S.N.
St. Mary's Hospital School of Nursing,
Huntington, West Virginia

CAROLE LABBY, R.N., B.S.N., M.S.
College of the Mainland,
Texas City, Texas

PATRICIA A. LADEWIG, R.N., B.S., M.S.N., N.P.
Loretto Heights College,
Denver, Colorado

ELAINE C. LAMBERT, R.N., M.S.N., C.C.R.N.
University of Tulsa,
Tulsa, Oklahoma

NANCY LATTERNER, R.N., A.A.S., B.S., M.A.
Nassau Community College,
Garden City, New York

JUNE LAWRY, R.N., B.S.N., M.Ed., M.S.N., C.P.N.P.
Maryland League of Nursing Board Reviewer,
Baltimore, Maryland

KAREN LEHMANN, R.N., B.S., M.S.
State University of New York at Farmingdale,
Farmingdale, New York

BONNIE B. LUNDQUIST, R.N., B.S.N., M.S.N.
Husson College;
Eastern Maine Medical Center,
Bangor, Maine

BARBARA C. MARTIN, R.N., B.S.N., M.S.
University of Tulsa,
Tulsa, Oklahoma

MARGARET MASSONI, R.N., B.S.N., M.S.N.
New York City Technical College,
Brooklyn, New York

JUDITH A. MCDONAGH, R.N., M.S.N., M.S.
Simmons College,
Boston, Massachusetts

KATHY MCSHANE, R.N., M.S.
Itawamba Junior College,
Fulton, Mississippi

CATHERINE MECHLING, R.N., B.S.N., M.Ed.
Citizens General Hospital School of Nursing,
New Kensington, Pennsylvania

DIANE MELANCON, R.N., A.D.N., B.S.N., M.S.N.
San Antonio College,
San Antonio, Texas

MARY DE MENESES, R.N. B.S.N., M.A., M.S., Ed.D
Southern Illinois University at Edwardsville,
Edwardsville, Illinois

RUTH ANN MILLER, R.N., B.S.N., M.S.N.Ed., Ph.D.
University of Pittsburgh,
Pittsburgh, Pennsylvania

JEANNE M. MILLETT, R.N., B.S., M.S., F.N.P., Ed.D.
Albany Medical Center Hospital;
Lifestar Regional Trauma System,
Albany, New York

MARILYN M. MOHR, R.N., B.S.N., M.S.N.
Lutheran Medical Center School of Nursing,
St. Louis, Missouri

RITA L. MONSEN, R.N., M.S.N., M.P.H.
Henderson State University,
Arkadelphia, Arkansas

ANNA P. MOORE, R.N., B.S.N., M.S.
Petersburg General Hospital School of Nursing,
Petersburg, Virginia

KAREN R. MOORE, R.N., B.S.N., M.S.N.
Cedar Crest College,
Allentown, Pennsylvania

THERESA A. MORAN, R.N., A.A.S., B.S., Ed.M.
Nassau Community College,
Garden, City, New York

ANN T. MULLER, R.N., M.S., M.Ed., Ph.D.
Private Practice,
Dallas, Texas

EILEEN NAHIGIAN, R.N., M.N.
Community College of Philadelphia,
Philadelphia, Pennsylvania

AYDA G. NAMBAYAN, R.N., B.S.N., M.Ed
University of Alabama,
Birmingham, Alabama

DORIS E. NICHOLAS, R.N., M.S., Ph.D.
Howard University,
Washington, D.C.

KATHLEEN M. NOKES, R.N., M.A.
Nursing Consultant,
New York, New York

NEIL J. NUGENT, A.A.S., B.S., M.B.A., M.S.W.
Nassau Community College,
Garden City, New York

PATRICIA A. NUTZ, R.N., B.S., B.S.N., M.A.
St. Francis Hospital School of Nursing,
New Castle, Pennsylvania

LEAH F. OAKLEY, R.N., A.D.N., B.S.N., M.S.N.
University of Alabama,
Huntsville, Alabama

MARGARET PARSONS, R.N., B.S.N., M.N.
Emory University,
Atlanta, Georgia

ELIZABETH T. PAYNE, R.N., B.S.N., M.S.N.
Henderson Community College,
Henderson, Kentucky

JOSEPH E. PELLICIA, B.A., M.A.
Nassau Community College,
Garden City, New York

NORMA NOLAN PINNELL, R.N., B.S.N., M.S.N.
Southern Illinois University at Edwardsville,
Edwardsville, Illinois

KAREN L. RADTKE, R.N., B.S.N., B.A., M.S.N.
St. Mary's College,
Minneapolis, Minnesota

BARBARA A. REDDING, R.N., M.S.N., Ed.D.
University of South Florida,
Tampa, Florida

LENORE D. REILLY, R.N., A.A.S., B.A., M.A.
Nassau Community College,
Garden City, New York

BRENDA RILEY, R.N., B.S., M.S.
Troy State University,
Troy, Alabama

LINDA OWEN RIMER, R.N., B.S.N., M.S.E.
University of Arkansas at Little Rock,
Little Rock, Arkansas

JOYCE A. ROBERSON, R.N., B.S.N., M.A., Ph.D.
Coe College,
Cedar Rapids, Iowa

JUDITH ROBINSON, R.N., B.S.N., M.S.E.
Baptist Memorial Hospital System,
School of Nursing, San Antonio, Texas

MARY ANN S. ROGERS, R.N., B.S.N., M.S.N.
Medical College of Georgia,
Augusta, Georgia

KATHLEEN S. ROSE, R.N., B.S.N.
Good Samaritan Hospital School of Nursing,
Cincinnati, Ohio

JANICE J. RUMFELT, R.N., M.S.N., R.N.C.
Southern Illinois University at Edwardsville,
Edwardsville, Illinois

DEBORAH LEKAN RUTLEDGE, R.N., M.S.N.
University of North Carolina,
Chapel Hill, North Carolina

MARY DAVIES SHANNAHAN, R.N., B.S.N., M.N., Ph.D.
Florida State University,
Tallahassee, Florida

CONNIE JOZWIAK SHIELDS R.N., B.S., M.S.
Niagara University,
Niagara University, New York

RAELENE V. SHIPPEE-RICE, R.N., B.S.N., M.S.
University of New Hampshire,
Durham, New Hampshire

CYNTHIA C. SMALL, R.N., B.S.N., M.S.N.
Lake Michigan College,
Benton Harbor, Michigan

MAXINE KAVEL SMATLAK, R.N., B.S.N., M.N., C.S.
Indiana University of Pennsylvania,
Indiana, Pennsylvania

ARLENE P. STEIN, R.N., B.S.N., M.S.N., Ph.D.
Weber State College,
Ogden, Utah

MARLENE K. STRADER, R.N., B.S.N., M.S.N.
Southern Illinois University at Edwardsville,
Edwardsville, Illinois

PATRICIA SZCZECH, R.N., B.S., M.A.
Ohio Wesleyan University,
Delaware, Ohio

PATRICIA R. TEASLEY, R.N., A.D.N., B.S.N., M.S.N., C.S.
Southern Union State Junior College,
Valley, Alabama

MARITA G. TITLER, R.N., M.A.
Coe College,
Cedar Rapids, Iowa

SR. JUDITH VANDERVEEN, R.N., B.S.N., M.A.
Washtenaw Community College,
Ann Arbor, Michigan

JUDITH A. VAN DOREN, R.N., B.S., M.Ed., M.S.N.
Good Samaritan Hospital School of Nursing,
Cincinnati, Ohio

CAROLYN H. WALTZER, R.N., B.S.N., B.A., M.A.
Parkersburg Community College,
Parkersburg, West Virginia

MARGARET T. WARREN, R.N., B.A., B.S., M.A., M.S.
Rockland Community College,
Suffern, New York

ALICE JEAN WILLIAMS, R.N., B.S., M.S.N., Ph.D.
MacMurray College,
Jacksonville, Illinois

DEBORAH WILLIAMS, R.N., A.S.N., B.A., M.S.N.
Western Kentucky University,
Bowling Green, Kentucky

SUE RODWELL WILLIAMS, R.D., M.R.Ed., M.P.H., Ph.D.
SRW Production Inc.,
Berkeley, California

FRANCES A. WOLLNER, R.N., B.S., B.S.N., M.N.
Niagara University,
Niagara University, New York

WANDA LEE WOOTON, R.N., B.S.N., M.A.Ed.
Eastern Kentucky University,
Richmond, Kentucky

JACQUELINE C. ZALUMAS, R.N., B.S.N., M.N.
Emory University,
Atlanta, Georgia

PATRICIA E. ZANDER, R.N., B.S.N., M.S.N., R.N.C.
Viterbo College,
La Crosse, Wisconsin

Preface

This book was developed to meet the requests of students for "still more questions with answers and rationales." We believe that, along with our other publications, **Mosby's Comprehensive Review of Nursing** and **Mosby's AssessTest,** this text completes the third leg of a strong tripod of study, self-evaluation, and review material on which students can base their study and review for both coursework and the NCLEX–RN.

The questions in the medical-surgical, maternity, pediatric, and psychiatric chapters and the two integrated comprehensive examinations incorporate material from the basic sciences, nutrition, pharmacology, and rehabilitation. We have presented the questions in traditional clinical groupings, for we believe that even in preparing for the NCLEX–RN, an integrated examination, most students will need to study all the distinct parts before attempting to put them together.

For every question in the clinical chapters, as well as the questions in the comprehensive examinations, the reasons why the incorrect answers are incorrect, as well as why the correct answer is correct, are included. In addition, each question has been analyzed as to the level of difficulty, the clinical area, the step in the nursing process, the area of client needs, and the category of concern (specific content).

All the questions in this book were developed by outstanding educators and practitioners of nursing. Initially the editorial panel reviewed all questions, selecting the most pertinent for inclusion in a mass field-testing project. Students graduating from baccalaureate, associate degree, and diploma nursing programs in various locations in the United States and Canada provided a diverse testing group. The results were statistically analyzed. This analysis was used to select questions for inclusion in this book and to determine each question's level of difficulty.

We would like to take this opportunity to express our sincere appreciation to our many colleagues for their contributions; to Edith Augustson for her careful processing of the manuscript; to our editors, Nancy Coon and Susan Epstein, for their assistance and support; and most of all to our families for their love, understanding, and encouragement.

Dolores F. Saxton
Patricia M. Nugent
Phyllis K. Pelikan
Selma R. Needleman

CONTENTS

CHAPTER 1

Preparing for the Licensure Examination

Introduction

Licensure examinations in the United States and Canada have been integrated and comprehensive for many years. Nursing candidates in both countries are required to answer questions that necessitate a recognition and understanding of the physiologic, biologic, and social sciences, as well as the specific nursing skills and abilities involved in a given client situation.

Both the United States and the Canadian tests contain objective multiple-choice questions. To answer the questions appropriately, a candidate needs to understand and correlate certain aspects of anatomy and physiology, the behavioral sciences, basic nursing, the effects of medications administered, the client's attitude toward illness, and other pertinent factors (e.g., legal responsibilities). Most questions are based on nursing situations similar to those with which candidates have had experience, because both the United States and Canada emphasize the nursing care of clients with representative common national health problems. Some questions, however, require candidates to apply basic principles and techniques to clinical situations with which they have had little if any actual experience.

To prepare adequately for an integrated comprehensive examination, it is necessary to understand the discrete parts that compose the universe under consideration. This is one of the major principles of learning on which our review and study materials have been developed.

Using this concept, this text first presents for each major clinical area questions that test the student's knowledge of principles and theories underlying nursing care in a variety of situations (acute, critical, and long term), in a variety of settings (acute care hospitals, nursing homes, and the community), and with a variety of nursing goals (preventive, curative, palliative, and restorative). The book concludes with two integrated comprehensive tests reflecting the licensing examinations. In other words, the questions require the student to cross clinical disciplines and respond to individual and specific needs associated with given health problems.

Answers to all of the questions, as well as rationales supporting the correct answers, are provided. Explanations are also presented to document why the other choices are inappropriate. Reviewing the rationales enables the student to verify information and reinforce knowledge.

How to Use This Book in Studying

A. Start in one clinical area. Answer all of the questions in the area. Record the answer by filling in the circle of the number you believe is correct. Do not worry if you select the same numbered answer repeatedly; there is usually no pattern to the answers.

B. As you answer each question, write a few words about why you think that answer was correct; in other words, justify why you selected the answer.

C. If you guess at an answer in this book, you should make a special mark to identify it. This will permit you to recognize areas that need further review. It will also help you to see how correct your "guessing" can be.

D. Tear out the sheets with answers and rationales for the area you are reviewing and compare your answers with those provided. If you answered the item correctly, check your reason for selecting the answer with the rationale presented. If you answered the item incorrectly, read the rationale to determine why the one you selected was incorrect. In addition, you should review the correct answer and rationale for each item answered incorrectly. If you still do not understand your mistake, look up the theory pertaining to these questions. You should carefully review all questions and rationales for items you identified as guesses, because you did not have mastery of the material being questioned.

E. Following the rationale for the correct answer you will find a letter—*a*, *b*, or *c*—in parentheses. These letters indicate the level of difficulty of the question and reflect the percentage of tested students answering the question correctly. These can serve as a guide in your studying. (See the sample questions on page 3.)

1. The letter *a* signifies that 75% or more—but less than 89%—of the students in the testing group answered the question correctly. Sample question 3 is an *a* level question.

2. The letter *b* signifies that 50% or more—but less than 75%—of the students in the testing group answered the question correctly. Sample questions 1 and 2 are *b* level questions.

3. The letter *c* signifies that more than 25% but less than 50% of the students in the testing group answered the question correctly. Sample questions 4 and 5 are *c* level questions.

4. Questions that 89% or more or 25% or less of the students in the testing group answered correctly were not included in the book.

F. In addition to the level of difficulty of the question, you will also find a grouping of letters that classify the question according to four categories: Clinical area; Nursing process; Client need; and Category of concern. This series of letters will always appear in the same order for each question in the book. The following descriptions and the five sample questions on p. (3) are presented to assist the reader in understanding and reviewing these classifications.

Clinical area *(reflects the specialized area of nursing knowledge)*

1. **Medicine (ME).** These questions include the care of adult clients who have health problems that do not require surgical intervention or invasive techniques. Sample question 1 is a *medical nursing* question.

2. **Surgery (SU).** These questions include care of adult clients with health problems that require surgical intervention or invasive techniques. Sample question 5 is a *surgical nursing* question.

3. **Maternity (OB).** These questions include the care of clients preparing for or experiencing childbirth. Sample question 2 is a *maternity nursing* question.

4. **Pediatrics (PE).** These questions include the care of clients from birth to young adulthood. Sample question 4 is a *pediatric nursing* question.

5. **Psychiatry (PS).** These questions include the care of clients experiencing emotional stress with or without overt psychiatric behavior in all settings. Sample question 3 is a *psychiatric nursing* question.

Phases of the nursing process *(reflects types of behaviors of the nurse)*

1. **Assessment (AS).** The assessment phase requires the nurse to obtain objective and subjective data from primary and secondary sources, to identify and group significant data, and to communicate this information to other members of the health team. The information necessary for making nursing decisions is obtained through assessment. Sample question 1 is an *assessment* question.

2. **Analysis (AN).** This phase requires the nurse to interpret data gathered during the assessment phase. A nursing diagnosis must be made, client and family needs identified, and both short-term and long-term goals set to meet the identified needs. Sample question 2 is an *analysis* question.

3. **Planning (PL).** The planning phase requires the nurse to design a regimen with the client and family to achieve goals set during the analysis phase. It also requires setting priorities for nursing intervention. Sample question 3 is a *planning* question.

4. **Implementation (IM).** The implementation phase requires the nurse to provide care designed during the planning phase. The client may be given total care or may be assisted and encouraged to perform activities of daily living or follow the regimen prescribed by the physician. Implementation also includes activities such as counseling, teaching, and supervising. Sample question 4 is an *implementation* question.

5. **Evaluation (EV).** This phase requires the nurse to determine the effectiveness of nursing care. The goals of care are reviewed, the client's response to intervention identified, and a consideration made as to whether the client has achieved the predetermined goals. Evaluation also includes appraisal of the client's compliance with the health plan. Sample question 5 is an *evaluation* question.

Client need *(reflects the health care need of the client that must be addressed by the nurse)*

1. **Support and promotion of physiologic and anatomic equilibrium (PA).** Meeting this need includes reducing risks that interfere with physiologic or anatomic integrity, promoting comfort and mobility, and providing basic care to assist, modify, or limit physiologic and anatomic adaptations. Sample questions 1 and 5 reflect this need.

2. **An environment that is safe and conducive to effective therapeutic care (TC).** The nurse must provide quality, goal-directed care that is coordinated, safe, and effective. Sample question 4 reflects this need.

3. **Education and other forms of health promotion to prevent, minimize, or correct actual or potential health problems (ED).** Fulfilling this need involves supporting optimal growth and development to provide for the achievement of the highest levels of functioning. This includes encouraging use of support systems and self-care directed toward promoting the prevention, recognition, and treatment of disease throughout the life cycle. Sample question 3 reflects this need.

4. **Support and promotion of psychosocial and emotional equilibrium (PE).** Addressing this need includes supporting individual emotional coping and adapting mechanisms to promote optimal emotional health while limiting or modifying those responses to crises that produce psychopathologic consequences. Sample question 2 reflects this need.

Category of concern *(reflects the specific content area within the broad clinical area from which the material in the question has been drawn)*

1. **Medical, Surgical, and Pediatric Nursing**
   Blood and immunity (BI)
   Cardiovascular (CV)
   Drug-related responses (DR)
   Emotional crisis related to health problems (EC)
   Endocrine (EN)
   Fluid and electrolyte (FE)
   Gastrointestinal (GI)
   Growth and development (GD)
   Integumentary (IT)
   Neuromuscular (NM)
   Respiratory (RE)
   Reproductive and genitourinary (RG)
   Skeletal (SK)

2. **Maternity Nursing**
   Drug-related responses (DR)
   Emotional crisis related to childbearing (EC)
   Fertility, sterility, and family planning (FS)
   High-risk newborn (HN)

High-risk pregnancy (HP)
Intrapartal period (IP)
Normal neonate (NN)
Postpartal period (PP)
Prenatal period (PN)

3. Psychiatric Nursing
Anxiety, somatoform, and dissociative disorders (AX)
Crisis situations (CS)
Disorders first evident before adulthood (BA)
Disorders of mood (MO)
Disorders of personality (PR)
Drug-related responses (DR)
Organic disorders (OR)
Schizophrenic disorders (SD)
Substance abuse (SA)
Therapeutic relationships (TR)

SAMPLE QUESTIONS:

1. On a routine physical, Philip Monroe is found to have a blood pressure of 150/96, and hypertension is suspected. In obtaining the health history, an early sign of hypertension that the nurse should expect Mr. Monroe to complain of is:
   ① Swollen ankles
   ② Recent weight loss
   ③ Palpitations of the heart
   ④ Early morning headaches
   [Correct answer is # 4. (b) (ME; AS; PA; CV)]

2. For a woman, identification with the parenting role begins:
   ① Early in life
   ② During adolescence
   ③ When pregnancy is confirmed
   ④ After the baby has been born
   [Correct answer is # 1. (b) (OB; AN; PE; EC)]

3. Michael Jones, age 19, has a history of an antisocial personality disorder. Mr. and Mrs. Jones tell the nurse that their son is very manipulative and causes havoc in their home. The nurse should include in the teaching plan ways that they can cope with their son by using an approach that is:
   ① Rigid
   ② Flexible
   ③ Accepting
   ④ Consistent
   [Correct answer is # 4. (a) (PS; PL; ED; PR)]

4. Margaret Webster, age 3, is admitted for surgery. When her mother leaves, she begins to sob. The nurse should:
   ① Tell her to be a big girl, her mother will be right back
   ② Put up the side rails on the crib and let her calm down by herself
   ③ Distract her with her teddy, expecting her to forget her mother has gone

   ④ Hold her and explain that her mother had to go but will return in the morning
   [Correct answer is # 3. (c) (PE; IM; TC; GD)]

5. Following a mastectomy, Ada Boles is prescribed tamoxifen (Nolvadex). The nurse knows that Mrs. Boles understands the teaching about this drug when she states, "I will:
   ① Drink 4 glasses of milk every day while I am taking this drug."
   ② Expect pain at the site of the tumor when I take this drug."
   ③ Take a stool softener every day while I am taking this medication."
   ④ Rise from a sitting position slowly when I am taking this medication."
   [Correct answer is # 2. (c) (SU; EV; PA; DR)]

G. A few days later, review the area again. If you miss the same question a second time, you need further study of the material.

H. After you have completed the clinical area questions, begin taking the comprehensive tests; they will assist you in applying knowledge and principles from the specific clinical area to any nursing situation. Take each of these examinations under conditions as closely approximating those of the licensure examination as possible.
   1. Arrange a quiet, uninterrupted, 1½ hour time span for each test in the comprehensive tests.
   2. Pace yourself during the testing period; allow about 1 minute per question.
   3. Do not rush.
   4. Answer every question.

I. To help analyze your mistakes on the comprehensive examinations and to provide a data base for making future study plans, two types of worksheets are included. One is designed to aid you in identifying and recording errors in the way you process information. The other is to help you identify and record gaps in knowledge. These worksheets follow the Answers and Rationales for each test on the Comprehensive Examinations and are on tear-out sheets.

J. After completing your worksheets, do the following:
   1. Use Worksheet 1 to identify the frequency with which you made particular errors. As you review material in class notes or study material such as *Mosby's Comprehensive Review of Nursing*, pay special attention to correcting your most common problems.
   2. Use Worksheet 2 to identify the topics you want to review. It might be helpful to set priorities; review the most difficult topics first so that you will have time to review them more than once.

K. Use this opportunity to learn from your mistakes.
   1. Because you receive immediate feedback on your performance, you have an excellent opportunity to learn from your mistakes. Answer every question. Do not leave any ques-

tions unanswered; use educated or pure guesses.

2. The mistakes you make on the questions in this book will be as valuable to you as the confident feeling you get from answering correctly.

Readiness for the Licensure Examination

A few individuals can improve their scores significantly by a highly concentrated period of study immediately before taking an examination. Most, however, profit by spreading their review over a much longer period of time. Cramming will not help. Identification of your own specific strengths and weaknesses should eliminate much of the anxiety of deciding what material to study by giving you a sense of direction and a means of setting priorities.

A. *Reduce stress*

Stress is a part of life. Although there is no way to prevent it, it is possible to reduce it by diffusing your emotional responses before stress gets the better of you. Controlling stress allows you to use it instead of being abused by it.

1. Talk it out, but try to talk it out with someone who is not as stressed as you are. This helps relieve the burden of coping alone and helps put things in perspective. Try talking with people who have had the same experience and understand what you are going through.

2. Obtain as much information as you can. **STUDY!!!**

3. Keep fit. Good nutrition, regular exercise, and ample sleep help.

4. Try relaxation exercises. Relaxation is essential to reduce stress.

5. Sort out the important things. Take stock of your strengths. Set realistic deadlines. Drop the non-essentials.

6. Spend time on yourself and your needs outside of nursing.

7. Be greedy and put yourself first. Be flexible with yourself. Do not set rigid, unmanageable goals.

8. Discover your positive defenses and use them.

B. *Manage test-taking time*

Since most examinations have specified time limits, you will need to pace yourself during the practice testing period, working as quickly and accurately as possible. It is helpful to estimate the time you can spend on each item and still complete the examination in the allotted time. You can obtain this figure by dividing the testing time by the number of items on the test. For example, with a 1½-hour (90-minute) testing period and 93 or 94 items, an average of 1 minute per item will be the appropriate pace.

Although certain questions will be more difficult than others and will require more time, spending too much time on these difficult items may compromise your overall score. Make a mark next to the item you cannot answer and go on. After you have answered all the questions you can answer easily, return to the marked items. Be sure to erase any extraneous marks near your answers. If time remains, it is useful to review all your answers, making sure you have marked them correctly.

Do not be pressured into finishing early. Do not rush! Students who achieve higher scores are typically those who use all the time available.

C. *Build test-taking confidence*

You should feel confident and competent if you have studied and reviewed the content to be tested and you are armed with methods for reading and answering questions. Your emotional state is vitally important when thinking about, preparing for, and taking any test. Think positively.

While you are taking the test, you may have problems with a question. Move on to another that you can answer. Anxiety about a difficult question may block the recall of familiar information required to answer other questions. Do not waste time and emotional energy when positive reinforcement and increased effectiveness can be gained by answering the questions you can manage comfortably.

If you come across a question containing material you have not reviewed, do not stop to think about gaps in your preparation. Move on and return to the question later. Questions that seem complicated at first glance can often be answered with the "educated guess." Remain calm and confident.

If you follow these suggestions, you will find that this practice test-taking experience, which is similar to the licensure examination, will give you confidence for the actual examination. After you have completed studying in this book, you may wish to take a simulated examination such as **Mosby's AssessTest** before you take the licensure examination. The **AssessTest** is a computer-scored, multiple-choice examination designed to test nursing knowledge and evaluate your ability to apply that knowledge in clinical situations. The extensive computer analysis of your performance, which is the most outstanding feature of this test, will help you design effective and efficient plans for further study and review.

Taking the Licensure Examination

In the United States, the licensure-examination for professional nursing is composed of approximately 372 multiple-choice questions, of which 300 are counted and 72+ are being pretested. The overall difficulty rate of the questions on the examination is between 65% and 75%.

All five steps of the nursing process are equally represented, with a variety of questions from each of the clinical areas. There appears to be a deemphasis in the areas of obstetric nursing and severe mental illness. There seems to be a greater emphasis on medical-surgical principles and interpersonal skills, especially communication. In the category of client health care needs, approximately 42% to 48% of the questions reflect support and promotion of physiologic and anatomic equilibrium; 25% to 31% reflect the need for a therapeutic environment; 12% to 18% reflect the need for education and health promotion; and 9% to 15% reflect the need for support and promotion of psychosocial and emotional equilibrium. The licensing examination is given over a 2-day period. The score is reported as pass or fail.

The most crucial requisite for doing well on the licensure examination is a sound understanding of the subject and a high level of reading comprehension. Determination to do well and a degree of confidence will further enhance the well-prepared individual's chance of earning a high score and achieving the recognition deserved.

At least three other requirements must be met if an individual's performance is to accurately reflect professional competence. First, the candidate must follow explicitly the directions given by the examiner and those printed at the beginning of each test, as well as any that refer to a specified group of questions. Second, the candidate must read each question carefully before deciding how to answer it. Third, the candidate must record the answers in the space and manner specified.

Some candidates find it helpful to glance over the entire test before starting to answer questions. This enables them to answer questions in the order most efficient and comfortable for them. Others find it better to go through the test answering all questions they are sure of first and then going back to the more difficult ones.

The score on the test is the number of questions answered correctly; there is no deduction for incorrect answers. You are not penalized for guessing. Do not leave an answer blank. You have a 1 in 4 (25%) chance of guessing the correct answer. Do not mark more than one answer for each question, because questions with more than one mark will be scored as incorrect. Remember; you do not have to answer all the questions correctly to pass.

Test-Taking Skills

Test-taking skills and techniques are not a substitute for good study habits or an adequate grasp of the content and abilities measured in an examination. Memorization is of little help because few questions are simple recall and most require the use of higher, more complex thought processes. If you have a thorough understanding of the knowledge measured in an examination, however, good test-taking skills will enhance your overall performance.

The question in its entirety is called a test item. The portion of the test item that poses the ques-

tion or problem is called the stem. Potential answers to the question or problem posed are called options. In well-constructed multiple-choice items there is only one correct answer among the options supplied; the incorrect options are called distractors. Remember that test questions are meant to measure your nursing knowledge. The items may be easy to read, but the answers to questions are not intended to be readily apparent. The questions draw on your ability to apply nursing knowledge from a variety of sources.

·Read Questions Carefully

Scores on written tests are strongly affected by reading ability. In answering a test item, you should begin by carefully reading the stem and then asking yourself the following questions:

What is the question really asking?

Are there any key words?

What information relevant to answering this question is included in the stem?

How would I ask this question in my own words?

How would I answer this question in my own words?

After you have answered these questions, carefully read the options and then ask yourself the following questions:

Is there an option that is similar to the one I thought of?

Is this option the best, most complete answer to the question?

Deal with the question as it is stated, without reading anything into it or making assumptions about it. Answer the question asked, not the one you would like to answer. For simple recall items the self-questioning process will usually be completed quickly. For more complex items the self-questioning process may take longer, but it should assist you in clarifying the item and selecting the best response.

·Identify Key Words

Certain key words in the stem, the options, or both should alert you to the need for caution in choosing your answer. Because few things in life are absolute without exception, avoid selecting answers that include words such as *always, never, all, every, only, must, no, except, and none,* since answers containing these key words are rarely correct. They place special limitations and qualifications on potentially correct answers. For example:

All of the following are services of the National Kidney Foundation except:

1. *Public education programs*
2. *Fund-raising affairs for research activities*
3. *Research about kidney disease*
4. *Identification of potential transplant recipients*

This stem contains two key words; *all* and *except.* They limit the correct answer choice to the one option that does not represent a service of the National Kidney Foundation. When *except, not,* or a phrase such as *all but one of the following* appears in the stem, the inappropriate option is the correct answer—in this instance, option 4. If the options in an item do not seem to make sense because more than one option is correct, reread the question; you may have missed one of the key words in the stem. Also be on guard when you see one of the key words in an option; it may limit the context in which such an option would be correct.

•Pay Attention to Specific Details

The well-written multiple-choice question is precisely stated, providing you with only the information needed to make the question or problem clear and specific. Careful reading of details in the stem can provide important clues to the correct option. For example:

Mr. Daniels is told that he will no longer be able to ingest alcohol if he wants to live. To effect a change in his behavior while he is in the hospital, the nurse should attempt to:

1. *Discuss the pathophysiology of the liver with him*
2. *Discuss his hopes and dreams for the future*
3. *Help Mr. Daniels set short-term dietary goals*
4. *Withhold approval until he agrees to stop drinking*

The specific clause *to effect a change in his behavior while he is in the hospital* is critical. Option 1 may be part of educating this client, but you would not expect a behavioral change observable in the hospital to emerge from this discussion. Option 2 is not really related to his alcoholism. Option 4 rejects the client, as well as his behavior instead of only his behavior. Option 3, the correct answer, could result in an observable behavioral change while the client is hospitalized; for example, he could define ways to achieve short-term goals relating to diet and alcohol while in the hospital.

•Eliminate Clearly Wrong or Incorrect Answers

Eliminate clearly incorrect, inappropriate, and unlikely answers to the question asked in the stem. By systematically eliminating distractors that are unlikely in the context of a given question, you increase the probability of selecting the correct answer. Eliminating obvious distractors also allows you more time to focus on the options that appear to be potentially sound answers to the question. For example:

The four levels of cognitive ability are:

1. *Medical nursing, surgical nursing, obstetric nursing, psychiatric nursing*
2. *Assessing, analyzing, applying, evaluating*
3. *Knowledge, analysis, assessing, comprehension*
4. *Knowledge, comprehension, application, analysis*

Option 1 is clearly inappropriate, since the choices are all clinical areas. Option 2 contains both cognitive levels and nursing behaviors, thus eliminating it from consideration. Both options 3 and 4 contain levels of cognitive ability; however, option 3 includes assessing, which is a nursing behavior. Therefore option 4 is correct. By reducing the plausible options, you reduce the material to consider and increase the probability of selecting the correct option.

•Identify Similar Options

When an item contains two or more options that are very similar in meaning, the successful test taker knows that all are correct, in which case it is a poor question, or that none is correct, which is more likely to be the case. The correct option will usually either include all the similar options or exclude them entirely. For example:

In teaching newly diagnosed diabetic clients about their condition, it is important to focus on:

1. *Dietary modifications*
2. *Use of diabetic nutritional exchange lists*
3. *Use of sugar substitutes*
4. *Their present understanding of diabetes*

Options 1, 2, and 3 deal only with the diabetic diet, involving no other aspect of diabetic teaching; it is impossible to select the most correct option because each represents equally plausible, though limited, answers to the question. Option 4 is the best choice, since it allows the other three options to be excluded and is most complete. As another example:

A child's intelligence is influenced by:

1. *Heredity and environment*
2. *Environment and experience*
3. *A variety of factors*
4. *Socioeconomic factors*

The most correct answer is option 3. It includes the material covered by the other options, eliminating the need for an impossible choice, since each of the other options is only partially correct.

•Identify Answer (Option) Components

When an answer contains two or more parts, you can reduce the number of potentially correct answers by identifying one part as incorrect. For example:

After a cholecystectomy the postoperative diet is usually:

1. *Low fat, high protein*
2. *Low fat, high calorie*
3. *High fat, low protein*
4. *High fat, low calorie*

If you know, for instance, that the diet after a cholecystectomy is usually low or moderate in fat, you can eliminate options 3 and 4 from consideration. If you know that the cholecystectomy client is most often overweight, you can eliminate option 2 from consideration. Therefore option 1 is correct.

•Identify Specific Determiners

When the options of a test item contain words that are identical or similar to words in the stem, the alert test taker recognizes the similarities as clues about the likely answer to the question. The stem word that clues you to a similar word in the option or that limits potential options is known as a specific determiner. For example:

The government agency responsible for administering the nursing practice act in each state is the:

  1. *Board of regents*
  2. *State nurses' association*
  3. *Board of nursing*
  4. *State hospital association*

Options 2 and 3 contain the closely related words *nurse* and *nursing*. The word *nursing*, used both in the stem and in item 3, is a clue to the correct answer.

•Identify Words In The Options That Are Closely Associated With Words In The Stem

Be alert to words in the options that may be closely associated with but not identical to a word or words in the stem. For example:

When a person develops symptoms of physical illness for which psychogenic factors act as causative agents, the resulting illness is classified as:

  1. *Dissociative*
  2. *Compensatory*
  3. *Psychophysiologic*
  4. *Reaction formation*

Option 3 ought to strike you are a likely answer, since it combines physical and psychologic factors, like those referred to in the stem.

•Watch For Grammatical Inconsistencies

If one or more of the options are not grammatically consistent with the stem, the alert test taker can frequently eliminate these distractors. The correct option must be consistent with the form of the question. For example, if the question demands a response in the singular, plural options usually can be safely eliminated. When the stem is in the form of an incomplete sentence, each option should complete the sentence in a grammatically correct way. For example:

Communicating with a client who is deaf will be facilitated by:

  1. *Use gestures*
  2. *Find out if he has a hearing aid*
  3. *Speaking loudly*
  4. *Facing the client while speaking*

Options 1 and 2 do not complete the sentence in a grammatically consistent way and can therefore be eliminated.

•Be Alert To Relevant Information From Earlier Questions

Occasionally information from one question may provide you with a clue for answering another. For example:

Mrs. Evans has a Cantor tube inserted for treatment of intestinal obstruction. Intestinal suction can result in excessive loss of:

  1. *Protein enzymes*
  2. *Energy carbohydrates*
  3. *Water and electrolytes*
  4. *Vitamins and minerals*

If you know that the correct answer to this question is option 3, it may help you to answer a later question. For example:

Critical assessment of Mrs. Evans while the Cantor tube is draining should include observation for:

  1. *Dehydration*
  2. *Nausea*
  3. *Edema*
  4. *Belching*

The correct answer is option 1. If you knew that excessive loss of water and electrolytes may lead to dehydration, you could have used the clue provided in the first question to assist you in answering the second question.

•Make Educated Guesses

When you are unsure about the correct answer to a question, it is better to make an educated guess than to not answer the question. You can generally eliminate one or more of the distractors by using partial knowledge and the methods just listed. The elimination process increases your chances of selecting the correct option from those remaining. Elimination of two distractors on a four-option multiple-choice item increases your probability of selecting the correct answer from 25% to 50%.

General Strategies

1. Develop a plan for study and stick to it. A good plan is to allow 1 week per clinical area.
2. As you study, identify your problem areas that need attention.
3. Avoid planning things that will add stress to your life between now and the time you take the comprehensive examination. Enough things will happen spontaneously; do not plan for them
4. Do not change your pattern of study. It has obviously contributed to your being here, so it worked. If you have studied alone, continue to study alone. If you have studied in a group, form a study group.
5. Practice timed tests and stick to their suggested time frame. You will have a little less than 1 minute per question on the examination (94 questions in 90 minutes).
6. Pace yourself during the testing period, and work as accurately as possible. Do not rush. Excessive

pressure on yourself early in the examination can result in early fade-out.

7. Move through the test rapidly, and answer all the questions that come easily. This gets these questions out of the way and builds your confidence. Although certain questions will be more difficult and will require more time, do not spend too much time on one question; this can compromise your overall score.

8. Make a mark next to questions you cannot answer and go on. After answering all the questions, go back to these items. Be sure to erase any extraneous marks you make.

9. If you find you tend to reread test answers and change the right ones to wrong ones, stop going back. If you find that going back helps you to correct wrong answers, by all means go back and review your answers. Your first answer is usually correct and should not be changed without reason.

10. Do not read information into questions, and avoid speculating. Reading into questions creates errors in judgment.

11. Make certain that the answer you select is reasonable and obtainable under ordinary circumstances and that the action can be carried out in the given situation.

12. Avoid selecting answers that state hospital rules or regulations as a reason or rationale for action.

13. Look for answers that focus on the client or are directed toward feelings.

14. If the question asks for an immediate action or response, all the answers may be correct, so base your selection on identified priorities for action.

15. Do not select answers that contain exceptions to the general rule, controversial material, or degrading responses.

16. Do not be pressured into finishing early. Use all the time necessary without pressuring yourself.

CHAPTER 2

Medical—Surgical Nursing Review Questions

Situation: Jen Bolin, an obese 22 year old, is admitted to the hospital after an automobile accident. She has a fractured hip and is taken to surgery for repair.

1. After surgery Ms. Bolin is to receive a piggyback of clindamycin phosphate (Cleocin) 300 mg in 50 ml of D5W. The piggyback is to infuse in 20 minutes. The drop factor of the IV set is 10 gtt/ml. The nurse should set the piggyback to flow at:
   ① 25 gtt/min
   ② 30 gtt/min
   ③ 35 gtt/min
   ④ 45 gtt/min
2. The day after surgery Ms. Bolin asks the nurse how she might lose weight. Before answering the nurse should bear in mind that long-term weight loss best occurs when:
   ① Fats are limited in the diet
   ② Eating patterns are altered
   ③ Carbohydrates are regulated
   ④ Exercise is part of the program
3. To motivate Ms. Bolin to eventually include aerobic exercises in her weight-reduction program, the nurse should discuss exercise and its relationship to weight loss. The nurse would know that this teaching was effective when Ms. Bolin says that exercise will:
   ① Increase her lean body mass
   ② Lower her metabolic rate
   ③ Decrease her appetite
   ④ Raise her heart rate
4. The physician orders non-weight bearing with crutches for Ms. Bolin. The nurse understands that before ambulation is begun, the most important activity to facilitate walking with crutches is:
   ① Exercising the triceps, finger flexors, and elbow extensors
   ② Sitting up in a chair to help strengthen back muscles
   ③ Keeping the unaffected leg in extension and abduction
   ④ Using the trapeze frequently to strengthen the biceps muscles
5. The nurse would recognize that Ms. Bolin understood the demonstration of crutch walking when she places her weight on:
   ① The palms of her hands and axillary regions
   ② Both feet placed wide apart
   ③ The palms of her hands
   ④ Her axillary regions

Situation: Jeremiah Ralph is a 45-year-old telephone repair man who is admitted because of mild chest pain. He is 5 feet, 7 inches tall and weighs 190 pounds. A myocardial infarct is diagnosed. Morphine sulphate, diazepam (Valium) and lidocaine are prescribed.

6. The physician orders 8 mg of morphine sulfate to be given by injection. The vial on hand is labeled 1 ml = 10 mg. The nurse should administer:
   ① 8 minims
   ② 10 minims
   ③ 12 minims
   ④ 15 minims
7. Mr. Ralph asks the nurse why he is receiving the injection of morphine. The nurse replies that it:
   ① Will help prevent fibrillation of the heart
   ② Relieves pain and prevents shock
   ③ Decreases anxiety and restlessness
   ④ Dilates coronary blood vessels
8. Oxygen by nasal cannula is prescribed for Mr. Ralph. The nurse plans to use safety precautions in the room because oxygen:
   ① Converts to an alternate form of matter
   ② Has unstable properties
   ③ Supports combustion
   ④ Is flammable
9. Isoenzyme laboratory studies are ordered. The isoenzyme test that is the most reliable early indicator of myocardial insult is:
   ① SGPT
   ② LDH
   ③ CPK
   ④ AST
10. An electrocardiogram is ordered. An early finding in the lead over the infarcted area would be:
    ① Disappearance of Q waves
    ② Elevated ST segments
    ③ Absence of P wave
    ④ Flattened T waves
11. Mr. Ralph, who had a myocardial infarction 2 days earlier, has just spent 5 minutes complaining to the nurse about numerous aspects of his hospital stay. The best initial nursing response would be to:
    ① Permit him to release his feelings and then promptly leave to allow him to regain his composure
    ② Refocus the conversation on his fears, frustrations, and anger about his condition

③ Explain how his being upset dangerously blocks his need for rest

④ Attempt to explain the purpose of different hospital routines

12. Several days after admission, Mr. Ralph develops pyrexia. The nurse monitors him for other adaptations related to the pyrexia, including:
① Dyspnea
② Chest pain
③ Elevated blood pressure
④ Increased pulse rate

13. Mr. Ralph asks the nurse, "What's the chance of having another heart attack if I watch my diet and stress levels carefully?" The most appropriate initial response would be for the nurse to:
① Suggest he discuss his feelings of vulnerability with his physician
② Tell him that he certainly needs to be especially careful in these areas
③ Avoid giving him direct information and help him explore his feelings
④ Recognize that he is frightened and suggest he talk with the psychiatric nurse

Situation: Angela Signelli, 60 years old, is having a workup for pernicious anemia.

14. A Schilling test is ordered for Mrs. Signelli. The nurse recognizes that the primary purpose of the Schilling test is to determine the client's ability to:
① Store vitamin B_{12}
② Digest vitamin B_{12}
③ Absorb vitamin B_{12}
④ Produce vitamin B_{12}

15. Pernicious anemia is confirmed, and the physician orders 0.2 mg of cyanocobalamin (vitamin B_{12}) IM. Available is a vial of the drug labeled 1 ml = 100 mcg. The nurse should administer:
① 0.5 ml
② 1.0 ml
③ 1.5 ml
④ 2.0 ml

16. When explaining the therapeutic regimen concerning vitamin B_{12} to Mrs. Signelli the nurse should tell her that:
① Oral tablets of vitamin B_{12} taken daily will control her symptoms
② Intramuscular injections are required daily for control
③ Intramuscular injections once a month will maintain control
④ Weekly Z-track injections provide needed control

17. The nurse knows that Mrs. Signelli understands the teaching regarding the vitamin B_{12} injections when she states that she must take it:
① When she feels fatigued
② During exacerbations of anemia

③ Until her symptoms subside
④ For the rest of her life

Situation: Archie Douglass, a 45-year-old actor, has recently had an abdominoperineal resection and colostomy.

18. Mr. Douglass accuses the nurse of being uncomfortable during a dressing change, because his "wound looks terrible." The nurse recognizes that the client is using the defense mechanism known as:
① Reaction formation
② Sublimation
③ Intellectualization
④ Projection

19. When preparing to teach Mr. Douglass how to irrigate his colostomy, the nurse should plan to perform the procedure:
① When Mr. Douglass would have normally had a bowel movement
② After Mr. Douglass accepts his altered body image
③ Before breakfast and morning care
④ At least 2 hours before visitors

20. When observing Mr. Douglass doing a return demonstration of the colostomy irrigation, the nurse knows that more teaching is required if he:
① Clamps off the flow of fluid when he feels uncomfortable
② Lubricates the tip of the catheter before inserting it into the stoma
③ Hangs the bag on a clothes hook on the bathroom door during fluid insertion
④ Discontinues the insertion of fluid after only 500 ml of fluid has been instilled

21. The problem occurring during colostomy irrigation at home that Mr. Douglass should be instructed to report to his physician is:
① Abdominal cramps during fluid inflow
② Difficulty in inserting the irrigating tube
③ Passage of flatus during expulsion of feces
④ Inabilty to complete the procedure in an hour

22. Mr. Douglass refuses to allow his wife to see the incision or stoma and ignores most of his dietary instructions. The nurse, on assessing this data, can assume that the client is experiencing:
① A reaction formation to his recent altered body image
② A difficult time accepting reality and is in a state of denial
③ Impotency due to the surgery and needs sexual counseling
④ Suicide thoughts and should be seen by a psychiatrist

23. The nurse continues to assist Mr. Douglass in following his diet. The nurse would know that dietary teaching had been effective when Mr. Douglass states that he will eat:

① Food low in fiber so that there is less stool
② Everything he ate before the operation but will avoid those foods that cause gas
③ Bland foods so that his intestines do not become irritated
④ Soft foods that are more easily digested and absorbed by the large intestines

Situation: Edmond Karp, 40 years old, is brought to the emergency room after the crash of his private plane. He has suffered multiple crushing wounds of the chest, abdomen, and legs. It is feared his right leg may have to be amputated.

24. When Mr. Karp arrives in the emergency room, the assessments that assume the greatest priority are:
① Level of consciousness and pupil size
② Abdominal contusions and other wounds
③ Pain, respiratory rate, and blood pressure
④ Quality of respirations and presence of pulses

25. Mr. Karp's respiratory status necessitates endotracheal intubation and positive pressure ventilation. The most immediate nursing intervention for him at this time would be to:
① Facilitate his verbal communication
② Maintain sterility of the ventilation system
③ Assess his response to the equipment
④ Prepare him for emergency surgery

26. A chest tube with water-seal drainage is inserted. Later, Mr. Karp's chest tube seems to be obstructed. The most appropriate nursing action would be to:
① Prepare for chest tube removal
② Milk the tube toward the collection container
③ Arrange for a stat chest x-ray film
④ Clamp the tube immediately

27. The observation that indicates a desired response to treatment of Mr. Karp's chest injury is:
① Increased breath sounds
② Constant bubbling in the drainage chamber
③ Crepitus detected on palpation of chest
④ Increased respiratory rate

28. In the evaluation of Mr. Karp's response to fluid replacement therapy, the observation that indicates adequate tissue perfusion to vital organs is:
① Urinary output of 30 ml in an hour
② Central venous pressure reading of 2 cm H_2O
③ Pulse rates of 120 and 110 in a 15-minute period
④ Blood pressure readings of 50/30 and 70/40 within 30 minutes

29. Twelve hours after Mr. Karp is transferred to the critical care unit, he begins to complain of increased abdominal pain in the left upper quadrant. A ruptured spleen is diagnosed, and he is scheduled for emergency splenectomy. In preparing Mr. Karp for surgery the nurse should emphasize in his teaching plan the:
① Complete safety of the procedure
② Expectation of postoperative bleeding
③ Risk of the procedure with his other injuries
④ Presence of abdominal drains for several days after surgery

30. Mr. Karp's chest injury improves, and his chest drainage is discontinued. To promote continued improvement in his respiratory status, the nurse should:
① Encourage bed rest with active and passive range-of-motion exercises
② Encourage frequent coughing and deep breathing
③ Turn him from side to side at least every 2 hours
④ Continue observing for dyspnea and crepitus

31. It has been decided that Mr. Karp's right leg must be amputated, and a below-the-knee amputation is performed. Three days postoperatively Mr. Karp is refusing to eat, talk, or perform any rehabilitative activities. The best initial nursing approach would be to:
① Give him explanations of why there is a need to quickly increase his activity
② Emphasize repeatedly that with a prosthesis he will be able to return to his normal life-style
③ Appear cheerful and noncritical regardless of his response to attempts at intervention
④ Accept and acknowledge that his withdrawal is an initially normal and necessary part of grieving

32. The key factor in accurately assessing how body image changes will be dealt with by the client is the:
① Extent of body change present
② Suddenness of the change
③ Obviousness of the change
④ Client's perception of the change

Situation: Henry King is diagnosed as having myelocytic leukemia and is admitted to the hospital for chemotherapy.

33. Mr. King discusses his recent diagnosis of leukemia by referring to statistics, facts, and figures. The nurse recognizes that Mr. King is using the defense mechanism known as:
① Reaction formation
② Sublimation
③ Intellectualization
④ Projection

34. Mr. King's laboratory results indicate bone marrow depression. The nurse should encourage Mr. King to:
    ① Increase his activity level and ambulate frequently
    ② Sleep with the head of his bed slightly elevated
    ③ Drink citrus juices frequently for nourishment
    ④ Use a soft toothbrush and electric razor
35. Mr. King receives a blood transfusion and develops flank pain, chills, fever, and hematuria. The nurse recognizes that Mr. King is probably experiencing:
    ① An anaphylactic transfusion reaction
    ② An allergic transfusion reaction
    ③ A hemolytic transfusion reaction
    ④ A pyrogenic transfusion reaction
36. Mr. King jokes about his leukemia even though he is becoming sicker and weaker. The nurse's most therapeutic response would be:
    ① "Your laughter is a cover for your fear."
    ② "He who laughs on the outside, cries on the inside."
    ③ "Why are you always laughing?"
    ④ "Does it help to joke about your illness?"
37. In dealing with a dying client such as Mr. King who is in the denial stage of grief, the best nursing approach is to:
    ① Agree with and encourage the client's denial
    ② Reassure the client that everything will be okay
    ③ Allow the denial but be available to discuss death
    ④ Leave the client alone to confront his loss
38. During an 8-hour shift Mr. King drinks two 6-ounce cups of tea and vomits 125 ml of fluid. During this 8-hour period his fluid balance would be:
    ① +55 ml
    ② +137 ml
    ③ +235 ml
    ④ +485 ml

Situation: Gregory Smith, age 67, is admitted to the coronary care unit with a diagnosis of left-sided congestive heart failure.

39. On assessment of Mr. Smith, the nurse should expect to find:
    ① Crushing chest pain
    ② Dyspnea on exertion
    ③ Extensive peripheral edema
    ④ Jugular vein distention
40. The physician orders a cardiac glycoside, a vasodilator, and furosemide (Lasix). The nurse understands that Lasix exerts its effects in the:
    ① Distal tubule
    ② Collecting duct
    ③ Glomerulus of the nephron
    ④ Ascending limb of Henle's loop
41. Mr. Smith weighed 210 pounds on admission to the hospital. After 2 days of diuretic therapy he weighs 205.5 pounds. The nurse could estimate that the amount of fluid he has lost is:
    ① 0.5 L
    ② 1.0 L
    ③ 2.0 L
    ④ 3.5 L
42. Mr. Smith has been receiving a cardiac glycoside, a diuretic, and a vasodilator drug. His apical pulse rate is 44, and he is on bed rest. The nurse concludes that his pulse rate is most likely a result of the:
    ① Diuretic
    ② Vasodilator
    ③ Bed-rest regimen
    ④ Cardiac glycoside
43. The diet ordered for Mr. Smith permits him to have 190 g of carbohydrates, 90 g of fat, and 100 g of protein. The nurse understands that this diet contains approximately:
    ① 2200 calories
    ② 2000 calories
    ③ 1800 calories
    ④ 1600 calories
44. After the acute phase of congestive failure, the nurse should expect the dietary management of Mr. Smith to include the restriction of:
    ① Magnesium
    ② Sodium
    ③ Potassium
    ④ Calcium

Situation: Henrick James, a traveling salesman, develops gastric bleeding and is hospitalized.

45. An important etiologic clue for the nurse to explore while taking Mr. James' history would be:
    ① The medications he has been taking
    ② Any recent foreign travel
    ③ His usual dietary pattern
    ④ The status of family relationships
46. In assessing Mr. James' abdomen, the nurse palpates the area directly above the umbilicus. This area is known as the:
    ① Iliac area
    ② Epigastric area
    ③ Hypogastric area
    ④ Suprasternal area
47. Once the bleeding is controlled, the physician orders individual dietary management. The meal pattern that would probably be most appropriate for Mr. James is:
    ① Three meals large enough to supply adequate energy
    ② Regular meals and snacks to limit gastric discomfort

③ Limited food and fluid intake when he has pain

④ A flexible plan according to his appetite

48. The physician prescribes cimetidine (Tagamet) and Maalox for Mr. James. The nurse should administer:
    ① One immediately before the other
    ② The drugs at least 1 hour apart
    ③ The two drugs simultaneously
    ④ The drugs together with milk or orange juice

49. Two years later, after several episodes of GI bleeding, Mr. James is admitted to the hospital for a gastrectomy. Following surgery, Mr. James has a nasogastric tube to low continuous suction. He begins to hyperventilate. The nurse should be aware that this pattern will alter his arterial blood gases by:
    ① Increasing HCO_3
    ② Decreasing P_{CO_2}
    ③ Decreasing pH
    ④ Decreasing P_{O_2}

50. IV fluids are ordered postoperatively for Mr. James. Routine postoperative intravenous fluids are designed to supply hydration and electolytes and only limited energy. Because 1 L of a 5% dextrose solution contains 50 g of sugar, 3 L per day would supply approximately:
    ① 400 kilocalories
    ② 600 kilocalories
    ③ 800 kilocalories
    ④ 1000 kilocalories

51. Thrombus formation is a danger for Mr. James as it is for all postoperative clients. The nurse should act independently to prevent this complication by:
    ① Encouraging adequate fluids
    ② Applying elastic stockings
    ③ Massaging gently with lotion
    ④ Performing in-bed exercises

Situation: Robert West, a 56-year-old construction worker, fell off the roof of a 2-story building and is brought to the hospital unconscious.

52. When assessing Mr. West the nurse would be most concerned if the assessment revealed:
    ① Reactive pupils
    ② A depressed fontanel
    ③ Bleeding from the ears
    ④ An elevated temperature

53. Mr. West is admitted to the intensive care area, IV fluids are instituted, and a Foley catheter is inserted. With an indwelling catheter, urinary infection is a potential danger. The nurse can best plan to avoid this problem by:
    ① Emptying the drainage bag frequently
    ② Collecting a weekly urine specimen
    ③ Maintaining the ordered hydration
    ④ Assessing urine specific gravity

54. The nurse performs full range of motion on Mr. West's extremities. When putting his ankle through range of motion the nurse must perform:
    ① Flexion, extension, and left and right rotation
    ② Abduction, flexion, adduction, and extension
    ③ Pronation, supination, rotation, and extension
    ④ Dorsiflexion, plantar flexion, eversion, and inversion

55. Mr. West has been in a coma for 2 months and is maintained on bed rest. The nurse understands that to prevent the effects of shearing force the head of the bed should be at an angle of:
    ① 30 degrees
    ② 45 degrees
    ③ 60 degrees
    ④ 90 degrees

Situation: Keith Jensen, age 62, is scheduled for a transurethral resection of the prostate in the morning.

56. As part of the preoperative teaching, the nurse should tell Mr. Jensen that after surgery:
    ① Urinary control may be permanently lost to some degree
    ② Urinary drainage will be dependent on a urethral catheter for 24 to 48 hours
    ③ Frequency and burning on urination will last while the cystotomy tube is in place
    ④ His ability to perform sexually will be permanently impaired

57. The transurethral resection of the prostate is performed. Following surgery, Mr. Jensen's nursing care should include:
    ① Changing the abdominal dressing
    ② Maintaining patency of the cystotomy tube
    ③ Maintaining patency of a three-way Foley catheter
    ④ Observing for hemorrhage and wound infection

58. In the early postoperative period following transurethral surgery, the most common complication the nurse should observe for is:
    ① Sepsis
    ② Hemorrhage
    ③ Leakage around the catheter
    ④ Urinary retention with overflow

59. Mr. Jensen's retention catheter is secured to his leg, causing slight traction of the inflatable balloon against the prostatic fossa. This is done to:
    ① Limit discomfort
    ② Provide hemostasis
    ③ Reduce bladder spasms
    ④ Promote urinary drainage

60. Twenty-four hours after surgery Mr. Jensen tells the nurse he has lower abdominal dis-

comfort. The nurse notes that catheter drainage has stopped. The nurse's initial action should be to:
① Irrigate the catheter with saline
② Milk the catheter tubing
③ Remove the catheter
④ Notify the physician

61. The nurse would know that Mr. Jensen understood his discharge teaching when he says, "I should:
① Get out of bed into a chair for several hours daily."
② Call the physician if my urinary stream decreases."
③ Attempt to void every 3 hours when I'm awake."
④ Avoid vigorous exercise for 6 months after surgery."

Situation: Lucy Parton is admitted to the surgical unit for a subtotal thyroidectomy. She has a history of Graves' disease.

62. When assessing Mrs. Parton, the nurse would expect to find:
① Lethargy, weight gain, and forgetfulness
② Weight loss, protruding eyeballs, and lethargy
③ Weight loss, exophthalmos, and restlessness
④ Constipation, dry skin, and weight gain

63. Mrs. Parton goes to surgery. In planning for Mrs. Parton's return the nurse should consider that in a subtotal thyroidectomy:
① The entire thyroid gland is removed
② A small part of the gland is left intact
③ One parathyroid gland is also removed
④ A portion of the thyroid and four parathyroids are removed

64. Before Mrs. Parton returns to her room, the nurse plans to set up emergency equipment, which should include:
① A crash cart with bed board
② A tracheostomy set and oxygen
③ An airway and rebreathing mask
④ Two ampules of sodium bicarbonate

65. When Mrs. Parton returns from surgery the nurse assess her for unilateral injury of the pharyngeal nerve every 30 to 60 minutes by:
① Observing for signs of tetany
② Checking her throat for swelling
③ Asking her to state her name out loud
④ Palpating the side of her neck for blood seepage

66. On Mrs. Parton's discharge the nurse teaches her to observe for signs of surgically induced hypothyroidism. The nurse would know that Mrs. Parton understands the teaching when she states she should notify the physician if she develops:
① Intolerance to heat
② Dry skin and fatigue
③ Progressive weight loss
④ Insomnia and excitability

67. Mrs. Parton's exophthalmos continues. The nurse teaches her how to reduce discomfort and prevent corneal ulceration. The nurse recognizes that Mrs. Parton understands the teaching when she states, "I should:
① Elevate the head of my bed at night."
② Avoid moving my extraocular muscles."
③ Avoid using a sleeping mask at night."
④ Avoid excessive blinking."

Situation: Joan Caffrey is a 37-year-old cook. She is admitted for treatment of partial and full-thickness burns of her entire right lower extremity and the anterior portion of her right upper extremity. Her respiratory status is compromised, and she is in pain and anxious.

68. Performing an immediate appraisal, using the rule of nines, the nurse estimates the percent of Mrs. Caffrey's body surface that is burned is:
① 4.5%
② 9%
③ 18%
④ 22.5%

69. The nurse applies mafenide acetate (Sulfamylon cream) to Mrs. Caffrey's burns as ordered by the physician. This medication will:
① Inhibit bacterial growth
② Relieve pain from the burn
③ Prevent scar tissue formation
④ Provide chemical debridement

70. Forty-eight hours after the injury the physician orders 2 liters of IV fluid to be administered q 12 h. The drop factor of the tubing is 10 gtt/ml. The nurse should set the flow to provide:
① 18 gtt/min
② 28 gtt/min
③ 32 gtt/min
④ 36 gtt/min

71. A temporary heterograft (pig skin) is used on some of Mrs. Caffrey's burns. These grafts will:
① Debride necrotic epithelium
② Be sutured in place for better adherence
③ Relieve pain and promote rapid epithelialization
④ Frequently be used concurrently with topical antimicrobials

72. Mrs. Caffrey has periodic episodes of dyspnea. The position that would provide for the greatest respiratory capacity would be the:
① Semi-Fowler's position
② Sims' position
③ Orthopneic position
④ Supine position

73. Ethylestrenol (Maxibolin), an anabolic steroid, is ordered for the treatment of the catabolic processes associated with Mrs. Caffrey's

burns. The nurse should observe her for signs of:
① Hyperglycemia
② Hyponatremia
③ Virilization
④ Lethargy

Situation: Jane Norcross, a 20-year-old college student, has been experiencing ptosis of the right eyelid, diplopia, and occasional dysphagia for several weeks. Because she also seems to have less endurance for her normal school and social activities, her mother takes her to their family physician for a checkup. Ms. Norcross is to undergo a neurologic workup because of a tentative diagnosis of myasthenia gravis.

74. Ms. Norcross is scheduled to have a series of diagnostic studies for myasthenia gravis, including a Tensilon test. In preparing her for this procedure, the nurse explains that her response to the medication will confirm the diagnosis if Tensilon produces:
① Brief exaggeration of symptoms
② Prolonged symptomatic improvement
③ Rapid but brief symptomatic improvement
④ Symptomatic improvement of just the ptosis

75. The initial nursing goal for Ms. Norcross during the diagnostic phase of her hospitalization would be to:
① Develop a teaching plan
② Facilitate psychologic adjustment
③ Maintain the present muscle strength
④ Prepare for the appearance of myasthenic crisis

76. The most significant initial nursing observations that need to be made about Ms. Norcross include her:
① Ability to chew and speak distinctly
② Degree of anxiety about her diagnosis
③ Ability to smile and to close her eyelids
④ Respiratory exchange and ability to swallow

77. Ms. Norcross' diagnosis is confirmed and pyridostigmine bromide (Mestinon) therapy is started. The Mestinon dosage is frequently changed during the first week. While the dosage is being adjusted, the nurse's priority intervention is to:
① Administer the medication exactly on time
② Administer the medication with food or milk
③ Evaluate the client's muscle strength hourly after administration
④ Evaluate the client's emotional side effects between doses

78. Ms. Norcross begins to experience increased difficulty in swallowing. To prevent aspiration of food, the nursing action that would be most effective would be to:

① Change her diet order from soft foods to clear liquids
② Place an emergency tracheostomy set in her room
③ Assess her respiratory status before and after meals
④ Coordinate her meal schedule with the peak effect of Mestinon

79. Ms. Norcross is concerned about her fluctuating physical condition and generalized weakness. In planning for Ms. Norcross' care it would be most important to:
① Have one of her parents stay with her
② Space her activities throughout the day
③ Restrict her activities and encourage bed rest
④ Teach her the limitations imposed by her disease

80. Because of inadequate symptomatic control with Mestinon, Ms. Norcross' physician begins long-term steroid therapy. When this type of therapy is being initiated, it is especially important to:
① Decrease the client's fluid intake to 1000 ml daily
② Increase the client's sodium intake
③ Place the client on reverse isolation
④ Observe the client for an exacerbation of symptoms

81. After a course of steroid therapy Ms. Norcross is scheduled for a thymectomy. In preparing her for surgery, the nurse should emphasize:
① A detailed explanation of the procedure
② The experimental nature of this procedure in myasthenia
③ The difficulty of predicting the degree of improvement after the operation
④ An explanation of the usual postoperative complications of a thymectomy

82. Ms. Norcross' surgery and immediate postoperative course are uneventful. As her condition is stabilizing, the nurse notes that she seems to be depressed. The nursing action that would be most appropriate at this point is:
① Talking with her about her prognosis and emphasizing things that she can do
② Reassuring her that she will feel better when her discharge date is set
③ Asking her physician to arrange for a psychologic consultation
④ Recognizing that depression often occurs after this surgery

Situation: Harriet Jenkins, 65 years old, has a history of hypertension for the past 10 years. She has mild dyspnea on exertion, and pedal edema.

83. The nurse recognizes that Mrs. Jenkins' dyspnea on exertion is probably:
① A result of left ventricular failure
② Associated with wheezing and coughing

③ A sign of advanced congestive heart failure

④ Accompanied by a rise in central venous pressure

84. Hydrochlorothiazide (HydroDIURIL) 50 mg bid is ordered for Mrs. Jenkins. The nurse would know that Mrs. Jenkins understands the side effects of HydroDIURIL when she says, "I should call the physician if I develop:
① Insomnia."
② A stuffy nose."
③ Increased thirst."
④ Generalized weakness."

85. The physician orders potassium supplements. The nurse recognizes that Mrs. Jenkins understands the teaching about potassium when she indicates that she should:
① Take the drug on an empty stomach
② Use salt substitutes with food
③ Report any abdominal distress
④ Increase the dosage if she has muscle cramps

86. The dietary practice that will help Mrs. Jenkins reduce her dietary intake of sodium is:
① Using an artificial sweetener in her coffee
② Using catsup for cooking and flavoring
③ Increasing her use of dairy products
④ Avoiding the use of carbonated beverages

87. The nurse suggests that Mrs. Jenkins, as all clients with chronic congestive heart failure, should:
① Take a hot bath before bedtime
② Avoid emotionally stressful situations when possible
③ Exercise daily until the pulse rate exceeds 100 per minute
④ Avoid sleeping in an air-conditioned room

88. The teaching plan for Mrs. Jenkins should include having the client:
① Sleep flat in bed
② Rest during the day
③ Follow a low-potassium diet
④ Take her pulse at least three times a day

89. Mrs. Jenkins arrives for another appointment and tells the nurse, "My feet are killing me. These shoes got so tight." The nurse's best initial action is to:
① Listen to the client's breath sounds
② Take the client's pulse rate
③ Notify the physician
④ Weigh the client

Situation: Saul King, a 61-year-old carpenter, is admitted to the hospital with upper right quadrant discomfort, jaundice, and a recent 29-pound weight loss. After a diagnostic workup, carcinoma of the pancreas is suspected and an exploratory laparotomy is scheduled.

90. Before surgery, meperidine (Demerol) is ordered for pain. Morphine sulfate is contraindicated for Mr. King because it:

① Causes respiratory excitement
② Stimulates pancreatic duct secretion
③ Causes spasm of the pancreatic ducts
④ Stimulates the sympathetic nervous system

91. The physician orders atropine sulfate preoperatively. After administering the atropine to Mr. King the nurse should be particularly observant for the occurrence of:
① Polyuria
② Diarrhea
③ Murmurs
④ Tachycardia

92. A Whipple procedure is performed on Mr. King. When Mr. King returns from surgery, the nurse should expect him to have a:
① Chest tube
② Intestinal tube
③ Nasogastric tube
④ Gastrostomy tube

93. After surgery Mr. King should be encouraged to turn from side to side and to carry out deep-breathing exercises. These activities are essential to prevent:
① Metabolic acidosis
② Metabolic alkalosis
③ Respiratory acidosis
④ Respiratory alkalosis

94. Mr. King's IV fluid orders for 24 hours are 1500 ml D5W followed by 1250 ml of NS. The IV tubing has a drop factor of 15 gtt/ml. To administer the required fluids, the nurse should set the drip rate at:
① 13 gtt/min
② 16 gtt/min
③ 29 gtt/min
④ 32 gtt/min

95. The physician orders cefazolin sodium (Kefzol) 375 mg IVPB every 8 hours. The vial of powder contains 500 mg of the drug. This must be reconstituted with 2 ml of 0.9% sodium chloride. In the resulting solution 1 ml equals 225 mg of Kefzol. The nurse should administer:
① 1.2 ml
② 2.2 ml
③ 20 minims
④ 25 minims

96. Oral pancreatic enzymes are prescribed for Mr. King. The nurse would know that the teaching about the enzymes was understood when Mr. King says, "I will take them:
① On arising each morning."
② An hour before meals."
③ With meals."
④ At bedtime."

97. Mrs. King asks the nurse about preparing meals for her husband. The statement the nurse should include in teaching about the diet would be:
① "Meals should be low fat because of inter-

ference with the fat digestion mechanism."

② "Meals should be restricted in protein because of compromised liver function."

③ "The diet should be low in calories to prevent taxing the diseased pancreas."

④ "There are no dietary restrictions; he may eat as desired."

98. The nurse is preparing Mr. King for discharge. A long-term complication that Mr. King must be made aware of is his hypoinsulinism. The nurse would know that he understands the teaching about hypoinsulinism when he indicates that he should seek medical supervision if he has:
① Oliguria
② Anorexia
③ Weight gain
④ Increased thirst

99. One month later Mr. King is readmitted with recurrent abdominal pain and fever. The diagnosis is fistula formation with chemical peritonitis. The nurse should place Mr. King in the:
① Supine position
② Right Sims' position
③ Semi-Fowler's position
④ Position that is most comfortable

Situation: Eloise Yoland is a 60-year-old widow living with her divorced drug-addicted daughter, Lynne Anne Stewart, and her seven grandchildren. Mrs. Yoland has been hospitalized for CHF and has a history of a myocardial infarction 1 year ago. On discharge from the hospital Mrs. Yoland was referred to the Visiting Nurse Association for monitoring of her cardiopulmonary status and for an evaluation of her home management and self-care.

100. Miss James, the public health nurse, visits the client in her home for the first time after making an appointment. She finds Mrs. Yoland in the kitchen feeding her 6-month-old granddaughter and preparing dinner for the rest of the family. A 14-year-old grandson, handicapped and in a wheelchair, is present. He says his mother is sleeping in the bedroom. The nurse should proceed by:
① Sitting down with Mrs. Yoland and exchanging identifying data and information
② Accepting coffee when offered by Mrs. Yoland and socializing for a few minutes
③ Asking Mrs. Yoland if there is a private place to examine her and take a health history
④ Asking Mrs. Yoland to show her around the apartment to establish environmental conditions

101. Mrs. Yoland confides to Miss James that she receives no help from her daughter, who seems run-down and disinterested in her own health, as well as the health of her family.

Mrs. Yoland tells Miss James that her daughter coughs a good deal and does a lot of sleeping. In this situation Miss James should pursue the daughter's condition for potential case finding because:
① Children younger than 14 are very susceptible to tuberculosis
② Deaths from tuberculosis have been generally on the increase
③ The incidence of tuberculosis has been dramatically rising
④ Aging clients with chronic illness are most adversely affected by tuberculosis

102. During the visit with Mrs. Yoland, Miss James observes that the 6-month-old granddaughter lies quietly in her crib, rarely smiles or vocalizes, and barely has her basic needs attended. Miss James should:
① Advise Mrs. Yoland that the child will be retarded if she is not stimulated
② Place an aide in the home to assist with chores and care for the infant
③ Encourage purchasing appropriate toys manufactured for the baby's age level
④ Ask the 14-year-old handicapped brother to pay more attention to his sister

103. Because of the ages of the children in the household, Miss James questions Mrs. Yoland about their immunization status. She informs Mrs. Yoland of the program of inoculations required by the public health law for school admission. To ensure immunity, children must receive at least:
① One dose of diphtheria toxoid; one dose of oral poliomyelitis, live measles, live rubella, and mumps vaccines
② Two doses of diphtheria toxoid and oral poliomyelitis vaccine; one dose of live measles, live rubella, and mumps vaccines
③ Three doses of diphtheria toxoid; two doses of oral poliomyelitis vaccine; one dose of live measles, live rubella, and mumps vaccines
④ Three doses of diphtheria toxoid; three doses of oral poliomyelitis vaccine; one dose of live measles, live rubella, and mumps vaccines

104. Further visits to the client disclose that the 14-year-old disabled grandson has experienced convulsions and that Mrs. Stewart, the child's mother, not only was unresponsive to his needs, but also failed to obtain needed medication or follow-up of medical attention. Mrs. Stewart also seems to provoke convulsive episodes by harsh verbal exchanges with the child. The nurse believes that intervention by an appropriate community resource is indicated. A referral should be made to:
① The Bureau of the Handicapped
② The Bureau of Child Welfare

③ The hospital pediatric unit

④ The outpatient clinic

105. Mrs. Stewart's respiratory status gets progressively worse, and she goes to the emergency room for medical attention. A chest x-ray film is obtained, a tentative diagnosis of tuberculosis is made, and she is admitted to the hospital. Mrs. Stewart's sputum smears for acid-fast bacillus (AFB) are positive, and she is placed on isolation. The nurse should anticipate the need to instruct her visitors to:

① Wear an Ultra-Filter mask when they are in her room

② Put on a gown and gloves before going into her room

③ Avoid contact with any objects present in her room

④ Limit contact with nonexposed family members

106. When teaching Mrs. Stewart about her recovery after discharge the nurse should reinforce that the treatment measure with the highest priority is:

① Having sufficient rest

② Getting plenty of fresh air

③ Changing her life-style

④ Consistently taking her medication

Situation: After a partial nephrectomy Brent Harris returns to the unit with a nephrostomy tube in place.

107. An acute, life-threatening complication that the nurse should assess Mr. Harris for in the early postoperative period is:

① Sepsis

② Renal failure

③ Hemorrhage

④ Paralytic ileus

108. The nurse's postoperative plan of care for Mr. Harris includes:

① Giving him a regular diet on the first postoperative day

② Turning him from his back to the operated side every 2 to 3 hours

③ Leaving the original dressing in place for at least the first 48 hours

④ Clamping the nephrostomy tube when he is out of bed

109. The observation about Mr. Harris' urinary output that the nurse should recognize as normal is that his:

① Hourly urine output will be less than 30 ml

② Urinary specific gravity will remain below 1.010

③ Urine will drain from the wound for several days

④ Urine will remain dark red with clots for several days

110. Mr. Harris still has residual obstruction to urine flow and is being discharged with the nephrostomy tube in place. The nurse should instruct him to:

① Irrigate the nephrostomy tube

② Change dressings frequently

③ Remain on bed rest at home

④ Limit his intake of fluids

111. Mr. Harris has been taught how to care for his nephrostomy tube and how to change his dressing. On the day of discharge he states, "I hope I can handle all this at home; it's a lot to remember." The best response by the nurse would be:

① "I'm sure you can do it!"

② "Oh, your wife can do it for you."

③ "You seem to be nervous about going home."

④ "Perhaps you can stay in the hospital another day."

Situation: Mary Kohl, 70 years old, comes to the Community Health Clinic complaining of increased thirst and appetite, and weight loss.

112. Diabetes mellitus is diagnosed, and the physician prescribes chlorpropamide (Diabinese). While taking this medication, Mrs. Kohl should be taught to observe for:

① Hypoglycemia

② Diabetic coma

③ Weight loss

④ Ketonuria

113. The nurse answers Mrs. Kohl's question about Diabinese by telling her it acts by:

① Stimulating the beta cells to produce insulin

② Stimulating the liver to release stored glycogen

③ Increasing glucose transport across the cell membrane

④ Lowering blood sugar in the absence of beta cell function

114. While the nurse is instructing Mrs. Kohl about the ordered 1800 calorie ADA diet, Mrs. Kohl says she does not like broccoli. The nurse suggests that she substitute:

① ⅓ cup of corn

② ½ cup of lima beans

③ ½ cup of green peas

④ ½ cup of green beans

115. When Mrs. Kohl is 73 years old she is admitted to the hospital for elective cataract surgery. Before surgery Mrs. Kohl asks the nurse, "How will my diabetes be managed during my hospitalization?" The best response by the nurse would be:

① "The anesthesiologist will take care of it."

② "What did your surgeon or the anesthetist tell you?"

③ "Your surgeon will write orders for fluids and insulin."

④ "I'm not quite certain I understand what you are asking."

116. Preoperative teaching for Mrs. Kohl should include the importance of:

① Remaining in bed for 48 hours

② Breathing and coughing deeply

③ Avoiding bending from the waist

④ Lying in the supine position for 12 hours

117. Postoperatively the nurse should provide for Mrs. Kohl's safety by:
   ① Putting the side rails up whenever she is in bed
   ② Darkening the room by closing the window shades
   ③ Applying a vest restraint until the dressing is removed
   ④ Immobilizing her head by placing a sandbag on each side

118. The physician orders 50 U of insulin to be added to Mrs. Kohl's IV of glucose and water. The nurse understands that the only insulin that can be used is:
   ① Lente insulin
   ② NPH insulin
   ③ Regular insulin
   ④ Ultralente insulin

119. After surgery Mrs. Kohl complains that she feels nauseated. The nurse should:
   ① Instruct her to deep breathe until the nausea subsides
   ② Explain that this is expected following surgery
   ③ Administer the antiemetic drug as ordered
   ④ Give her some dry crackers to eat

120. Mrs. Kohl administers her own eyedrops before discharge. The nurse approves her technique when she:
   ① Squeezes her eye shut after instilling the eye drops
   ② Raises her upper eyelid with gentle traction
   ③ Places the drops on the cornea of the eye
   ④ Holds the dropper tip above the eye

Situation: Sally Anders has been diagnosed as having nodular poorly differentiated lymphocytic lymphoma (NLPD). Following treatment with a chemotherapeutic protocol called COP that includes vincristine (Oncovin), cyclophosphamide (Cytoxan), and prednisone, radiation therapy is planned.

121. Mrs. Anders comes for her first radiation treatment. As the nurse prepares her for the therapy the client states, "I'm so discouraged," and starts to cry. The nurse should:
   ① Leave her alone so that she can regain her composure
   ② State, "It's difficult to deal with your diagnosis and treatment."
   ③ Complete the preparation and tell her, "We can talk about this later."
   ④ Explain the therapy and reiterate that it will cause only a little discomfort

122. Mrs. Anders' discouragement continues during radiation therapy because of the long time required for treatment and its side effects. In assisting her to plan for the future, the nurse should emphasize that:
   ① A positive outlook can influence the outcome of cancer therapy
   ② The prognosis for NLPD is more favorable than for other types
   ③ Her feelings are normal and will lessen with time
   ④ Antidepressant medication can be prescribed

123. Mrs. Anders develops pancytopenia during the course of chemotherapy. Mrs. Anders asks the nurse why this has occurred. The nurse should explain that:
   ① Dehydration caused by nausea, vomiting, and diarrhea results in hemoconcentration
   ② Steroid hormones have a depressant effect on the spleen and bone marrow
   ③ Lymph node activity is depressed by the radiation therapy and chemotherapy
   ④ Normal cells are also susceptible to the effects of chemotherapeutic drugs

124. Because of the complication of pancytopenia, the nurse should plan to teach Mrs. Anders to:
   ① Begin a program of aggressive, strict mouth care
   ② Avoid traumatic injuries and exposure to infection
   ③ Increase her oral fluid intake to a minimum of 3000 ml daily
   ④ Report any unusual muscle cramps or tingling sensations in the extremities

Situation: Melinda Carl has had a variety of vague complaints for the past 6 months. The physician suspects multiple sclerosis and plans a complete neurologic assessment.

125. When testing the trigeminal nerve, the nurse should expect the physician to evaluate:
   ① Ocular muscle movement
   ② Shrugging of the shoulders
   ③ Smiling and frowning
   ④ Corneal sensation

126. During the office visit, the nurse might expect Mrs. Carl to complain about the most common initial symptom associated with multiple sclerosis, which is:
   ① Diarrhea
   ② Headaches
   ③ Skin infections
   ④ Visual disturbances

127. Approximately 1 year later multiple sclerosis is confirmed and Mrs. Carl is informed that it is a chronic progressive neurologic condition. Mrs. Carl asks the nurse, "Will I experience pain?" The nurse's best response would be:
   ① "Tell me about your fears regarding pain."
   ② "Analgesics will be ordered to control the pain."

③ "Let's make a list of the things you need to ask your doctor."

④ "Pain is not a characteristic symptom of this disease process."

128. Mrs. Carl is obviously upset with the diagnosis and asks, "Am I going to die?" The nurse's best response would be:
① "Most individuals with your disease live a normal life span."
② "Is your family here? I would like to explain your disease to all of you."
③ "The prognosis is variable; most individuals experience remissions and exacerbations."
④ "Why don't you speak with your doctor who can give you more details about your disease?"

129. During an exacerbation Mrs. Carl complains of urinary urgency and frequency. The initial nursing measure should be to:
① Initiate a regimen to monitor urinary output
② Develop a plan to ensure high fluid intake
③ Begin teaching self-catheterization
④ Palpate the suprapubic area

130. A tentative diagnosis of cystitis is made, pending laboratory results. The nurse recognizes that *Escherichia coli* is a common causative agent in cystitis. The reason for this is that it is:
① A particularly virulent bacteria
② Commonly found in the kidneys
③ Usually found in the intestinal tract
④ A competitor with *Candida* for host sites

131. Mrs. Carl has decided to become a total vegetarian (vegand) and wishes to plan her diet to ensure adequate protein quality. In guiding her, the nurse would indicate that she should:
① Add milk to grains to provide complete proteins
② Use eggs with plant foods to provide essential amino acids
③ Plan a careful mixture of plant proteins to provide a balance of amino acids
④ Add cheese to grains and beans to increase the quality of the protein consumed

Situation: Frank Link, a 38-year-old stock broker, is admitted to the hospital with a tentative diagnosis of peptic ulcer.

132. When performing the initial history and physical assessment the nurse would expect him to describe the pain as:
① Located in the right shoulder and preceded by nausea
② Gnawing epigastric pain or boring pain in the back
③ Sudden, sharp abdominal pain, increasing in intensity

④ Heartburn and substernal discomfort when lying down

133. Mr. Link's ulcer is confirmed by a gastroscopy and upper GI series. The physician orders ranitidine (Zantac) 150 mg bid with meals. The nurse should check this order with the physician because:
① This drug is usually given on an empty stomach
② Zantac may be given by a variety of routes
③ Zantac is contraindicated for peptic ulcer
④ This is less than the recommended dose

134. Mr. Link has bathroom privileges. He is becoming irritable and asks the nurse if it is really necessary that he stay in bed so much. The nurse's best reply would be:
① "Why do you want to be out of bed?"
② "Yes. Bed rest is part of ulcer therapy."
③ "Not always. Ask your doctor to change the order."
④ "Rest will help your body direct energy to healing."

135. Later in the evening Mr. Link vomits his undigested antacids and complains of severe epigastric pain. The nursing assessment reveals an absence of bowel sounds, pulse rate of 134, and shallow respirations of 32 per minute. In addition to calling the physician, the nurse should:
① Place the client in the Trendelenburg position
② Ask the client if he has had red or black stools
③ Start O_2 per nasal cannula at 3 to 4 L per minute
④ Keep the client npo in preparation for possible surgery

136. Mr. Link's condition worsens, and a subtotal gastrectomy (Billroth I) is performed. Mr. Link recovers from surgery and begins to eat more food in varied forms. After meals he experiences a cramping discomfort and a rapid pulse with waves of weakness, which are frequently followed by nausea and vomiting. The nurse recognizes that this response is known as the "dumping syndrome" and is caused by:
① A slowed passage of food dumping into the small intestine
② A rapid passage of dilute food mixture into the small intestine
③ Rapid passage of hyperosmolar food solution into the small intestine
④ Food that is less concentrated than surrounding extracellular fluid entering the small intestine

137. About 2 hours after his initial postmeal attack, Mr. Link experiences a second period of discomfort, feeling somewhat "shaky." This later follow-up effect, which is precipitated by the dumping syndrome, is caused by:

① Mild hypoglycemia from an overproduction of insulin that occurs in response to the postprandial blood glucose rise

② Hyperglycemia from a rapidly absorbed glucose load, which overwhelms the insulin-adjusting mechanism

③ The increased fat content and larger amount of seasoned food, creating digestive discomfort

④ The increased use of simple carbohydrates in meals, creating a more prolonged glucose rise

Situation: Simon Irving, who is 73 years old and has Type I diabetes mellitus, complains of hematuria and urinary hesitancy. After a complete workup, prostatic cancer is diagnosed. He is to be admitted to the hospital in 1 week for a suprapubic prostatectomy.

138. In answer to Mr. Irving's question, the nurse explains that a suprapubic prostatectomy differs from other surgical procedures of the prostate in that:
    ① An indwelling catheter is not required after surgery
    ② An incision is made directly into the urinary bladder
    ③ The postoperative convalescent period is shorter
    ④ A major complication, that of sexual impotence, may occur

139. The night before surgery the anesthesiologist orders meperidine hydrochloride 100 mg IM preoperatively. The priority nursing action would be to:
    ① Raise the side rails after administering the medication
    ② Administer the preoperative medication as ordered
    ③ Determine if the client is allergic to meperidine
    ④ Question the anesthesiologist about the order

140. Four hours after surgery, Mr. Irving's blood glucose level is elevated. The nurse should expect to:
    ① Administer an oral hypoglycemic
    ② Decrease the rate of the intravenous infusion
    ③ Give supplemental doses of regular insulin
    ④ Institute urine glucose monitoring

141. Preoperatively Mr. Irving's insulin requirements were elevated but well controlled. Postoperatively the nurse would anticipate that his insulin requirements will:
    ① Decrease immediately
    ② Fluctuate widely
    ③ Increase sharply
    ④ Remain elevated

142. The nurse understands that Mr. Irving's plan of care must include the prevention of postoperative deep vein thrombosis. This can be

achieved by increasing the:
    ① Coagulability of the blood
    ② Velocity of the venous return
    ③ Effectiveness of internal respiration
    ④ Oxygen-carrying capacity of the blood

143. The nurse is concerned with the prevention of postoperative thrombosis for Mr. Irving because the majority of pulmonary emboli begin as deep vein thromboses of the:
    ① Calf of the leg
    ② Thoracic cavity
    ③ Pelvis and thighs
    ④ Extremities and abdomen

144. To prevent bleeding after surgery, Mr. Irving should be instructed to avoid straining on defecation. The nurse knows that he understands the related teaching when he says he must increase his intake of:
    ① Milk products
    ② Ripe bananas
    ③ Creamed potatoes
    ④ Green vegetables

Situation: Sally Spring fractured her left hip as a result of a fall in the kitchen. The fractured hip and osteoporosis are confirmed by x-ray films.

145. The most observable changes caused by osteoporosis will occur in:
    ① Facial bones
    ② The long bones
    ③ The vertebral column
    ④ Joints of the hands and feet

146. The physician applies Buck's extension (traction) until surgery can be performed to replace the head of the femur with a prosthesis. When checking Mrs. Spring's Buck's extension, the nurse should be aware that:
    ① Tape must cover the malleoli to adequately secure the weights to the leg
    ② The moleskin is placed on the anterior and posterior aspects of the leg
    ③ Weights above 8 pounds will cause skin damage
    ④ The spreader bar should fit snugly around the foot

147. After surgery to replace the head of the femur, an incentive spirometer is ordered. The nurse would recognize that Mrs. Spring is using the spirometer correctly when she:
    ① Inhaled deeply, sealed her lips around the mouthpiece, and exhaled
    ② Coughed twice before inhaling deeply through the mouthpiece
    ③ Inhaled deeply through the mouthpiece, relaxed, and then exhaled
    ④ Used the incentive spirometer for 10 consecutive breaths per hour

148. After 10 days Mrs. Spring is permitted to sit for short periods. When getting her out of bed the nurse should place her in a:
    ① Soft armchair with her left leg straight out in front

② Firm armchair with her left leg elevated on a stool

③ Firm chair with her left foot flat on the floor's surface

④ Soft chair with enough pillows to keep the hip at a right angle

149. Mrs. Spring refuses to go to her twice-a-day sessions in physical therapy. The nurse might best approach this problem by:

① Planning a conference with the client, the physical therapist, and the nurse to discuss Mrs. Spring's feelings

② Assuring the client that she will receive pain medication before going to physical therapy

③ Being the client's advocate and asking the physician if therapy can be decreased to once daily

④ Having Mrs. Spring observe the progress of a more cooperative client with the same problem

150. Mrs. Spring is finally discharged from the hospital. The nurse knows that Mrs. Spring can best limit further progression of her osteoporosis by:

① Increasing her consumption of milk and milk products

② Increasing her consumption of eggs and cheese

③ Taking supplemental magnesium and vitamin E

④ Taking supplemental calcium and vitamin D

151. During a follow-up visit, Mrs. Spring asks when she can resume her daily walks. The nurse bases the answer on the knowledge that after surgery:

① Partial weight-bearing and positional restrictions will be in effect for 2 months

② Partial weight-bearing restrictions will be enforced for at least 12 weeks

③ Full weight-bearing is usually restored after 4 months

④ Full weight-bearing is usually permitted after 6 weeks

Situation: Ting Whang is admitted for diagnosis and treatment of a lesion in the right lung. A bronchoscopy is performed.

152. When Mr. Whang returns from the bronchoscopy, the nurse should withhold food and fluid for several hours to prevent:

① Abdominal distention

② Aspiration of food

③ Dysphasia and dyspepsia

④ Projectile vomiting

153. Cancer of the lung is diagnosed, and a pneumonectomy is performed. When inspecting Mr. Whang's dressing, the nurse observes some puffiness of the tissue around the area. When the area is palpated, the tissue feels spongy and crackles. In charting, the nurse should describe this observation as:

① Chest distention

② Crepitus

③ Pitting edema

④ Stridor

154. The physician orders Mr. Whang's IV fluids to be delivered at 80 ml/hour. To adjust the drip rate the nurse must know the:

① Total volume of fluid in the IV bag

② Size of the needle or catheter in the vein

③ Drops per milliliter delivered by the infusion setup

④ Diameter of the tubing being used to instill the fluid

155. On the first postoperative day Mr. Whang suddenly sits straight up in bed. His respirations are labored, and he is making a crowing sound. His skin is pale, cool, and moist. Immediately the nurse should:

① Notify the physician

② Check the chest tube for patency

③ Auscultate the left lung

④ Inspect the incision for bleeding

156. When turning Mr. Whang the nurse should plan to use the:

① Supine position or right side-lying position

② Supine position until the chest tube is removed

③ Right side-lying or left side-lying position

④ High-Fowler's position or supine position

157. Irradiation to the chest wall is prescribed for Mr. Whang on an outpatient basis. In teaching Mr. Whang skin care, the nurse should emphasize:

① Massaging 4 times a day to increase circulation

② Frequent washing to remove desquamated cells

③ Keeping the skin dry and protected from abrasions

④ Using skin lotion twice daily to keep the skin supple

158. Mr. Whang develops increased respiratory secretions because of the radiation therapy. When teaching him postural drainage, the nurse should explain that he will know that it is effective when he:

① Is free of rales

② Is able to expectorate saliva

③ Can breathe deeply

④ Demonstrates a productive cough

159. Mr. Whang's serum albumin is 2.8 g/100 ml. The nurse should evaluate client teaching as successful when Mr. Whang says that for lunch he is going to have:

① Clear beef broth

② Fruit salad

③ Sliced turkey

④ Spinach salad

160. Mr. Whang is cautioned to avoid vitamin D toxicity while increasing his protein intake. The nurse would know he understands the teaching when he tells his wife he must increase his intake of:
    ① Cottage cheese custard
    ② Powdered whole milk
    ③ Fruit and eggnog
    ④ Tofu products

Situation: Andrea Becker, a teacher, is hospitalized with cramping abdominal pain noted especially after eating. She has a history of hypertension and elevated serum cholesterol for which she has been taking chlorothiazide (Diuril) and cholestyramine (Questran) for the past 9 months.

161. The characteristics that would alert the nurse that a client is at increased risk of developing gallbladder disease would be:
    ① Female, under the age of 40, family history of gallstones
    ② Male, over the age of 40, low serum cholesterol level
    ③ Male, under the age of 40, past history of hepatitis
    ④ Female, over the age of 40, obese

162. Mrs. Becker is to undergo an oral cholecystogram in the morning. As part of the preparation for this test the nurse should tell her:
    ① The test will be administered on 2 successive days
    ② The contrast medium in the pills may cause constipation
    ③ Any stones present will be readily visible on the x-ray film
    ④ A low-fat supper should be eaten the night before the test

163. The presence of gallstones is confirmed, and a cholecystectomy is scheduled. Before the cholecystectomy, nutritional deficiencies and excesses should be corrected. Based on her history, a nutritional assessment should be conducted to determine if Mrs. Becker:
    ① Is deficient in vitamins A, D, and K
    ② Consumes excessive amounts of protein
    ③ Consumes adequate amounts of dietary fiber
    ④ Has excessive levels of potassium and folic acid

164. Before the cholecystectomy the physician orders a modified diet. The nurse understands that with cholecystitis:
    ① Soft-textured foods are used to reduce the digestive burden
    ② Low-cholesterol foods are used to avoid further formation of gallstones
    ③ Fat is decreased to avoid stimulation of the cholecystokinin mechanism for bile release
    ④ Increased protein and kilocalories are needed to promote tissue healing and provide energy

165. Mrs. Becker undergoes a cholecystectomy with common duct exploration. In the immediate postoperative period, the nursing action that should assume the highest priority is:
    ① Encouraging Mrs. Becker to take adequate fluids by mouth
    ② Encouraging Mrs. Becker to cough and deep breathe
    ③ Changing Mrs. Becker's dressing at least bid
    ④ Irrigating Mrs. Becker's T-tube frequently

166. The finding that would most significantly indicate that a client is hypertensive is:
    ① An extended Korotkoff sound
    ② A regular pulse of 92 beats per minute
    ③ A systolic pressure ranging from 150 to 160 mmHg
    ④ A diastolic pressure that remains greater than 90 mmHg

167. Mrs. Becker is to be released from the hospital on her previous regimen of Diuril and Questran. The nurse should instruct Mrs. Becker to:
    ① Avoid eating fruits and vegetables because they limit the liver's effect on digestion
    ② Take protein supplements to promote healing and speed her recovery
    ③ Alter her diet to compensate for the nutrient effects of her medications
    ④ Return to her normal eating habits once she is home

Situation: Rodney Flack is admitted to the hospital for fever of unknown origin. He has recently experienced an unexplained weight loss and a series of respiratory infections. Mr. Flack is accompanied to the unit by his life partner, Jack Kemper. AIDS-related complex (ARC) is suspected.

168. The nurse knows that a positive diagnosis for the disease of AIDS is made based on a positive HIV antibody test and:
    ① A history of high-risk sexual behaviors
    ② A positive ELISA and Western blot test
    ③ The presence of weight loss and high fever
    ④ The presence of an associated opportunistic infection

169. When taking Mr. Flack's blood pressure, the nurse must:
    ① Wear clean gloves
    ② Use barrier techniques
    ③ Wear a mask and gown
    ④ Wash hands thoroughly

170. Mr. Flack is receiving Azidothymidine (AZT). It is most important for the nurse to monitor his:
    ① Cardiac enzymes
    ② Serum electrolytes
    ③ HIV antibody levels
    ④ Complete blood cell count

171. Mr. Flack is diagnosed as having AIDS-related complex (ARC). In comparison to acquired immunodeficiency syndrome, AIDS-related complex is:
① More physiologically debilitating
② Caused by a more virulent organism
③ Not associated with opportunistic infections
④ Less frequently transmitted by blood contact

172. The nursing staff has a team conference on AIDS and discusses the routes of transmission of the human immunodeficiency virus (HIV). The discussion reveals that an individual has no risk of exposure to the human immunodeficiency virus when that individual:
① Uses a condom each time there is sexual intercourse
② Limits sexual contact to those without HIV antibodies
③ Makes a donation of a pint of whole blood
④ Has intercourse with just the spouse

173. Mr. Flack's diagnosis of ARC would be changed to AIDS if he developed:
① Enlarged lymph nodes
② Weight loss
③ Purplish skin lesions
④ Leukocytosis

174. Three weeks later Mr. Flack experiences a spike in temperature and develops shortness of breath that progresses to respiratory arrest. Based on a Do Not Resuscitate (DNR) order, which he signed on admission, Mr. Flack is not resuscitated. A true statement about the legal aspects of a DNR order would be:
① Once the order has been signed, it remains in force for the entire hospitalization
② The status of the DNR order is contingent on the policies of the institution
③ The decision not to resuscitate resides with the client's physician
④ Age is an important factor in the decision not to resuscitate

Situation: Sara Raymond, 23 years old, is admitted for a diagnostic workup with complaints of frequent loose, watery stools; anorexia; and malaise. Ms. Raymond has lost considerable weight over the past month and is constantly tired.

175. On receiving the reports of Ms. Raymond's blood work, the nurse notes findings indicative of leukocytosis and an elevated sedimentation rate. The nurse recognizes that Ms. Raymond's presenting symptoms in conjunction with these findings could be indicative of:
① Poor dietary practices that have resulted in an alteration of bowel function

② Systemic responses of the body to a localized inflammatory process
③ An emotional response that has resulted in physical symptoms
④ The consistent, long-term use of an irritant-type laxative

176. Prednisone, an adrenal steroid, is ordered, and the nurse teaches Ms. Raymond about the drug when giving her the first dose. The nurse should stress that this drug:
① Is relatively slow in effecting a response but is effective in reducing symptoms
② Is not curative but does cause a suppression of the inflammatory process
③ Will protect her from getting an infection while she is taking it
④ May decrease her appetite, causing her to lose weight

177. Ms. Raymond is diagnosed as having colitis. She inquires as to whether surgery will ever be necessary. When teaching Ms. Raymond about the disease and its treatment, the nurse should emphasize that:
① Medical treatment for colitis is curative, and surgery is not required
② Surgery for colitis is considered only as a last resort for most clients
③ Surgery for colitis is done early in the course of the disease for most clients
④ Medical treatment is all that will be needed if the client can acquire some emotional stability

178. The physician orders total parenteral nutrition (TPN) 1L q 12 hours for 2 days to aid recovery. The primary nursing responsibility should be to monitor Ms. Raymond's:
① Electrolytes
② Urinary output
③ Administration rate
④ Urine glucose levels

179. The nurse is aware that total parenteral nutrition is a more desirable therapy than just intravenous fluids for Ms. Raymond. The nurse understands that clients receiving only IV fluids lose weight because of:
① Lack of bulk in the diet
② Deficient carbohydrate intake
③ Insufficient intake of water-soluble vitamins
④ Increased concentrations of electrolytes in cells

180. In preparing Ms. Raymond to go home with TPN the nurse should help her plan:
① Which days will be used for administration
② For professional help to administer the TPN
③ For daily insertion of the administration tubing
④ A schedule of administration around normal activity

181. Ms. Raymond develops an infection at the catheter insertion site. The nurse uses the term *iatrogenic* when describing this infection because it resulted from:
    ① The client's developmental level
    ② Inadequate dietary patterns
    ③ A therapeutic procedure
    ④ Poor physical hygiene

Situation: Bruce Edwards is admitted with severe left flank pain, nausea, and hematuria. The tentative diagnosis is a ureteral calculus.

182. When Mr. Edwards is first admitted, the initial nursing action should be to:
    ① Obtain a urine specimen for culture
    ② Administer prescribed analgesics
    ③ Increase his fluid intake
    ④ Strain all urine output

183. When taking the admitting history, the nurse would expect Mr. Edwards to report:
    ① Boring pain in the left flank
    ② Pain that intensifies on urination
    ③ Pain that is dull and constant in the costovertebral angle
    ④ Spasmodic pain on the left side radiating to the suprapubis

184. Mr. Edwards is scheduled for an intravenous pyelogram (IVP). The nurse explains to Mr. Edwards that on the day before the IVP he must:
    ① Eat a fat-free dinner
    ② Drink a large amount of fluids
    ③ Omit dinner and limit beverages
    ④ Take a laxative before going to bed

185. Mr. Edwards' serum calcium is elevated, and the IVP confirms the presence of a ureteral calculus. If Mr. Edwards' blood test indicated an elevated purine instead of an elevated calcium level, the nurse would recognize that the stone would probably be composed of:
    ① Struvite
    ② Cystine
    ③ Uric acid
    ④ Oxalate

186. Later that evening, Mr. Edwards' urinary output is much less than his intake. When it is noted that his bladder is not distended, the nurse should suspect the development of:
    ① Oliguria
    ② Hydroureter
    ③ Renal shutdown
    ④ Urethral obstruction

187. A ureterolithotomy is immediately scheduled to remove the stone located in the proximal portion of the ureter. The nurse prepares Mr. Edwards for the postsurgical period by informing him that:
    ① A dressing will be present in the flank area
    ② Surgery will be performed transurethrally

③ A suprapubic catheter will be in place
④ The left ureter will be removed

188. Before Mr. Edwards' discharge the nurse discusses the need to avoid urinary tract infections. The nurse knows that Mr. Edwards understands the signs of infection when he says he will report:
    ① Pain radiating to the external genitalia
    ② Urgency or frequency of urination
    ③ The inability to maintain an erection
    ④ An increase in alkalinity or acidity of urine

189. To facilitate micturition the nurse should instruct Mr. Edwards to:
    ① Assume the normal position for voiding
    ② Wash his hands after voiding
    ③ Drink cranberry juice daily
    ④ Use a urinal for voiding

Situation: Eli Watson, with a 20-year history of excessive alcohol use, is admitted to the hospital with jaundice and ascites.

190. A priority nursing action during the first 48 hours after Mr. Watson's admission will be to:
    ① Monitor his vital signs
    ② Increase his fluid intake
    ③ Improve his nutritional status
    ④ Identify his reasons for drinking

191. The nurse, aware of Mr. Watson's 20-year history of excessive alcohol use, would expect his physical assessment to reveal a:
    ① Type A hepatitis
    ② Low blood ammonia
    ③ Small liver with a rough surface
    ④ High fever with a generalized rash

192. Mr. Watson reports that his gums bleed spontaneously. In addition, the nurse notes small hemorrhagic lesions on his face. The nurse recognizes that Mr. Watson needs additional:
    ① Vitamin A
    ② Bile salts
    ③ Vitamin K
    ④ Folic acid

193. The physician schedules a paracentesis. To prepare Mr. Watson for the abdominal paracentesis the nurse should:
    ① Instruct him to empty his bladder
    ② Encourage him to drink fluids
    ③ Shave and prep his abdomen
    ④ Medicate him for pain

194. Mr. Watson complains of severe pruritus. To relieve his discomfort, the nurse would expect the physician to order:
    ① Sponge baths with alcohol
    ② Applications of talcum powder
    ③ Baths with sodium bicarbonate solution
    ④ Liberal applications of baby oil to the involved areas

195. Mr. Watson develops bronchitis, and IPPB

treatments and potassium iodide (SSKI) 300 mg are ordered. Before administering this drug, the nurse should:
① Restrict the client's oral fluid intake
② Dilute it with milk or fruit juice
③ Determine the client's apical pulse
④ Administer the ordered IPPB treatment

Situation: Larry Short, a 55-year-old mailman, has a cerebral vascular accident while delivering mail in the snow. He is brought to the emergency room with right-sided hemiplegia, and a left intracerebral hemorrhage is suspected.

196. The physician orders aminocaproic acid (Amicar Elixir) 4 grams po for Mr. Short. The bottle is labeled 250 mg/ml. The nurse should administer:
① 0.016 ml
② 0.16 ml
③ 1.6 ml
④ 16 ml

197. Dexamethasone (Decadron) is ordered for the early management of Mr. Short's cerebral edema. This treatment is effective because it:
① Acts as a hyperosmotic diuretic
② Increases tissue resistance to infection
③ Reduces the inflammatory response of tissues
④ Decreases the formation of cerebral spinal fluid

198. During the time Mr. Short is receiving the Decadron, the nurse should observe for the development of a negative side effect by:
① Monitoring deep tendon reflexes
② Measuring blood glucose levels
③ Culturing respiratory secretions
④ Auscultating for bowel sounds

199. The neuromuscular status and decreased mobility of Mr. Short must be assessed early. It is important for the nurse to consider any restrictions or abnormalities that are observed because:
① Disuse hypertrophy of the muscles will eventually result
② Shortening and eventual atrophy of the muscles will occur
③ Rigid extension can occur, making therapy painful and difficult
④ Decreased movement on the affected side predisposes to infection

200. Mrs. Short tells the nurse that her sister had a CVA and was receiving anticoagulant therapy. She asks why anticoagulant therapy is not being given to Mr. Short. The nurse explains that in this situation anticoagulant therapy:
① Will be started if necessary to enhance circulation
② May be necessary to prevent pulmonary thrombosis
③ Is contraindicated because bleeding would be increased
④ Is contraindicated because it would mask signs and symptoms

201. Mr. Short manifests hemianopsia as a result of his CVA. The nurse should:
① Instruct Mr. Short to scan his surroundings
② Correct Mr. Short's misuse of equipment
③ Provide tactile stimulation to Mr. Short's affected extremities
④ Teach Mr. Short to look at the position of his right extremities

202. Mr. Short is discharged. On a follow-up visit Mrs. Short explains that Mr. Short cries easily and without provocation. She asks why he is so emotionally labile. The nurse should explain that:
① He can remember only depressing events from the past
② He feels guilty about the demands he is making on his family
③ This is a way of getting attention and the behavior should be ignored
④ This behavior is a common response over which he has very little control

203. Several months after discharge Mr. Short is readmitted with aphasia. He is awake but oriented only to person. A bruit is heard over his left carotid artery, and his pulse is irregular. The nurse is aware that complete occlusion of the branches of the middle cerebral artery resulting in aphasia may occur because of:
① Emboli associated with atrial fibrillation
② A history of hypertensive disease
③ Inappropriate paroxysmal neural discharge
④ Developmental defects of the arterial wall

204. Mrs. Short asks, "Will Larry's speech ever return?" The nurse should respond:
① "You will have to ask your doctor."
② "It should return to normal by discharge."
③ "It is hard to say how much improvement he will have."
④ "This will probably be the extent of his speech from now on."

205. For Mrs. Short to help Mr. Short regain as much speech function as possible, the nurse should instruct her to:
① Speak louder than usual to him when she visits
② Give positive reinforcement for correct communication
③ Tell him to use the correct words when speaking
④ Encourage him to talk and be patient with his efforts

Situation: Joan Herrick has partial-thickness burns on her chest, abdomen, and right leg from a fire at her workplace.

206. When Mrs. Herrick arrives in the emergency room the nurse's first responsibility should be to:
① Evaluate whether heat inhalation occurred
② Carefully remove all of Mrs. Herrick's clothes
③ Apply sterile saline dressings on all burned surfaces
④ Determine the extent of the burns, using the rule of nines

207. In the evaluation of Mrs. Herrick's condition, an assessment that would indicate potential respiratory obstruction is:
① Deep breathing
② Abdominal breathing
③ Hoarse quality to the voice
④ Pink-tinged, frothy sputum

208. Mrs. Herrick's second-degree, or partial-thickness burns differ from third-degree, or full-thickness burns in that with second-degree burns the burned area will:
① Have to be grafted before it can heal
② Be painful, reddened, and have blisters
③ Have total destruction of the epidermis and dermis
④ Take months of extensive treatment before healing

209. The physician orders a low dosage of narcotic to relieve Mrs. Herrick's pain. The nurse recognizes that the preferred mode of administration is:
① Oral
② Rectal
③ Intravenous
④ Intramuscular

210. Mrs. Herrick has a nasogastric tube, a central venous line, and a Foley catheter inserted. Management of fluid and electrolytes is accomplished by the administration of a balanced salt solution (Ringer's solution), water, and albumin. The physician orders albumin intravenously. When this solution is given, the nurse is aware that body water will shift from the:
① Interstitial compartment to the extracellular compartment
② Extracellular compartment to the intracellular compartment
③ Intracellular compartment to the extracellular compartment
④ Intravascular compartment to the interstitial compartment

211. The nurse is aware that the shift of body fluids associated with the administration of albumin occurs by the process of:
① Active transport
② Diffusion
③ Osmosis
④ Filtration

212. The nurse, in assessing the adequacy of Mrs. Herrick's fluid replacement during the first 2 to 3 days, would be aware that the most significant data would be obtained from recording:
① Weights every day
② Urinary output every hour
③ Blood pressure every 15 minutes
④ Central venous pressure every 2 hours

213. Mrs. Herrick's arterial blood gases (ABGs) show a Po$_2$ of 89 mmHg; a Pco$_2$ of 35 mmHg; and a pH of 7.37. These findings indicate Mrs. Herrick is in:
① Fluid balance
② Metabolic acidosis
③ Acid-base balance
④ Oxygen depletion

214. The method of treatment chosen for Mrs. Herrick's burns is the exposure method with application of mafenide (Sulfamylon) bid. When applying this medication the nurse should plan to:
① Use medical asepsis
② Give ordered pain medication
③ Apply a dry sterile dressing
④ Monitor liver function studies

215. When formulating Mrs. Herrick's plan of care concerning exercising to prevent deformities and contractures, the nurse should plan to begin routine range-of-motion exercises when Mrs. Herrick's:
① Pain has lessened
② Vital signs are stable
③ Skin grafts are healed
④ Emotional status stabilizes

Situation: George Manson, age 43, is admitted to the hospital with a diagnosis of cancer of the sigmoid colon. An abdominoperineal resection with a permanent colostomy is planned.

216. Before surgery a low-residue diet is ordered for Mr. Manson. The nurse explains that this is necessary to:
① Lower the bacterial count in the GI tract
② Limit production of gas in the intestine
③ Prevent irritation of the lining of the intestine
④ Reduce the amount of stool in the large bowel

217. Mr. Manson returns from surgery with a permanent colostomy. During the first 24 hours the colostomy does not drain. The nurse should realize this is a result of:
① Intestinal edema following surgery
② The absence of gastrointestinal motility
③ A presurgical decrease in fluid intake
④ Proper functioning of the gastric decompression

218. Mr. Manson is to receive D5RL 850 ml every 8 hours. The drop factor of the tubing is 10 gtt/ml. The nurse should set the flow to provide:

① 12 gtt/min
② 18 gtt/min
③ 24 gtt/min
④ 36 gtt/min

219. One week after surgery Mr. Manson develops an infection of the abdominal incision. He overhears the nurses say that he has a nosocomial infection. Mr. Manson asks the nurse what this means. The nurse should reply:
① "As a result of medical treatment, you have developed a secondary infection."
② "This is a highly contagious infection requiring reverse isolation."
③ "You acquired the infection after being admitted to the hospital."
④ "The infection you had before hospitalization has flared up."

220. Cefoperazone sodium (Cefobid) 250 mg is ordered for Mr. Manson. A vial containing 1 g of the powdered form of the drug must be reconstituted with 2.8 ml of diluent to form a withdrawable volume of 3 ml. Using this solution, the nurse should administer:
① 8 minims
② 10 minims
③ 12 minims
④ 17 minims

221. The physician places Mr. Manson on strict isolation. After being taught about isolation, Mr. Manson is seen sneaking out of his room to make telephone calls on the public phone. The most effective nursing intervention would be to:
① Ensure regular visits by staff members
② Explore what isolation means to the client
③ Report the situation to the infection control nurse
④ Reteach the entire isolation procedure to Mr. Manson

222. Mr. Manson is almost ready for discharge. A primary nursing goal before Mr. Manson is sent home should be to:
① Evaluate his ability to care for the colostomy
② Coax him into caring for the colostomy by himself
③ Ensure that he understands the limitations in his diet
④ Have him change the dry sterile dressing on the incision alone

223. Discharge instructions include irrigation of the colostomy when at home. The nurse is aware he understands the teaching when he states he will contact his physician and report:
① The occurrence of abdominal cramping while the solution is running in
② Any difficulty in inserting the irrigating tube in the stoma
③ The expulsion of flatus while the fluid is running out
④ Any problems in completing the procedure in 1 hour

Situation: Howard Bell, age 54, has noticed a tremor of his extremities and comes to the neurologic clinic for evaluation. When assisting him in walking to the examining room, the nurse notes that Mr. Bell exhibits the characteristic gait associated with Parkinson's disease.

224. When recording on Mr. Bell's chart, the nurse would describe this gait as:
① Shuffling
② Ataxic
③ Scissoring
④ Spastic

225. When performing the history and physical examination, the nurse assesses Mr. Bell for:
① A recent increase in appetite and weight gain
② A low-pitched, monotonous voice
③ Frequent bouts of diarrhea
④ Hyperextension of the neck

226. During the assessment, the nurse notes additional evidence of Mr. Bell's altered neural function, which would be:
① Tremors of the hand on movement
② Leaning toward the affected side
③ Blank facies or lack of expression
④ Hyperextension of the affected extremity

227. Mr. Bell states he has had a problem with elimination. The nurse should encourage Mr. Bell to:
① Increase residue in his diet
② Take cathartics regularly
③ Decrease his fluid intake
④ Eat a banana daily

228. Levodopa is prescribed for Mr. Bell. The sign or symptom that would be unrelated to the administration of levodopa would be:
① Nausea
② Anorexia
③ Bradycardia
④ Mental changes

Situation: Frank Romano, age 26, is admitted for repair of bilateral inguinal hernias under general anesthesia.

229. Before surgery the nurse would assess the client for signs that strangulation may have occurred. An early sign of strangulation would be:
① Increased flatus
② Projectile vomiting
③ Sharp abdominal pain
④ Decreased bowel sounds

230. Preoperatively the nurse should teach the client that postoperatively the client will:
① Have a nasogastric tube in his nose
② Have a portable wound drainage system
③ Turn and change his position every 2 hours
④ Perform coughing and deep-breathing exercises

231. Preoperatively the physician orders meperidine (Demerol) and atropine sulfate. A sign

that the client has an overdose of atropine would be:
① Respiratory depression
② Extreme hypotension
③ Nausea and vomiting
④ Severe tachycardia

232. After the bilateral herniorrhaphy the client should be observed for the development of:
① Thrombophlebitis
② A hydrocele
③ Urinary retention
④ Paralytic ileus

233. The client's scrotum becomes swollen and painful. The nurse should:
① Assist the client with a sitz bath
② Apply warm soaks to the scrotum
③ Elevate the scrotum using a soft support
④ Prepare for a possible incision and drainage

Situation: Neal Kemp, a 39-year-old corporate executive, is 5 feet, 10 inches tall, weighs 180 pounds, and has a blood pressure of 150/100. His lipid panel shows triglycerides 160, high-density lipoprotein (HDL) cholesterol 70, and low-density lipoprotein (LDL) cholesterol 218. His total cholesterol level is 320.

234. To help reduce the client's risk factors for heart disease, in discussing his diet the nurse should teach him to:
① Increase the ratio of complex carbohydrates
② Decrease the amount of fat-binding fiber
③ Decrease the amount of unsaturated fat
④ Avoid eating between meals

235. Mr. Kemp appears discouraged and says, "Well, I guess I'd better cut out all the fat and cholesterol in my diet." The nurse's most appropriate response would be:
① "Well yes, that would certainly lower the amount of your blood fats."
② "That's good, but be sure to compensate by adding more proteins and carbohydrates."
③ "You need some fat to supply a necessary fatty acid, so it's mainly just a need for cutting down the amount."
④ "You need some cholesterol in your diet because your body cannot manufacture it, so just avoid excessive amounts."

236. Mr. Kemp is placed on the Prudent Diet proposed by the American Heart Association. The caloric distribution of this diet includes:
① 45% fat (15% saturated), 40% carbohydrate (20% complex), 15% protein
② 10% fat (5% saturated), 80% carbohydrate (50% complex), 10% protein
③ 30% fat (<10% saturated), 50% carbohydrate (35% complex), 20% protein
④ 50% fat (20% saturated), 20% carbohydrate, 30% protein

Situation: Leland Howard had a myocardial infarction when he was 48 years old and has been taking digoxin and warfarin sodium (Coumadin) for the last 6 months. He becomes progressively short of breath and goes to his physician, who immediately admits him to the hospital with severe congestive heart failure.

237. On Mr. Howard's admission, when assessing him for signs of congestive heart failure, the nurse should expect to note:
① A pleural friction rub
② Neck vein distention
③ A slowed pulse rate
④ Increasing hypotension

238. The physician adjusts Mr. Howard's dosages of digoxin and coumadin. The antidote for coumadin that the nurse should keep in the client's medicine drawer is:
① Protamine sulfate
② Vitamin K
③ Fibrinogen
④ Prothrombin

239. The nurse should suspect that Mr. Howard is experiencing denial when he:
① Expresses displeasure with his activity program
② Refuses to discuss his condition with his wife
③ Lacks an emotional response to his illness
④ Attempts to minimize his illness

240. Mr. Howard is to continue to take digoxin (Lanoxin) after discharge from the hospital. The nurse would know he understands the teaching concerning digoxin when he states, "I should:
① Not eat foods high in potassium."
② Check my pulse rate and rhythm daily."
③ Adjust my dosage according to my activities."
④ Increase my intake of vitamin K."

241. A year later Mr. Howard is again hospitalized for CHF. He has pulmonary edema and is admitted to the intensive care unit. When assessing Mr. Howard, the nurse should expect:
① Rales at the base of each lung
② A decreased blood pressure
③ Radiating anterior chest pain
④ A pulse that is weak and rapid

242. Mr. Howard has a Swan-Ganz catheter inserted for monitoring cardiovascular status. With the Swan-Ganz catheter the most accurate measurement of Mr. Howard's left ventricular pressure would be the:
① Right atrial pressure
② Cardiac output by thermodilution
③ Pulmonary artery diastolic pressure
④ Pulmonary capillary wedge pressure

243. Because Mr. Howard is now receiving Heparin, the potential complication of hemorrhage may occur. In the event of excessive bleeding, the nurse should be prepared to administer:
① Vitamin K
② Panheparin

③ Warfarin sodium
④ Protamine sulfate

Situation: Andrew Bogen has a 10-year history of self-diagnosed gastritis that has gotten progressively more severe in the last 6 months. This increased discomfort precipitated a recent visit to the physician, and the physician diagnosed a peptic ulcer.

244. The nurse, when teaching Mr. Bogen about his diet, also instructs him to report any stools that appear:
① Frothy
② Ribbon shaped
③ Pale or clay colored
④ Dark brown or black

245. Mr. Bogen develops severe epigastric pain and shocklike symptoms. He is brought to the emergency room, stabilized, and sent to the operating room for a subtotal gastrectomy because of a perforated gastric ulcer. Postoperatively he has a nasogastric tube to low suction and IV fluids. Three hours after surgery he complains of nausea and abdominal pain, his abdomen appears distended, and there are no bowel sounds. Considering the type of surgery and the orders for pain medication and irrigation of the NG tube, the nurse should first:
① Give the prn pain medication
② Notify the physician of absent bowel sounds
③ Irrigate the nasogastric tube
④ Check stools and gastric drainage for blood

246. In the evening of the day of surgery, the nurse notes bright red blood in Mr. Bogen's nasogastric drainage. The nurse should:
① Clamp the nasogastric tube and call the physician
② Continue to monitor the drainage from the tube and record the observations
③ Gently irrigate the tube with 30 ml normal saline
④ Reduce the pressure on the suction and record observations of the drainage

247. The physician orders 1250 ml of IV fluid every 8 hours. The drop factor of the tubing is 15 gtt/ml. The nurse should set the flow to provide:
① 36 gtt/min
② 39 gtt/min
③ 40 gtt/min
④ 42 gtt/min

248. The day before discharge, Mr. Bogen complains of perspiring and having epigastric discomfort about a half hour after eating lunch. The symptoms disappear within a few minutes. Mr. Bogen understands the nurse's teaching when he states that these symptoms can be prevented by:

① Eating small, low-carbohydrate meals
② Resting before and after each meal
③ Avoiding spicy, gas-forming meals
④ Increasing fluids with each meal

249. Mrs. Bogen joins her husband for a discharge conference with the nurse. This is helpful because in addition to diet planning, Mr. and Mrs. Bogen need to work together to plan:
① Methods of avoiding pernicious anemia after gastric surgery
② To deal with long-term complications following surgery
③ Ways of dealing with stress in their environment
④ To maximize changes in his life-style

Situation: Michael Maloney, age 70 years, cut his leg on a rusty fence 2 weeks ago. He has been a heavy smoker all his adult life. He is admitted to the hospital for intravenous antibiotic therapy and an incision and drainage of an abscess that developed at the site of the laceration. In addition, osteomyelitis is suspected.

250. The nurse should begin teaching wound care to Mr. Maloney:
① During the first dressing change
② On the first postoperative day
③ A few days before discharge
④ In the preoperative period

251. Mr. Maloney is to have an incision and drainage of the abscess with debridement of the infected bone. When planning for his postoperative care the nurse knows that:
① He will be allowed out of bed after the first day
② Septicemia is a common postoperative complication
③ His leg will be immobilized in a cast or splint
④ Frequent range-of-motion exercises will be needed

252. The physician orders 1200 mg of an antibiotic, to be added to 50 ml D5W qid IVPB via a Heplock. The vial contains 5 g of powdered antibiotic to which 12 ml of diluent is to be added. The resulting solution contains 1 gram of drug per 3 ml. The nurse should use:
① 0.7 ml
② 1.2 ml
③ 2.9 ml
④ 3.6 ml

253. The nurse on the unit tells Mr. Maloney that the nurse epidemiologist will visit him daily. Mr. Maloney asks what the nurse epidemiologist does. The nurse could correctly explain the role by saying: "The nurse epidemiologist:
① Decides what antibiotics should be prescribed for infections."
② Is responsible for doing cultures of all infections and drainages."

③ Helps physicians and hospital personnel to control infections."

④ Works in the laboratory to identify bacteria that are causing infection."

254. Mr. Maloney is placed on a high-calorie, high-protein diet. In light of his history of smoking he should also be encouraged to eat foods high in:
① Vitamin B_{12}
② Vitamin C
③ Thiamin
④ Niacin

255. Mr. Maloney is to be discharged to complete his recuperation at home. Oxacillin sodium (Bactocill) 500 mg every 6 hours is ordered by the physician. The nurse would know that Mr. Maloney understands the teaching about Oxacillin when he says:
① "I will take the medication with meals."
② "I should drink a glass of milk with each pill."
③ "I should drink at least six glasses of water every day."
④ "I will take the medication 1 hour before or 2 hours after meals."

Situation: Marguerite Ramirez, a 65-year-old obese woman, has had gout for several years and has been taking allopurinol (Zyloprim). She comes to the physician complaining of being tired all the time. Her test reveals hyperglycemia, and the physician tells her she has Type II diabetes, which does not require insulin. She will be managed on an ADA diet and exercise.

256. Because Mrs. Ramirez has Type II diabetes mellitus, the nurse should expect her laboratory studies to reveal:
① Ketones in the blood but not in the urine
② Glucose in the urine but not in the blood
③ Urine negative for ketones and 4+ for glucose
④ Urine and blood positive for both glucose and ketones

257. Mrs. Ramirez asks about the use of alcohol or special "dietetic" food in her diet. She should be taught that:
① Alcohol can be used with its calories accounted for in the diet
② Alcohol should not be used in cooking because it adds too many calories
③ Special "dietetic" foods are needed because many regular foods cannot be used
④ Unlimited amounts of sugar substitutes such as aspartame can be used as desired

258. Mrs. Ramirez travels frequently and asks how to plan her diet during trips. The nurse's most appropriate response would be:
① "You can order diabetic foods on most airlines and in restaurants."
② "You should plan your food ahead and carry it with you from home."

③ "Make regular food choices, wherever you are, following your food plan."
④ "You can monitor your blood sugar level frequently and can eat accordingly."

259. Mrs. Ramirez is monitored regularly at the endocrine clinic at the community hospital. When she consistently demonstrates an elevated serum glucose, the physician orders chlorpropamide (Diabinese) in addition to her routine dose of Zyloprim. At a follow-up visit Mrs. Ramirez states, "I've been fainting and sweating a lot in the past week." The nurse should realize that the:
① Diabinese should be changed to insulin
② Diabinese dosage may have to be reduced
③ Zyloprim and Diabinese should be alternated daily
④ Zyloprim should be eliminated from her medication regimen

260. Mrs. Ramirez develops a nonhealing ulcer of the right lower extremity and complains of leg cramps after walking short distances. Mrs. Ramirez asks the nurse what causes these leg pains. The nurse's best response would be:
① "Pain occurs in the legs while walking because there is a lack of oxygen to the muscles."
② "Pressure occurs in the legs because of vasodilation and pooling of blood in the extremity."
③ "Muscle weakness occurs in the legs because of a lack of exercise."
④ "Edema and cyanosis occur in the legs because they are dependent."

261. The physician prescribes a progressive exercise program that includes walking. The nurse should tell Mrs. Ramirez that if she develops leg cramps while she is walking, she should:
① Take one aspirin twice a day
② Stop and rest until the pain resolves
③ Walk more slowly while pain is present
④ Take one nitroglycerine tablet sublingually

262. Medical management of the ulcer and a graft to the ulcer fail. Mrs. Ramirez is scheduled for a below-the-knee amputation of the right leg. Legally, Mrs. Ramirez may not sign the operative consent if she has:
① Ambivalent feelings regarding the operation
② Just been medicated with a sedative
③ Not discussed alternatives with two physicians
④ Not had a complete history and physical examination

263. Mrs. Ramirez' serum glucose rises. The physician orders finger sticks for serum glucose measurements ac and hs with regular insulin coverage. A serum glucose measurement reveals that Mrs. Ramirez requires 30 U of reg-

ular insulin. The nurse has regular insulin U 100 but no insulin syringe. The nurse should administer:
① 3 minims
② 5 minims
③ 7 minims
④ 9 minims

264. Immediately after surgery Mrs. Ramirez awakens and begins screaming while feeling for her lower right leg. The nurse should:
① Leave the client alone to provide time for privacy
② Allow the client to ventilate her feelings
③ Encourage frequent family visits for distraction
④ Administer medication to promote sleep

265. Mrs. Ramirez begins to experience extreme discomfort in the area where the limb once was. An appropriate nursing diagnosis at this time would be:
① Hopelessness related to life-style changes
② Ineffective coping mechanisms
③ Sensory-perceptual alterations
④ Pain related to amputation

266. Mrs. Ramirez' stump is snugly bandaged during the postoperative period. The main purpose of this is to:
① Promote secretion drainage
② Prevent injury to the stump
③ Prevent suture line infection
④ Promote stump shrinkage

267. The nurse raises Mrs. Ramirez' bedside rails at night. An alteration of the environment through the use of side rails may affect the psychologic status of Mrs. Ramirez, resulting in:
① A sense of security
② The prevention of falls
③ Increased independence
④ An alteration in proprioception

268. Mrs. Ramirez' serum glucose remains elevated, and the physician plans to discharge her with insulin coverage based on glucose stick levels. She will also have to perform stump care and learn how to use a prosthesis. Teaching for clients such as Mrs. Ramirez, who have sustained a major loss, is often most satisfactorily done during the acceptance or adaptation stage. The rationale is that clients in this stage are:
① Less anxious and more aware of reality and therefore are ready to learn
② Less angry and are therefore more compliant and easier to deal with
③ At the peak of mental anguish and therefore are open to change
④ Ready for discharge and therefore are in need of preparation

269. Mrs. Ramirez is extremely obese. Because she must administer her own insulin at home, the nurse should teach her to:
① Spread the tissue and inject at a 45 degree angle

② Spread the tissue and inject at a 90 degree angle
③ Bunch the tissue and inject at a 45 degree angle
④ Bunch the tissue and inject at a 60 degree angle

Situation: Enid Cohen, 60 years old, has come to the clinic with a painful swelling of the distal joint of the ring finger. A tentative diagnosis of rheumatoid arthritis is made.

270. During a subsequent clinic visit Mrs. Cohen tells the nurse, "I'm so confused. The doctor said I probably have arthritis, but my lab tests were negative. I don't see how that can be when I'm always so uncomfortable." The nurse's best response would be:
① "It might help if you try not to think about your discomfort."
② "Don't let that upset you; eventually the tests will be positive."
③ "Laboratory tests are often negative in the early stages of arthritis."
④ "Did the doctor say that the laboratory tests were going to be repeated?"

271. Mrs. Cohen returns for the laboratory checkup. She tells the nurse that she has been taking aspirin to reduce her pain and it has helped. The client says the arthritis has moved to her ears because she has buzzing in the ears. The nurse recognizes that ringing in the ears may be:
① Caused by an accumulation of cerumen in the ear
② Evidence of eighth cranial nerve involvement
③ A result of the aging process
④ A symptom of otitis media

272. Except for the rheumatoid arthritis, Mrs. Cohen is in good health. She asks the nurse if she should be taking some multivitamin and mineral supplements. The best response by the nurse is:
① "Absolutely! They are a necessity as you get older."
② "Older people usually do need more vitamins, especially vitamin A."
③ "There is no evidence that healthy older adults require added nutrient supplements."
④ "If you took the supplement, you could cut down on your food and help keep your weight down."

273. Mrs. Cohen tells the nurse that she read about a vitamin that may be related to aging because of its relationship to the structure of cell walls. The nurse should recognize that Mrs. Cohen is referring to:
① Vitamin A
② Vitamin C

③ Vitamin E
④ Vitamin B₁ (thiamine)

274. Several years later Mrs. Cohen is admitted to the hospital for a total hip replacement. The nurse's preoperative teaching plan for the early postoperative period should include instructions related to:
① Hip flexion of 90 degrees on the operative side
② Turning 45 degrees onto the operative side
③ Abduction of the operative hip
④ Adduction of the operative hip

275. When assisting Mrs. Cohen onto the bedpan on the first postoperative day, the nurse should instruct her to:
① Turn toward the operative side
② Flex both knees and slowly lift the pelvis
③ Extend both legs and pull on the trapeze to lift the pelvis
④ Flex the nonoperative knee and pull on the trapeze to lift the pelvis

276. On the fourth postoperative day Mrs. Cohen appears angry and very restless and says, "I can't stand this another minute. There's a wrinkle in my sheet and my water is warm." She changes position frequently and does not maintain eye contact with the nurse. The best initial interpretation of Mrs. Cohen's behavior is that it indicates:
① Severe discomfort in the hip
② An increased level of anxiety
③ Anger at the poor nursing care
④ Frustration with the need for leg abduction

277. The nurse responds, "Now Mrs. Cohen, let me get you some cold water and your pain pill, and you'll be much better." The nurse's approach demonstrates the:
① Use of problem identification and clarification
② Inappropriate use of the data presented
③ Introduction of the needs approach
④ Empathetic recognition of anxiety

Situation: Carol Point was recently diagnosed with Graves' disease (hyperthyroidism).

278. When assessing Ms. Point the nurse would expect to find a history of:
① Diaphoresis
② Menorrhagia
③ Dry, brittle hair
④ Sensitivity to cold

279. Ms. Point is very anxious and complains of feeling dizzy and light-headed and of having tingling sensations of the fingertips and around the lips. Her respirations are shallow and very rapid (40 per minute). The nurse should attribute these symptoms to:
① Eupnea
② Hyperventilation

③ Kussmaul respirations
④ Carbon dioxide intoxication

280. Intervention for Ms. Point should be:
① Administration of oxygen
② Reassurance and use of a rebreathing mask
③ Intermittent positive pressure breathing (IPPB)
④ An intravenous infusion of fluid containing bicarbonate ions

281. Based on Ms. Point's symptoms, the nurse should expect the client's laboratory values to reflect:
① A decreased pH, decreased Pco₂
② A decreased pH, elevated Pco₂
③ An elevated pH, decreased Pco₂
④ An elevated pH, elevated Pco₂

282. Ms. Point's hyperventilation resolves. The nurse obtains the client's vital signs and auscultates her lungs. The description that would be used for the soft swishing sounds of normal breathing heard when the nurse auscultates Ms. Point's chest is:
① Diminished breath sounds
② Vesicular breath sounds
③ Adventitious sounds
④ Fine crepitant rales

283. Ms. Point is acutely ill. She tells the nurse, "I know I'm going to die. I'm very sick." The best response by the nurse would be:
① "Tell me why you feel you are going to die."
② "I can understand how you feel, but people do not die from this problem."
③ "If you would like, I will call your family and tell them to come to the hospital."
④ "You must feel very sick and frightened."

284. The nurse performs preoperative teaching related to a subtotal thyroidectomy. The nurse would know that the client understands the teaching about the local effects of general anesthesia when she says that immediately after surgery she will experience:
① Difficulty in swallowing
② Paroxysmal hiccoughs
③ Transient headaches
④ Feelings of chilliness

285. When planning care for Ms. Point in the first 24 hours after surgery, the nurse should include:
① Checking the back and sides of the operative dressing
② Supporting her head during mild range-of-motion exercises
③ Encouraging the client to ventilate her feelings about the surgery
④ Advising the client that she can resume her normal activities immediately

Situation: Jim Sinclair comes to the emergency room complaining of nausea, vomiting, headache, and "flu-like" symptoms. The nurse notes slight jaundice of the sclera. Mr. Sinclair is admitted to the hospital with a diagnosis of possible hepatitis A.

286. Blood and enteric precautions are ordered for Mr. Sinclair. The isolation procedures that must be followed are:
     ① A private room is required, and the door must be kept closed
     ② Persons entering the room must wear a gown, mask, and gloves
     ③ Linens must be double bagged, and gloves must be worn when handling the bedpan
     ④ Gowns and gloves must be worn only when handling the client's soiled linen, dishes, or utensils

287. The nurse takes a history from Mr. Sinclair. The information from the history that is most likely linked to hepatitis A is:
     ① Being exposed to arsenic compounds at work
     ② Working in a hemodialysis unit of a hospital
     ③ Washing dishes at a local restaurant
     ④ Working for a local plumber

288. Mr. Sinclair expresses concern over the change in color of his skin. The nurse should recognize that this color change is due to:
     ① Stimulation of the liver to produce an excess quantity of bile pigments
     ② The inability of the liver to remove normal amounts of bilirubin from the blood
     ③ Increased destruction of red blood cells during the acute phase of the disease
     ④ Decreased prothrombin levels, leading to multiple sites of intradermal bleeding

289. Mr. Sinclair is to be discharged to continue his recovery at home. The nurse should expect that the diet the physician will order will be:
     ① Low calorie, high protein, low carbohydrate, low fat
     ② High calorie, low protein, high carbohydrate, high fat
     ③ Low calorie, low protein, low carbohydrate, moderate fat
     ④ High calorie, high protein, high carbohydrate, moderate fat

290. Mrs. Sinclair states that there is only one bathroom in their home and she is worried that other members of the family could get hepatitis. The nurse's best reply would be:
     ① "I suggest that you buy a commode exclusively for Mr. Sinclair's use."
     ② "There is no problem with Mr. Sinclair sharing the same bathroom with everyone."
     ③ "Mr. Sinclair may use the same bathroom, but you need to use disposable toilet covers."
     ④ "It is important that all family members wash their hands after using the bathroom."

Situation: Ruth Wool, 32 years old, comes to the physician complaining of fatigue, shortness of breath, and swelling of her hands. She has a history of rheumatic fever.

291. During auscultation of the heart, the nurse would expect the first heart sound (S_1) to be the loudest at the:
     ① Apex of the heart
     ② Right lateral border
     ③ Left lateral border
     ④ Base of the heart

292. When auscultating Mrs. Wool's heart the nurse understands that the first heart sound is produced by the closure of the:
     ① Aortic and tricuspid valves
     ② Aortic and pulmonic valves
     ③ Mitral and pulmonic valves
     ④ Mitral and tricuspid valves

293. The physician prescribes furosemide (Lasix) 40 mg qd in conjunction with digoxin (Lanoxin). The nurse recognizes that potassium supplements are essential with this combination of drugs because:
     ① Lasix requires adequate serum potassium to promote diuresis
     ② Digitalis toxicity occurs rapidly in the presence of hypokalemia
     ③ Potassium is destroyed by the liver as digoxin is detoxified
     ④ Digitalis causes significant potassium depletion

294. Mrs. Wool's symptoms persist, and cardiac catheterization of the heart via the femoral artery is scheduled. An ECG is performed before the cardiac catheterization, and hypokalemia is suspected. The physician can confirm the presence of hypokalemia by:
     ① Blood cultures times 3
     ② A complete blood count
     ③ A serum electrolyte level
     ④ An x-ray film of long bones

295. When preparing Mrs. Wool for the cardiac catheterization, the nurse should advise her that:
     ① The procedure will take 15 minutes
     ② She will be npo 6 to 8 hours before the procedure
     ③ Ambulation will be permitted within 1 hour after the procedure
     ④ Complete sedation will be maintained throughout the procedure

296. Before the cardiac catheterization the nurse should assess and mark the location of pedal pulses with a ballpoint pen on Mrs. Wool's feet to:
     ① Establish baseline data
     ② Identify the site for arterial cannulation
     ③ Assess the extent of any residual edema
     ④ Check the effectiveness of venous return

297. Mrs. Wool returns from the cardiac catheterization with a pressure dressing over the

right groin. She is to be flat in bed for 6 hours with her leg straight. These measures are important to prevent:
① Infiltration of radiopaque dye into tissue
② Bleeding at the arterial puncture site
③ Headache and disorientation
④ Orthostatic hypotension

298. For the first several hours following the cardiac catheterization, the nursing action that would be essential is:
① Keeping the head of the bed elevated 45 degrees
② Encouraging coughing and deep breathing every 2 hours
③ Monitoring the apical pulse and blood pressure frequently
④ Checking the temperature every hour until it returns to normal

299. Mrs. Wool is found to have a valvular defect, and open heart surgery is performed. The client is transferred to the recovery room with mediastinal and pleural chest tubes. The nurse knows that a pleural tube connected to closed water-seal drainage is functioning properly when the fluid in the water-seal chamber of the drainage system:
① Bubbles vigorously on inspiration
② Contains many small air bubbles
③ Rises with inspiration and falls with expiration
④ Remains at a consistent level during the respiratory cycle.

300. Mrs. Wool develops an atrial dysrhythmia, and the physician orders 1000 mcg of procainamide (Pronestyl) IV per minute. The directions state 500 mg of the drug should be added to 500 ml of D5W. The IV set has a drop factor of 60 gtt/ml. To administer the medication correctly the nurse should set the flow rate at:
① 30 gtt/min
② 60 gtt/min
③ 90 gtt/min
④ 120 gtt/min

Situation: Virginia Penn comes to the emergency room with severe epigastric pain. The physician in the emergency room rules out cardiac and gastric problems and makes the tentative diagnosis of cholecystitis. She is instructed to make an appointment with her private physician for a more definitive diagnostic workup.

301. When providing instructions for discharge from the emergency room, the recommendation that would produce the most valuable information for Mrs. Penn's physician would be:
① "Keep a journal related to your pain."
② "Save all stool and urine for inspection."
③ "Follow the doctor's orders exactly without question."

④ "Keep a record of the amount of fluid you drink daily."

302. When Mrs. Penn visits her physician the next day the nurse performs an initial history and physical assessment and asks Mrs. Penn to make a list of the foods that upset her. Considering the tentative diagnosis of cholecystitis, the foods that are most likely to be included on the list are:
① Nuts and popcorn
② Meatloaf and baked potato
③ Chocolate and boiled shrimp
④ Fried chicken and buttered corn

303. The physician orders a gallbladder x-ray film (cholecystogram), and Mrs. Penn is given instructions regarding preparation for the examination. On the morning of the examination the nurse would postpone the test if Mrs. Penn stated she:
① Swallowed some water when she brushed her teeth
② Had slight diarrhea the night before the test
③ Vomited the tablets of radiopaque dye
④ Ate a fat-free meal for supper

304. Mrs. Penn's diagnostic workup indicates cholelithiasis, and a cholecystectomy is performed. The physician orders IV fluids and gentamicin sulfate (Garamycin) 100 mg IVPB q 8 h. The nurse hangs the piggyback gentamicin higher than the primary IV bag. When the piggyback bag is empty, Mrs. Penn observes air in the tubing of the IVPB and she becomes frightened. The nurse should explain that:
① Air in the tubing, even if it got into the vein, would not be fatal unless it was a large amount
② The gentamicin and now the air are flowing into the large IV bag not into the venous system directly
③ The solution from the large IV bag will begin to flow when the solution from the smaller bag ceases to flow
④ The clamps on the tubing leading from both bags can be closed for a few minutes to prevent air from entering the vein

305. The physician orders peak and trough levels of the gentamicin. For peak levels the nurse should have the laboratory obtain a blood sample from Mrs. Penn:
① Between 30 to 60 minutes after the IVPB
② Halfway between 2 IVPB administrations
③ Immediately before administering the IVPB
④ Any time it is convenient for the client and laboratory

306. Two days after surgery Mrs. Penn's temperature is normal. The physician orders a clear liquid diet and OOB ad lib. After lunch Mrs. Penn complains of dizziness when she gets up to go to the bathroom. The nurse should

recognize that the dizziness is probably related to:
① Bed rest
② The liquid diet
③ The gentamicin
④ Postanesthesia hypotension

307. Mrs. Penn's bile drainage has been prolonged and she complains of raw, excoriated skin around the T-tube. After assessing the skin the nurse should plan to:
① Reinforce the dressings when they are wet
② Cleanse the area with an antiseptic solution
③ Use a skin barrier around the T-tube exit site
④ Change the type of adhesive tape used on the dressing

308. Because of the prolonged bile drainage, Mrs. Penn may develop symptoms related to a lack of fat-soluble vitamins, such as:
① Easy bruising
② Muscle twitching
③ Excessive jaundice
④ Tingling of the fingers

309. Mrs. Penn asks if she will be able to eat anything she wants. The nurse would recognize that Mrs. Penn understands the dietary teaching when she tells her husband:
① "I will need to avoid fatty foods for the rest of my life."
② "I should not eat those foods that upset me before I had surgery."
③ "Most people can tolerate a regular diet after this type of surgery."
④ "Most people need to eat a high-protein diet for several months after surgery."

Situation: Len Moyes comes to the eye clinic with persistent dull eye pain. Chronic glaucoma is diagnosed.

310. When performing the nursing history, a symptom of chronic glaucoma that the nurse should expect is complaints of:
① Flashes of light
② Intolerance to light
③ Seeing floating specks
④ Loss of peripheral vision

311. When the nurse is caring for Mr. Moyes, the eye drops the nurse should expect to administer would be:
① Pilocarpine hydrochloride (Pilocarpine)
② Atropine sulfate (Atropisol)
③ Cyclopentolate (Cyclogyl)
④ Tetracaine (Pontocaine)

312. Mr. Moyes is scheduled for eye surgery. The nurse would know that he understands the preoperative teaching about the first 24 hours after surgery when he says that he should:
① Elevate the head of the bed
② Move around freely in bed
③ Cough and deep breathe
④ Lie on the unaffected side

313. Despite therapy, Mr. Moyes becomes blind. The nurse should be aware that sensory restriction can:
① Heighten the client's ability to make decisions
② Increase the use of daydreaming and fantasy
③ Lead to the use of permanent neurotic behaviors
④ Decrease the client's restlessness and lethargy

Situation: Tracy Allen, a 29-year-old computer programer with a husband and 2 young children, comes to the emergency room complaining of epigastric pain and nausea. She has been vomiting for 3 days. Her respirations are shallow, her skin is dry and flushed, and she acts weak and lethargic.

314. The following laboratory data is noted: a plasma pH of 7.51; a Pco_2 of 50 mmHg; an HCO_3 of 58 mEq/L; a Cl of 55 mEq/L; a K of 3.8 mEq/L. The nurse recognizes that the collected data indicates:
① Hyperchloremia
② Metabolic alkalosis
③ Respiratory acidosis
④ Hyperkalemia

315. Mrs. Allen's clinical symptoms indicate a possible gastric ulcer. Considering her symptoms and her laboratory results, the primary nursing diagnosis for Mrs. Allen is:
① Pain related to hypersecretion of gastric acids
② Potential for injury related to weakness
③ Impaired gas exchange related to pain
④ Actual fluid volume deficit related to vomiting

316. Mrs. Allen has a gastroscopy. Following the gastroscopy the nurse should assess for return of the gag reflex by:
① Instructing the client to breathe deeply and cough gently
② Observing for when the client spits out the airway
③ Giving a small amount of water using a syringe
④ Touching the pharynx with a tongue depressor

317. A gastric ulcer is confirmed, and Mrs. Allen is scheduled for a subtotal gastrectomy. The operating room nurse knows that the ability the client will lose last during the induction of anesthesia is:
① Respiratory movement
② Consciousness
③ Corneal reflex
④ Gag reflex

318. Immediately after the surgery Mrs. Allen returns to the surgical unit. The nurse irrigates

the nasogastric tube and notes small blood clots in the return. The nurse should:
① Clamp the nasogastric tube
② Irrigate the tube with iced saline
③ Consider this a normal event
④ Notify the physician of this finding

319. On the third postoperative day, Mrs. Allen complains of severe abdominal pain. The nurse palpates her abdomen and notes rigidity. The nurse should first:
① Administer the prescribed analgesic
② Assist the client to ambulate
③ Assess the client's vital signs
④ Encourage the use of the spirometer

320. The physician orders 2 units of blood to be infused. Before blood administration the nurse's highest priority should be:
① Obtaining a consent for the blood transfusion
② Allowing the blood to reach room temperature
③ Monitoring the hemoglobin and hematocrit levels
④ Determining proper typing and cross-matching of blood

321. When administering blood, it is important for the nurse to:
① Administer each unit within a 6-hour period
② Use a volume control infusion pump to administer the blood
③ Run the blood at a slower rate during the first 5 to 10 minutes
④ Draw blood samples from the client immediately after each unit is transfused

322. Halfway through the first unit of blood, Mrs. Allen complains of lumbar pain. The nurse should:
① Increase the flow of normal saline
② Assess the pain further
③ Stop the transfusion
④ Obtain vital signs

323. Mrs. Allen had to return to surgery to repair the suture line and is now having an uneventful recovery. To determine when Mrs. Allen can begin oral feedings after surgery, the nurse must assess for the:
① Occurrence of dumping syndrome
② Stabilization of hematocrit
③ Extent of incisional pain
④ Presence of flatulence

324. Before discharge, Mrs. Allen asks what to do if she experiences epigastric pain. The nurse would know that the teaching was effective when Mrs. Allen says she should:
① Increase her food intake
② Take aspirin with milk
③ Eliminate fluids with meals
④ Take an antacid preparation

Situation: Pierre Jaques is a 56-year-old garage mechanic. Over the past few months his family has no-

ticed that he has had an increased appetite, has been drinking an excess of fluid, and has been urinating frequently at night. The physician diagnoses non-insulin-dependent diabetes mellitus (NIDDM).

325. When obtaining a health history the nurse should expect Mr. Jaques to mention symptoms associated with the classic signs of diabetes mellitus, which are:
① Polydipsia, nocturia, weight loss
② Polyphagia, confusion, polyuria
③ Polydipsia, polyphagia, polyuria
④ Polydipsia, polyuria, irritability

326. After completing an assessment of Mr. Jaques, the nurse concludes that he has a knowledge deficit related to diabetes mellitus. Based on the conclusion that Mr. Jaques is motivated to learn and will comprehend information, a teaching priority should be for him to learn how to:
① Identify hypoglycemia and hyperglycemia
② Perform urine testing
③ Administer insulin
④ Care for his feet

327. While hospitalized, Mr. Jaques is able to provide for his own care. The nurse notices on daily assessments that he is picking at calluses on his feet. The nurse should immediately:
① Warn him of the danger of infection
② Suggest he wear white cotton socks
③ Check his shoes for proper fit in the area of the calluses
④ Demonstrate and teach the importance of proper foot care

328. The nurse teaches Mr. Jaques about the treatment of hypoglycemia. The nurse recognizes that the client understands the teaching when he says that if he becomes hypoglycemic he will ingest:
① Peanut butter crackers and a glass of milk
② Chocolate candy and a banana
③ A slice of bread and sugar
④ Hard candy and fruit juice

329. Mr. Jaques is taking one tolbutamide (Orinase) tablet daily. He asks if he should take an extra pill before exercise. The nurse should reply:
① "You will need to decrease exercise."
② "Exercise decreases your body's need for insulin."
③ "An extra pill will help your body use glucose correctly."
④ "Your diet and medicine will not be affected by exercise."

330. Mr. Jaques calls the physician's office because he is experiencing symptoms of the flu. He is concerned about his diabetes and inquires about the need for special care. The nurse should advise him to:
① Take his medication, drink warm fluids, and perform a fingerstick for glucose ac and hs

② Eat as much as possible, increase fluid intake, and call the office again the next day

③ Skip his oral hypoglycemic agent, drink plenty of fluids, and stay in bed

④ Avoid food, drink clear liquids, take his temperature, and stay in bed

331. Several years later Mr. Jaques is admitted with a large leg ulcer, and a femoral angiogram is scheduled. After the angiogram the nurse should:
① Have the client void within 2 hours
② Elevate the foot of the bed for 36 hours
③ Provide passive ROM to the extremities
④ Apply pressure to the catheter insertion site

332. Mr. Jaques has a femoral-popliteal bypass graft. When assessing the client's vital signs, the nurse finds that his blood pressure is 200/110. The nurse should notify the physician immediately because the:
① Graft could rupture
② Client is hypovolemic
③ Graft may occlude
④ Client is anaphylactic

333. The nurse provides discharge teaching. The nurse is aware that the teaching was effective when Mr. Jaques understands that he should:
① Sit in a hot tub for 25 minutes bid
② Elevate the foot of his bed at night
③ Massage his calves gently every day
④ Assess the color and pulses of his legs

Situation: Justine Andrews, 21 years old, is seen by a physician for weight loss and fatigue. Physical examination reveals a slight enlargement of her cervical lymph nodes.

334. Ms. Andrews states that she had a low-grade fever. To assess possible causes for the fever, it would be most appropriate for the nurse to initially ask:
① "When did you first notice that your temperature had gone up?"
② "Have you been exposed recently to anyone with an infection?"
③ "Do you have a sore throat at the present time?"
④ "Have you been sexually active lately?"

335. One afternoon the nurse overhears Ms. Andrews having an argument with her boyfriend. A while later Ms. Andrews complains to the nurse that dinner is always late and the meals are terrible. The nurse recognizes that the defense mechanism Ms. Andrews is using is:
① Dissociation
② Intellectualization
③ Projection
④ Displacement

336. Although upset by Ms. Andrew's complaints, the nurse ignores them and attempts to divert the conversation. Immediately following this exchange, the nurse discusses with a friend the various stages of development of young adults. The defense mechanism the nurse is using is:
① Intellectualization
② Identification
③ Substitution
④ Sublimation

337. Ms. Andrews is diagnosed as having Hodgkin's disease stage III A with a grossly involved spleen. She is scheduled for a splenectomy. After the nurse performs preoperative teaching, Ms. Andrews appears very anxious. The best approach for the nurse to use at this time would be to:
① Allow the client to regress at this time and let her rest quietly
② State simply that she seems anxious and ask her if she would like to talk for a while
③ Consider her reaction an unconscious response and inquire about her relations with her mother
④ Consider that anxiety prevented the client from understanding and repeat the information in simpler terms

338. The physician has also decided to use total nodal irradiation in conjunction with MOPP therapy. Ms. Andrews tells the nurse she wants to have children and is quite concerned that the radiation therapy includes the pelvic nodal areas. When questioned about this, the nurse should refer Ms. Andrews to the physician, because the nurse should be aware that:
① The ovaries can be surgically moved and placed in a shielded area
② The radiation used is not radical enough to destroy ovarian function
③ Intense radiation to the area always causes permanent sterilization
④ Ovarian function will be temporarily destroyed but will return in about 6 months

339. Ms. Andrews has the splenectomy. The consideration that is of primary importance after a splenectomy is:
① Early ambulation
② Pulmonary embolism
③ Adequate lung aeration
④ Postoperative hemorrhage

340. During an interview with Ms. Andrews' parents, the nurse notices that Mr. Andrews continually defends and makes excuses for all of his daughter's actions, whereas her mother seems to feel Ms. Andrews is just lazy and that there is nothing wrong with her that she couldn't fight with some effort. The nurse recognizes that the Andrews family probably relates by using the mechanism known as:
① Coalitions
② Resignation
③ Scapegoating
④ Reaction formation

341. Ms. Andrews is started on MOPP therapy.

Mechlorethamine HCl (Mustargen) is given IV. With this drug Ms. Andrews is most likely to develop:
① Neurologic dyskinesia
② Urinary incontinence
③ Transient nausea
④ Hair loss

342. Ms. Andrews enters a remission and remains symptom free for 6 months when a relapse occurs. Ms. Andrews is diagnosed at stage IV. The therapy option the nurse should expect to be implemented at this time is:
① Surgical removal of the affected nodes
② Radiation with chemotherapy
③ Combination chemotherapy
④ Radiation therapy

343. Ms. Andrews is to receive the ABVD chemotherapeutic regimen. Doxorubicin (Adriamycin) is given IV. The major life threatening side effect of Adriamycin that the nurse should assess Ms. Andrews for is:
① Ulcerative stomatitis
② Pulmonary fibrosis
③ Cardiotoxicity
④ Pancytopenia

Situation: Susan Marte, 45 years old, develops acute glomerulonephritis following a streptococcal infection.

344. When performing the health assessment the nurse would expect Mrs. Marte to report a history of:
① An increased appetite
② A recent weight loss
③ Mild headache
④ Nocturia

345. Mrs. Marte complains of thirst. The nurse should offer her:
① Hard candy
② A cup of broth
③ A milk shake
④ Ginger ale

346. To prevent future attacks of glomerulonephritis, the nurse should instruct Mrs. Marte to:
① Seek early treatment for respiratory infections
② Continue the same restrictions on fluid intake
③ Avoid situations that involve physical activity
④ Take showers instead of bubble baths

347. Mrs. Marte has extensive glomerular scarring and eventually develops chronic renal failure. She has been on hemodialysis for 2 years. She relates to the nurse in dialysis in an angry, critical manner and is frequently noncompliant with medications and diet. The nurse can best intervene by first understanding that the client's behavior is most likely:

① An effort to maintain life to the fullest extent possible
② A defense against underlying depression and fear
③ A constructive method of accepting reality
④ An attempt to punish the nursing staff

348. Mrs. Marte is accepted for a transplant and is placed on a waiting list. She attends a group educational program for potential transplant candidates. Mrs. Marte asks the nurse where her new kidney will be placed. The nurse answers:
① "It will replace your right kidney because it has a longer renal vein, making transplant easier."
② "The kidney that is the most diseased is removed and replaced with the new one."
③ "It will be placed in the right lower quadrant, and your kidney will not be removed."
④ "It is up to the surgeon as to which kidney is replaced with the new one."

349. In addition to the kidney transplant, Mrs. Marte is taught to expect:
① A colonoscopy
② An appendectomy
③ A partial gastric resection
④ An intravenous cystogram

350. Mrs. Marte has an emergency admission because a donor kidney is found. The surgery goes well, and she is transferred from the recovery room to the ICU. The nurse plans to measure Mrs. Marte's urinary output every:
① 15 minutes
② 30 minutes
③ Hour
④ 2 hours

351. The most important test used to determine if Mrs. Marte's new kidney is working is the:
① 24-hour output
② White blood cell count
③ Serum creatinine
④ Renal scan

352. As the nurse assesses Mrs. Marte's kidney function after surgery, the components of urine will be monitored. Essential to this process is the knowledge that the normal kidney filters a number of blood components, and urine should not contain:
① Urea nitrogen
② Large proteins
③ Sodium chloride
④ Potassium chloride

353. Mrs. Marte is taught the signs of transplant rejection. The nurse would know that the teaching was effective when Mrs. Marte says that a sign of rejection would be:
① Weight loss
② A subnormal temperature
③ An increased urinary output
④ An elevated blood pressure

354. In planning discharge teaching for Mrs.

Marte the nurse should explain the drug regimen that will be needed to prevent rejection of the kidney. The drugs of choice usually include:
  ① Ancef, methotrexate, and citric acid
  ② Lasix, neomycin, and cyclosporine (Sand-immune)
  ③ Methylprednisolone, (Solu-Medrol), Dilantin, and insulin
  ④ Prednisone, cyclophosphamide (Cytoxan) and azathioprine (Imuran)

355. Mrs. Marte develops leukopenia 3 weeks after surgery. The nurse should be aware that the leukopenia is probably caused by:
  ① The antirejection medications
  ② Rejection of the kidney
  ③ High creatinine levels
  ④ A bacterial infection

Situation: Samuel Burns, age 27, is tested for tuberculosis as part of a screening physical for his job. The Mantoux test is used, and he returns to the health office to have it read.

356. The nurse notes 12 mm of induration at the site of the test and explains to Mr. Burns that:
  ① His results indicate a need for further tests, including a chest x-ray film examination
  ② His skin tests are inconclusive and will have to be repeated in 6 weeks
  ③ The test used was for screening, and a Tine test will now be given
  ④ The test result was negative, and no follow-up is needed

357. To make a definitive diagnosis of tuberculosis, the nurse understands that the physician must order a:
  ① Sputum sample for acid-fast testing
  ② Pulmonary function test
  ③ Tuberculin skin test
  ④ Chest x-ray film

358. Tuberculosis is confirmed, and Mr. Burns is placed on isoniazid (INH) and rifampin (Rifadin). He says, "I've never had to take so much antibiotic for an infection before." The nurse explains:
  ① "Your infection is well advanced and needs aggressive therapy."
  ② "You'll need only one medication when you get better."
  ③ "This type of organism is difficult to destroy."
  ④ "Rifampin prevents side effects of INH."

359. Before Mr. Burns starts the rifampin therapy, the nurse explains its purpose and side effects to Mr. Burns. The nurse knows the teaching was effective when Mr. Burns states:
  ① "It's normal for my urine to be orange colored from this medication."

  ② "A skin rash is normal with rifampin and is nothing to worry about."
  ③ "I will drink large amounts of fluid while I am taking this medicine."
  ④ "I will have my hearing tested while I am taking this medicine."

360. Vitamin B_6 is prescribed along with isoniazid. The nurse explains that this vitamin is used because it:
  ① Improves the nutritional status of the client
  ② Enhances the tuberculostatic effect of isoniazid
  ③ Accelerates destruction of dormant tubercular bacilli
  ④ Counteracts the peripheral neuritis that isoniazid may cause

361. Mr. Burns is seen 1 month later in the pulmonary clinic. After completing the assessment the nurse evaluates the findings and recognizes that prompt intervention is required for his:
  ① Weight gain of 5 pounds
  ② Temperature of 96.8° F
  ③ Orange stools
  ④ Yellow sclera

Situation: Carrie Robinson, while driving home from work after the evening shift as a nursing assistant, is hit by another car. She sustains multiple injuries and is taken to the emergency room via ambulance.

362. An x-ray film of Mrs. Robinson's arm reveals a comminuted fracture of the left radial bone. The nurse understands that with a comminuted fracture:
  ① There is a break in the skin and the bone is protruding
  ② Splintering has occurred on one side and bending on the other
  ③ The bone has broken into several fragments, but the skin is intact
  ④ The bone is broken into two parts, and the skin may or may not be broken

363. Mrs. Robinson also has a fracture of the right tibia, and a cast is applied. The physician orders bed rest with the right leg elevated and Tylenol with codeine for pain. After cast application, to assess for damage to major blood vessels from the fractured tibia, the nurse should monitor the client for:
  ① Increased skin temperature of the foot
  ② A decreased dorsalis pedis pulse
  ③ An increased blood pressure
  ④ Swelling of the right thigh

364. After casting of the arm and leg, Mrs. Robinson is admitted overnight for observation. The next morning she complains that she is seeing frequent flashes of light. The nurse should suspect:
  ① A cerebral concussion
  ② A detached retina

③ Acute glaucoma
④ Scleroderma

365. Mrs. Robinson is scheduled for surgery to alleviate the cause of the "flashing light" sensation. The nurse explains that the procedure employed involves the use of:
① Radiation
② Burr holes
③ Dermabrasion
④ Laser technique

366. Three days after the cast is applied Mrs. Robinson states that she has a burning pain over her ankle. The cast over the ankle feels warm to the touch, and the pain is not relieved when Mrs. Robinson changes her position. The nurse's priority action would be to:
① Obtain an order for an antibiotic
② Administer the Tylenol with codeine for pain
③ Explain that it is a typical response to a cast
④ Report the client's complaint to the physician

367. Mrs. Robinson is to be discharged. When discussing pain management with Mrs. Robinson, the nurse should advise her to take the Tylenol with codeine:
① Just as a last resort
② Before she goes to sleep
③ As the pain becomes intense
④ When she begins to get uncomfortable

368. Mrs. Robinson is discharged to recuperate at home. Eight weeks later, after the leg cast is removed, Mrs. Robinson should be instructed to:
① Put her leg through a full range of motion once daily
② Elevate her leg when sitting for long periods of time
③ Cleanse the leg by scrubbing with a brisk motion
④ Report any discomfort or stiffness of the ankle

Situation: Cristy Cort, 46 years old, is 5 feet 5 inches tall and weighs 310 lbs. She comes to the emergency room complaining of nausea and vomiting and severe colicky pains in the right upper quadrant that are usually aggravated by an intake of fatty foods.

369. Mrs. Cort is admitted to the surgical unit, and intravenous fluids are ordered. Mrs. Cort is to receive 100 ml D5W at 90 ml per hour. If the drop factor is 15 gtt/ml, the nurse should set the drip rate at:
① 15 gtt/min
② 23 gtt/min
③ 25 gtt/min
④ 30 gtt/min

370. Following a diagnostic workup, cholelithiasis and a hiatal hernia are confirmed and a cholecystectomy is scheduled. Atropine is to be given preoperatively. The nurse should specifically assess for the presence of glaucoma before administering this medication because it causes:
① Increased intraocular pressure
② Pupillary constriction
③ Increased heart rate
④ Deviation of the eye

371. Mrs. Cort returns from surgery with a T-tube in place. Immediately after the cholecystectomy the position that would be most comfortable is:
① Sims'
② Supine
③ Side-lying
④ Low Fowler's

372. The nurse is aware that Mrs. Cort's T-tube has been inserted to:
① Facilitate bile drainage while the common duct is edematous
② Prevent postoperative infection at the site of the incision
③ Drain blood and pus from the operative site
④ Divert the bile flow to the cystic duct

373. Mrs. Cort is placed on a progressive postsurgical diet. This diet is characterized by progressive alterations in the:
① Caloric content of food
② Nutritional value of food
③ Texture and digestability of food
④ Variety of food and fluids included

374. The nurse observes another nurse changing Mrs. Cort's sterile dressing. The nurse changing the dressing uses the same pair of clean gloves to remove the soiled dressing and apply the new dressing. The observing nurse's initial action should be to:
① Discuss the incident with the nurse
② File an incident report about the action
③ Offer to demonstrate the proper technique
④ Report the individual to the nursing supervisor

375. Individual nurses are responsible for their own professional actions. In addition, a hospital can be held legally responsible for the actions of a nurse employed by the hospital under the doctrine of:
① In loco parentis
② Respondeat superior
③ The state's department of health
④ The American Hospital Association's Review Board

376. Mrs. Cort asks about her hiatal hernia and how she can best prevent esophageal reflux. The nurse's best response would be:
① "Drink several glasses of fluid during each of your meals."
② "Reduce your caloric intake to foster weight reduction."
③ "Lie down after eating to help your digestion."
④ "Divide fats equally among your meals."

Situation: Janet Marris, age 62, is diagnosed as having hypertension. The physician orders digoxin (Lanoxin), furosemide (Lasix), and a 2 g sodium diet.

377. When talking with Mrs. Marris about her recent symptoms, the nurse would expect her to report experiencing the most common symptom associated with hypertension, which is:
① Flushed face
② Nosebleeds
③ Headache
④ Fatigue

378. Mrs. Marris is being taught to restrict her intake of sodium. She would demonstrate her understanding about foods low in sodium when she indicates she can eat:
① Shredded wheat cereal
② Carrot and celery sticks
③ A bologna sandwich
④ Broiled scallops

379. Mrs. Marris is taught about Lasix. In assessing her understanding of the side effects of Lasix, the nurse should expect Mrs. Marris to:
① Wear dark glasses
② Avoid lying flat in bed
③ Avoid eating citrus fruits
④ Change her position slowly

380. Because Mrs. Marris is receiving Lasix, at each clinic visit the nurse should assess her for:
① Hyporeflexia
② Tinnitus
③ Bronchospasm
④ Xanthopsia

381. Mrs. Marris has recently been having episodes of headache and double vision and has had two nosebleeds. She comes to the emergency room when the third nosebleed occurs. Her blood pressure is 260/120. She is admitted to medical intensive care. Lasix 20 mg IV is given and a nitroprusside (Nipride) infusion is begun. Within minutes Mrs. Marris' BP is 160/94. Nipride decreases blood pressure by:
① Relaxing venous and arterial muscles
② Increasing peripheral resistance
③ Increasing cardiac output
④ Decreasing the heart rate

382. Mrs. Marris' blood pressure is controlled, and she is sent to the medical unit with orders for a 2 g sodium 1600 calorie ADA diet. Mrs. Marris complains about the bland food and refuses to eat her dinner. The nurse should first:
① Explain that she will eventually have to accept this diet
② Urge her to eat to get accustomed to the diet she must eat at home
③ Provide her with several packets of lemon juice and one packet of salt
④ Ask her what she usually includes in her diet at home

383. Mrs. Marris is to be discharged on propranolol HCl (Inderal) and digoxin (Lanoxin). The nurse should be aware that Inderal, when administered with Lanoxin, may:
① Produce headache
② Potentiate bradycardia
③ Increase blood pressure
④ Stimulate nodal conduction

384. On the evening before discharge Mrs. Marris has another hypertensive crisis and has a cerebral vascular accident. Initially, the nurse should place her in a:
① Supine position
② Contour position
③ Side-lying position
④ Slight Trendelenburg position

385. Initially Mrs. Marris' pupils are equal and reactive to light. Later the nurse assesses that Mrs. Marris' right pupil is reacting more slowly than her left and her systolic blood pressure begins to rise. The nurse recognizes that these adaptations are suggestive of:
① Spinal shock
② Hypovolemic shock
③ Transtentorial herniation
④ Increasing intracranial pressure

Situation: Greg Davis has had symptoms of gastritis for years. When self-management is unsuccessful, he goes to the physician for diagnostic studies, and extensive carcinoma of the stomach is diagnosed. Mr. Davis is admitted for gastric surgery.

386. Mr. Davis questions why the diagnosis took so long. The nurse's explanation is based on the knowledge that carcinoma of the stomach is:
① Difficult to accurately diagnose until late in the disease process
② Painful in early stages and often misdiagnosed as myocardial infarction
③ Usually diagnosed following the discovery of enlarged lymph nodes in the epigastric area
④ Rarely diagnosed early because the symptoms are usually nonspecific until late in the disease

387. An esophagojejunostomy is scheduled. When preparing Mr. Davis for the surgery, the nurse should include information about the possibility that:
① The Trendelenburg position will be used on the first day after surgery
② Complete bed rest may be necessary for 48 hours after surgery
③ A chest tube will be in place in addition to a nasogastric tube
④ Liquids by mouth may be permitted the evening after surgery

388. As the nurse is preparing Mr. Davis for bed the evening before surgery, Mr. Davis says, "I really don't think this is cancer at all. I'll bet

they won't find anything." The nurse's most appropriate initial response would be:
1. "I can understand why you'd like to believe that."
2. "I hope you're right, but the tests do indicate cancer."
3. "It must be difficult to be facing such serious surgery."
4. "You think the doctor may have made a wrong diagnosis?"

389. Mr. Davis has the esophagojejunostomy. He returns to his room with a nasogastric tube in place. Twelve hours after surgery the nurse notes large amounts of bloody drainage from the nasogastric tube. The nurse should:
1. Instill 30 ml of iced normal saline into the tube
2. Clamp the tube and call the physician immediately
3. Report the type and quantity of drainage to the physician
4. Continue to monitor the drainage and record the observations

390. The pathology report describes the tumor removed during surgery as "well-differentiated, grade I." After this finding is discussed with Mr. and Mrs. Davis by the physician, the nurse should:
1. Be supportive and assist the Davises to prepare for a rapidly advancing terminal outcome
2. Teach the Davises how to observe for the development of a primary lesion at another site
3. Support a positive outlook, because the tumor cells showed little dysplasia
4. Provide statistics about the 5-year survival for this type of cancer

391. Before Mr. Davis' discharge, the nurse discusses his diet with both Mr. and Mrs. Davis. The nurse knows Mr. Davis' dietary needs are understood by them when they state they will plan:
1. To gradually resume their normal eating routine and diet
2. Five or six small meals for Mr. Davis every day, limiting bulk
3. A diet of blenderized foods for Mr. Davis for an indefinite period
4. A diet high in carbohydrates, proteins, and fats to replace lost nutrients

392. Mrs. Davis is concerned about her husband's health in the future. She asks if this cancer will spread. The nurse recognizes that Mrs. Davis is looking for reassurance but knows that stomach cancers are most likely to metastasize to the:
1. Lymph nodes and blood
2. Pancreas and brain
3. Bone and brain
4. Liver and lung

393. The nurse should also plan to include in Mr. Davis' discharge teaching the need for:
1. Daily replacement therapy of pancreatic enzymes
2. Monthly injections of iron dextran (Inferon)
3. Regular daily use of a stool softener
4. Weekly injections of vitamin B_{12}

Situation: Ryan Beacon, 60 years old, has a history of chronic obstructive pulmonary disease (COPD). He is admitted because of pleural effusion.

394. A right-sided thoracentesis is planned. The nurse knows that:
1. A thoracentesis is generally followed by instillation of a sclerosing agent
2. A thoracentesis is usually contraindicated in clients with a history of COPD
3. The rapid removal of large amounts of pleural fluid may precipitate cardiovascular collapse
4. The client usually has a temporary increase in dyspnea immediately following the procedure

395. When assessing a client with pleural effusion the nurse should expect to find:
1. Increased resonance with percussion of the involved area
2. Reduced or absent breath sounds at the base of the lung
3. Deviation of the trachea toward the involved site
4. Moist rales at the base of the lungs

396. When caring for Mr. Beacon the nurse should plan to:
1. Assess him for signs of pneumonia
2. Administer pain medication frequently
3. Administer medication to suppress his cough
4. Limit fluid intake to prevent pulmonary edema

397. After discharge, Mr. Beacon returns to the physician's office for a follow-up visit. The nurse would suspect a recurrence of pleural effusion when Mr. Beacon says:
1. "I've been coughing up larger amounts of thicker mucus for the last 2 days."
2. "I get a sharp, stabbing pain when I take a deep breath."
3. "During the night I sometimes have a fever and chills."
4. "At night I can only breathe well if I sit up."

398. Mr. Beacon is readmitted to the ambulatory care unit for another thoracentesis. Immediately after the procedure his right lung collapses. A chest tube is inserted and attached to a three-chamber closed drainage system. The nurse knows that the chest tube is functioning properly when fluid:
1. Rises in the tube of the waterseal chamber on inspiration

② Is bubbling vigorously in the suction control chamber

③ Is bubbling gently in the chest drainage chamber

④ Remains constant in the chest drainage chamber

399. Mr. Beacon should be observed for early indications of respiratory acidosis, which include:
① Lightheadedness
② Restlessness
③ Bradycardia
④ Bradypnea

400. When assessing Mr. Beacon's arterial blood gases the nurse would know that he was in compensated respiratory acidosis when his pH is 7.34 and his:
① PO_2 is 80 mmHg
② PCO_2 is 60 mmHg
③ HCO_3 is 50 mEq/L
④ Serum potassium is 4 mEq/L

401. The nurse is aware that Mr. Beacon understands the instructions about an appropriate breathing technique for COPD when he:
① Inhales through his mouth
② Increases his respiratory rate
③ Holds his breath for a second at the end of inspiration
④ Progressively increases the length of the inspiratory phase

402. Mr. Beacon's liver becomes enlarged. The nurse understands that this results from:
① Liver hypoxia
② Hepatic acidosis
③ Esophageal varices
④ Portal hypertension

Situation: Norma Willow, a 28-year-old secretary, has morning stiffness lasting 30 minutes to 2 hours. She also has swollen, painful joints of the hands and feet. A diagnosis of rheumatoid arthritis is made, and aspirin 10 grains po four times a day is prescribed.

403. Mrs. Willow asks the nurse about ways to decrease morning stiffness. The nurse should suggest:
① Planning a 15-minute rest break periodically
② Taking a hot tub bath or shower in the morning
③ Avoiding excessive physical stress and fatigue
④ Wearing loose, warm clothing

404. Mrs. Willow is admitted to the hospital 3 months later for an acute episode of rheumatoid arthritis. During the admission interview, the nurse observes that Mrs. Willow's finger joints are swollen. The nurse understands that the swelling is most likely related to:
① Inflammation in the joints' synovial lining
② Formation of bony spurs on the joint surfaces

③ Edema resulting from the body's autoimmunity
④ Escaped fluid from the capillaries, increasing interstitial fluids

405. The physician orders ibuprofen (Motrin) 800 mg po tid. The nurse teaches Mrs. Willow about the side effects of Motrin. The nurse would know the teaching was effective when Mrs. Willow:
① Recognizes that she must balance periods of exercise with rest
② Understands she must take the drug between meals
③ Makes an appointment for blood work in 1 month
④ Says she should make position changes slowly

406. As the acute episode subsides, range of motion is ordered for Mrs. Willow. The nurse avoids applying direct pressure to a joint because it may precipitate:
① Pain
② Swelling
③ Nodule formation
④ Tophaceous deposits

Situation: John Craig, a 26-year-old college student, is admitted to the hospital with a history of severe cramping and violent diarrhea of 2 days duration. The tentative diagnosis made by the physician is salmonellosis.

407. Relevant data to gather from Mr. Craig on admission to the hospital is a history of:
① Rectal cancer in his family
② His food intake for the past 24 hours
③ Any recent extreme emotional stress
④ An upper respiratory infection in the past 10 days

408. Enteric precautions for salmonellosis include:
① Isolation in a private room
② Double bagging laundry
③ Limiting visiting hours
④ Wearing a mask

409. The diagnosis of salmonellosis is confirmed by a:
① CBC
② Urinalysis
③ Stool culture
④ Febrile agglutinin test

410. The treatment for salmonellosis includes administration of:
① Antispasmodics
② Antidiarrheics
③ Electrolytes
④ Antacids

411. Blood work is ordered. The medical diagnosis is metabolic acidosis. In metabolic acidosis the:
① pH of the blood is increased
② Plasma bicarbonates are increased
③ Excess hydrogen ions are excreted in the urine

④ Respiratory center in the medulla is depressed

412. Mr. Craig improves and is taught how to prevent food poisoning in the future. The nurse evaluates that Mr. Craig understands the teaching when he says:
① "Cooked food should be cooled before being put into the refrigerator."
② "Poultry should be stuffed and then refrigerated before cooking."
③ "Once most food is cooked it does not need to be refrigerated."
④ "All meats and cream-based foods need to be refrigerated."

Situation: Mark Brown, 18 years old, is admitted to the emergency room in a semicomatose state. His father states the client has been "healthy" but has had the flu for 2 days. This morning he vomited, complained of severe abdominal pain, and became very lethargic. A diagnosis of diabetic ketoacidosis is made by Mr. Brown's physician based on the physical examination and a blood glucose level of 600 mg/100 ml.

413. The nurse understands that Mr. Brown's elevated ketone level is caused by the incomplete oxidation of:
① Carbohydrates
② Potassium
③ Protein
④ Fats

414. Mr. Brown's serum potassium level is 5.4 mEq/L. When monitoring the ECG tracing, the nurse would expect to observe:
① Abnormal P waves and depressed T waves
② Peaked T waves and widened QRS complexes
③ Abnormal Q waves and prolonged S-T segments
④ Peaked P waves and an increased number of T waves

415. Mr. Brown is receiving intravenous therapy for rehydration and insulin. He complains of tingling and numbness of his fingers and toes. He is short of breath and the cardiac monitor shows the appearance of a U wave. The nurse should recognize that these symptoms indicate:
① Hyponatremia
② Hypoglycemia
③ Hypercalcemia
④ Hypokalemia

416. Mr. Brown states he hates asparagus, broccoli, and mushrooms. When reviewing the exchange list with him, the nurse would know that Mr. Brown understood the exchange diet when, in their place, he selected:
① Corn, lima beans, or dried peas
② Baked beans, potatoes, or parsnips
③ Corn muffin, corn chips, or pretzels
④ String beans, beets, or carrots

417. Mr. Brown receives NPH insulin every morning at 8 AM. The nurse recognizes that he understands the action of this insulin when he says he should be alert for signs of hypoglycemia between:
① 10 AM and 12 Noon
② 2 PM and 4 PM
③ 4 PM and 6 PM
④ 8 PM and 10 PM

418. Mr. Brown is in a self-care teaching group. The nurse has confidence that he is able to recognize hypoglycemia when he drinks orange juice and eats a slice of bread when he feels:
① Nervous and weak
② Thirsty and nauseated
③ Flushed and short of breath
④ Abdominal cramping and has a headache

Situation: Carol Oxford, 26 years old, comes to the physician because she has been experiencing fatigue and double vision. After performing a thorough physical examination the physician suspects myasthenia gravis.

419. When talking with Ms. Oxford the nurse would expect her to report that:
① The symptoms seem more severe in the evening
② Her strength increases with progressive activity
③ The longer she rests, the weaker she feels
④ Her level of fatigue has been constant

420. When talking with Ms. Oxford further the nurse observes that the client has:
① Nonintention tremors of the extremities
② Intention tremors of the hands
③ Difficulty swallowing saliva
④ Problems with cognition

421. The nurse recognizes that the most specific diagnostic test that the physician can perform for myasthenia gravis is:
① Electromyography (EMG)
② A thorough history and physical assessment
③ The pyridostigmine (Mestinon) test
④ The edrophonium chloride (Tensilon) test

422. The physician orders neostigmine (Prostigmin). The nurse would know that Ms. Oxford understands the teaching about this drug when she says:
① "The drug should be taken between meals to promote absorption."
② "I should take the drug at the exact time specified by the doctor."
③ "The peak action of the drug occurs 3 to 4 hours after ingestion."
④ "I should keep the drug in a tight container in the refrigerator."

423. Several months later Ms. Oxford is admitted to the emergency room in crisis. To distinguish between myasthenic crisis and cholin-

ergic crisis the nurse should prepare to administer:
① Atropine sulfate
② Protamine sulfate
③ Naloxone (Narcan)
④ Edrophonium chloride (Tensilon)

424. The priority nursing diagnosis for Ms. Oxford while she is in crisis is:
① Activity intolerance
② Impaired physical mobility
③ Ineffective breathing pattern
④ Sensory-perceptual alteration: visual

425. Ms. Oxford's crisis is resolved with therapy, and she is stabilized at her previous level of functioning. When assessing Ms. Oxford the nurse should expect:
① Dramatic worsening in muscle strength with anticholinesterase drugs
② Involvement of the distal muscles rather than the proximal muscles
③ Fluctuating weakness of muscles enervated by the cranial nerves
④ Partial improvement of muscle strength with mild exercise

426. The nurse reinforces previous teaching about myasthenia gravis with Ms. Oxford. The nurse would evaluate that the teaching was effective when Ms. Oxford recognizes that she should:
① Plan activities for later in the day
② Avoid people with respiratory infections
③ Eat meals in a semirecumbent position
④ Take muscle relaxants when she is under stress

Situation: Ellen Miro, who is 42 years old and premenopausal, has been performing breast self-examination every month for several years ever since her sister had a mastectomy.

427. To perform breast self-examination correctly, Mrs. Miro should be examining her breasts:
① When she ovulates
② The first of every month
③ The day her menses begins
④ Three days after her menses ends

428. When performing breast self-examination Mrs. Miro should be:
① Squeezing the nipples to check for discharge
② Using the right hand to examine the right breast
③ Placing a pillow under the shoulder opposite the side being examined
④ Pressing the palm of the hand against the breast to compress it to the chest wall

429. Mrs. Miro calls the local women's health center for an appointment for mammography. Mrs. Miro should be told that:
① The room will be darkened throughout the procedure
② Each breast will be firmly compressed between 2 plates

③ Food and fluid must be avoided for 6 hours before the test
④ She does not need mammography until she is 50 years old

430. The physician identifies an area of density on the mammograph and sends Mrs. Miro to a surgeon for a needle biopsy. The nurse knows that after hearing the instruction about the needle biopsy, Mrs. Miro understands the teaching when she tells her husband:
① "The lump will be removed, and a frozen section will be examined."
② "Fluid will be drawn out of the lump and examined under a microscope."
③ "A dye marker will be injected around the tumor during mammography."
④ "A needle-shaped piece of the tissue will be surgically removed and examined."

431. Mrs. Miro is diagnosed as having cancer of the right breast, and she is admitted to the hospital for a modified radical mastectomy. While being admitted by the nurse, Mrs. Miro has tears in her eyes and her chin is quivering. In a shaky voice she says, "I can't believe this is happening." The nurse's best response would be:
① "You can't believe this is happening?"
② "This must be a very scary time for you."
③ "Do you have any questions at this time?"
④ "Cancer of the breast has a high cure rate."

432. Mrs. Miro returns to her room after surgery with an incisional dressing and two portable wound drainage systems exiting from the operative site. The nurse recognizes that the principle underlying the function of a portable drainage system is:
① Gravity
② Osmosis
③ Active transport
④ Negative pressure

433. Mrs. Miro is to receive adjuvant chemotherapy. The nurse teaches her that alopecia is a side effect of chemotherapy. The most important fact that Mrs. Miro should be told is that the occurrence of alopecia is:
① Usually rare
② Never permanent
③ Frequently prolonged
④ Sometimes preventable

Situation: At the age of 58, Roland Johnson, who lives alone, develops degenerative joint disease of the vertebral column.

434. Mr. Johnson is taught to turn himself from his back to his side keeping his spine straight. The least effort will be exerted if he does this by crossing his arm over his chest and:
① Crossing his ankles and turning with both legs straight

② Bending his top knee to the side to which he is turning

③ Flexing his bottom knee to the side to which he wishes to turn

④ Pulling himself to one side by using his night table

435. Mr. Johnson develops a herniated nucleus pulposus at L4-5, and a laminectomy is scheduled. The night before surgery Mr. Johnson has been extremely demanding and has made frequent requests for about 2 hours. An empathetic nurse might best show understanding by saying:
① "You are being demanding tonight."
② "You are facing a rough day tomorrow."
③ "Don't be so concerned; we'll take good care of you."
④ "I know how scared you are, but this is routine surgery."

436. Mr. Johnson's surgery is successful, and he is receiving a skeletal muscle relaxant that he must continue to take at home. The nurse recognizes that no further health teaching is necessary when Mr. Johnson says:
① "I'll take an extra dose of the medication before I do anything active."
② "If the medication upsets my stomach, I'll take it with milk."
③ "If the medication makes me sleepy, I'll stop taking it."
④ "I'm going to take the medication 3 hours after meals."

437. When preparing Mr. Johnson for discharge the nurse would know that he did not understand the health teaching when he says, "I should:
① Sleep on a firm mattress to support my back."
② Spend most of the day sitting in a straight-back chair."
③ Avoid lifting heavy objects until the doctor tells me I can."
④ Put a pillow under my knees when sleeping on my back."

438. Mr. Johnson is to wear a back brace when he is home. The nurse should include in the teaching plan instructions to:
① Use the brace when his back feels tired
② Apply the brace before getting out of bed
③ Put the brace on while in the sitting position
④ Wear the brace when performing twisting exercises

Situation: As the result of a routine annual physical examination, the physician diagnoses that Sheila Berger has an abdominal aortic aneurysm. She is immediately admitted to the hospital, and surgery is scheduled for the next morning.

439. When performing the admission assessment the nurse should expect:
① A palpable pulsating abdominal mass

② A pattern of visible peristaltic waves
③ Cyanosis and symptoms of shock
④ Severe radiating abdominal pain

440. During the evening Mrs. Berger suddenly develops symptoms of shock. The nurse should:
① Administer the prescribed sedative
② Notify the physician immediately
③ Give the client nothing by mouth
④ Prepare for blood transfusions

441. Shock associated with an abdominal aneurysm is called:
① Vasogenic shock
② Neurogenic shock
③ Cardiogenic shock
④ Hypovolemic shock

442. Mrs. Berger is taken to surgery, and the aneurysm is resected and replaced with a graft. When she arrives in the recovery room she is still in shock. The nursing priority should be:
① Placing her in the Trendelenburg position
② Putting several warm blankets on her
③ Monitoring her hourly urine output
④ Assessing her respiratory status

443. When performing further assessments on Mrs. Berger the nurse should expect to note:
① Hypertension
② Tachycardia
③ Bradypnea
④ Polyuria

444. The nurse should assess Mrs. Berger's laboratory values, especially the arterial blood gases, because people in profound shock will develop:
① Respiratory alkalosis
② Metabolic acidosis
③ Decreased PCO_2
④ Hypokalemia

445. Mrs. Berger's hematocrit is 20%. The nurse should anticipate that the physician will order:
① High molecular dextran
② Blood replacement
③ Serum albumin
④ Ringer's lactate

446. Mrs. Berger develops peritonitis and sepsis. On assessment the nurse should expect to find:
① Leukopenia
② Bradycardia
③ Abdominal rigidity
④ Increased bowel sounds

Situation: A nurse stops at the scene of an accident and finds a man, Jean Valcon, with a deep laceration on his hand, a fractured arm and leg, and abdominal pain.

447. The nurse wraps Mr. Valcon's hand in a soiled cloth and drives him to the nearest hospital. The nurse is:
① Negligent and can be sued for malpractice
② Practicing under guidelines of the Nurse Practice Act

③ Protected for these actions, in most states, by the Good Samaritan Law

④ Treating a health problem that can and should be handled by a physician

448. Mr. Valcon is admitted to the hospital from the emergency room with a fractured arm and leg, which are casted; a lacerated hand, which is sutured; and bladder trauma. The physician inserts an indwelling urinary catheter and initiates a continuous bladder irrigation. When planning care for a client with a continuous bladder irrigation the nurse should:

① Irrigate with saline tid

② Measure output hourly

③ Monitor specific gravity

④ Exclude irrigant from the output

449. The physician orders bed rest. The nurse is aware that the most beneficial method of preventing skin breakdown while Mr. Valcon is confined to bed is to:

① Encourage independent movement

② Promote passive range of motion

③ Use a sheepskin pad on the bed

④ Massage his skin with cream

450. Mr. Valcon is a self-employed fisherman, has no hospitalization insurance, and is very worried about the medical bills. As he is describing the accident to a friend, he becomes very restless, and his pulse and respirations increase sharply. It is most important for the nurse to recognize that his symptoms are probably related to:

① A parasympathetic nervous system response to anxiety

② Delayed psychologic response to trauma

③ Bleeding from undiscovered injury

④ His method of seeking sympathy

451. Because of Mr. Valcon's multiple physical injuries and emotional concerns, he is at high risk to develop a stress (Curling's) ulcer. The nurse should know that stress ulcers are usually evidenced by:

① Sudden massive hemorrhage

② A gradual drop in hematocrit

③ Melena for several days

④ Unexplained shock

452. The physician orders Maalox and cimetidine (Tagamet). Mr. Valcon asks why he is receiving these medications. The nurse's best response would be:

① "They're what your doctor ordered to calm your stomach."

② "They're ordered for all clients with multiple trauma."

③ "They limit acidity in the stomach and intestine."

④ "They decrease irritability of the bowel."

453. After 3 days of bed rest and therapy with Maalox and cimetidine, Mr. Valcon complains of diarrhea. The nurse recognizes that the diarrhea is most likely caused by:

① Diet alterations

② The cimetidine

③ The Maalox

④ Bed rest

Situation: Ted Baxter is admitted with a diagnosis of cancer of the pancreas. An extensive revision of the head of the pancreas is performed.

454. After surgery, to decrease the chance of hemorrhage of the operative site the nurse should:

① Keep the client in the supine position

② Maintain patency of the nasogastric tube

③ Replace fat-soluble vitamins as necessary

④ Administer the ordered tube feeding slowly

455. Postoperatively Mr. Baxter's nutritional and fluid regimen will be influenced by the remaining amount of functioning pancreatic tissue. Considering both the exocrine and endocrine functions of the pancreas, Mr. Baxter's postoperative regimen would primarily include managing the intake of:

① Alcohol and caffeine

② Vitamins and minerals

③ Fluids and electrolytes

④ Fats and carbohydrates

456. Total parenteral nutrition is instituted via a central venous infusion route. During the fourth hour of the first infusion Mr. Baxter complains of nausea, fatigue, and a headache. His hourly urine is twice the amount of the previous hour. The nurse should call the physician and:

① Increase fluids via a peripheral IV route and give analgesics for the headache

② Prepare Mr. Baxter for immediate surgery for possible bowel obstruction

③ Slow the infusion and check the serum glucose level

④ Stop the infusion and cover the insertion site

457. Mr. Baxter is aware of the terminal nature of his illness. Behaviors that would indicate that he is accepting the fact of his impending death are:

① Alternately crying and talking openly about death

② Getting second, third, and fourth medical opinions

③ Making out his will and planning a visit to a good friend

④ Refusing to follow treatments and stating, "I'm going to die anyway."

458. Mr. Baxter decides to donate his eyes for organ transplantation after he dies. Statutes that address organ transplantation attempt to prevent abuse by:

① Permitting active euthanasia when necessary

② Preventing children from giving organs to others

③ Allowing physicians to control both donor and recipient

④ Requiring participating institutions to have review boards

Situation: Kim Meyer, 19 years of age, visits the health center at her college because she feels nervous, irritable, and extremely tired. She complains that although she eats large amounts of food she is still losing weight.

459. In giving the health history Miss Meyer complains of feeling hot and having frequent bouts of diarrhea. The nurse observes that Miss Meyer has a fine hand tremor, her reactions to external stimuli are exaggerated, and her face has a wide-eyed expression. The laboratory tests that might be ordered to determine what may be causing Miss Meyer's symptoms are the:
① T_3 and T_4
② PTT and PT
③ VDRL and CBC
④ Serum barbiturate levels

460. A diagnosis of hyperthyroidism is made by the physician, and Miss Meyer is treated first with propylthiouracil. When teaching Miss Meyer about this medication, the nurse should include the information that:
① Her symptoms may not subside for several days or weeks after the start of therapy
② She should take the medication between meals so that it is more readily absorbed
③ She should take the medication with milk so that it does not cause gastric irritation
④ This medication will have to be taken for the rest of her life

461. Miss Meyer is scheduled to have a partial thyroidectomy. When providing preoperative teaching for the postoperative period, the nurse should teach Miss Meyer to:
① Cough and deep breathe every 2 hours
② Perform range-of-motion activities of the head and neck
③ Support the head with the hands when changing position
④ Apply gentle pressure against the incision when swallowing

462. After Miss Meyer's thyroidectomy the nurse should observe for possible complications. If Miss Meyer experiences tingling and numbness of the fingers and toes, muscle twitching, or muscle spasms, the client may be:
① In hypovolemic shock
② In thyroid crisis
③ Hypocalcemic
④ Hypokalemic

463. Miss Meyer should be observed for the possible complication of thyroid crisis after surgery. This complication is evidenced by:
① An increased temperature and pulse rate
② A decreased pulse rate and respirations

③ A decreased blood pressure
④ An increased pulse deficit

464. When preparing Miss Meyer for discharge, the nurse should inform her of the signs of hypothyroidism. The nurse would be aware that Miss Meyer understands the teaching when she says she should call her physician if she develops:
① Weight gain and tachycardia
② Dry skin and an intolerance to cold
③ Muscle cramping and sluggishness
④ Fatigue and an increased pulse rate

465. Miss Meyer does not understand how she could develop hypothyroidism when she has hyperthyroidism. The nurse should base the response on the knowledge that:
① Hypothyroidism is a gradual slowing of the body's function
② There will be a decrease in pituitary thyroid-stimulating hormone
③ There is less thyroid tissue to supply thyroid hormone after surgery
④ Atrophy of tissue remaining after surgery reduces secretion of thyroid hormones

Situation: Clare Benson, 50 years old, has been excessively fatigued and anorexic. When she notices a perceptible weight loss, she visits her physician. After diagnostic tests, chronic myelogenous leukemia (CML) is diagnosed and Mrs. Benson enters the hospital for chemotherapy.

466. Mrs. Benson is receiving chlorambucil (Leukeran). When assessing for complications of alkylating agents, the nurse should be alert for:
① Leukopenia and thrombocytopenia
② Fluid retention and hyperglycemia
③ Feminization or masculinization
④ Stomatitis and nausea

467. Mrs. Benson is receiving busulfan (Myleran) to treat her leukemia. Specific nursing intervention should include:
① Emphasizing that the disease will be cured with this treatment
② Administering medications IM and increasing activity level
③ Serving hot liquids, such as broths or tea, with each meal
④ Giving frequent oral hygiene and increasing oral fluids

468. When Mrs. Benson develops a temperature of 101° F, the physician is notified. Aspirin 500 mg q4h prn is ordered. The nurse should:
① Ask the physician for an antacid order
② Question the type of antipyretic ordered
③ Question the dosage ordered by the physician
④ Withhold aspirin until her temperature reaches 102° F

Situation: Allen Rogers, a 62-year-old engineering consultant, has had an inguinal hernia for years. It becomes incarcerated, and he is admitted to the hospital for surgery. He has a past history of thrombophlebitis and varicosities of the lower extremities.

469. Mr. Rogers' past medical history and present diagnosis indicate to the nurse that a primary responsibility following surgery is to:
① Get him OOB twice daily
② Raise the foot of the bed
③ Maintain body alignment with firm support of the extremities
④ Encourage him to turn often and to exercise his legs regularly

470. Mr. Rogers travels a great deal, making many cross-continent or cross-Atlantic trips. He confides to the nurse that he is concerned because his legs swell on long flights. The nurse should advise him to:
① Relax in a reclining position
② Sit upright with his legs extended
③ Walk about the cabin at least once every hour
④ Sit in any position that relieves pressure on the legs

471. Mr. Rogers is apprehensive about the possibility of a clot reaching his heart and causing sudden death. The nurse's initial intervention should be to:
① Clarify his misconception
② Explain preventive measures
③ Teach recognition of early symptoms
④ Encourage discussion of his concern

472. Before Mr. Rogers' discharge the nurse teaches him about exercising to prevent venous stasis. For best results, the nurse should:
① Demonstrate specific exercises
② Suggest frequent moving of the legs
③ Advise against sitting for prolonged periods
④ Suggest that he change his position frequently

473. Mr. Rogers asks how future attacks of thrombophlebitis can best be prevented. The nurse should teach him to:
① Follow the program of exercises
② Take prophylactic anticoagulants
③ Apply warm soaks to his legs daily
④ Apply elastic stockings before arising

Situation: Bob Parks, 60 years old, is diagnosed as having chronic angina pectoris. The physician prescribes isosorbide dinitrate (Sorbitrate) 10 mg prn tid and a nitroglycerine transdermal disc once a day.

474. Mr. Parks asks the nurse why he is taking the Sorbitrate. The nurse's best response would be:
① "It allows more oxygen to get to the heart tissue."
② "It increases the force of contraction of the heart."

③ "It suppresses irritability in the ventricles."
④ "It prevents the blood from clotting."

475. When teaching Mr. Parks about Sorbitrate, the nurse should plan to include instructions about how to prevent:
① Bradycardia
② Respiratory distress
③ Postural hypotension
④ Constipation

476. Several weeks later Mr. Parks is brought into the emergency room with an apparent heart attack. To determine the status of Mr. Parks' carotid pulse, the nurse should palpate:
① At the anterior neck lateral to the trachea
② At the base of the neck along the clavicle
③ Immediately below the mandible
④ In the lateral neck region

477. One of the major manifestations of a heart attack is a decrease in the conductive energy provided to the heart. The nurse understands that the existing action potential is in direct relationship to the:
① Heart rate
② Refractory period
③ Pulmonary pressure
④ Strength of contraction

478. Mr. Parks remains hospitalized because his vital signs are unstable. He experiences a noticeably decreased pulse pressure. The nurse should immediately recognize this as a possible indication of:
① Decreased force of contraction
② Increased cardiac sufficiency
③ Hyperactivity of the heart
④ Increased blood volume

479. The nurse notes premature ventricular contractions (PVCs) on Mr. Parks' cardiac monitor and recognizes that these complexes are a sign of:
① Atrial fibrillation
② Cardiac irritability
③ Impending heart block
④ Ventricular tachycardia

480. It is determined that Mr. Parks will require implantation of a permanent pacemaker to assist the function of his heart. In response to Mr. Parks' inquiries as to why this is necessary, the nurse's best response would be:
① "It shocks the AV node to contract."
② "It will cause a normal heartbeat to occur."
③ "It will work the valves of your heart better."
④ "It will slow down the heart to a more normal rate."

481. The nurse recognizes that a pacemaker was indicated because Mr. Parks was experiencing:
① Angina
② Chest pain

③ Heart block

④ Tachycardia

482. Mrs. Parks arrives at the cardiac care unit and is informed about Mr. Parks' need for a pacemaker. She is worried that her husband could accidently become electrocuted. The nurse's best response would be:

① "The voltage emitted is not strong enough to electrocute him."

② "Pacemakers are pretested for safety before being inserted."

③ "The new technology prevents electrocution from occurring."

④ "No one has been electrocuted yet by a pacemaker."

Situation: Harrison Wills, age 70, comes to the clinic with complaints of anorexia, alternating episodes of constipation and diarrhea, blood-streaked stools, and a 10-pound weight loss in 1 month.

483. The physician orders three stool specimens for occult blood. To ensure valid test results the nurse would instruct Mr. Wills to:

① Avoid eating red meat before testing

② Test the specimen while it is still warm

③ Discard the first stool of the day and use the next three stools

④ Take three specimens from different sections of the fecal sample

484. Following a proctosigmoidoscopy and biopsy, rectal cancer is confirmed, and an abdominoperineal resection and colostomy are scheduled. The nurse recognizes that the physician will need the client to sign a consent for a:

① Permanent sigmoid colostomy

② Permanent ascending colostomy

③ Temporary double-barrel colostomy

④ Temporary transverse loop colostomy

485. The physician discusses the surgical procedure with Mr. Wills. After the physician leaves, Mr. Wills tells the nurse that he is pleased only minor surgery is necessary. The nurse recognizes that Mr. Wills' reaction is an example of:

① Regression

② Repudiation

③ Reconciliation

④ Reflection

486. Three days later, after further explanation of the effects of the surgery, Mr. Wills remarks to the nurse, "It will be difficult for my wife to care for a helpless old man." Mr. Wills' comments regarding himself are an example of Erikson's conflict of:

① Initiative vs guilt

② Integrity vs despair

③ Industry vs inferiority

④ Generativity vs stagnation

487. Preoperatively, the anesthesiologist orders meperidine hydrocholoride (Demerol) 50 mg IM and atropine sulfate 0.8 mg IM. On hand is a vial of atropine containing 0.4 mg/ml. The amount of atropine the nurse should administer is:

① 0.2 ml

② 0.5 ml

③ 2.0 ml

④ 2.4 ml

488. Mr. Wills' surgery is performed, and he is to receive the following intravenous fluids over 24 hours: 1000 ml D5W; 0.5 liter normal saline; 1500 ml D5NS. In addition, an antibiotic piggyback in 50 ml D5W is ordered every 8 hours. The nurse calculates that Mr. Wills' IV fluid intake for 24 hours will be:

① 3150 ml

② 3200 ml

③ 3650 ml

④ 3750 ml

489. Several days after surgery, the physician orders colostomy irrigations for Mr. Wills. The nurse should explain that the primary purpose of the irrigation is to:

① Limit the amount of fluid lost from the intestine

② Decrease the amount of flatus in the bowel

③ Establish a regular elimination schedule

④ Prevent straining at passage of stool

490. For colostomy teaching to be effective for Mr. Wills, the nurse must first:

① Begin with simple written instructions concerning his care

② Wait until he has accepted the change in his body image

③ Assess barriers to learning ostomy care

④ Wait until a family member is present

491. To promote perineal wound healing, the nurse should encourage Mr. Wills to assume the:

① Knee-chest position

② Left or right Sims' position

③ Dorsal recumbent position

④ Left or right side-lying position

492. The nurse plans to teach Mr. Wills to irrigate his colostomy when the:

① Perineal wound heals and the client can sit comfortably on the commode

② Client can lie on his side comfortably, about the third postoperative day

③ Abdominal incision is closed and contamination is no longer a danger

④ Stool starts to become formed, around the seventh postoperative day

Situation: Grant Redick, a 60-year-old widower who lives with his daughter, has had insulin-dependent diabetes mellitus for several years. His typical blood glucose level is 130 mg/100 ml. At 7:30 every morning he takes 40 units of NPH and 20 units of regular insulin. At 1:00 PM as he is preparing to eat lunch, he collapses with intense chest pain. He is admitted to the hospital with a suspected heart attack.

493. In reviewing the events prior to his admission the nurse suspects he may also be hypoglycemic. If this has occurred, the nurse would expect his blood glucose to be:
① About 100 mg/100 ml
② Between 50 and 70 mg/100 ml
③ Between 100 and 120 mg/100 ml
④ At least 20 mg/100 ml below the norm

494. Mr. Redick's serum glucose drops to 30 mg/100 ml and insulin shock is diagnosed. The nurse understands the reason for the development of acute hypoglycemia in Mr. Redick is that:
① The stress brought on by his chest pain increases the use of glucose available to him
② Glycogenolysis was accelerated when he failed to eat his lunch after taking NPH insulin
③ Glucose levels that are controlled by insulin drop more quickly than those controlled by oral antidiabetics
④ His body became sensitive to the prescribed dose of insulin after long use, and the blood glucose dropped erratically

495. When assessing the client who is experiencing hypoglycemia, the nurse should expect to find:
① Increased respirations
② Warm, dry skin
③ Tachycardia
④ Lethargy

496. Besides the individual such as Mr. Redick who has Type I diabetes, the nurse is aware that acute hypoglycemia can also develop in the client who is diagnosed with:
① Hypertension
② Liver disease
③ Type II diabetes
④ Hyperthyroidism

497. Mr. Redick's blood glucose level is stabilized, but his chest pain persists. Blood is drawn for cardiac enzymes because a myocardial infarction is strongly suspected. He is admitted to the cardiac intensive care unit, where a circulatory access is instituted. Mr. Redick's ECG tracing reveals multiple PVCs. The physician orders Lidocaine 1.5 mg per minute. The nurse adds 500 mg of Lidocaine to 100 ml of D5W. The drop factor of the IV set is 60 gtt/ml. To administer the correct amount of medication the nurse should set the IV at:
① 18 gtt/minute
② 14 gtt/minute
③ 12 gtt/minute
④ 10 gtt/minute

498. Mr. Redick's chest pain continues. The nursing intervention that would be most effective in relieving his pain would be to administer the ordered:
① Oxygen per nasal cannula
② Nitroglycerine sublingually
③ Morphine sulfate 2 mg IV push titrated
④ Lidocaine hydrochloride 50 mg IV bolus

499. With administration of lidocaine, a serious side effect that must be reported to the physician immediately is:
① Hypertension
② Tachycardia
③ Anorexia
④ Tremor

500. Mr. Redick is digitalized, and a nitroglycerine patch is ordered. The nurse recognizes that the purpose of the nitroglycerine is to decrease:
① Preload of the heart, thereby reducing cardiac workload
② Pulse rate, thereby strengthening cardiac contractility
③ Cardiac output, thereby reducing cardiac work load
④ Peripheral resistance by dilating coronary arteries

501. When administering the ordered digoxin (Lanoxin) 0.25 mg po qd, the nurse should:
① Give it with orange juice
② Monitor for dysrhythmias
③ Withhold it if the apical pulse is 90
④ Administer it 1 hour after the AM insulin

502. Because a client with a myocardial infarction can develop left ventricular failure, the nurse should assess Mr. Redick for:
① Right upper quadrant tenderness
② Paroxysmal nocturnal dyspnea
③ Anorexia and weight loss
④ Distended neck veins

503. Mr. Redick develops left ventricular failure that progresses to right ventricular failure, which produces ascites and severe respiratory distress. The physician orders a paracentesis. Before the procedure, the nurse should instruct Mr. Redick to:
① Empty his bladder
② Eat foods low in fat
③ Be npo for 24 hours
④ Remain in the supine position

504. During the evening after the paracentesis, the nurse finds Mr. Redick smoking incessantly. He also seems very anxious. The best nursing approach is to:
① Offer him a back rub
② Administer the ordered narcotic
③ Reinforce the physician's explanation of the procedure
④ Discuss his concerns and give him the ordered hypnotic

Situation: Terry Spoke, 21 years old, sustained a vertebral fracture at the T1 level as a result of diving into shallow water.

505. On admission to the emergency room a detailed neurologic assessment is performed. The nurse would expect to find:

① Difficulty breathing and a flaccid diaphragm
② Loss of pain sensation in the hands
③ Normal biceps reflexes in the arm
④ Inability to move the lower arm

506. The nurse is aware that autonomic dysreflexia is a complication in some spinal cord injuries. The nurse plans to observe for signs of this problem in Mr. Spoke because:
① His injury has resulted in loss of all reflexes
② He has had a partial transection of the cord
③ His injury is above the sixth thoracic vertebra
④ He has flaccid paralysis of his lower extremities

507. The nurse is aware that Mr. Spoke is developing autonomic dysreflexia when it is observed that he has:
① Flaccid paralysis and numbness
② Absence of sweating and pyrexia
③ Escalating tachycardia and shock
④ Paroxysmal hypertension and bradycardia

508. During the first week, Mr. Spoke and the nurse identify a short-term goal. An appropriate short-term goal would be, "Mr. Spoke will:
① Carry out personal hygiene activities."
② Perform independent ambulation."
③ Consider alternate life-styles."
④ Understand his limitations."

509. Mr. Spoke is recuperating, and he wants to use a wheelchair. In preparation for this activity he should be taught:
① Leg lifts to prevent hip contractures
② Push-ups to strengthen arm muscles
③ Balancing exercises to promote equilibrium
④ Quadriceps-setting exercises to maintain muscle tone

510. In light of Mr. Spoke's developmental level, he will most likely have difficulty with:
① Differentiating himself from the environment
② Developing meaningful relationships
③ Identifying with the male role
④ Mastering his environment

Situation: Ed Long is admitted with cellulitus of the left leg and a temperature of 103° F. He has a history of non–insulin-dependent diabetes mellitus. The physician orders IV antibiotics.

511. Before instituting the prescribed antimicrobial therapy, the nurse should:
① Determine if he has any allergies
② Measure the amount of swelling in his leg
③ Apply a warm, moist dressing over the area
④ Obtain the results of the culture and sensitivity tests

512. Mr. Long has a diminished urine output. The nurse should recognize that this is probably the result of:
① A normal compensatory response to fever
② Nephrotoxicity from antimicrobial agents
③ Bacterial invasion of the kidneys
④ A declining blood pressure

513. The physician orders bed rest. The nurse understands that the primary purpose of bed rest is to:
① Decrease catabolism to promote healing at the site of injury
② Lower the metabolic rate in an attempt to help reduce the fever
③ Reduce the energy demands on the body in the presence of infection
④ Limit muscle contractions that would force causative organisms into the blood stream

514. The nurse teaches Mr. Long how to provide self-care to prevent future infections in his feet. The nurse recognizes that the teaching was effective when Mr. Long says, "I should:
① Massage my feet and legs with oil or lotion."
② Apply heat intermittently to my feet and legs."
③ Eat foods high in kilocalories of protein and carbohydrates."
④ Control my diabetes through diet, exercise, and medication."

Situation: Anita Roth, the mother of five children, has had a history of severe varicose veins.

515. During a recent office visit to her gynecologist, Mrs. Roth asks the nurse to explain what causes varicose veins. The nurse's best response would be, "They are caused by:
① Abnormal configurations of the vascular system."
② Atherosclerotic plaque formation in the veins."
③ Decreased pressure within the deep veins."
④ Incompetent valves of superficial veins."

516. When collecting data about Mrs. Roth's legs, the nurse should expect her to report:
① Calf pain on dorsiflexion of the foot
② Intermittent claudication of the legs
③ Hematomas of the lower extremities
④ A feeling of heaviness in both legs

517. When assessing Mrs. Roth's lower extremities the nurse should expect to find:
① Pallor
② Ankle edema
③ Yellowed toenails
④ Diminished pedal pulses

518. Mrs. Roth is referred by the gynecologist to a surgeon, and a bilateral ligation and stripping of the varicose veins is scheduled. When obtaining the informed consent the nurse should explain that the surgery involves:
① Removing the dilated saphenous veins

② Cleaning out plaque from within the vessels

③ Anastomosing superficial veins to deep veins

④ Injecting a sclerosing agent into the affected veins

519. To prevent thrombus formation after surgery, the nurse should plan to:
    ① Have Mrs. Roth dangle her legs frequently
    ② Keep the bed gatched to elevate Mrs. Roth's knees
    ③ Change the elastic bandage on Mrs. Roth's legs twice a day
    ④ Encourage Mrs. Roth to ambulate with assistance as needed

Situation: Charles Harold is admitted to the hospital with severe pain in the left upper quadrant, abdominal distention, and nausea and vomiting. A diagnosis of acute pancreatitis is made.

520. Mr. Harold is npo. Total parenteral nutrition is prescribed. The most accurate explanation the nurse can give Mr. Harold regarding reasons for his receiving hyperalimentation is:
    ① "It is the easiest method for the staff to administer needed nutrition."
    ② "It is the safest method for meeting your nutritional requirements."
    ③ "It will satisfy your desire for food without the discomfort associated with eating."
    ④ "It will meet your nutritional needs without causing the discomfort associated with eating."

521. The nurse can assist the physician with the safe insertion of the central venous catheter by instructing Mr. Harold to:
    ① Void 15 minutes before the procedure is started
    ② Maintain npo status for 2 hours before the procedure
    ③ Breathe out slowly and use the "purse-lip" breathing technique
    ④ Breathe deeply, hold the breath, and bear down with his mouth closed

522. The medication order that should be questioned by the nurse if it is prescribed for Mr. Harold is:
    ① Tagamet
    ② Phenergan
    ③ Morphine sulfate
    ④ Meperedine hydrochloride

523. Six hours after the parenteral hyperalimentation is started, Mr. Harold's blood glucose is 240 mg/100 ml. The nurse recognizes that the primary cause for Mr. Harold's elevated blood glucose is probably related to:
    ① An infusion that is flowing too rapidly
    ② The prescribed solution being too concentrated
    ③ An infusion too slow to meet total nutritional needs

④ A normal response to the initial infusion of solution

524. The equipment that will be used by the nurse during the intravenous site care for Mr. Harold is:
    ① Double sterile gloves
    ② Gown and sterile gloves
    ③ Mask and sterile gloves
    ④ Mask, gown, and sterile gloves

525. If Mr. Harold develops steatorrhea, the nurse should describe his stool as:
    ① Clay colored and pasty
    ② Black and blood-streaked
    ③ Bulky and foul smelling
    ④ Dry and rock-hard

Situation: Richard Gregg, a 41-year-old Vietnam veteran, went to his physician for a routine physical examination before starting a new job. A chest x-ray film reveals a lesion in the right upper lobe.

526. When the office nurse obtains a history from Mr. Gregg the information that supports the physician's tentative diagnosis of pulmonary tuberculosis is:
    ① Frothy sputum and fever
    ② Night sweats and service in Vietnam
    ③ Dry cough and pulmonary congestion
    ④ Productive cough and engorgement of neck veins

527. A tuberculin skin test with purified protein derivative of tuberculin (PPD) is performed on Mr. Gregg. The nurse tells him to make an appointment so that the test can be read in:
    ① 3 days
    ② 5 days
    ③ 7 days
    ④ 10 days

528. The nurse should teach Mr. Gregg that the sputum specimens he must supply should be:
    ① Refrigerated until brought to the laboratory
    ② Copius in amount for adequate testing
    ③ Collected in the early morning hours
    ④ Coughed up from deep in the lungs

529. Tuberculosis is diagnosed, and one of the drugs the physician orders is pyrazinamide. The nurse evaluates that the teaching concerning the drug was effective when Mr. Gregg says he will:
    ① Drink at least 2 quarts of fluid a day
    ② Take the medication 2 hours after each meal
    ③ Report any changes in vision to the physician
    ④ Expect a discoloration of urine, sweat, and tears

530. The nurse tells Mr. Gregg he needs to maintain optimal nutrition and explains that his diet should:
    ① Contain liquid protein supplements
    ② Be low in calories but high in carbohydrates

③ Be made of frequent small high-calorie meals

④ Contain foods high in calories and low in protein

531. Mr. Gregg is treated on an outpatient basis. To help control the spread of the disease he should be instructed to:
① Have visitors sit at least 8 feet away from him
② Keep his personal articles away from the rest of his family
③ Not put his dishes in the dishwasher with the rest of the family's dishes
④ Open the windows slightly to allow a good airflow throughout the house

Situation: Paul Summer is admitted to the intensive care unit with a diagnosis of adult respiratory distress syndrome.

532. When assessing Mr. Summer, the nurse should expect to find:
① Hypertension
② Tenacious sputum
③ Altered mental status
④ Slowed rate of breathing

533. Mr. Summer is placed on a ventilator. Because hyperventilation can occur when mechanical ventilation is used, the nurse should monitor Mr. Summer for signs of:
① Respiratory alkalosis
② Metabolic acidosis
③ Hypercapnia
④ Hypoxia

534. A tracheostomy is performed. After the procedure Mr. Summer should be placed in the:
① Semi-Fowler's position
② High-Fowler's position
③ Orthopneic position
④ Supine position

535. Mr. Summer begins to "fight" the respirator, and the physician orders pancuronium bromide (Pavulon). The most important nursing action for a client receiving Pavulon is to:
① Decrease anxiety
② Monitor skin integrity
③ Promote urinary output
④ Maintain mechanical ventilation

536. The nurse knows that a high-volume, low-pressure tracheostomy cuff is used primarily to prevent:
① Lung infection
② Leakage of air
③ Mucosal necrosis
④ Tracheal secretion

Situation: A nurse works in the sexually transmitted disease (STD) clinic, seeing a variety of clients each day.

537. Nineteen-year-old Jay Breen comes to the clinic because he has a discharge from his penis. The physician suspects gonorrhea and orders a culture and sensitivity test to assist with the diagnosis. To obtain the culture the nurse should:
① Instruct the client to provide a semen specimen
② Swab the discharge as it appears on the prepuce
③ Obtain a mucosal scraping from the anterior urethra
④ Teach the client how to obtain a clean catch specimen of urine

538. Mr. Breen's sexual partner comes to the clinic to be examined. She tells the nurse she has had anal sex. The nurse should assess for:
① Melena
② Anal itching
③ Constipation
④ Ribbon shaped stools

539. Holly Greely, also a client of the STD clinic, has been diagnosed as having early syphilis. The nurse understands that an early symptom would be:
① Flat wart-like plaques around the vagina and anus.
② An indurated painless nodule on the vulva that begins to drain
③ Glistening patches in the mouth covered with a yellow exudate
④ A maculopapular rash on the palms of the hands and soles of the feet

540. Ms. Greely tells the nurse that she must have caught syphilis from a toilet seat. The nurse knows that this cannot be true because the causative agent of syphilis is:
① Immobilized by body contact
② Chelated by wood and plastic
③ Destroyed by warmth and moisture
④ Inactivated when exposed to dryness

541. The physician orders penicillin G benzathine suspension (Bicillin L-A) 2.45 million units for Ms. Greely. The drug is available in a multidose vial of 10 ml in which 1 ml = 300,000 units. The nurse should administer:
① 0.008 ml
② 0.8 ml
③ 8.2 ml
④ 8.8 ml

542. Peter Daily, a 53-year-old homeless person, is referred from the emergency room to the STD clinic because the physician suspects that the client has late-stage syphilis. The statement by Mr. Daily that would support this diagnosis is:
① "I'm having trouble keeping my balance."
② "I've been losing a lot of hair lately."
③ "I have sores all over my mouth."
④ "I noticed a wart on my penis."

Situation: Janet Collins has gallstones, and the physician attempts to dissolve the stones with methyl tertiary butyl ether (MTBE) via a transhepatic catheter.

543. After the procedure Mrs. Collins should be placed in the:

① Right side-lying position to prevent localized bleeding
② Left Sims' position to prevent pressure on
the operative site
③ Supine position to evenly distribute the
chemical in the gallbladder
④ High-Fowler's position to prevent operative edema and facilitate respirations

544. This procedure did not totally dissolve the
stones, and an extracorporeal shock wave
lithotripsy is scheduled. Preoperative teaching should include the information that:
① Narcotics will be available for postoperative pain
② A fever is a common response to this intervention
③ Heart palpitations frequently occur after
the procedure
④ Analgesics and anesthetics are not necessary during the procedure

545. Mrs. Collins' sister, Barbara Holden, develops a gallstone that becomes lodged in the
common bile duct. The physician schedules
an endoscopic sphincterotomy. Preoperative
teaching should include information that for
the procedure she will:
① Have spinal anesthesia
② Have general anesthesia
③ Receive an epidural block
④ Receive intravenous diazepam (Valium)

Situation: Sean Byrne, 64 years old, has been attending the neurologic clinic because of progressive
carotid and cerebral atherosclerosis. He has a history
of transient ischemic attacks (TIAs)

546. The nurse understands that TIAs are:
① Ischemic attacks that result in progressive
neurologic deterioration
② Periods of alternating exacerbations and
remissions

③ Transient attacks caused by multiple
small emboli
④ Temporary episodes of neurologic dysfunction

547. Atherosclerotic plaques are identified, and after discussion with Mr. Byrne a right carotid
endarterectomy is performed. Two hours after surgery Mr. Byrne demonstrates progressive hypotension. The nurse should:
① Increase the IV flow rate
② Raise the head of the bed
③ Notify the physician immediately
④ Position the client in slight Trendelenburg

548. Cranial nerve dysfunction is a complication
of an endarterectomy. To monitor for this
complication the nurse should assess for:
① Labored breathing
② Edema of the neck
③ Difficulty in swallowing
④ Alteration in blood pressure

549. One month after the endarterectomy the physician instructs Mr. Byrne to take 5 grains of
aspirin a day. The nurse evaluates that Mr.
Byrne understands the reason for taking this
drug when he says it will:
① Limit the inflammation around his incision
② Help to prevent further clogging of his arteries
③ Lower the slight fever he has had since
surgery
④ Reduce the discomfort he feels at the surgical site

550. The physician orders docusate sodium (Co-
lace) every day. The nurse recognizes that
this drug is ordered specifically to:
① Lubricate the feces and GI tract
② Create an osmotic effect in the GI tract
③ Lower the surface tension in the GI tract
④ Stimulate the motor activity of the GI
tract

CHAPTER 3

Psychiatric–Mental Health Nursing Review Questions

Situation: Lucy Hines, a 17-year-old student, weighs 78 pounds and is 5 feet 6 inches tall. She is admitted to the hospital because of weight loss and malnutrition. Ms. Hines is diagnosed as having anorexia nervosa.

1. The nurse is aware that anorexia nervosa is usually precipitated by:
   ① An inaccurate perception of hunger stimuli and a struggle between dependence and independence
   ② The acting out of aggressive impulses, which results in feelings of hopelessness
   ③ The inability to deal with being the center of attention in the family and a desire for independence
   ④ An unconscious wish to punish a parent who tries to dominate the adolescent's life

2. After Ms. Hines' physical condition is stabilized, the psychiatrist, in conjunction with the client and her parents, decides to institute a behavior modification program for Ms. Hines. The nurse is aware that a major component of behavior modification is that it:
   ① Decreases necessary restrictions
   ② Rewards positive behavior
   ③ Reduces anxiety-producing situations
   ④ Deconditions fear of weight gain

3. The nurse interviews Ms. Hines to obtain information for the nursing history. Ms. Hines' history is likely to reveal:
   ① A close, supportive mother-daughter relationship
   ② Low achievement in school, with little concern for grades
   ③ Satisfaction with and a desire to maintain present weight
   ④ A strong desire to improve her self-image

4. Mr. and Mrs. Hines are very upset about their daughter's diagnosis and treatment plan. The best intervention by the nurse when Ms. Hines' parents ask if they may bring food in to her is to state:
   ① "It is important that you bring in whatever you think she'll eat."
   ② "While in the hospital she should eat the hospital food."
   ③ "For now, allow the hospital staff to handle her food needs."
   ④ "Your concerns about food contribute to her problem."

5. When interacting with Ms. Hines the nurse should:
   ① Show empathy
   ② Maintain control
   ③ Focus on dietary nutrition
   ④ Set and maintain limits

6. When Ms. Hines starts to discuss food and eating, the nurse should plan to:
   ① Let her talk about food as long as she wants, but limit discussion about her eating
   ② Use her current interest in food to encourage her to increase her intake
   ③ Listen closely to determine her favorite foods and secure these foods for her
   ④ Tell her gently but firmly to direct all discussion of food to the dietician

7. In talking with one of the day nurses, Ms. Hines states that the day nurses give better care and are nicer than the night nurse. Ms. Hines also asks a question that the nurse is aware was answered by the night nurse. The nurse should recognize that Ms. Hines:
   ① Needs assistance in exploring and verbalizing her feelings about the night nurse
   ② Has negative feelings about the night nurse and the nurse should be informed of her feelings
   ③ Is attempting to divide the staff and her behavior should be reported to the other staff members
   ④ Is trying to develop a bond of trust with a staff member that should be encouraged

Situation: Peter Tompson is brought to the hospital by the police after he appeared at his workplace and threatened several fellow employees with a knife. He tells the admitting nurse that his boss and co-workers have been trying to poison his lunches for several months. He explains that they dislike him because he is an important advisor to the President of the United States.

8. In establishing a nursing care plan the nurse should understand that Mr. Tompson's delusion that he is an important government advisor is most likely related to:
   ① A psychotic loss of touch with his real identity
   ② An attempt to compensate for feelings of depression about his problems
   ③ An attempt at wish fulfillment created to manipulate others
   ④ A need to feel a sense of importance and control over his environment

9. The nurse who is planning to establish a trusting relationship with Mr. Tompson should begin by:
   ① Sitting on the ward and observing his behavior throughout the day
   ② Being available on the ward frequently but waiting for him to approach
   ③ Seeking him out frequently to spend long blocks of time with him
   ④ Calling him into the office to establish a contract for regular therapy sessions

10. Mr. Tompson refuses to eat, stating, "The food is poisoned." The nurse should:
    ① Ask him what foods he likes so that they can be ordered for him
    ② Accompany him to the cafeteria and taste his food to show him it is not poisoned
    ③ Encourage him to go to the cafeteria and select those foods he feels safe eating
    ④ Encourage his family to bring his favorite foods from home

11. The physician orders haloperidol (Haldol) concentrate 10 mg po bid for Mr. Tompson, who is also receiving phenytoin (Dilantin) for control of his epilepsy. In planning Mr. Tompson's care the nurse should be aware that anticonvulsants may interact with Haldol to:
    ① Mask its therapeutic effect
    ② Potentiate its CNS depressant effect
    ③ Interfere with its absorption
    ④ Enhance its rate of metabolism

12. Forty-eight hours after starting the Haldol regimen, Mr. Tompson is observed standing by the nurses' station with his neck arched sharply backward. The nurse should recognize that Mr. Tompson:
    ① Needs to have the dosage increased because his psychotic behavior is not lessening
    ② Is experiencing temporary side effects that usually disappear after several days
    ③ Is having pseudoparkinsonian side effects and needs to have his medication adjusted
    ④ Needs immediate treatment and is experiencing an acute dystonic reaction to the drug

Situation: Damon Watson, a 42-year-old veteran, has a long history of alcohol abuse. When Mr. Watson returned from military service he graduated from college and taught history at the elementary school level for several years. His teaching contract was not renewed because of budgetary cuts, and simultaneously his alcohol consumption increased. Mr. Watson lives with his mother, who works several days per week to supplement her fixed income. Mr. Watson's father, who was also an alcoholic, died 10 years ago of cancer.

13. Mr. Watson seeks help for his drinking problem in one of the local hospitals. The major underlying factor for his success in an alcohol treatment program will be his:
    ① Family
    ② Motivation
    ③ Psychiatrist
    ④ Self-esteem

14. The nurse understands that Mr. Watson ingests alcohol primarily because he:
    ① Has no other coping mechanism
    ② Lacks the motivation to stop
    ③ Enjoys the associated socialization
    ④ Is dependent on it

15. To give Mr. Watson greater responsibility for self-control, the nurse should initially plan to:
    ① Confront him with his substance abuse
    ② Administer medications according to the prescribed schedule
    ③ Tell him about the detoxification program
    ④ Assist him to identify and adopt more healthful coping patterns

16. Two days after admission to the program, Mr. Watson tells the nurse, "I don't know why I came here." The nurse's best response would be:
    ① "You did admit yourself into the program."
    ② "Don't you remember why you decided to come here?"
    ③ "You realize you are trying to avoid your problem."
    ④ "You feel you don't need this program."

17. Mr. Watson has been informed that he has extensive liver damage. He is told that he has approximately 1 year to live if alcohol abuse persists. He is intensely depressed and one evening leaves the hospital and returns drunk. The nurse is aware that Mr. Watson's behavior suggests that he:
    ① Cannot associate his increasing depression and lack of fulfillment to his heavy use of alcohol
    ② Does not trust the judgment of the health professionals because he feels well physically
    ③ Believes that he inherited the disease of alcoholism from his father and cannot stop drinking
    ④ Wants to punish his mother for his physical and emotional discomfort and cause her pain

18. Mr. Watson has been in the hospital for a week. He tells the nurse that he feels better and will probably not require any further treatment. In evaluating Mr. Watson's progress the nurse would recognize that:
    ① Mr. Watson lacks insight about the emotional aspects of his illness and most likely needs continued supervision
    ② Mr. Watson has accepted his illness and now needs to use his willpower to resist the alcohol

③ As long as Mr. Watson's family remains supportive, he will probably not use alcohol again

④ The physician must be notified of his statement so that aversion therapy can be started before Mr. Watson's discharge

19. Therapy has helped Mr. Watson make a fairly satisfactory adjustment during his time in the hospital. He will continue to receive therapy on an outpatient basis and will be discharged with the drug disulfiram (Antabuse). The nurse should caution Mr. Watson to avoid using:
① Undecaffeinated coffee and strong tea
② White sugars and vinegars
③ Suntan lotions and oils
④ Elixirs and liniments

Situation: Myra Beal, 79 years old, is admitted to a nursing home from the general hospital. She is often confused and quite forgetful. Her diagnosis is dementia of the Alzheimer type.

20. Mrs. Beal has been in the nursing home for several days. This morning she is going to join a group of residents in recreational therapy. The nurse notes that Mrs. Beal has laid out several dresses on her bed but has not changed from her nightclothes. It would be most helpful for the nurse to:
① Help Mrs. Beal select appropriate attire and offer her assistance in getting dressed
② Remind Mrs. Beal to dress more quickly to avoid delaying the other residents
③ Help Mrs. Beal dress and tell her what time the residents are expected at the activity
④ Allow Mrs. Beal as much time as she needs but explain that she is too late to attend this activity

21. Mrs. Beal hoards leftover food from her meal tray, along with other seemingly valueless articles, and stuffs them in her dress pockets and sweater "so the others won't steal them." The nurse should plan to:
① Remove unsafe and soiled articles from Mrs. Beal's belongings during the night
② Tell Mrs. Beal that the staff is required to keep harmful objects out of reach in the resident's closet
③ Give Mrs. Beal a small bag in which to place selected personal articles and food of her own choosing
④ Explain to Mrs. Beal why the nursing home's policy for cleanliness and safety must be followed

22. In planning activities for Mrs. Beal the nurse should:
① Provide familiar activities that Mrs. Beal can successfully complete
② Plan varied activities that will keep Mrs. Beal occupied

③ Make sure that Mrs. Beal actively participates in the unit's daily activities
④ Offer challenging activities to maintain Mrs. Beal's contact with reality

23. Mrs. Beal likes to talk about her youth and at times has a tendency to confabulate. The nurse should recognize that this behavior serves to:
① Prevent regression
② Attract the attention of others
③ Reminisce about achievements
④ Increase self-esteem

24. Mrs. Beal frequently talks about "the good old days at the ranch" where she was born. On the basis of an understanding of Mrs. Beal's diagnosis, the nurse's most appropriate action at this time would be to:
① Gently remind Mrs. Beal that those "good old days" are past and she should think about the present
② Allow Mrs. Beal to reminisce about her past, and listen with interest to her stories
③ Involve Mrs. Beal in interesting diversional activities in a small group
④ Introduce Mrs. Beal to other residents her age so that they can mutually share their past experiences

Situation: Thomas Hill is a 32-year-old client on the psychiatric unit who sits alone most of the day. No other clients ever seem to go near Mr. Hill. On close observation, the nurse notices that Mr. Hill's musculature is very tense and that his eyes continually dart around the room.

25. The nurse, deciding to establish a relationship with Mr. Hill, approaches him. When the nurse gets approximately 3 feet from Mr. Hill, he lets out a string of profanity and says, "Leave me alone; I don't want to talk to you!" The most appropriate response for the nurse to make at this time would be:
① "Mr. Hill, I don't like it when you talk like that. Are you trying to push me away?"
② "I'll leave for now, Mr. Hill, but I'll be back later."
③ "Why do you feel the need to greet me in this way?"
④ "Mr. Hill, do not talk to me like that. I am here to spend time with you."

26. Several mornings later, the nurse finds Mr. Hill curled up in the fetal position in the corner of the dayroom. The most accurate evaluation of his behavior would be that he is:
① Feeling more anxious today
② Physically ill and experiencing abdominal discomfort
③ Tired and probably did not sleep well last night
④ Attempting to hide from the nurse

27. The most appropriate intervention for the nurse to take after finding Mr. Hill in the fetal position would be to:

① Tap him gently on the shoulder and say, "I'm here to spend time with you Mr. Hill."

② Go to him and say, "I'll be waiting for you by the table and chairs, Mr. Hill."

③ Sit down beside him on the floor and say, "I'm here to spend time with you, Mr. Hill."

④ Leave him alone because he is too regressed to benefit from talking with the nurse

28. One morning Mr. Hill tells the nurse, "My legs are turning to rubber because I have an incurable disease called schizophrenia." The nurse recognizes that this is an example of:

① Paranoid thinking
② Autistic verbalization
③ Depersonalization
④ Hallucination

29. In responding to Mr. Hill's statement about his legs it would be most appropriate for the nurse to state:

① "That's a rather unusual sensation."
② "Mr. Hill, your legs look fine to me."
③ "When did this first start, Mr. Hill?"
④ "That must be a frightening way to feel."

30. The staff could interpret that Mr. Hill has established some trust in the nurse who has been seeing him regularly if he:

① Attends morning meeting every day for 1 week
② Plays bingo with the nurse and other clients each day
③ Demonstrates decreased muscle tension and is able to maintain direct eye contact
④ Acts out until he requires seclusion on each day that the particular nurse is not available

Situation: Gerry Kune is remanded to the psychiatric unit by the court for observation. She was arrested and charged with abusing her youngest son, 2-year-old Gary, who has been admitted to the pediatric intensive care unit in critical condition with a fractured skull and other injuries resulting from a beating.

31. In approaching Mrs. Kune, the nurse, Sally Winthrop, should expect her to:

① Deny beating Gary
② Express concern for her son Gary
③ Ask where her three other children are
④ Avoid talking about the situation completely

32. In speaking with Mrs. Kune, Mrs. Winthrop should expect her to:

① Ask how she may get permission to visit Gary on the pediatric unit
② Offer a detailed explanation of how Gary was injured
③ Attempt to rationalize and explain her behavior
④ Reveal an overwhelming feeling that her children are worthless

33. One morning before work Mrs. Winthrop becomes very angry with her daughter, and both mother and daughter end the argument in tears. At the hospital Mrs. Winthrop is again assigned to care for Mrs. Kune and finds she has difficulty spending time with her. Mrs. Winthrop tells another nurse about the argument and states, "Mrs. Kune makes me feel very uncomfortable today." The best explanation of what is happening with Mrs. Winthrop is that she:

① Is beginning to question her own potential for abuse
② Is experiencing guilt that is causing her to be ineffective
③ Has identified with a client of the same sex
④ Would have difficulty caring for any client today

34. The most therapeutic response by the other nurse would be:

① "You're a wonderful mother. Everything will be okay. Teenagers can really drive you to distraction."
② "Why don't you bring home a surprise for your daughter? It will make you both feel better."
③ "Sometimes we find it difficult to live up to our own expectations of ourselves."
④ "You can't compare yourself to that client. After all, you didn't beat your child."

35. Having worked through her own problems, Mrs. Winthrop may best assist Mrs. Kune to alter her behavior toward Gary by helping her to:

① Ignore his negative, nondestructive behavior and support his acceptable behavior
② Learn what behavior is appropriate for a 2-year-old child
③ Identify the specific ways in which his behavior provokes frustration in her
④ Learn appropriate ways of punishing Gary for his behavior

36. Gary is reported to be improving rapidly, and Mrs. Winthrop decides to go to the pediatric unit to visit him. She should expect Gary to:

① Smile readily at anyone who enters the room
② Pay little attention to her standing at the bedside
③ Begin to cry and scream as she nears his bedside
④ Be wary of physical contact initiated by anyone

Situation: Robert Diamond, a 62-year-old accountant, has an inoperable occipital lobe tumor. Both he and his wife Pearl have been informed of the diagnosis and prognosis.

37. Mr. Diamond has been experiencing rather frightening visual hallucinations, especially when he is alone. The nurse can best help Mr. Diamond cope with these hallucinations by planning to:
    ① Suggest that he not be alone and work out a schedule for visitors
    ② Have his wife remain with him until the hallucinations stop
    ③ Suggest that he turn on the radio or television when he is alone
    ④ Move him to a four-bed room closer to the nurse's station

38. The nurse recognizes that characteristic behavior in the initial stage of a client's coping with dying often includes:
    ① Asking for additional medical consultation
    ② Pressing the call button as soon as the nurse leaves
    ③ Criticizing medical care
    ④ Sleeping for long periods

39. Mrs. Diamond, who is employed as a legal secretary, tells the nurse that although she wants to visit her husband daily, she can visit only twice per week because she works and has to take care of the house and their cat and dog. The nurse assesses that her statement demonstrates the use of the defense mechanism known as:
    ① Sublimation
    ② Rationalization
    ③ Projection
    ④ Compensation

40. Mrs. Diamond tells the nurse that she knows that her husband is asking the nurses to leave his pain medication on his bedside table and she fears he is saving it up for a suicide attempt. The nurse knows that many of the staff members have mixed feelings about the client's terminal status and prolonged pain. The nurse uses an approach that is ethically sound by:
    ① Reporting the information and Mrs. Diamond's concern to the supervisor and letting the supervisor handle it
    ② Speaking to all of the nurses and telling them not to leave the medication at the bedside
    ③ Asking the head nurse to handle the problems of the client's medication and the staff's feelings
    ④ Suggesting a nursing conference be held to discuss staff feelings, as well as the medication problem

41. The nurse recognizes that at this time to assist Mr. and Mrs. Diamond in dealing with their feelings about his terminal illness, it would be important to:
    ① Help Mr. and Mrs. Diamond to express their feelings about his terminal illness to each other

    ② Place Mr. and Mrs. Diamond in a couples' therapy group that deals with the terminal illness of one partner
    ③ Encourage Mr. and Mrs. Diamond to verbalize their feelings to a therapist during their individual therapy sessions
    ④ Refer Mr. Diamond to the psychotherapist for assistance in dealing with his anger about death

Situation: David Quinn, a 15-year-old with an 11-year history of multiple foster home placements, is admitted to an adolescent unit for evaluation. He has a long history of drug abuse, stealing, refusal to comply with rules, and an inability to get along in any setting.

42. When collecting data related to David's lifestyle, the nurse may be prevented from accurately listening to what he is saying by:
    ① The pressure of inadequate time to complete care
    ② The client's disease process
    ③ Personal cultural beliefs
    ④ A personal need to secure information

43. Lately windows in the recreation room have been found broken on numerous occasions, and after group discussion, another adolescent indicates he has seen David breaking windows. The nurse, using assertive intervention instead of aggressive confrontation, should:
    ① Knock on the door of David's room, and ask if he would like to come out and talk about the situation
    ② Approach David when he is alone and, after making eye contact, inquire about his involvement in these incidents
    ③ Use a trusting approach, implying that the staff doubts his involvement but requests his denial for the record
    ④ Confront him openly in the group, using a controlled voice and maintaining direct eye contact with him

44. The most appropriate plan of care for David at this time would be for the nurse to:
    ① Allow him as much freedom as possible, setting few rules and providing minimal structure
    ② Behave in a moralistic, punitive manner toward him when he does not follow rules
    ③ Act as a role model for mature behavior and provide a very structured setting
    ④ Provide activities that ensure immediate gratification, as well as social stimulation

Situation: Phil and Irene Ferris, a devout couple in their late twenties, are very happy to be expecting a child that they have been praying for since their marriage. When Mrs. Ferris delivers, she is disappointed that the baby is a boy. However, Mr. Ferris is very pleased. On the second day after delivery, when the baby is brought to Mrs. Ferris, she seems far away as though she is daydreaming. The nurse calls her name, and Mrs. Ferris states, "I don't have a baby. I have sinned." She proceeds to rock her empty arms.

45. The nurse recognizes that the precipitating factor for Mrs. Ferris' emotional reaction is probably her:
① Desire for a baby girl
② Husband's behavior
③ Religious upbringing
④ Alteration in role

46. Mrs. Ferris continues to be apathetic and exhibits an inappropriate affect. A diagnosis of acute schizophrenic reaction is made. A characteristic symptom the nurse would expect to observe in Mrs. Ferris' communication or behavior is:
① Absence of self-criticism
② Suicidal preoccupation
③ Abstract and logical deductions
④ Autistic magical thinking

47. While the nurse is assisting with morning care, Mrs. Ferris suddenly throws off the covers and starts shouting, "My body is disintegrating; I am being pinched." The term that best describes Mrs. Ferris' behavior is:
① Depersonalization
② Ideas of reference
③ Loose association
④ Paranoid ideation

48. Mrs. Ferris is transferred to a psychiatric unit when her behavior becomes increasingly bizarre. When obtaining a history from Mrs. Ferris' family, the nurse would expect to find that her premorbid behavior included:
① Depression and anxiety
② Extroversion and inflated self-esteem
③ Irritability and circumstantiality
④ Suspiciousness and introversion

49. When assessing Mrs. Ferris the nurse recognizes that the potential for recovery is better in a client whose history reveals the:
① Presence of a family history of schizophrenia
② Presence of many poorly defined prepsychotic symptoms
③ Slow and insidious onset of the illness
④ Occurrence of a precipitating event

50. When helping Mrs. Ferris select foods for breakfast, the most therapeutic question for the nurse to ask would be:
① "What kind of foods do you like?"
② "Which of these foods do you want?"
③ "Do you want boiled or scrambled eggs?"
④ "How do you want your eggs fixed today?"

51. Mrs. Ferris, like many clients with schizophrenia, often experiences opposing emotions simultaneously. The nurse recognizes this phenomenon as:
① Inappropriate affect
② Ambivalence

③ Loose associations
④ Double bind

Situation: Flora Wilson is admitted to the psychiatric unit with a diagnosis of severe depression.

52. One morning Mrs. Wilson states to the nurse, "God is punishing me for my past sins." The nurse's best response would be:
① "God is punishing you for your sins, Mrs. Wilson?"
② "Why do you think that, Mrs. Wilson?"
③ "You really must feel upset about this."
④ "If you feel this way, you should talk to your clergyman."

53. The best initial approach to take with a self-accusatory, guilt-ridden client like Mrs. Wilson is to:
① Redirect the client whenever a negative topic is mentioned
② Medicate the client when these thoughts are expressed
③ Accept the client's statements as personal beliefs
④ Contradict the client's persecutory delusions

54. In working with Mrs. Wilson the nurse should initially:
① Attempt to keep her occupied
② Keep the surroundings bright and gay
③ Accept what she says
④ Try to keep her from talking too much

55. When the nurse sees Mrs. Wilson sitting alone in the dayroom, the best action would be to approach her and say:
① "May I sit with you for a while?"
② "Do you mind if I sit and talk to you?"
③ "Call me if you would like to talk."
④ "I'll be sitting with you for a while today."

56. When caring for the depressed client the nurse usually has the most difficulty dealing with the:
① Negative nonverbal responses
② Contagious quality of depression
③ Client's lack of energy
④ Client's psychomotor retardation

57. In planning continuing care for Mrs. Wilson the nurse should include:
① Making all decisions for her to relieve her of this responsibility
② Offering her the opportunity to make some decisions
③ Encouraging her to decide how she wants to spend her time
④ Allowing her time by herself so she can decide what she would like to do

58. The nurse identifies establishing trust as a major nursing goal for Mrs. Wilson. This goal can best be accomplished by:
① Spending the day with Mrs. Wilson
② Waiting for Mrs. Wilson to initiate conversation

③ Asking Mrs. Wilson at least one question daily

④ Spending short periods of time with Mrs. Wilson every day

59. Mrs. Wilson is still extremely depressed, and her physician orders a tricyclic antidepressant, imipramine hydrochloride (Tofranil), for her. Mrs. Wilson asks the nurse what the medication will do. The nurse's best response would be:
① "You will really begin to feel much better after taking this medication for 2 to 3 days."
② "This medication will help you forget why you are depressed."
③ "The medication will help increase your appetite and make you feel better."
④ "When you take this along with phenelzine sulfate (Nardil), you'll feel less depressed."

Situation: Julie Ames, 7 years of age, has been diagnosed as having acute myelogenous leukemia. Before Julie's admission to the hospital, the diagnosis and prognosis were discussed by the physician and Mr. and Mrs. Ames.

60. While Mr. and Mrs. Ames are sitting in the lounge after visiting Julie they have a serious argument over something trivial. The nurse should help them recognize that they are using the defense mechanism of:
① Projection
② Compensation
③ Denial
④ Displacement

61. The nurse plans to use family therapy as a means of assisting the family to cope with Julie's illness. The nurse's basis for this choice is that:
① It is more time efficient to deal with the whole family together
② It will prevent the parents from deceiving each other about the true nature of Julie's condition
③ The entire family is involved because they can be perceived as victims
④ The nurse can control manipulation and alliances better by using this mode of intervention

62. The nurse should always take the time to keep a client's family informed about what is happening to the client. The main reason for this action is that informed families:
① Decrease the client's anxiety
② Frequently cause less nursing problems
③ Are more relaxed and at ease with the client
④ Are better equipped to undertake necessary family role changes

63. Julie is demanding of her parents and the staff. She asks for many privileges the other children on the unit do not have, such as

staying up later to watch television and eating candy. The staff knows she does not have too much longer to live. The nurse can best help the staff cope with Julie's demands by encouraging them to:
① Give her as many extra treats as possible because she is dying
② Set reasonable limits to help Julie and her family become more secure and content
③ Give her some extra treats so that they will feel less anxiety after her death
④ Recognize that the dying child has unique needs and that special privileges can provide the necessary security

64. When Mr. and Mrs. Ames visit, Julie continues to play and ignore their presence. Mr. and Mrs. Ames state they are upset by her behavior. The nurse informs them that Julie's behavior is common among hospitalized children and tells them this is called:
① Denial
② Undoing
③ Repression
④ Sublimation

65. The head nurse gives permission to the hospital's inservice division to use Julie's chart in a nursing seminar on the care of children with leukemia. The nurse believes releasing the information will help other nurses give better care to children like Julie. The legal right of the client that was violated is the right to:
① Freedom
② Respectful care
③ Privacy
④ Informed consent

66. Julie's condition deteriorates and she is now comatose. Mr. and Mrs. Ames state that a relative said they should not allow her to be resuscitated and they feel unsure about this. The response by the nurse that would best demonstrate a recognition of the ethical issues involved is:
① "You should discuss this thoroughly with your doctor and then with your religious advisor."
② "The final decision must be made by you and your physician, but it is important to talk about it."
③ "Have you talked to your doctor about this yet? I'll be happy to page him."
④ "Let me tell you about the implications of a no-code; then you can decide."

67. After speaking with Mr. and Mrs. Ames, the physician gives a no-code order verbally but refuses to put it in writing. The nurse should:
① Follow the order as given by the physician
② Refuse to follow the order, unless the nursing supervisor approves it
③ Ask the physician to write the order in pencil on the client's Kardex before leaving

④ Determine whether the family is in accord with the physician and follow hospital policy

Situation: Ruth Birch, a 41-year-old single executive secretary, experiences an overwhelming impulse to count and arrange the rubber bands and paper clips in her desk. She believes something dreadful will happen if she does not carry out the ritual. She becomes increasingly guilty and unhappy about her reduced work efficiency and makes an appointment with a nurse therapist in a community mental health clinic.

68. In regard to Ms. Birch's symptoms, the nurse is aware that:
    ① Her symptoms are a displacement of general anxiety onto an unrelated specific fear
    ② She is able to consciously control her symptoms although this raises her anxiety level
    ③ Compulsive rituals are useful in our society as long as they can be controlled
    ④ Compulsive rituals serve to control anxiety resulting from unconscious impulses

69. Ms. Birch tells the nurse, "I am spending 30 minutes counting each time, starting in the morning, and my boss is getting very upset. What should I do?" The nurse could best suggest that she:
    ① Substitute another activity at home, such as counting her shoes or other objects
    ② Limit her counting activity to only 20 minutes each time
    ③ Arrive at work 30 minutes early each morning for counting
    ④ Talk with her boss and ask for tolerance because she is under psychiatric treatment

70. Ms. Birch states, "I feel so guilty. None of this makes any sense. My boss must really think I'm crazy." The most therapeutic response by the nurse would be:
    ① "Guilt serves no useful purpose. It just helps you stay stuck where you are."
    ② "Your behavior is bizarre, but it serves a useful purpose in your life."
    ③ "I'm sure your boss understands that you can't help this behavior right now."
    ④ "You're concerned about what other people are thinking about you."

Situation: Joyce Silver, recently admitted to the hospital, is pacing the floor and acting aloof and suspicious. According to her husband, whom she recently married, she laughed In a silly manner when told her father was critically injured, and she has had difficulty with her colleagues at work, accusing them of sabotage. Mrs. Silver has stated that she is being controlled by others.

71. The nurse, to be most helpful to Mrs. Silver, should first:

① Obtain a complete copy of her history
② Meet with Mr. Silver to learn why she was admitted
③ Review a textbook description of the schizophrenic client
④ Observe and evaluate her behavior in terms of her needs

72. The central problem the nurse might face with Mrs. Silver is her:
    ① High anxiety and suspicious feelings
    ② Continuous pacing
    ③ Relationship with her father
    ④ Concern about working with others

73. A break with reality, such as the one experienced by Mrs. Silver, requires that the nurse first realize that:
    ① The client believes what she has undergone and is experiencing
    ② The family must cooperate in the maintenance of the psychotherapeutic plan
    ③ Electroconvulsive therapy produces remission in most clients with schizophrenia
    ④ Extended institutional care is a necessary part of the treatment modality

74. When Mrs. Silver talks about being controlled by others, the nurse should:
    ① Arrange an interesting daily schedule for her
    ② Express disbelief about her delusion
    ③ Respond to the verbal content of the delusion
    ④ Respond to the feeling, tone, or theme of the delusion

75. Mrs. Silver, watching the nurse pour the juice for her medication from a nearly empty pitcher, screams, "That juice is no good. It's poisoned." The nurse should:
    ① Assure Mrs. Silver that the juice is not poisoned
    ② Pour her a glass of juice from a full pitcher
    ③ Remark, "You sound frightened, Mrs. Silver."
    ④ Take a drink of the juice to show her that it is okay

Situation: Blanche Henderson, 26 years old, is admitted to the psychiatric unit with a diagnosis of mood disorder—manic episode. She is brought in by her husband, who states that she was fine until 3 days before admission. At that time she decided to plan a huge high school reunion and began calling all her classmates. Her speech became louder, more rapid, and insulting when her idea was not greeted with enthusiasm. Yesterday she went on a shopping spree and charged clothing worth $7000. This morning she went into her husband's office and began reorganizing his files. She became quite agitated, and Mr. Henderson brought her to the emergency room.

76. In assessing Mrs. Henderson, the nurse is aware that the manic episode is in reality an:

① Attempt to block unconscious feelings of depression
② Incorrect interpretation of environmental stimuli
③ Exaggerated response to an elating situation
④ Uncontrolled acting out of uncensored id drives

77. The nurse realizes that in the care of an elated client such as Mrs. Henderson the environment is very important. The nurse should therefore:
① Put bright drapes in her room to help cheer her up
② Assign her to a room with other clients so that she can have company
③ Assign her to a room near the dayroom to provide access to activities
④ Place her in a private room to provide a quiet atmosphere

78. On the unit Mrs. Henderson is elated and sarcastic. She is constantly cursing and using foul language. She has the other clients on the unit terrified. The nurse should:
① Demand that she stop what she is doing
② Firmly tell her that her behavior is unacceptable
③ Ask her what is bothering her
④ Increase her medication or have additional medication ordered

79. In caring for Mrs. Henderson the nurse must be aware of the client's physical needs. This is particularly important because:
① The danger of exhaustion is always present for Mrs. Henderson
② Mrs. Henderson may gain too much weight from overeating
③ Left alone, Mrs. Henderson will withdraw to her room
④ Mrs. Henderson has difficulty making her needs known

80. Encouragement and praise should be given to Mrs. Henderson to help her increase her feelings of self-esteem. When she has behaved well, the best way to let her know the staff is aware of her improvement is for the nurse to say:
① "Your behavior today was much better than yesterday."
② "Everyone likes you better when you behave like this."
③ "I knew you could behave."
④ "You behaved well today."

81. Mrs. Henderson is receiving lithium carbonate. She complains of diarrhea, tremors, and drowsiness. The nurse should:
① Get an order for a stimulant
② Withhold the medication
③ Make certain Mrs. Henderson stays on her special diet
④ Decrease Mrs. Henderson's fluid intake to 2000 ml daily

82. Several weeks later Mrs. Henderson is to be discharged on a regimen of lithium carbonate. In the teaching plan for discharge the nurse should include:
① Advising her to watch her diet carefully
② Suggesting that she take the pills with milk
③ Reminding her that she must have a CBC done once per month
④ Encouraging her to have her blood levels checked as ordered

Situation: Patty Jefferies, 3 years old, has been brought by her parents to the mental health clinic on the advice of her nursery school teacher, who has noticed some problems with Patty's behavior. Patty is found to have a pervasive developmental autistic disorder.

83. With the diagnosis of possible autism, the nurse would find it most unusual for Patty to demonstrate:
① An interest in music
② A responsiveness to her parents
③ An attachment to odd objects
④ Ritualistic behavior

84. Mr. and Mrs. Jefferies begin family therapy with a nurse therapist. Mr. Jefferies states that they wish to share their religion with the therapist. The nurse should:
① Plan for a mutual discussion of religious beliefs
② Keep the sessions focused on the family's concerns
③ Invite the family minister to a therapy session
④ Limit Mr. Jefferies' discussion of religion

Situation: Jane Thomas, 7 years old, was admitted to the hospital after an explosion at school. She died soon after admission. Mr. and Mrs. Thomas arrive at the hospital a few minutes later.

85. After being told what had happened, Mr. and Mrs. Thomas ask the nurse if they can see their daughter. The best response by the nurse would be:
① "It's best to wait a while."
② "I will take you in to see her now."
③ "Would you like to wait until the physician can be with you?"
④ "It will be less traumatic if you wait and see her at the funeral home."

86. Mrs. Thomas tells the nurse that Jane was just getting over chickenpox and did not want to go to school but she insisted that Jane go. Mrs. Thomas cries bitterly and says Jane's death is her fault. The nurse should realize that perceiving a death as preventable will most often influence the grieving process in that:
① It causes the mourner to experience a pathologic grief reaction

② The grieving process may progress to a psychiatric illness

③ Bereavement may be of greater intensity and duration

④ The loss may be easier to understand and to accept

87. The initial nursing intervention for the significant others during the shock phase of a grief reaction should be focused on:
① Presenting full reality of the loss to the individuals
② Mobilizing the individuals' support systems
③ Staying with the individuals involved
④ Directing the individuals' activities at this time

Situation: Ida Kitt, age 55, is admitted to the acute care unit of a psychiatric hospital. Her husband states that she has gradually become withdrawn over the last month, refusing to bathe or change clothes, eating little, failing to go to work, and sleeping only 3 to 4 hours per night. This evening Mr. Kitt heard a shot from the basement and found Mrs. Kitt bleeding from a superficial chest wound.

88. Mrs. Kitt does not respond to any of the nurse's questions. To assess Mrs. Kitt's current potential for suicide, the nurse should:
① Ask Mrs. Kitt why she feels like killing herself
② Observe Mrs. Kitt for scars on her wrists or other signs of previous attempts
③ Ask Mr. Kitt about any previous suicidal attempts or threats by Mrs. Kitt
④ Determine if there is a family history of suicide

89. Mrs. Kitt is placed on one-to-one observation. A short-term goal specific for Mrs. Kitt's nursing care needs is that:
① Within 3 days she will understand the continued presence of a staff member
② Within 2 days she will go for a walk on the grounds with other clients
③ Within 3 days she will verbally accept responsibility for her actions
④ Within 2 days she will understand why she wanted to hurt herself

90. To further assess Mrs. Kitt's suicidal potential the nurse should be especially alert to her expression of:
① Frustration and fear of death
② Anger and resentment
③ Anxiety and loneliness
④ Helplessness and hopelessness

91. On Mrs. Kitt's fifth day in the hospital, the nurse observes that Mrs. Kitt remains lying on her bed when the clients are called to the dining room for lunch. To encourage Mrs. Kitt to eat the nurse should:
① Bring a tray to her room and leave it without comment

② Tell Mrs. Kitt, "I will accompany you to the dining room."
③ Provide information about the importance of eating to maintain health
④ Tell Mrs. Kitt, "All clients are expected to go to the dining room for meals."

92. One day, the nurse sits by Mrs. Kitt's bed and states, "I will be spending some time with you today." Mrs. Kitt responds angrily, "Go talk to someone else. They need you more." The most therapeutic response by the nurse would be:
① "I will be spending the next 15 minutes with you, Mrs. Kitt."
② "I'll go, but I will be back tomorrow."
③ "Why are you angry with me, Mrs. Kitt?"
④ "Don't say that, Mrs. Kitt. You are important too."

93. In communicating with Mrs. Kitt the nurse uses silence. When silence is used in therapeutic communication, clients should feel:
① Unhurried to answer
② The nurse is thinking
③ It is their turn to talk
④ There is nothing more to say

94. Mrs. Kitt's methods of coping are maladaptive. The nurse can best help her develop more healthful coping mechanisms by:
① Promoting interpersonal relationships with peers
② Allowing her to assume responsibility for decisions
③ Setting realistic limits on her maladaptive behavior
④ Providing a stress-free environment for the client

95. Mrs. Kitt is prescribed amitriptyline hydrochloride (Elavil) twice a day. The nurse would expect to observe a therapeutic response to this medication in:
① 30 minutes to 2 hours
② 12 to 24 hours
③ 1 to 3 days
④ 1 to 3 weeks

96. Mrs. Kitt is being discharged. In conversation, she tells the nurse that she is planning to retire from her job next year. The nurse can best respond to Mrs. Kitt by recognizing that retirement is:
① A developmental task of tremendous significance
② Damaging to both self-image and self-esteem
③ Always emotionally associated with the concept of aging
④ Eagerly anticipated by the majority of older people

Situation: Sam Early, 28 years old, enters the emergency room, stating, "My wife is having another affair and is now trying to kill me." He is dressed in a dirty shirt and jeans, wears no shoes, has on a pair of sunglasses, and smells of body odor. Mrs. Early has consistently denied her husband's charges and has threatened to leave him if he does not get help.

97. Mr. Early's symptoms are most typical of:
① Paranoid schizophrenia
② Paranoid disorder
③ Shared paranoia
④ Paranoid personality disorder

98. Mr. Early is admitted to the psychiatric unit of the hospital. During the admission procedure, Mr. Early refuses to answer the nurse's questions, stating, "You are in a conspiracy to kill me." The nurse understands that his feelings are related to his:
① Need for attention
② Low self-esteem
③ Need to be alone
④ Lack of acceptance

99. The nurse recognizes that Mr. Early's accusations are an example of:
① A hallucination
② A delusion
③ An idea of reference
④ A neologism

100. In planning care for Mr. Early the nurse should realize the importance of:
① Providing him with activities in which he can succeed
② Reducing all stress so that he can relax
③ Giving him difficult tasks to stimulate him
④ Not placing any demands on him at all

101. One afternoon the nurse notes Mr. Early rushing down the hall of the unit, rapidly hitting his fist against the wall as he goes. The best nursing action at this time would be to:
① Immediately summon staff assistance to enable administration of medication prescribed for Mr. Early's agitation
② Forcefully use additional staff members to subdue Mr. Early and stop his acting-out behavior
③ Attempt to approach Mr. Early in a nonthreatening manner to determine the basis for his agitation
④ Observe Mr. Early to see if this behavior escalates and may involve harm to other clients or staff

102. Mr. Early is scheduled to begin group therapy. He refuses to attend. The nurse should:
① Tell him that he must attend the meeting
② Have another client ask him to reconsider
③ Insist that he join to help him socialize
④ Accept his decision without discussion

103. Mr. Early tells the nurse about his wife's extramarital affairs. The nurse should:
① Listen to what he is saying
② Tell him that his wife loves him
③ Ask him to explain how he knows this
④ Refuse to listen to his stories

104. A long-term nursing objective for Mr. Early would be to help him develop:
① Faith in his wife
② Better self-control
③ Feelings of self-worth
④ Insight into his behavior

105. When Mr. Early's condition improves, the physician suggests giving him a 1-day pass. Mrs. Early is very nervous about the pass and worries about what she will do if he starts to "act up." The nurse's best intervention at this time would be to:
① Have the social worker talk with Mrs. Early
② Cancel the pass until Mrs. Early is reassured
③ Have Mr. Early promise Mrs. Early that he will behave
④ Discuss this concern with Mr. and Mrs. Early together

Situation: Nancy Paul, a recently married 22-year-old, is brought to the trauma center by the police. She had been robbed, beaten, raped, and sodomized.

106. Mrs. Paul, although very anxious and tearful, appears in control. The physician orders diazepam (Valium) 5 mg po prn for agitation. The nurse should administer this medication when the:
① Client requests something to calm her
② Nurse determines the client's anxiety is increasing
③ Physician is ready to do a vaginal examination
④ Client's crying and trembling increase

107. Mr. Paul arrives at the hospital after being called by the police. After reassuring him about his wife's condition, the nurse should give priority to:
① Making him comfortable until the physician has finished examining Mrs. Paul
② Discussing with him his own feelings about the situation
③ Calling the rape counselor in to immediately meet with Mrs. Paul
④ Helping him to understand how Mrs. Paul feels about the situation

108. Mr. Paul is extremely upset and his conversation is pressured and rambling. A therapeutic technique that the nurse can use when a client's communication rambles is:
① Touch
② Focusing
③ Silence
④ Summarizing

Situation: Lola West, a 41-year-old housewife, has a history of heavy drinking for 5 years. She finally but belligerently consented to being admitted to the hospital's detoxification unit when her husband threatened to divorce her and take custody of their teenage son.

109. On admission, Mrs. West states to the nurse, Hank James, "Both my husband and my son give me plenty of reason to worry." The defense mechanism, common among alcoholics, that is exemplified in Mrs. West's statement is:
   ① Denial
   ② Projection
   ③ Displacement
   ④ Compensation

110. Within a few hours of alcohol withdrawal, Mr. James should assess Mrs. West for the presence of:
   ① Irritability, heightened alertness, jerky movements
   ② Disorientation, paranoia, tachycardia
   ③ Tremors, fever, severe diaphoresis
   ④ Yawning, anxiety, convulsions

111. On the third day of hospitalization Mrs. West develops delirium tremens. When she is experiencing hallucinations, it would be most appropriate for Mr. James to:
   ① Pretend that he also senses the imaginary things Mrs. West is telling him about and do what she asks
   ② Ask Mrs. West to describe the sensation, then assure her it is caused by the alcohol
   ③ Tell Mrs. West that he does not sense or perceive the same things that seem to frighten her
   ④ Do nothing, because Mrs. West may just be having vivid dreams or nightmares

112. In addition to hydration during delirium tremens, the physician prescribes parenteral administration of chlorpromazine (Thorazine) for Mrs. West. Mr. James understands that chlorpromazine is given during detoxification primarily to:
   ① Reduce the anxiety-tremor state and prevent more serious withdrawal symptoms
   ② Quiet Mrs. West and enable her to cooperate and accept treatments more readily
   ③ Enable Mrs. West to sleep and eat better during periods of agitation
   ④ Prevent physical injury to Mrs. West when she has convulsions

113. To prevent life-threatening complications resulting from the administration of chlorpromazine (Thorazine), it is important that Mr. James:
   ① Provide adequate restraint
   ② Monitor her vital signs
   ③ Watch her for extrapyramidal side effects
   ④ Provide measures against photosensitivity

114. Mr. West is upset that Mrs. West's delirium tremens persist for the second day. The initial response by Mr. James that would be most appropriate is:

   ① "Are you afraid that your wife may die? I assure you that very few alcoholics die during the detoxification process."
   ② "The staff is making Mrs. West comfortable while she is undergoing the withdrawal process. Your wife will not feel pain."
   ③ "This is normal, Mr. West. I suggest that you go home because there is nothing you can do to help at this time."
   ④ "I see that you are very worried. Medications are being used to lessen Mrs. West's discomforts."

115. Mrs. West is placed on a diet high in vitamin B₁ (thiamine). Mr. James would know that Mrs. West understands her diet when she states, "I will select something for each meal from among:
   ① Lean pork, organ meat, and nuts."
   ② Leafy and green vegetables and citrus fruits."
   ③ Poultry, milk products, and eggs."
   ④ Fish, aged cheese, and breads."

116. Mrs. West has been in the detoxification unit for 5 days. One evening she complains of numbness and tingling in her feet and legs. At this time it be would be most appropriate for Mr. James to:
   ① Gently massage Mrs. West's lower extremities with a light lotion
   ② Emphasize the need to rest and to keep the lower extremities elevated
   ③ Use mechanical aids to keep bed sheets off Mrs. West's lower extremities
   ④ Observe for the progression of symptoms and monitor the pedal pulses frequently

117. One evening Mr. West asks to talk with Mr. James. He relates that he is concerned about Mrs. West's behavior if she returns to drinking and states, "When she drinks it really disrupts family life, and I'm not sure how to handle it." Mr. James' best response would be:
   ① "Help her avoid embarrassment by making excuses for her when she cannot function."
   ② "Try to maintain a normal home environment for you and your son."
   ③ "Search the house regularly for hidden alcohol, and accompany her when she goes out."
   ④ "Include her in the family's activities even when she has been drinking."

Situation: Carl White, 60 years old, has been hospitalized on a medical unit for various aches and pains he has been experiencing for several weeks. He feels depressed and tense and is unable to sleep at night.

118. In talking with Mr. White the nurse finds that his wife died 8 months ago and he has

not adjusted to the loss. In caring for Mr. White the nurse should:

① Ask the internist for a psychiatric consultation for Mr. White as soon as possible
② Continue the discussion of his wife's death
③ Focus on teaching him relaxation techniques
④ Explain why he needs to recognize his ambivalence toward his wife

119. Mr. White says, "What's the use in talking? I'd rather be dead. I can't go on without my wife." The best response by the nurse would be:

① "You'd rather be dead?"
② "Tell me what death means to you."
③ "Are you thinking about killing yourself?"
④ "I can understand why you feel that way."

120. The nurse recognizes that the suicidal risk for Mr. White is greatest:

① When his depression is most severe
② Before any type of treatment is started
③ As he loses interest in the environment
④ As the depression begins to improve

121. The nurse makes the nursing diagnosis of dysfunctional grieving associated with the loss of his wife. The nurse uses this diagnosis because of Mr. White's:

① Prolonged period of grief and mourning after his wife's death
② Difficulty in expressing his loss
③ Inability to talk about his loss
④ Inability to sleep and the presence of symptoms of depression

Situation: The nurse is at the rape intervention clinic when Fran Kraus, a rape victim, calls, saying, "I've got to talk to someone or I'll go crazy. I should not have dated him."

122. Before effectively responding to Ms. Kraus, it is essential that the nurse:

① Be aware of any personal bias about rape
② Know some myths and facts about rape
③ Call for assistance from the psychiatrist
④ Get the client's full name and address

123. Ms. Kraus arrives at the clinic alone, tearful, but generally calm. In assessing Ms. Kraus' condition, it is important for the nurse to identify Ms. Kraus':

① Support network
② Knowledge of rape victimology
③ Ability to relate the facts
④ Sexual background

124. Three weeks later Ms. Kraus admits herself to the hospital because of intense feelings of unrest, inability to sleep, and frequent episodes of panic. She tells the nurse, "I admitted myself because I think I'm going crazy." The nurse should recognize Ms. Kraus' remark as a:

① Reflection of her insightfulness
② Plea for support

③ Symptom of depression
④ Test of the nurse's trustworthiness

125. One morning Ms. Kraus is pacing the floor. The nurse approaches her in an attempt to alleviate her anxious feelings. The most therapeutic question by the nurse would be:

① "Shall we sit and talk about your feelings?"
② "Are you feeling upset right now?"
③ "Would you like to go to the gym and work out?"
④ "Would you like me to walk with you?"

126. The nurse is aware that nursing intervention for clients with anxiety disorders should include:

① Promoting the suppression of anger and hostility by the client
② Limiting the involvement of the client's family during the acute phase
③ Promoting the verbalization of feelings by the client
④ Insisting that the client accept the role of psychologic factors

127. At times, Ms. Kraus' anxiety level is so high that it blocks communication and the nurse is unsure of what is being said. To clarify understanding, the nurse states, "Let's see whether we both mean the same thing." This is an example of the technique of:

① Making observations
② Reflecting feelings
③ Attempting to place a sequence
④ Seeking consensual validation

Situation: Mike Zenkel has been admitted to the psychiatric unit. His diagnosis is schizophrenia, undifferentiated type.

128. The nurse should be aware that the defense mechanism Mr. Zenkel would most probably exhibit is:

① Rationalization
② Repression
③ Regression
④ Projection

129. Noticing Mr. Zenkel sitting in the corner smiling and talking to himself the nurse realizes that he is hallucinating. The nurse should:

① Ask him why he is smiling
② Tell him it is not good for him to talk to himself
③ Invite him to join in watching television
④ Leave him alone until he stops talking

130. When speaking with Mr. Zenkel the nurse notices that he keeps interjecting sentences that have nothing to do with his main thoughts. He asks whether the nurse understands. The nurse should reply:

① "You aren't making any sense; let's talk about something else."

② "I'd like to understand what you are saying, but you are too confused now."

③ "Why don't you take a rest, and then we can talk again later this afternoon."

④ "I'd like to understand what you are saying, but I'm having difficulty following you."

131. Mr. Zenkel tells the nurse he hears a man speaking to him from the corner of the room. He asks whether the nurse hears him too. The nurse should respond:

① "No, I don't hear him, but it must make you uncomfortable to hear him."

② "No one is in the corner of the room. Can't you see that?"

③ "What is he saying to you Mr. Zenkel? Does it make any sense?"

④ "Yes, I hear him, but I can't understand what he is saying."

132. In addition to hallucinating, Mr. Zenkel yells and curses throughout the day. The nurse should:

① Be willing to explain the meaning of the behavior to Mr. Zenkel

② Isolate Mr. Zenkel until the behavior stops

③ Become aware of what the behavior means to Mr. Zenkel

④ Ignore the behavior exhibited by Mr. Zenkel

133. Chlorpromazine hydrochloride (Thorazine) 300 mg tid is prescribed for Mr. Zenkel, who is going home on a weekend pass. The nurse informs him that he should:

① Not need to take the medication during the time he is at home

② Take all his medication early in the day to be sure he does not forget it

③ Not drink any alcoholic beverages during the time he is taking this medication

④ Reduce the dosage of the medication if he feels better at home

134. The nurse is aware that phenothiazines such as chlorpromazine hydrochloride (Thorazine) are most effective when the client exhibits:

① Excited depressed behavior

② Withdrawn secretive behavior

③ Manic assaultive behavior

④ Excited overactive behavior

135. Mr. Zenkel returns from the weekend at home, and the nurse notices that his sclera look yellow. The nurse's initial action should be to:

① Reduce the dosage of the medication

② Omit the medication

③ Give the medication with milk

④ Tell him this symptom will disappear

Situation: Judy Herman, a 29-year-old attorney, is admitted to a psychiatric facility. For 2 weeks before admission, she spent hours each day performing a complicated handwashing ritual. Her hands are raw and bloody.

136. The nurse recognizes that Ms. Herman's handwashing ritual represents a conflict with dirt, which is often associated with:

① Gender identity, with the ritual done to avoid homosexual panic

② Initiative, with the ritual done to rebel against autonomy

③ Aggression, with the ritual done to control rage

④ Freedom, with the ritual done to remain dependent

137. On her second day on the unit, Ms. Herman misses breakfast because of her handwashing ritual. During the early period of Ms. Herman's hospitalization it would be most therapeutic for the nurse to:

① Encourage her to interrupt her rituals for meals at the scheduled times

② Allow her to choose between eating breakfast or completing the ritual

③ Wake her early so that she can complete the ritual before breakfast is served

④ Prevent her from beginning the ritual until after breakfast is served

138. Ms. Herman is prescribed Valium, which she refuses to take because of fear of addiction. Initially the nurse should:

① Provide Ms. Herman with information about Valium

② Speak with the physician regarding a change in medication

③ Further assess Ms. Herman's knowledge and feelings about Valium

④ Have the physician speak to her about the safety of this drug

Situation: Sheila Kaye, an evening nurse in the surgical intensive care unit, notes that a number of clients do not seem to be responding to meperidine hydrochloride (Demerol) that has been administered for pain. In checking the clients' charts and the narcotic register, Ms. Kaye finds that Ruth Oaks, the nurse assigned to medications, has signed for all of the Demerol injections.

139. Later that evening Ms. Kaye finds Ms. Oaks in the nurses' lounge dozing. When Ms. Oaks is awakened, her speech is slurred and she appears somewhat uncoordinated and drugged. Ms. Kaye should:

① Tell Ms. Oaks that she knows she has been stealing the Demerol

② Ask the other staff members if they have noticed anything unusual

③ Call the nursing supervisor and ask for help in confronting Ms. Oaks

④ Arrange to secretly observe Ms. Oaks the next time she administers Demerol

140. It is determined that Ms. Oaks has a drug abuse problem. As an initial intervention, Ms. Oaks should be:

① Dismissed from her job immediately

② Counseled by the staff psychiatrist

③ Forced to promise she will abstain from drugs

④ Referred to the employee assistance program

141. Ms. Kaye is aware that the use of opiates creates:
① Psychologic addiction, tolerance, and physical addiction
② Physical addiction, tolerance, but no psychologic addiction
③ Physical addiction, psychologic addiction, but no tolerance
④ Psychologic addiction, tolerance, but no physical addiction

142. At a staff meeting the question of Ms. Oaks' returning to work after a drug rehabilitation program is discussed. Ms. Kaye helps the staff to decide that the best way to handle her return would be to:
① Avoid mentioning her problem unless she brings up the topic
② Assign another nurse to keep her under close observation
③ Offer her support in a direct, straightforward manner
④ Limit her assignments to administration of only non-narcotic medications

143. At the meeting one nurse states, "I don't know why we are wasting time on that woman. We all know she will go back to drugs as soon as the pressures increase." Ms. Kaye's best response would be:
① "Since you have such strong negative feelings, I don't think you should be assigned to work with Ms. Oaks."
② "I know it's hard, but it's our professional obligation to work with her."
③ "It's important for us to share our feelings about staff members with problems."
④ "I guess you feel somewhat guilty that you failed to recognize that Ms. Oaks was addicted."

Situation: Kara Wright is a 50-year-old homemaker. During the last 6 months, her husband of 30 years has been made president of his company and their children have both married. She is brought to the hospital with a history of weight loss, crying spells, restlessness, early morning insomnia, sitting in one place staring into space, and picking at her skin.

144. From Mrs. Wright's history, the nurse should realize she is demonstrating the classic symptoms associated with:
① Involutional induced reactions
② Bipolar mood disorders
③ Major depression, melancholic type
④ Mood-incongruent manic disorders

145. The first priority for the nurse is helping Mrs. Wright to:
① Investigate new leisure activities
② Feel comfortable with the nurse

③ Initiate conversations about feelings
④ Participate in small-group activities

146. In planning activities for Mrs. Wright the nurse finds her very resistive and complaining about her inabilities and worthlessness. The best approach by the nurse would be to:
① Involve Mrs. Wright in activities in which she will be assured of success
② Listen to Mrs. Wright and delay the planned activity for another time
③ Schedule activities for Mrs. Wright that she can implement independently
④ Encourage Mrs. Wright to select an activity in which she has some interest

147. When assessing Mrs. Wright's premorbid personality characteristics the nurse would not expect to find that she demonstrated:
① Rigidity
② Overmeticulousness
③ Stubbornness
④ Diverse interests

Situation: Bob Dolan, a 21-year-old high school dropout, is admitted with a diagnosis of acute schizophrenia. He has been experiencing hallucinations and delusions.

148. Mr. Dolan's family relates that one day he looked at a linen sheet on a clothesline and thought it was a ghost. The nurse recognizes that this was:
① An illusion
② A hallucination
③ A delusion
④ A confabulation

149. When asking the family about the onset of Mr. Dolan's problems the nurse would expect that his difficulties began in:
① Early childhood
② Late childhood
③ Puberty
④ Adolescence

150. Mr. Dolan states that he cannot eat because someone has taken his stomach. The nurse recognizes this as an example of:
① An illusion
② Depersonalization
③ A somatic delusion
④ A hallucination

151. To deal with Mr. Dolan's hallucinations therapeutically the nurse plans to:
① Reinforce his perceptual distortions until he develops new defenses
② Provide an unstructured environment and assign him to a private room
③ Avoid helping him make connections between anxiety-producing situations and hallucinations
④ Distract his attention by providing a competing stimulus that is stronger than the hallucination

152. After Mr. Dolan has been hospitalized for 2 weeks, the nurse feels he is ready to begin

participating in therapeutic activities. The nurse should initially suggest:
① Watching television in the dayroom
② Drawing or painting with the nurse
③ Participating on the softball team
④ Attending a class on medications

Situation: Isabella Wiern, 82 years old, is admitted to a skilled-nursing home. She is quite confused and often does not recognize her children.

153. Mrs. Wiern appears slovenly, often soiling her clothing with excreta or urine. The nurse can best manage her problem by:
① Toileting her at least once every 2 hours
② Supervising bathroom activities closely
③ Explaining how offensive her behavior is to others
④ Putting her into orientation therapy

154. Mrs. Wiern's family tells the nurse that she has suffered some memory loss in the last few years. They say that she is sensitive about not being able to remember and tries to cover up this loss to avoid embarrassment. When attempting to increase Mrs. Wiern's self-esteem the nurse should try to avoid discussing events that require memory of her:
① Married life
② Recent days
③ Young adulthood
④ Work years

155. During her first month in the nursing home, Mrs. Wiern demonstrates numerous behaviors related to disorientation and cognitive impairment. The nurse's plan for care should continue to take into consideration the:
① Realistic ability of the client to perform without becoming frustrated
② Assessment of the client's orientation to time, place, and person
③ Identification of stressors that appear to precipitate the client's disruptive behavior
④ Fact that her impairment will increase until adjustment to the home is accomplished

Situation: Athea Cris, 18 years old, seeks help at a crisis intervention clinic. She appears very anxious, and states to the nurse, "I came back to the city 2 months ago. I had been a freshman in college in Missouri. The instructors were dumb and the kids acted like babies. I am more mature than most of them. We had nothing in common. When I failed biology, I had it. I was a psychiatric aide for 6 weeks. I got into trouble because the staff's thinking was archaic. I tried waiting on tables but got fired. The boss said I was nasty to the customers. They were the nasty ones. I don't have one friend here. Now I can't even pay my rent. If people were nicer, I wouldn't be in this mess."

156. In relation to crisis theory, Ms. Cris' stressful events can be seen as:

① Age related and frequent
② Experiential
③ Usually non-crisis producing
④ Situational and maturational

157. According to crisis theory, the minimal long-term goal in crisis intervention is:
① Restoration of the original functioning level
② Relief of acute symptoms
③ Relief of panic-level anxiety
④ Reorganization and reordering of personality

158. According to Erikson, an individual who fails to master the maturational crisis of adolescence will most often:
① Use drugs and alcohol to escape
② Experience role confusion
③ Rebel at all parental orders
④ Be interpersonally isolated

159. A constructive and lengthy method of confronting the stress of adolescence and preventing a negative and unhealthy developmental outcome is:
① Sublimation through schoolwork
② Adherence to all peer standards
③ Role experimentation
④ Development of dependency on parents

160. The most critical factor for the nurse to determine during crisis intervention is the client's:
① Available situational supports
② Underlying unconscious conflict
③ Willingness to restructure personality
④ Developmental history

161. When intervening in a crisis situation, the initial concern of the nurse is:
① What the precipitating factor was
② Whether the individual can go back to daily activities
③ How the individual is affecting others
④ How the client will deal with successive crises

162. Situational crises are usually resolved in a period of:
① 1 to 4 days
② 2 to 3 weeks
③ 1 to 2 months
④ 2 to 6 months

Situation: Andrew Marshall, 42 years old, is brought to the psychiatric unit by his parents and a sister who states, "He's just not himself since his wife died 2 years ago. He has no interests and doesn't care for himself any more, just sitting alone at home when he's not working."

163. The nurse completes a history and physical assessment of Mr. Marshall, particularly noting that he has lost a significant amount of weight, has poor eye contact, and appears sad. The most important assessment for the nurse to explore with Mr. Marshall at this time is:

① Feelings about his wife's death
② Whether he has considered suicide recently
③ What seems to be making him sad
④ His relationship with his deceased wife

164. The nurse discusses the plan of care with Mr. Marshall. The nurse recognizes it would be most helpful to:
    ① Involve him in group outdoor games each morning
    ② Encourage him to interact with female clients and staff
    ③ Encourage him to talk about and plan for his future
    ④ Talk with him about his wife and the details of her death

165. Mr. Marshall attends group therapy in which the nurse is a co-leader. During one session, another client talks about his wife leaving and his feeling of abandonment. When the members are leaving the session, the nurse notices that tears are running down Mr. Marshall's face. Considering his problems, the nurse should:
    ① Ask the group members to return and discuss Mr. Marshall's feelings
    ② Observe Mr. Marshall's behavior carefully during the next several hours
    ③ Go to Mr. Marshall's room and ask him to discuss his thoughts and feelings
    ④ Ask another client to stay and spend time talking with Marshall

166. Mr. Marshall has been severely depressed and suicidal for almost 2 months. As he becomes more energized and communicative the nurse should:
    ① Continue to check him at regular intervals
    ② Recognize that his suicidal potential has decreased
    ③ Increase the vigilance of the suicidal precautions
    ④ Encourage his participation in group activities

167. The nurse should recognize that Mr. Marshall has an increased suicidal potential when he exhibits:
    ① Persistent severe anxiety and increased somatic complaints
    ② Sleep and appetite disturbances with his history of suicidal ideation
    ③ Severe depression and a preoccupation with religion
    ④ Withdrawal from reality with a history of suicidal threats

Situation: Sadie Roy, 84 years old, has been a widow for 20 years. She comes to the community health center with a vague list of complaints. Her only child, a son, died at birth. She has lived alone since her husband's death and performs all of her own daily tasks of living. She has had a very active social life in the past but has outlived many of her friends and family members. Mrs. Roy states, "I still like living alone and have no difficulty keeping occupied."

168. When taking Mrs. Roy's health history, it is important for the nurse to ask:
    ① "Do you feel all alone?"
    ② "Do you still miss your husband?"
    ③ "What unfulfilled hopes do you have?"
    ④ "How did you feel when your son died?"

169. Mrs. Roy states, "I really don't need anyone to talk to, the TV is my best friend." The nurse recognizes that Mrs. Roy is using the defense mechanism known as:
    ① Displacement
    ② Projection
    ③ Denial
    ④ Sublimation

170. The initial intervention strategy that is of primary importance in counseling Mrs. Roy is:
    ① Helping her to secure assistance with cleaning and shopping
    ② Setting clear goals and time limitations for visits with the nurse
    ③ Writing down and repeating important information for her use
    ④ Maintaining her routine and supporting her usual habits

171. The change in Mrs. Roy's behavior that would indicate that the nurse should reassess any current plan of care would be the development of:
    ① Additional complaints
    ② Hypochondriasis
    ③ Increased socialization
    ④ Confusion

Situation: Susan Sims, a nurse on the mental health unit, has been assigned to work with Tom Brown, a 21-year-old college student who was admitted the previous night. Mr. Brown has never used mental health services before.

172. Ms. Sims' most appropriate initial approach to Mr. Brown would be:
    ① "Hi, Tom; I've been assigned to care for you today."
    ② "Good morning, Mr. Brown. I am Susan Sims, a registered nurse assigned to the mental health unit."
    ③ "Good morning, Tom. I see you were admitted last night. Tell me what brought you to our unit."
    ④ "Hello, Mr. Brown. I'm Susan Sims."

173. Mr. Brown looks briefly at Ms. Sims but does not respond to her greeting. Ms. Sims' most appropriate action would be to state:
    ① "Mr. Brown, I guess you would rather be alone for now; I will return later so we can talk."
    ② "Mr. Brown, I am talking to you. Are you having trouble understanding what I am saying?"

③ "Mr. Brown, I am here to tell you about the services available to you on the mental health unit and to offer you my help."

④ "Mr. Brown, this is the mental health unit of the hospital. We have many services to offer. Let me tell you about them."

174. Mr. Brown quietly listens to Ms. Sims' explanation of the services and activities available. He looks around the unit and states, "So this is where they keep the crazies." Ms. Sims' most appropriate initial response would be:
① "No, that is not correct. Let me explain the purpose of a mental health unit."
② "Some people feel that way. Let's talk about mental health."
③ "These people are sick Mr. Brown. They are not crazy."
④ "Are you feeling that a person has to be crazy to need mental health services?"

175. Ms. Sims' response was based on her awareness that value clarification is a technique useful in therapeutic communication in that it helps:
① Alter clients' poor values to make them more socially acceptable
② Make clients aware of their personal values
③ Assist clients in making correct decisions related to their health
④ Provide information related to clients' needs

176. The nurse tells Mr. Brown that talking with staff is part of the therapy program. Mr. Brown responds, "I don't see how talking to you can possibly help." The nurse's most appropriate response would be:
① "I can see how you would feel that way now, but hopefully you'll change your mind."
② "Hopefully, I can help you sort out your thoughts and feelings so you can better understand them."
③ "The one-to-one relationship has proved very helpful for others. Why don't you give it a try?"
④ "You will never know if it is helpful or not unless you are willing to give it a try."

177. A reasonable short-term nursing goal for Mr. Brown, who is functioning below the optimal level of mental health, would be to help him become better able to:
① Confront his inadequacies in interpersonal relations and be more sociable
② Take actions that will increase his satisfaction with his relationships with others
③ Discuss his feelings regarding significant others and his life experiences
④ Understand the dynamics behind his inadequate interpersonal relations

178. Ms. Sims plans to teach Mr. Brown to use more healthy coping behaviors that can be consciously used to reduce anxiety, including:
① Repression, intellectualization, reading
② Exercise, talking to friends, suppression
③ Eating, dissociation, fantasy
④ Sublimation, fantasy, rationalization

179. Mr. Brown asks Ms. Sims for a date. It is most likely that:
① Ms. Sims may have been acting unprofessionally toward Mr. Brown
② Mr. Brown misinterpreted Ms. Sims' friendliness
③ Ms. Sims may have led Mr. Brown on
④ Mr. Brown may be trying to protect a threatened sexual identity

180. Ms. Sims can best handle the answering of personal questions asked by Mr. Brown in any phase of the nurse-client relationship by:
① Providing brief truthful answers and redirecting the focus of conversation
② Offering an honest, brief expression of her views on the subject raised
③ Reviewing the positive and negative aspects of the subject
④ Gently reminding Mr. Brown that her feelings are not his concern

Situation: Inez Gomez, a 65-year-old who emigrated from Cuba 25 years ago, is admitted with a history of depression. She speaks little English and has few outside interests. Since she separated from her husband 11 years ago, she has lived with her daughter and son-in-law who both work. Mrs. Gomez cares for their child, Marie, age 13. Marie is beginning to spend more time with her friends, and Mrs. Gomez states that she feels she "is useless and unneeded."

181. According to Erikson, Mrs. Gomez is in the developmental stage of:
① Initiative vs guilt
② Integrity vs despair
③ Intimacy vs isolation
④ Identity vs role diffusion

182. For Mrs. Gomez to successfully complete the tasks of this stage, she should:
① Feel a sense of satisfaction when reflecting back on her productive life
② Look to recapture opportunities that were not started or completed
③ Redefine her role in society and offer something of value
④ Invest her creative energies in promoting social welfare

183. Mrs. Gomez is a member of the Cuban community. This is important because the nurse must:
① Offer a therapeutic regimen compatible with the life-style of the family
② Ensure that the nurse's biases are understood by the family
③ Make plans to counteract Mrs. Gomez' misconceptions of family practice

④ Recognize that Mrs. Gomez' responses will be different from those of other clients

184. The nurse recognizes that Mrs. Gomez' life before coming to this country:
① Has little impact on her life today
② Affects all of her inherited traits
③ Is important in assessing her values
④ Established forever how she would interact

Situation: John Gilbert, a single 22-year-old, is admitted with a diagnosis of acute schizophrenia, undifferentiated type. He has become increasingly agitated, neglects his personal hygiene, eats and sleeps poorly, and hears voices that threaten him and accuse him of perverted sex acts.

185. Mr. Gilbert's family ask about the treatment of schizophrenia. The nurse, before responding, recalls that:
① Insight therapy has proved to be highly successful in the treatment of clients with schizophrenia
② Electroconvulsive therapy is more effective in treating schizophrenia than mood disorders
③ Family therapy has not proved to be effective in the treatment of clients with schizophrenia
④ Drug therapy, while not treating the underlying problem, reduces the symptoms of acute schizophrenia

186. In planning activities for Mr. Gilbert the nurse should recognize that it would be most therapeutic for him to:
① Go for a walk with the nurse
② Watch a movie with other clients
③ Play solitaire by himself in the dayroom
④ Play cards with a group of clients

187. Mr. Gilbert claims the voices he hears are clearly telling him what actions and decisions to make. It would be most therapeutic for the nurse to:
① Begin talking to Mr. Gilbert when he is hearing the voices
② Demonstrate to Mr. Gilbert that his perceptions are wrong
③ Recognize that Mr. Gilbert must be frightened by the voices
④ Play soft music when Mr. Gilbert starts hearing voices

188. To plan Mr. Gilbert's care the nurse should recognize that his delusions are a defense against his underlying feelings of:
① Aggression
② Persecution
③ Inferiority
④ Guilt

189. Mr. Gilbert is prescribed chlorpromazine (Thorazine). In teaching him about this drug the nurse should emphasize that:

① He should never drive while taking this drug
② A sunscreen must be used outdoors on a year-round basis
③ This drug will indirectly control his essential hypertension
④ He will feel increased energy while taking this drug

190. Mr. Gilbert is discharged on a regimen of Thorazine. Eight weeks later he calls the nurse to say he has suddenly developed a sore throat and has a high fever. The nurse, recognizing the drug's effects, evaluates Mr. Gilbert's complaints and tells him to:
① Continue the medication, drink fluids, take aspirin, and see his physician if his condition has not improved in a few days
② Stop the medication immediately and see his physician when an appointment is available
③ Skip the medication and, if his physician cannot see him today, go to the emergency room for evaluation
④ Stay in bed, force fluids, take aspirin, and skip the next two scheduled doses of Thorazine

Situation: Hal Arno, 54 years old, had been a successful real estate agent until 18 months ago. At that time he became forgetful, irritable, and antisocial. He frequently embarrassed others by his obscene speech and gestures. After he is found disoriented and seminaked walking down a street, he is brought to the hospital. A diagnosis of Alzheimer's disease is made.

191. On admission to the unit, Mr. Arno expresses fear and anxiety about his new surroundings. Considering Mr. Arno's diagnosis, the best approach to this type of response would be for the nurse to:
① Explain the nature of the unit and tell Mr. Arno why he is there
② Reassure Mr. Arno by the frequent presence of staff
③ Initiate a program of planned interaction and activity
④ Explore in depth the reasons for his concerns

192. Mrs. Arno appears tired and angry on her first visit with her husband. As she is leaving she says to the unit nurse in a sarcastic tone, "Let's see what you can do with him." The nurse's most therapeutic response would be:
① "I don't understand what you mean by that comment."
② "It must have been very difficult to care for him."
③ "We have experience in caring for clients such as your husband."
④ "It's too bad you didn't realize you needed help to care for him."

193. Treatment of Mr. Arno at this stage in his illness is mainly directed toward:
① Rechanneling his excessive energies
② Managing his somewhat bizarre behaviors
③ Preventing further deterioration of his condition
④ Restricting all gross motor activity to prevent injury

Situation: Irene Karl, a staff nurse on a medical-surgical unit, has been assigned to have daily one-to-one interactions with a number of clients. Ms. Karl decides to review some basic principles of the one-to-one relationship to prepare for her assignment.

194. Before making an initial contact with her clients, Ms. Karl decides to review their individual medical records. This phase of the nurse-client relationship could best be referred to as the:
① Orientation phase
② Preinteraction phase
③ Working phase
④ Termination phase

195. Ms. Karl is aware that clients in the working phase of the nurse-client relationship:
① Frequently exhibit testing behaviors such as flirtation and lateness
② Accept limits and initiate topics for discussion
③ Often focus the conversation on the nurse
④ May repress emotionally charged material to avoid shocking the group

196. Margaret Janey, one of the clients, is exhibiting withdrawn patterns of behavior. Ms. Karl is aware that this type of behavior eventually produces feelings of:
① Anger
② Loneliness
③ Repression
④ Paranoia

197. In caring for Mrs. Janey, Ms. Karl recognizes that withdrawn behavior may temporarily provide a:
① Defense against anxiety
② Time to collect personal resources
③ Time for internal problem solving
④ Basis for emotional growth

Situation: Kevin Smythe is admitted to the psychiatric unit wearing a soiled tuxedo and bright facial makeup. During the first 24 hours he paces continually, laughing loudly. When approached by the nurse, he refuses to cooperate with any requests, shouting, "I am in charge. I give the orders!"

198. The nurse recognizes that Mr. Smythe's manic symptoms are:
① A response to an imagined loss
② An attempt to ward off depression
③ The fulfillment of innate desires
④ An uncontrollable urge to relate

199. Mr. Smythe is demanding and active. The nurse's major objective should be to:
① Point out reality through continued communication
② Broaden his contacts with other clients and staff
③ Help lessen his feelings of guilt and rejection
④ Maintain a supportive, structured environment

200. The psychiatrist orders lithium carbonate, 600 mg po tid, for Mr. Smythe. The nurse would be aware that Mr. Smythe understood the teaching about the side effects of this drug when he states, "I will call my doctor immediately if I notice any:
① Sensitivity to bright light or sun."
② Fine hand tremors or slurred speech."
③ Impotence or breast enlargement."
④ Inability to urinate or difficulty when urinating."

201. The physician plans to have Mr. Smythe continue on a regimen of lithium after discharge. The nurse would recognize that Mr. Smythe understood the medication plan when he states, "I know that this medication:
① May need to be taken for the rest of my life."
② Must be increased at the first sign of a manic episode."
③ Should be stopped if illness is suspected."
④ Rarely causes serious side effects when taken correctly."

Situation: Beth Ellison, a 7-year-old third grader, is brought to the clinic by her mother, Jean Ellison. Mrs. Ellison tells the nurse that Beth, her only child, has been having trouble in school since she and Mr. Ellison separated 6 months ago. Beth's teacher told Mrs. Ellison that Beth no longer associates with her friends, has difficulty concentrating, and is falling behind in her schoolwork.

202. Mrs. Ellison reports that lately Beth has not been eating her dinner and she sometimes hears Beth crying in her room. The nurse realizes that Beth:
① Would probably be happier living with her father
② Probably blames herself for her parents' breakup
③ Is working through her feelings of loss
④ Feels different from her classmates

203. When assessing mental status in a child Beth's age, it is most important for the nurse to:
① Listen to the parent's description of the child's behavior
② Engage the child in a discussion about feelings
③ Use direct questions to determine the child's mental ability

④ Compare the child's functioning from one time with another

204. The nurse is aware that a child experiencing emotional problems would probably exhibit:
① Passive and deliberate behavior
② Overinvolvement with her peer group
③ Impaired ability to reality test
④ A mild to moderate level of anxiety

205. It is decided that Beth would probably benefit most from family therapy. The nurse plans that the first group session will include:
① Mr. and Mrs. Ellison and Beth
② Mrs. Ellison and Beth
③ Mr. and Mrs. Ellison
④ Mrs. Ellison, Beth, and her teacher

Situation: Saul Taylor, a 76-year-old widower, is admitted to the hospital for a bunionectomy. Mr. Taylor has a history of hypertension and at the time of admission his blood pressure is found to be 180/102.

206. When the nurse asks Mr. Taylor if he has been taking any medications, he replies, "I took the pills my doctor prescribed for a few weeks, but I didn't feel any different. So I decided I'd just take them if I felt sick." The best initial response by the nurse would be:
① "I'm glad to hear you felt well enough to stop the medication."
② "You must be quite frightened about having high blood pressure."
③ "I think we should talk to the physician about a plan of treatment you can follow."
④ "You really should try to take your medication; the doctor felt it was needed."

207. The nurse becomes aware of Mr. Taylor's feeling of loneliness when he states, "I only have a few friends. My daughter lives in another state and couldn't care whether I live or die. She doesn't even know I'm hospitalized." The nurse recognizes that Mr. Taylor's communication is probably a:
① Manipulative attempt to persuade the nurse to call his daughter
② Request for information about community social support groups
③ Call for help to prevent acting out of suicidal thoughts
④ Clue to depression that is blocking his motivation for self-care

208. When planning care for Mr. Taylor the nurse is aware that normal aging has little effect on a client's:
① Sense of taste or smell
② Gastrointestinal motility
③ Muscle or motor strength
④ Ability to handle life's stresses

209. The nurse's role in maintaining or promoting the health of the older adult should be based on the principle that:

① Some of the physiologic changes that occur as a result of aging are reversible
② There is a strong correlation between successful retirement and good health
③ Thoughts of impending death are frequent and depressing to most older adults
④ Older adults can better accept the dependent state often caused by chronic illness

210. After Mr. Taylor works with the nurse for a period, he says he always enjoyed working and playing with children. During discharge planning the nurse recommends that Mr. Taylor look into the volunteer Foster Grandparent Program in his area. The nurse recognizes that this type of activity may help Mr. Taylor to:
① Forget his problems when he sees the problems of others
② Take better care of himself if he feels needed by someone
③ Be able to find new acquaintances with similar interests
④ Be motivated to become involved with younger people

Situation: The nurse on the pediatric unit is planning care designed to help several children better adapt to illness and hospitalization.

211. The nurse is aware that according to Erikson, increased vulnerability to anxiety in response to separations or impending separations from significant others results from failure to complete the developmental task called:
① Autonomy
② Identity
③ Trust
④ Initiative

212. The nurse knows that Erikson identified the developmental tasks of the school-age child from 6 to 12 years as:
① Initiative vs guilt
② Industry vs inferiority
③ Breaking away vs staying at home
④ Psychosexual impulses vs psychosexual development

213. The parents of 3-year-old Sally O'Hara have been unable to visit her since she was admitted to the hospital. Sally has become quiet and withdrawn. To best help Sally at this time the nurse should:
① Bring Sally a doll or stuffed animal to cuddle
② Encourage Sally to play games with the other children
③ Assign the same nurse to care for Sally whenever possible
④ Contact her parents and tell them to immediately come to visit

214. Gail Bond, 3½ years old, begins screaming and kicking when the laboratory technician

comes to draw her blood. The nurse recognizes that this reaction is due primarily to Gail's:
① Fear of loss of control
② Inability to localize pain
③ Fear of intrusive procedures
④ Past experience with this procedure

215. Harry Banes, 7 years old, wakes up crying because he has wet his bed. It would be most appropriate for the nurse to:
① Change his bed while he changes his pajamas
② Allow him to change his own bed and pajamas
③ Take him to the bathroom and change his pajamas
④ Remind him that he must call for the nurse the next time

216. Just before 8-year-old Mark Lyne's physical examination by the physician, the nurse can best meet Mark's developmental needs by:
① Allowing him to handle the examination equipment
② Explaining exactly what will happen during the examination
③ Having him talk to a child who has recently had an examination
④ Arranging to have one of his parents present during the examination

217. Jim McDonald, 9 years old, was admitted with a fractured femur. He has just been told he must stay in the hospital in traction for at least a month. The nurse finds him crying and unwilling to talk. At this time, the nurse should give the highest priority to:
① Giving him privacy and allowing him to cry
② Telling him that his injury will not be permanent
③ Trying to distract him to prevent embarrassment
④ Arranging for him to have a tutor begin immediately

Situation: Kyle Thompkins tells the nurse in the health service department at his college that his girlfriend's period is late and they both think she is pregnant.

218. Mr. Thompkins, with a broad smile on his face, says to the nurse loudly and angrily, "If she is pregnant, I will drop out of school, marry her, and get a full-time job." The nurse's best initial assessment of Mr. Thompkins' verbal and nonverbal behavior would be that they are:
① Consistent
② Incongruent
③ Uniform
④ Appropriate

219. When talking about his decision to get married, Mr. Thompkins says, "It's really the best decision. It is important for a child to

have two parents." The nurse realizes that Mr. Thompkins is using the defense mechanism known as:
① Displacement
② Introspection
③ Intellectualization
④ Projection

220. The nurse recognizes that Mr. Thompkins is attempting to cope with the situation. The most basic therapeutic tool used by the nurse to assist a client's psychologic coping is the:
① Self
② Milieu
③ Helping process
④ Client's intellect

221. In an attempt to remain objective and support Mr. Thompkins during this experience, the nurse uses imagination and determination to project the self into the client's emotions. The nurse accomplishes this by using the technique known as:
① Acceptance
② Empathy
③ Projection
④ Sympathy

222. It is most helpful to the nurse who is attempting to apply the principles of positive mental health to understand that:
① Emotionally ill people can empathize easily with others
② Emotionally healthy people function optimally in all settings
③ A sense of mastery of self and environment are crucial to emotional health
④ Mental illness is always characterized by observable signs or socially inappropriate behavior

Situation: Henry Cole, 10 years old, is admitted to a child psychiatric unit with the diagnosis of attention deficit disorder with hyperactivity. He has a history of school failure and destructive acting out. Henry, the youngest of three children, is identified by both his parents and his siblings as the family problem. Riva and Stanley Cole state, "Henry's behavior has resulted in our having severe marital problems. We are only staying together for the sake of the children."

223. The nurse would be correct in identifying the family's pattern of relating to Henry as:
① Overburdening
② Patronizing
③ Scapegoating
④ Controlling

224. To help Henry develop a trusting relationship the nurse should:
① Initiate limit setting and explain the unit's rules
② Implement daily 30-minute one-to-one interactions
③ Inquire as to Henry's feelings about his parents

④ Offer support and emphasize safety in play activities

225. Henry is started on a behavior modification program. One day he is playing a game with his peers and becomes frustrated when he begins to lose. He kicks the other children under the table and calls them names. The nurse, using the most appropriate behavior modification technique, should:
① Engage Henry in a conversation about good sportsmanship
② Ignore Henry's behavior with the intent of extinguishing it
③ Negatively reinforce Henry by taking two of his tokens
④ Require Henry to have a time-out and regain control

226. After 1 month on the unit, Henry is asked to leave the group therapy session because of his disruptiveness. He begins to cry as he is led out. The nurse's best approach at this time would be to:
① Send Henry for a time-out in his bedroom
② Engage Henry in a talk about his school day
③ Offer an interpretation of his self-defeating behavior
④ Provide nurturance by sharing a snack and a glass of milk

227. The nurse is aware that a child's psychiatric symptoms usually occur as a result of:
① Family pathology
② Rejection by the parents
③ Authoritarian parenting style
④ Overbearing overprotectiveness

228. Henry is to be discharged in a couple of weeks. In preparation for Henry's discharge it is most important for the nurse to plan to:
① Establish, maintain, and/or enforce limits on his behavior
② Help Henry begin to terminate his relationship with the staff
③ Schedule a home visit and a community trip with his family
④ Meet with Henry's teacher to review Henry's needs

Situation: Ruth Inez, 32 years old, is admitted to the hospital for the third time with a diagnosis of schizophrenic disorder, paranoid type. Her first admission was 3 years ago. The nurse notes that her clothes are very soiled and disheveled and she appears not to have bathed recently. Her parents report that she has refused to leave the house for the past month.

229. In taking the nursing history, the nurse asks Ms. Inez why she came to the hospital. Ms. Inez states, "They lied about me. They said I murdered my mother. You killed her. She died before I was born." The nurse recognizes that Ms. Inez is experiencing:
① Persecutory delusions
② Auditory hallucinations

③ Ideas of grandeur
④ Confusing illusions

230. The nurse could best respond to Ms. Inez' statement by saying:
① "I just saw your mother and she is doing fine."
② "Tell me more about your concerns for your mother."
③ "You are having very frightening thoughts at this time."
④ "We'll put you in a private room where you will be safe."

231. Ms. Inez refuses to remove her clothing. To best meet the client's needs the nurse should:
① Get assistance and remove her clothing to meet her basic hygiene needs
② Tell her she will look more attractive in clean clothes to increase her self-esteem
③ Allow her to wait and change when she is ready to help her maintain her identity
④ Provide her with two outfits to assist her to make a simple decision

232. Ms. Inez tells the nurse that the voices have told her that she is in danger. She states, "They told me I would only be safe if I stay in this room, wear these clothes, and avoid stepping on the cracks between the floor tiles." The nurse's best initial response to this statement would be:
① "Don't worry. You're safe here. The door is locked. I won't let anyone hurt you."
② "I know these voices are real to you, but I want you to know that I do not hear them."
③ "You need to leave this room and get your mind occupied so the voices don't bother you."
④ "Tell me more about the voices. Are they men or women? How many voices are there?"

233. The nurse is aware that a common nursing diagnosis for clients with a schizophrenic disorder is:
① Social isolation related to impaired ability to trust
② Sleep disturbances related to impaired thinking ability
③ Potential for violence directed at others and related to hallucinations
④ Impaired mobility related to fear of loss of control of hostile impulses

234. After treatment, Ms. Inez improves and is scheduled to go home on a weekend pass. Mr. and Mrs. Inez tell the nurse they are concerned about how to respond if "Ruth starts to act crazy." It would be most therapeutic for the nurse to:
① Refer Mr. and Mrs. Inez to a self-help group for the parents of schizophrenic clients
② Reassure Mr. and Mrs. Inez that Ms. Inez is improved and is unlikely to act out

③ Teach Mr. and Mrs. Inez how to respond to Ms. Inez' bizarre behavior

④ Meet with Mr. and Mrs. Inez and Ms. Inez together to discuss their mutual concerns

Situation: Tony Patter, an overweight 12-year-old, is brought to the clinic by his parents, Rose and John Patter. Mr. Patter states, "You got to do something to help him. Just look at his size." Tony is 5 feet tall and weighs 145 pounds. Mr. Patter reports Tony has few friends and spends most of his time watching television and eating. He is an average student but does not like school. His only sibling is a 19-year-old brother who is a college basketball star.

235. Tony tells the nurse that he dislikes school because his classmates tease him about his weight. He states rather sadly, "I'm always last when they choose up sides in gym." The nurse's most therapeutic response would be:
① "Won't it be great when you lose weight and can do better in gym?"
② "That hurts a lot when you want to be liked."
③ "Have you tried letting them know how that makes you feel?"
④ "Not everybody's a great athlete. You have other strengths."

236. Mr. and Mrs. Patter tell the nurse that they are concerned that Tony feels inferior to his successful brother. They ask the nurse what they can do about this problem. The nurse should:
① Suggest that they give Tony recognition for his own strong points
② Advise them to tell Tony to view his brother's success as a challenge
③ Suggest that they seem to be creating a problem where none exists
④ Tell them to avoid talking about the brother's accomplishments

237. The nurse, along with Tony and Mr. and Mrs. Patter, sets bolstering Tony's self-esteem as a high-priority goal. The nursing action that would contribute to the achievement of this goal would be:
① Encouraging Tony to talk about his pride in his brother
② Suggesting that Mrs. Patter give him lots of hugs and cuddling
③ Urging Tony to join a neighborhood basketball team
④ Supporting Tony's interest in getting a newspaper route

238. The nurse would evaluate that the plan for Tony was effective when, 3 months later, Mrs. Patter reports that Tony:
① Asks her to prepare his favorite dessert
② Seems to be doing average work in school
③ Has joined a dirt bicycle club that meets at the school
④ Imitates his brother's manner of speech and dress

Situation: Barry Lydon, 45 years old, is admitted because of severe rectal bleeding. He has a long history of ulcerative colitis. His physician has informed him that he may need an ileostomy, and he is very concerned about this possibility.

239. The nursing staff on the unit has found Mr. Lydon to be an angry, demanding person. One day the nurse's aide tells the nurse, "I've had it with that man and his demands. I'm not going in there again." The nurse's best response to the aide's statement would be:
① "Just ignore him and get on with the rest of your work. Let someone else take a turn."
② "You need to try to be patient with him. He's going through a lot right now."
③ "He's frightened and taking it out on the staff. Let's think how we can approach him."
④ "I'll talk with him and see if I can figure out the best way for us to handle this."

240. Mr. Lydon calls out to every nursing staff member who passes his door and asks them to do something for him. The nurse can best manage this behavior by:
① Informing him that one staff member of his choice will come in frequently to see if he has any requests
② Closing the door to his room so he cannot see the staff members as they pass by
③ Assigning a variety of staff members to take turns going into his room to see if he has any requests
④ Assigning one staff member to approach him regularly and spend time talking with him

241. The nurse could evaluate that the staff's approach to Mr. Lydon was effective if he:
① No longer calls nursing staff for assistance
② Apologizes for disrupting the unit's routine
③ Discusses his concerns about his condition
④ Understands the reasons for his frequent calls

242. One day Mr. Lydon says to the nurse, "If I have to have this surgery, I know my wife will never come near me." The nurse's best initial response would be, "You're:
① Concerned that your wife will reject you."
② Probably underestimating her love for you."
③ Wondering about the effect on your sexual relations."
④ Worried that the surgery will change how others see you."

Situation: The nurse is scheduled to be the co-leader of a therapy group to be formed in the mental health clinic.

243. In planning for the first meeting, the nurse must first consider the:
① Number of clients in the group

② Needs of the clients being included

③ Diagnoses of the clients being included

④ Socioeconomic status of the clients in the group

244. During the first meeting of the group, the members become quite uncomfortable. The nurse notes frequent periods of silence, tense laughter, and a good deal of nervous movement in the group. The nurse would assess that these responses:

① Are expected group behaviors because relationships are not yet established

② Require active leader intervention to relieve symptoms of obvious stress

③ Indicate unhealthy group processes with an unwillingness to relate openly

④ Should be pointed out and discussed so that members will not become too uncomfortable

245. To further develop trust among group members the nurse plans to:

① Have group members reveal some personal information about themselves

② Bring up for discussion the need for and the importance of trusting each other

③ Reveal some personal data as a role model for trusting behavior

④ Remind group members about the need for confidentiality in the group

246. The nurse would be aware that the group has reached the working stage when the members:

① Appear happy in their group interactions

② Say and do what is expected and wanted by the others

③ Focus on a wide variety of needs and concerns

④ Show concern for the feelings of the group leaders

247. During the working phase, Irene Novak, one of the group members, becomes tearful after being told by another member that she needs to change her behavior. The nurse evaluates that Ms. Novak:

① Has had her feelings hurt by this response

② Is angry about the confrontation with another member

③ Feels too fragile to be challenged at this time

④ Has been depressed about this aspect of her behavior

248. Another member, Donald King, tends to monopolize the group discussions, and no one has confronted his behavior. The nurse could best handle this situation by:

① Ignoring his behavior because Mr. King may become upset if confronted

② Encouraging other members of the group to do more talking by calling on various silent members

③ Saying to him, "Mr. King, you use too much of the time in our sessions."

④ Saying to the group, "I'm wondering why the group is so willing to let Mr. King do so much of the talking."

249. At one session Ralph Erik, another member, using a teasing manner, makes several negative remarks about the nurse's appearance and behavior. The nurse could best respond by saying to:

① The group, "What do you think Mr. Erik is trying to tell me?"

② The group, "Do you think Mr. Erik's behavior is appropriate today?"

③ Mr. Erik, "You seem very interested in my appearance and behavior. What's this all about?"

④ Mr. Erik, "I cannot just sit here and let you talk about me this way. What have I done to make you angry?"

250. At another session Judy Gage tearfully tells the other members that she lost her job as a receptionist during the past week. It would be most appropriate for the nurse to:

① Ask her to look at the reasons this may have occurred

② Quietly observe how the group responds to her statement

③ Suggest she check the help wanted advertisements in the local paper

④ Request that the group help her see how she may have precipitated the dismissal

251. Another member, Peggy Lang, states with a smile, "Things haven't gone well in my life this week either." It would be most appropriate for the nurse to:

① Make note of the incongruity of her message but remain silent

② Ask her to share what has been happening in her life this week

③ Say, "Mrs. Lang, you say things have been bad, yet you are smiling."

④ Comment, "This seems to have been a bad week for a number of group members."

Situation: Mark Victor, 30 years old, received multiple stab wounds to the abdomen during a fight. After surgical repair, Mr. Victor is admitted to ICU. The nurse notes that Mr. Victor's pain does not seem to be relieved by the prescribed IM meperidine (Demerol) injections he is receiving, because he is continually asking for additional medication. The nurse observes recent needle marks and scars on both his arms. Although Mr. Victor denies it, opiate use is suspected.

252. Because of the tentative diagnosis of opiate addiction, the nurse should assess Mr. Victor for signs of withdrawal. These signs would include:

① Lacrimation, vomiting, drowsiness

② Nausea, dilated pupils, constipation

③ Muscle aches, pupillary constriction, yawning

④ Rhinorrhea, convulsions, subnormal temperature

253. The nurse is aware that opiates are used because the individual most frequently:
① Desires to become independent
② Wants to fit in with the peer group
③ Attempts to blur reality and reduce stress
④ Enjoys the social interrelationships that occur

254. The nurse recognizes that Mr. Victor's failure to achieve pain relief from the Demerol injections indicates that he is experiencing the phenomenon of:
① Psychologic addiction
② Physical addiction
③ Habituation
④ Tolerance

255. Opiate addiction is confirmed. After a visit from several friends the nurse finds Mr. Victor in a deep sleep, unresponsive to attempts to arouse him. The nurse assesses his vital signs and would evaluate that an overdose of opiates had occurred if the findings showed a:
① Blood pressure of 70/40, a pulse of 120, and respirations of 10
② Blood pressure of 120/80, a pulse of 84, and respirations of 20
③ Blood pressure of 140/90, a pulse of 76, and respirations of 28
④ Blood pressure of 180/100, a pulse of 72, and respirations of 18

256. Because of the symptoms demonstrated, the nurse would expect the physician to order:
① Methadone
② Amphetamine
③ Naloxone
④ Epinephrine

257. The nurse, in planning care for Mr. Victor after he recovers from the overdose, should take into consideration that his underlying problem is a feeling of:
① Inferiority with strong dependency needs
② Anger with an overwhelming need for independence
③ Guilt with a rejection of reality
④ Hostility with a need for acceptance

Situation: Kay Andrews, an emaciated 13-year-old only child from an upper-class family, faints when doing calisthenics in the school gymnasium. In the emergency room she is found to be 5 feet 3 inches tall and weighs 78 pounds. Her father, Ron Andrews, who was called to the school and accompanied Kay in the ambulance, states that Kay rarely eats and is always exercising. Her weight has dropped from 108 pounds in the past 6 months. The admitting diagnosis is starvation secondary to anorexia nervosa.

258. The nursing intervention that should receive the highest priority in the period immediately following Kay's admission would be:

① Providing her with adequate rest and nutrition
② Obtaining more data about her exercise program
③ Completing an assessment of her mental status
④ Monitoring her fluid and electrolyte balance

259. The nurse is aware that a major health problem associated with severe anorexia nervosa is:
① Endocrine imbalance resulting in amenorrhea
② Cardiac arrhythmias resulting in cardiac arrest
③ Protein depletion resulting in muscle wasting
④ Glucose intolerance resulting in hypoglycemia

260. During Kay's admission to the unit, the nurse finds a bottle of assorted pills in her handbag. Kay tells the nurse they are antacids she takes for stomach pain. The best initial response by the nurse would be:
① "Tell me more about these stomach pains."
② "These pills don't look like antacids."
③ "Some girls take pills to lose weight."
④ "Let's talk about your drug use."

261. The multidisciplinary team decides to employ a behavior modification approach to Kay's problem. A planned nursing intervention that would follow this approach would be to:
① Have the client role play her interaction with her parents
② Restrict the client to her room until she gains 2 pounds
③ Provide the client with a high-calorie, high-protein diet
④ Force the client to talk about her favorite foods for 1 hour each day

262. The nurse notes that Kay telephones home just before each mealtime. She ignores the reminder to eat and continues talking until the other clients are finished eating. She then refuses to eat "cold food." The nurse should:
① Insist that Kay eat the cold food
② Revoke her telephone privileges
③ Schedule a family meeting to discuss the problem
④ Hang up the telephone when meals are served

263. The nurse could evaluate that the nursing plan was effective when Kay:
① Contacts her family frequently by telephone between meals
② Begins reading and clipping recipes from magazines
③ Arrives on time for meals without being called
④ Organizes an aerobic group for the clients

Situation: Alice Farley, 32 years old, is admitted to the hospital with a diagnosis of depression that has not responded to tricyclic antidepressants or outpatient ECT. Her husband Larry states, "She spends most of her time crying and blaming herself for all the problems of the world. This has been going on for months now."

264. The physician orders tranylcypromine sulfate (Parnate) for Mrs. Farley. The nurse would be aware that Mrs. Farley understood the teaching about the drug when the client states, "While taking the medicine I should avoid eating:
① Fish."
② Red meat."
③ Citrus fruit."
④ Chocolate."

265. The nurse should teach Mrs. Farley that failure to adhere to the dietary restrictions can result in:
① Hyperglycemic episodes
② Bradycardia
③ Hypertensive crisis
④ Syncope

Situation: Lyle Klein, 68 years old, has metastatic carcinoma and has been told by his physician that he has only 1 or 2 months to live.

266. The nurse enters Mr. Klein's room after the physician leaves and finds Mr. Klein crying. The nurse's action should take into consideration that:
① Crying releases tension, which frees the energy for coping
② Nurses should not interfere with a client's behavior and defenses
③ Crying relieves depression and helps the client face reality
④ Accepting a client's crying maintains and strengthens the nurse-client bond

267. Mr. Klein tells the nurse that he believes the physician has made an error and that he does not have cancer and is not going to die. The nurse evaluates that Mr. Klein is experiencing the stage of death and dying known as:
① Shock
② Bargaining
③ Anger
④ Acceptance

268. Two weeks later Mr. Klein tells the nurse that all he wants is to pass his high school equivalency test before he dies. He asks the nurse if this is possible. The nurse's best approach would be to:
① Refocus the conversation on the things Mr. Klein has already accomplished in his life
② Attempt to get Mr. Klein to see that his wish is too taxing and somewhat unrealistic
③ Suggest to Mr. Klein that he use this en-

ergy to work through his unexpressed anger at dying
④ Set up a study schedule with Mr. Klein and offer to work with him in preparing for the test

269. The nurse's response to Mr. Klein's desire to pass his high school equivalency test is based on an awareness of the fact that:
① Conversations and activities should focus on pleasant experiences
② Clients should be encouraged to set meaningful goals for themselves
③ Activities that support the client's denial should not be encouraged
④ The energies expended on such an activity would not justify the outcome

270. Mr. Klein dies, and his grieving wife says to the nurse, "We should have spent more time together. I always felt the children's needs came first." The nurse recognizes that Mrs. Klein is experiencing:
① Ambivalent feelings about him
② Displaced anger
③ Normal feelings of guilt
④ Shame for past behaviors

271. Mr. Klein's daughters ask the nurse if they can get some tranquilizers for their mother. They feel it will help her get through the next few weeks. The nurse is aware that tranquilizers are rarely ordered for individuals undergoing acute grief because they:
① Extend the period of denial and suppress normal mourning
② Magnify depression and increase the risk of suicide
③ Cause lethargy and prevent the return to interpersonal activity
④ Suppress the brain activity needed to prevent depression

Situation: Gloria George, 18 years old, is admitted to the hospital after taking 20 tablets of diazepam (Valium). In obtaining the history the nurse learns that Ms. George had been arrested for selling cocaine and is out on bail. She tells the nurse that she took the pills because she is worried about going to jail. Her diagnosis is antisocial personality disorder.

272. One evening during visiting hours, the nurse discovers Ms. George smoking in her room with two young men. By the odor, the nurse knows they are smoking marijuana. When confronted, Ms. George responds, "I'm celebrating. Didn't you hear? I went to trial today and just got put on probation. Don't you think I have reason to celebrate?" The nurse's best response would be:
① "Why don't you and your friends come out and join the other clients and their visitors?"
② "You were lucky you just got probation, so don't get right back into trouble."

③ "I understand your relief about the trial, but pot smoking is against the rules."

④ "If you can't follow the rules against pot smoking, your visiting privileges will be cancelled."

273. Ms. George spends a great deal of time with Brian Henry, another adolescent client on the unit. One day the nurse's aide enters Ms. George's room and finds them in her bed. Later the aide reports the incident to the nurse. The nurse should:
① Assign a staff member to observe both clients every 15 minutes
② Call a ward meeting to talk about sexual activity among all the clients
③ Arrange a discussion with both Ms. George and Mr. Henry
④ Lock the bedroom doors to keep clients within view of the staff

274. The nurse could evaluate that nursing action had been successful when Ms. George:

① Promises to never take drugs again
② Discusses her need to seduce men
③ Identifies the feeling underlying her behavior
④ Recognizes the need to conform to society's norms

275. Ms. George plans to live with her parents after discharge. Helen and Harold George request advice on how to respond to their daughter's behavior. The nurse tells them it would be most therapeutic for them to:
① Discuss her behavior with her and encourage her to develop self-control
② Set clear limits, explain the consequences of disregarding them, and firmly and consistently apply them
③ Avoid setting expectations for her behavior and react to each situation as it arises
④ Help her find new friends and encourage her to get a job and assume responsibility for herself.

CHAPTER 4

Pediatric Nursing Review Questions

Situation: Billy Budd, 6 years old, has been complaining of malaise, lethargy, and weakness. His appetite has also been poor for several days, and his urine is dark colored. When he complains of a headache, his mother brings him to the local pediatric clinic.

1. When taking a nursing history, the nurse asks Mrs. Budd if Billy has had a:
   ① Recent loss of at least 2 pounds
   ② Streptococcal infection within the last 2 weeks
   ③ Rash on his palms and feet within the last 3 weeks
   ④ Pain in his shoulders and knees
2. Acute glomerulonephritis is diagnosed, and Billy is admitted to the pediatric unit. The nursing action that has priority is:
   ① Assessing for dysuria
   ② Monitoring blood pressure
   ③ Testing vomitus for occult blood
   ④ Observing for jaundice
3. An additional finding the nurse should expect on assessment of Billy is:
   ① An increase in urine volume
   ② The presence of periorbital edema
   ③ A decrease in joint mobility
   ④ The occurrence of an intermittent fever
4. Billy is admitted before lunch. The nurse should anticipate that the physician will order a diet low in:
   ① Glucose
   ② Fat
   ③ KCl
   ④ Protein
5. Billy is found to be hypertensive. The nurse expects the physician to initially order:
   ① Hydralazine (Apresoline)
   ② Diazapam (Valium)
   ③ Phenytoin (Dilantin)
   ④ Digoxin (Lanoxin)

Situation: Three-month-old Terry Pane, who has a history of diarrhea of 36 hours' duration, is admitted to the pediatric unit. He is diagnosed as having gastroenteritis and dehydration. Terry is placed on enteric precautions.

6. In assessing the infant with diarrhea, the nurse should expect to find:
   ① Resilient skin turgor
   ② A bulging fontanel
   ③ Marked restlessness
   ④ Decreased urinary output
7. When assessing Terry, the nurse would expect to find a:

① Specific gravity of 1.014
② Urinary output of 50 ml/hr
③ Depressed anterior fontanel
④ History of allergies to various foods

8. The nurse understands that the magnitude of Terry's fluid loss is best ascertained by:
   ① Comparing his pre-illness weight with current weight
   ② Noting the elevation of his hematocrit level
   ③ Evaluating his skin turgor carefully
   ④ Assessing the moistness of his mucous membranes
9. The physician orders multielectrolyte solution (MES) 150 ml per kg of body weight per 24 hours for Terry, who weighs 13 pounds. The nurse is aware that Terry's intake of MES should be:
   ① 500 ml/24hr
   ② 750 ml/24hr
   ③ 885 ml/24hr
   ④ 965 ml/24hr
10. Terry is receiving IV fluids via a scalp vein. The nurse should:
    ① Check his pupils for reaction every hour
    ② Observe behind his ear and occiput for infiltration
    ③ Explain to the parents why they cannot hold him now
    ④ Restrain Terry's arms and legs while not with him
11. Mr. and Mrs. Pane want to be involved with Terry's care. The nurse realizes that they understand the teaching about the maintenance of enteric precautions when they state, "We should:
    ① Wear a mask when we are holding Terry."
    ② Close the door of his room most of the time."
    ③ Wear gloves each time we change his diaper."
    ④ Weigh his diaper each time we change him."
12. The best method of assessing Terry's response to treatment for dehydration is for the nurse to:
    ① Measure his abdominal girth
    ② Weigh him at the same time daily
    ③ Assess the color of his stools
    ④ Monitor his skin turgor frequently
13. Once the severe effects of dehydration are under control, the physician orders Lactinex granules (lactobacilli) to:
    ① Recolonize the normal flora of the gastrointestinal tract

② Relieve the pain of gas in the gastrointestinal tract
③ Relieve the pain caused by gastric hyperacidity
④ Diminish inflammatory mucosal edema

14. As 3-month-old Terry responds to therapy and shows an interest in playing, the nurse appropriately provides him with a:
① Push-pull toy
② Stuffed animal
③ Large plastic ball
④ Metallic mirror

Situation: Lawrence Hill, age 2 years, has just been diagnosed as having hemophilia A. His mother is distraught. She is 3 months pregnant with a second child.

15. Mrs. Hill asks the nurse what the chances are that her second child will have hemophilia. The nurse answers:
① "There is a 25% chance the baby will be affected."
② "There is a 75% chance the baby will be affected."
③ "There is no chance the baby will be affected."
④ "There is a 50% chance the baby will be affected."

16. The most common area for bleeding to develop in a child with hemophilia is the:
① Brain
② Pericardium
③ Abdomen
④ Joints

17. Lawrence is placed in a room with 2-year-old Andrew. The nurse observes that each is actively engaged in his own play. The nurse realizes that this is a characteristic of this age-group and it is called:
① Parallel play
② Group play
③ Cooperative play
④ Dramatic play

Situation: Penny Ryan, 13 years old, comes to the emergency room with an elevated temperature, nuchal rigidity, and vomiting. A diagnosis of meningococcal meningitis is made.

18. When admitting this client to the unit, the nurse is aware that isolation:
① Of any kind is not required
② Will be required for 7 days
③ Is required during the incubation period
④ Is required for 24 to 72 hours after onset of antibiotic therapy

19. The purpose of isolation for a client with an infectious disease is to:
① Separate the infected client from noninfected persons
② Interrupt the infectious process as quickly as possible

③ Prevent nosocomial infection during the hospitalized period
④ Protect clients with a decreased resistance to infection

20. Three days later, Penny, now afebrile and asymptomatic, appears very sad and cries frequently. To assist Penny to verbalize her thoughts and feelings the nurse should:
① Ask Penny directly what is troubling her
② Encourage Mr. and Mrs. Ryan to talk to her
③ Show Penny some photos of hospitalized children and ask her to tell stories about them
④ Have Penny watch videotapes about sick children and answer her questions after she sees them

Situation: Bobby Gregory, 2 weeks old, has been diagnosed as HIV positive.

21. Caring for an infant who is HIV positive can best be accomplished in:
① The home environment
② An extended care facility
③ The pediatric unit
④ A critical care unit

22. Later, Bobby is admitted to the hospital with the diagnosis of AIDS (acquired immunodeficiency syndrome). The nurse should immediately institute:
① Enteric precautions
② Strict isolation
③ Reverse isolation
④ Body secretion precautions

23. Mrs. Gregory asks for suggestions for toys for her son, who is now 8 months old. The nurse knows Mrs. Gregory needs additional discussion of appropriate toys for 8-month-old Gregory when she states she will buy him a:
① Stuffed animal
② Hanging mobile
③ Book with textures
④ Play telephone

Situation: Fifteen-year-old David Adrian has leukemia. He is admitted to the hospital out of remission and will require chemotherapy. He has a 7-year-old brother at home.

24. David is prescribed prednisone and vincristine. He complains of constipation. The most probable cause for the constipation is:
① Leukemic mass obstructing the bowel
② Enlarged spleen obstructing the bowel
③ Side effect of the vincristine
④ Toxic effect of the prednisone

25. In discussing his condition with David, the nurse should keep in mind that a 15-year-old will:
① Be most bothered by having to limit activities
② Be preoccupied by concerns about missed schoolwork

③ Feel dependent and enjoy the "sick role"
④ Feel different because of an altered body image

26. David's 7-year-old brother develops chickenpox. The nurse plans the discharge teaching based on the knowledge that:
① Chickenpox can be fatal to clients with leukemia
② Clients receiving prednisone are immune to chickenpox
③ David need not worry if he receives immmunization before discharge
④ David can go home as long as he avoids direct contact with his brother

Situation: Jane Grey, 3 years old, is brought to the emergency room with severe burns of the lower arms and hands. The emergency room nurse notes many bruises on the child's body. Jane's right eye is swollen shut. The parents indicate Jane struck the side of a table with her eye. Jane is crying and is fearful as the nurse approaches to examine her.

27. Extensive eschar formation is present on Jane's arms. A priority nursing action is to:
① Check radial pulses
② Enforce respiratory isolation
③ Perform range of motion
④ Remove blisters
28. When assessing the family dynamics of a suspected abusing family, the nurse would be surprised to observe that the:
① Child has many unexplained old injuries, scars, and bruises
② Parents offer consistent, detailed stories about the injuries
③ Parents provide little emotional support to the child
④ Child cringes and appears unduly afraid when approached
29. The nurse is aware that abusing parents:
① Often have been raised with little discipline
② Are mature independent individuals
③ Are aware of the abilites of young children
④ Have few available personal resources
30. The physician orders an antibiotic IM for Jane. To be most therapeutic when giving an injection to a toddler such as Jane, the nurse should approach her and say:
① "I brought another nurse along to help me give your medicine."
② "Are you afraid of having a shot because of the pain?"
③ "I know this might hurt, but it's important that you hold still."
④ "Be a big girl and we can be done real quick."
31. Screening for hearing loss should be planned for if the antibiotic prescribed for Jane is:
① Penicillin
② Tetracycline

③ Streptomycin
④ Chloramphenicol

Situation: Daniel James is admitted to the nursery from the delivery room after a difficult delivery.

32. As the nurse examines Daniel, a positive Ortolani's sign is detected. This is indicated by:
① A broadening of the perineum
② An apparent shortening of one leg
③ An audible click on hip manipulation
④ A unilateral droop of the hip
33. Daniel has congenital hip dysplasia. Before Daniel is discharged the nurse should teach Mr. and Mrs. James that hip dislocation can be avoided if Daniel is:
① Tightly swaddled in blankets
② Carried straddling the hip
③ Periodically strapped to a cradleboard
④ Placed in an infant seat on a set schedule
34. When Daniel is 6 months old, he is placed in a hip spica cast for treatment of the congenital hip dysplasia. In planning home care with Mr. and Mrs. James, the nurse should stress that:
① No special precautions will be necessary when diapering him
② The entire cast should be wrapped in plastic wrap to prevent soiling
③ The edges of the cast in the perineal area should be covered with plastic wrap
④ Baby oil and powder should be used liberally around the diaper area
35. At 18 months of age when Daniel visits the clinic, it is discovered that he is anemic. Considering his diagnosis, age, and dietary needs, the nurse should suggest that Mrs. James feed him:
① Bread pudding with raisins
② Fresh seedless grapes
③ A slice of pumpkin pie
④ An entire sliced apple

Situation: Ronald Taft, 1 month old, is admitted to the hospital with a diagnosis of hydrocephalus.

36. Because of the admission diagnosis, the abnormal finding the nurse would expect to observe during assessment of Ronald would be that:
① He is unable to support his head and shoulders while prone
② His anterior fontanel is tense on palpation
③ His head circumference is larger than his chest circumference
④ He demonstrates poor eye-muscle coordination
37. Ronald is scheduled for surgery and a ventriculoperitoneal (VP) shunt is to be inserted. A short-term preoperative goal for Ronald would be to:
① Keep him as comfortable as possible to limit his crying

② Establish and maintain a strict fixed feeding schedule to ensure hydration

③ Use a thick head bandage to protect his head from injury

④ Provide a wide variety of play objects to maintain age-appropriate stimulation

38. Preoperatively, after teaching Mr. and Mrs. Taft, the nurse can evaluate their understanding of the immediate postoperative positioning when they state, "We will avoid putting pressure on Ronald's valve site by positioning him:
① In the position that provides him the most comfort."
② On his back with a small support beneath his neck."
③ Flat with a small support against the right side of his head and back."
④ On his abdomen with a small support against the left side of his head."

39. On the day after surgery Ronald's temperature rises to 103° F. The nurse should first notify the physician and then:
① Recheck the temperature in 2 hours
② Record the temperature on Ronald's chart
③ Remove any excess clothing from Ronald
④ Sponge Ronald with tepid alcohol

Situation: Naomi Rice brings her 6-year-old daughter, Gail, to the local clinic because Gail has been complaining of rectal itching, especially at night. Intestinal infestation with *Enterobius vermicularis* (pinworm) is suspected.

40. The nurse can assist in confirming Gail's diagnosis by:
① Instructing Mrs. Rice to do an anal Scotch tape test early in the morning
② Asking Mrs. Rice to collect stools for 3 consecutive days for culture
③ Assisting Mrs. Rice to schedule hypersensitivity tests of Gail's blood serum
④ Having Mrs. Rice bring in Gail's stools for visual examination for 3 days

41. Pyrvinium pamoate (Povan) is prescribed for Gail. The nurse should tell Mrs. Rice and Gail that:
① Rectal itching will be relieved rapidly once the drug is started
② Gail is the only family member who will need treatment
③ The drug will color stools bright red and stain clothing
④ A single course of treatment is usually adequate to control the problem

Situation: Theresa Lane, 9 months old, was admitted to the pediatric unit because of failure to thrive. She is the youngest of three children whose mother was abandoned by their father shortly before Theresa was born.

42. When the admission procedure is over, Theresa's mother begins to leave. In view of the diagnosis, when Theresa's mother is leaving, the nurse would expect Theresa to react by:
① Clinging to her mother and expressing fear of the nurse
② Crying at first but then letting the nurse hold and comfort her
③ Sustaining eye contact with her mother and refusing the nurse's arms
④ Readily allowing the nurse to take her but remaining stiff while being held

43. After a few days of tube feedings, the nurse notes that Theresa's skin and mucous membranes have become dry. The nurse verifies that Theresa has retained all her feedings but her urinary output is consistently 250 ml less than her intake. She has lost a pound since admission. The nurse should:
① Recognize underhydration and call the physician to increase her fluid intake
② Realize this is probably normal for babies and infants with failure to thrive
③ Increase the intravenous flow of half-normal saline and call the physician
④ Recognize undernutrition and call the physician to increase the caloric intake

44. To help Theresa retain her tube feedings and avoid aspiration, the nurse should place her in the:
① Supine position with her head turned
② Prone position
③ Left side-lying position
④ Semi-Fowler's position

Situation: Four-year-old Fred Blake is diagnosed as having undescended testicles and is admitted for surgery.

45. The nurse understands that early surgery is needed in children with undescended testicles because:
① Maturation of the testes starts at about age 7
② Early surgery produces less psychologic damage
③ The puboscrotal ring is more elastic at this age
④ Future malignancy may be prevented

46. The nurse explains to Mr. and Mrs. Blake that uncorrected bilateral cryptorchidism can cause:
① Hydrocele
② Varicocele
③ Epididymitis
④ Sterility

47. Specific preoperative teaching before an orchiopexy in a child of Fred's age should include a:
① Demonstration of the use of the abdominal binder
② Doll with an intravenous tube in the arm
③ Picture of a boy with a bandage on his lower abdomen

④ Doll with a rubber band stretched from perineum to thigh

48. Fred is given scopolamine (Hyoscine) before surgery. The side effect the nurse should expect after administering this medication is:
① Postural hypotension
② Hyperpnea and hyperventilation
③ Confusion and hallucinations
④ Decreased heartbeat

49. To assess any discomfort that Fred is having postoperatively, the nurse should know that the most reliable indicator of pain in a 4-year-old is:
① Decreased heart rate
② Verbal reports of pain
③ Changes in behavior
④ Crying and sobbing

50. To ensure maintenance of nitrogen balance after surgery, the best food the nurse could order for Fred would be:
① Chicken soup
② A bacon sandwich
③ A hamburger on a bun
④ Cut up orange slices

Situation: Rose Noille, 20 months old, develops diarrhea after her visit to the well-baby clinic. Her mother Irene Noille calls the clinic to ask the nurse about the diarrhea.

51. Mrs. Noille requests information to help her care for Rose at home. The nurse advises her to:
① Put Rose to bed, hold all oral feedings, observe her carefully, and call back in 4 hours
② Wrap Rose snugly, give sugar water, and bring her in to see the physician immediately
③ Allow Rose to continue her normal activities, hold all feeding for 24 hours, and call back tomorrow
④ Continue to feed Rose as usual, make an appointment with the receptionist, and bring her to see the physician

52. Rose's diarrhea persists for 3 days, and she is admitted to the pediatric unit with a diagnosis of severe dehydration. The blood gas report that would most likely reflect the acid-base imbalance found when Rose is admitted is:
① pH of 7.50 and P_{CO_2} of 34
② pH of 7.20 and P_{CO_2} of 20
③ pH of 7.23 and P_{CO_2} of 70
④ pH of 7.56 and P_{CO_2} of 20

53. Initial assessment of Rose by the nurse should reveal:
① Stools that are frothy
② A weak, decreased pulse
③ Bulging of the occipital fontanel
④ An elevated urine specific gravity

54. The physiologic compensatory mechanism that is activated to counteract the effects of Rose's acid-base imbalance is:
① Renal retention of H^+
② Elevated temperature
③ Increased respirations
④ Profuse diaphoresis

55. Rose has been receiving water and electrolyte infant formula (Pedialyte), which she tolerates well. As the diarrhea subsides, her diet is advanced to soft foods. A food that would be contraindicated is:
① Mashed bananas
② Animal crackers
③ Strained carrots
④ Creamed soup

Situation: John Lemel, 4 years old, is admitted to the pediatric unit with nephrotic syndrome. His parents, Ida and Henry Lemel, are with him.

56. On John's admission, the nurse should assess for:
① Flushed, ruddy complexion
② Dark, frothy urine output
③ Severe lethargy
④ Chronic hypertension

57. When admitting John, the nurse assigns him to a room with a:
① 2-year-old boy with croup
② 3-year-old boy with impetigo
③ 4-year-old girl with conjunctivitis
④ 5-year-old girl with a fractured femur

58. When planning care for John, the nurse includes:
① A diet low in carbohydrates and protein
② Restriction of fluids to 500 ml each shift
③ Provision of meticulous skin care
④ A laboratory test for blood type and cross-match

59. The nurse realizes that Mr. and Mrs. Lemel need further instruction for discharge when they state:
① "We know we need to test John's urine for specific gravity."
② "We will look at John's eyelids every morning."
③ "We will ignore any weight gain of John's since it's normal."
④ "We will give John his prednisone with meals or milk."

60. The nurse has been teaching Mr. and Mrs. Lemel about urine testing at home. The statement by them that alerts the nurse to the fact that the teaching has been effective is:
① "We will discard the first urine before we test for acetone."
② "John is old enough to learn how to test his own urine."
③ "We should notify the doctor if there is protein in the urine."
④ "We realize his urine will show a false positive if it is cloudy."

61. A few years later, John, who has chronic renal failure, is admitted to the hospital critically ill. John develops Cheyne-Stokes respirations and the nurse suspects an increasing acid-base balance related to:
    ① Respiratory alkalosis from overbreathing and excess carbon dioxide output
    ② Metabolic alkalosis from an increase in base bicarbonate due to his primary health problem
    ③ Respiratory acidosis from impeded breathing and the retention of carbon dioxide
    ④ Metabolic acidosis from the concentration of cations in body fluids, which displace bicarbonate

Situation: Cynthia Wood, a 13-year-old girl with Down's syndrome, is being admitted for application of a spica cast for multiple fractures that resulted from an automobile accident.

62. The nurse understands that the genetic cause of Down's syndrome is an:
    ① Autosomal recessive gene
    ② Intrauterine infection
    ③ X-linked chromosome
    ④ Extra chromosome

63. The nurse should recognize that the most common serious anomaly associated with Down's syndrome is:
    ① Congenital heart disease
    ② Hepatic defects
    ③ Renal disease
    ④ Endocrine gland malfunction

64. Before Cynthia's discharge the nurse teaches Mr. and Mrs. Wood to care for her at home. The nurse emphasizes that the correct way to turn Cynthia while she has the cast on is to:
    ① Log-roll her body as one unit
    ② Use the cross bar between her legs
    ③ Have her assist by using the overhead trapeze
    ④ Tell her to sit up and help in changing her position

Situation: The nurse assesses 3-year-old Jason Holder, who has developed a rash after a day of mild fever, sneezing, and coughing.

65. The symptoms that would most probably lead the nurse to suspect that Jason has rubella are:
    ① Enlargement of the posterior cervical and postauricular nodes
    ② Koplik's spots on the soft palate and buccal mucosa
    ③ Conjunctivitis and sensitivity to light
    ④ Severe headache and nuchal rigidity

66. In implementing transmission barriers while Jason's rash persists, the nurse should give greatest consideration to suggesting that Jason be isolated from his unimmunized:
    ① 3-year-old girl friend who lives next door
    ② 18-year-old female cousin who has recently married
    ③ 13-year-old aunt who had rubeola as a toddler
    ④ 20-year-old brother who is living at home

Situation: Eric Van Dyke, 18 months old, suddenly develops a left earache, slight nasal congestion, and high fever. At the pediatrician's office his parents, Elissa and Allen Van Dyke, are informed that for the second time their son has developed a middle ear infection.

67. The nurse knows that among infants and children otitis media is considered the most common:
    ① Bacterial infection
    ② Rickettsial infection
    ③ Fungal infection
    ④ Viral infection

68. Mr. and Mrs. Van Dyke are anxious to know why Eric has another episode of suppurative otitis media. In replying the nurse should explain the:
    ① Functional difference between an infant's eustachian tube and that of an older child
    ② Difference between the size of the middle ear cavity in infants and older children
    ③ Structural difference between the eustachian tube of younger and older children
    ④ Immunologic difference between the young child and the adult

69. Benzocaine (Auralgan) eardrops are prescribed to relieve Eric's earache. To ensure that the Auralgan is correctly instilled by Mr. and Mrs. Van Dyke, the nurse should teach them to:
    ① Straighten the auditory canal by pulling the earlobe up and back
    ② Apply medicated ear wicks tightly before instilling the Auralgan
    ③ Cleanse the ear canal by pulling the pinna up and down
    ④ Straighten the auditory canal by pulling the pinna down and back

70. Eric's severe earache persists despite the Auralgan instillation and a few doses of ampicillin (Polycillin N). He returns to the pediatrician's office, where a myringotomy is performed. When explaining the myringotomy procedure to Mr. and Mrs. Van Dyke, the nurse should emphasize that the incision:
    ① Widens the perforation in the eardrum to allow for drainage
    ② Often results in permanent perforation of the tympanic membrane
    ③ Takes several days to heal and frequently leaves a scar
    ④ Provides immediate relief of pressure in the middle ear

71. The most important nursing responsibility during the myringotomy procedure is to:
    ① Have his mother stay and hold Eric in her arms

② Keep Eric restrained and completely immobilized
③ Collect the aspirated drainage in a culture tube
④ Maintain the continuous flow of local anesthetic

72. To help Mrs. Van Dyke promote the effectiveness of Eric's myringotomy, the nurse should suggest that Mrs. Van Dyke:
① Position Eric with his affected ear down
② Keep Eric flat on his back
③ Position Eric with his affected ear uppermost
④ Observe Eric for bleeding from the operative site

73. The nurse discusses the expected effects of myringotomy and any local manifestation of complications with Mr. and Mrs. Van Dyke. The occurrences that should be reported at once are:
① Mild or moderate hearing loss
② Lack of drainage and increased pain
③ Bleeding and diminished pain
④ Low-grade temperature and headache

74. The nurse is aware that children of Eric's age (1½ years) who have normal hearing have usually acquired a vocabulary sufficient to enable them to communicate by:
① Making babbling sounds
② Pointing and grunting
③ Using at least six words
④ Using complete sentences

Situation: Perry Makela, 6 months old, is admitted to the hospital with a diagnosis of bronchiolitis.

75. In making an assessment of Perry, the nurse would expect:
① A decreased heart rate
② A prolonged expiratory phase
③ Increased breath sounds
④ Intercostal and subcostal retractions

76. Based on the problems associated with bronchiolitis, the treatment of choice for Perry should consist of:
① Adequate hydration, bronchodilators
② Croupette, adequate hydration
③ Croupette, broad spectrum antibiotics
④ Postural drainage, corticosteroids

77. The nurse organizes Perry's care to allow for uninterrupted periods of rest. This plan is:
① Appropriate because this action promotes decreased oxygen demands
② Appropriate because the cool mist helps to maintain hydration status
③ Inappropriate because frequent assessment by auscultation is required
④ Inappropriate because constant care is necessary in the acute stage

78. An important nursing measure for Perry is:
① Promoting stimulating activities that meet his developmental needs
② Making frequent observations of his skin color, anterior fontanel, and vital signs

③ Discouraging visits from his parents during the acute phase of the illness to conserve his energy
④ Keeping him on strict isolation and using a gown, cap, mask, and gloves when giving him any care

79. When Perry is able to tolerate a regular diet, the nurse should plan to feed him:
① Bananas, sweet potatoes, ham, and formula
② Pears, green beans, turkey, and whole milk
③ Peaches, corn, cottage cheese, and whole milk
④ Applesauce, carrots, chicken, and formula

80. As Perry's condition improves, the nurse needs to provide toys for him. The most appropriate toys for a 6-month-old infant would be:
① Soft stuffed animals
② Wooden blocks
③ Push-pull toys
④ Shape matching toys

81. While caring for Perry, the nurse should observe for the presence of the reflex called:
① Extrusion
② Startle
③ Tonic neck
④ Babinski

82. To plan nursing care for Perry, the nurse needs to have an understanding of the growth and development process of children. With this in mind the nurse would expect Perry to be able to:
① Sit alone, display pincer grasp, wave bye-bye
② Turn completely over, sit momentarily without support, reach to be picked up
③ Crawl, transfer toy from one hand to the other, display fear of strangers
④ Pull himself to a standing position, release a toy by choice, play peek-a-boo

Situation: John Lane, a 10-year-old recently diagnosed diabetic, is hit in the head with a baseball bat during Little League practice. He is brought to the emergency room by ambulance accompanied by his parents, Polly and Harold Lane. He is found to have a pronounced swelling in the center of the forehead and is admitted for further observation because intracranial bleeding is suspected. His blood pressure and pulse rate on admission are 90/60 and 60, respectively.

83. Surgery is scheduled. Mr. and Mrs. Lane express concern about the surgery because their son has diabetes. The nurse is aware that for a client who is diabetic:
① The greatest danger during the surgical procedure is from diabetic ketoacidosis
② The stress of surgery causes a rise in blood glucose levels during the postoperative period

③ Urine test results provide the best gauge of diabetic control after the surgery

④ If insulin was not required before surgery it generally will not be required in the postoperative period

84. A craniotomy is performed, and a hematoma is extracted. When John returns from the recovery room, the nurse positions him in a semi-Fowler's position to:
   ① Decrease the cardiac work load and facilitate oxygenation after surgery
   ② Increase cranial drainage and prevent accumulation of fluid
   ③ Reduce subdural pressure and promote reaction from anesthesia
   ④ Decrease pressure on the diaphragm and increase thoracic expansion

85. Mannitol (Osmitrol) is ordered for John after the surgery, and Mr. and Mrs. Lane ask why it is being given to their son. The nurse explains that its purpose is to:
   ① Reduce the amount of glucose in the urine
   ② Increase the filtration rate of the bladder
   ③ Relieve cerebral pressure following surgery
   ④ Decrease the peripheral retention of fluid

86. The day after surgery John's temperature is 103° F. Aspirin suppositories, an antibiotic, and tepid sponge baths are ordered to decrease the temperature. The nurse understands that:
   ① A slight fever is to be expected after any surgery
   ② An excess of viscid secretions has caused inadequate respiratory ventilation
   ③ Anyone with diabetes will develop an infection after surgery
   ④ Edema after the surgery often causes pressure on the hypothalamus

87. John recovers from his surgery with no residual defects and is soon to be discharged. The nurse suspects that there may be a problem with family dynamics when Mrs. Lane states:
   ① "We want to encourage John to do as much as he can for himself."
   ② "We know John is special and we'll have to go easy on the discipline for him."
   ③ "We know John and the rest of the family are in for a lot of ups and downs over the years."
   ④ "We really hope John can still be in the Boy Scouts and participate in Little League baseball."

88. Before discharge the nurse institutes a teaching schedule to help John and his parents cope with his diabetes. When teaching John to administer his own insulin, the nurse should teach him to:
   ① Give the insulin injections primarily in the opposite arm or either leg
   ② Shake the bottle of insulin thoroughly before drawing the dose

③ Briskly rub the injection site for a minute after giving the injection

④ Always wash his hands before preparing the insulin injection

89. The nurse includes prevention of infection, especially of the extremities, in the teaching program. The nurse should emphasize to John and his parents the importance of:
   ① Treating minor cuts immediately with a strong antiseptic such as iodine
   ② Drying the feet thoroughly after a bath by rubbing vigorously with a towel
   ③ Inspecting both feet frequently and carefully
   ④ Soaking the feet at least once daily in hot water

Situation: Kent Collins, 2½ years old, has a fractured femur and is in Bryant's traction.

90. After giving him morning care, the nurse checks the traction to be sure that the hip angle is maintained at:
   ① 45 degrees
   ② 60 degrees
   ③ 90 degrees
   ④ 180 degrees

91. Nursing care specific for a child in Bryant's traction should include:
   ① Checking the sites of pins for bleeding or infection
   ② Applying topical or antibiotic ointment as ordered
   ③ Assessing that the elastic bandages are not too loose or too tight
   ④ Removing the bandages daily to lubricate the skin

92. Kent communicates in two- or three-word phrases. When his parents discuss the accident, Kent says, "Bad, bad tree." The nurse understands that he is within the cognitive developmental norm of Piaget's:
   ① Sensorimotor development
   ② Preconceptual operations
   ③ Concrete operations
   ④ Concept of reversibility

Situation: Marc Goldstein, 5 years old, is admitted to the hospital with unusual weight loss and severe anorexia. Wilms' tumor, an embryoma of the kidney, is diagnosed. A nephrectomy is performed, and chemotherapy with dactinomycin (Cosmegen) and doxorubicin (Adriamycin) is started.

93. In light of the Cosmegen therapy, the intervention the nurse should plan to include in Marc's plan of care is:
   ① Administering aspirin for pain
   ② Using an anesthetic mouthwash
   ③ Serving citrus juices with meals
   ④ Providing age-appropriate books

94. Marc is to receive 500 ml of D5NS and 250 ml RL over 24 hours. The tubing delivers 60 gtt/ml. The nurse should set the flow to provide:

① 11 gtt/min
② 21 gtt/min
③ 31 gtt/min
④ 41 gtt/min

95. In considering the side effects of Marc's drug therapy, the nurse can suggest to him and his parents that he:
① Wear a baseball cap
② Dress in light clothing
③ Eat three large meals
④ Avoid dairy products

Situation: Lillie and Frank Carlino have 4 children, Tommy age 16, Mario age 9, Anthony age 4, and Salvatore age 2. Mr. Carlino earns $12,000 a year, and they are living at the edge of poverty. The public health nurse makes weekly home visits to assess the status and care of Mario, who has cystic fibrosis.

96. When caring for a family that is economically deprived, the nurse should understand that the characteristic most common to those living in poverty is:
① Long-term feelings of powerlessness
② A willingness to postpone gratification
③ Open and direct expressions of anger
④ Compliance with health recommendations

97. When performing an assessment of Mario, the nurse should be aware that the adaptations of cystic fibrosis are related to the:
① Cilia of the respiratory tract
② Sweat glands
③ Endocrine glands
④ Mucus-secreting glands

98. The nurse evaluates that Mario's pancreatic enzyme replacement is inadequate when Mario complains of:
① Anorexia
② Constipation
③ Abdominal cramping
④ Sudden weight gain

99. The nurse reviews cystic fibrosis and its treatment with Mario. An explanation most suitable to Mario's stage of development would be:
① "Your medication is scheduled at this time because your doctor has prescribed it this way."
② "The postural drainage will help you feel better."
③ "Your mucus is thick because cystic fibrosis interferes with how your mucous glands work."
④ "The dietician says this meal schedule is best for you."

100. Mrs. Carlino tells the nurse that her son Tommy is a football player in high school and that he said he needs more thiamine in his diet to give him more energy. She asks what foods contain thiamine. The nurse's best response would be:

① Fruits
② Green vegetables
③ Eggs
④ Whole or enriched grains

101. The nurse asks Mrs. Carlino if she has any other questions. Mrs. Carlino tells the nurse that she is also worried about Salvatore, age 2, because he refuses to eat and hardly touches his meals. Considering a toddler's food and feeding needs the nurse should teach Mrs. Carlino that:
① The child's normal struggle for independence at this age often involves refusal of food, but he will eat the amount he needs
② His energy requirements during the toddler stage are so high that he needs more calories to meet them
③ His growth rate is increased at the age of 2 years, so he needs more protein per unit of body size
④ Because he often refuses food, prepare more of only a few foods that he really likes and avoid snacks between meals

102. While the nurse is talking with Mrs. Carlino, Anthony, age 4, quietly interrupts the conversation. Anthony is obviously shy and stutters. The nurse is aware that stuttering is considered:
① A normal characteristic for a preschooler
② An indication of a serious permanent impairment
③ An indication of a delay in neural development
④ The result of a serious emotional problem

103. Mrs. Carlino asks what they can do about Anthony's stuttering. When discussing how to handle his stuttering, the nurse should include a suggestion to:
① Stop him and tell him to think before starting again and to speak slowly
② Avoid looking directly at Anthony while he is having difficulty finding words
③ Help Anthony by supplying the correct word when he is experiencing a block
④ Identify situations that increase stuttering and avoid or ignore the hesitancy

104. The public health nurse has been visiting the Carlino family weekly. When working with a family as the unit of service the nurse should consider that:
① Separating health problems from other aspects of this family's life is essential to help them
② Assessing each member of this family is not necessary to plan the care for the family as a whole
③ Certain members of the family may be capable of providing more support than the nurse can
④ Values, beliefs, and attitudes held by the family have limited influence on how they will perceive assistance

Situation: Regina Sharpe brings her 2-year-old son, Alvin, to the pediatric clinic because he has been irritable, lethargic, and pale. He has had abdominal cramps and vomited this morning. After a thorough physical examination, Alvin is admitted to the pediatric unit with lead poisoning (plumbism).

105. The nurse should be aware that a high level of lead in the blood leads to:
    ① Marked anemia
    ② Increased urination
    ③ Severe malnutrition
    ④ Liver damage

106. Developmentally, young children such as Alvin are at risk for lead poisoning primarily because:
    ① Their vascular system is very fragile
    ② They have a high level of oral activity
    ③ Lead is easily available to them
    ④ Motor vehicle pollution has increased

107. The nursing diagnosis that is used most commonly with children with lead poisoning is:
    ① Potential for injury
    ② Alteration in nutrition
    ③ Alteration in comfort
    ④ Unilateral neglect

108. Alvin has a lead level of 50 µg per 100 ml and requires chelation therapy. Priority nursing care for children prescribed edetate calcium disodium (Calcium EDTA), a chelating agent, should include:
    ① Careful monitoring of intake and output
    ② Providing a high-protein diet
    ③ Scrupulous care of the skin
    ④ Drawing blood daily for liver function tests

109. In addition to removing lead from the blood, chelation therapy predisposes the child to:
    ① Hyperkalemia
    ② Hypocalcemia
    ③ Hypoglycemia
    ④ Anemia

Situation: Tom and Jane Franklyn's 16-month-old son Charlie appeared to be recovering from varicella (chickenpox) when he began vomiting and became increasingly lethargic. He is brought to the emergency room and is admitted to the pediatric unit.

110. Charlie is diagnosed as possibly having Reye's syndrome. The nurse caring for him must be alert for manifestations of Reye's syndrome, such as:
    ① Bleeding and ecchymosis from liver involvement
    ② A macular rash on the face and trunk
    ③ Bladder distention and overflow
    ④ Marked periorbital edema from renal shutdown

111. The physician orders 700 ml of IV fluid over 24 hours. The IV tubing has a drop factor of 60 gtt/ml. The nurse should set the flow to provide:

① 15 gtt/min
② 20 gtt/min
③ 29 gtt/min
④ 34 gtt/min

112. Charlie has been in the hospital for 3 weeks and seems increasingly withdrawn and mute. It would be most appropriate for the nurse to:
    ① Assign different nurses to be with him to provide sensory stimuli
    ② Encourage the parents to stay with him as much as possible
    ③ Move him in with other children
    ④ Provide him with distracting toys

Situation: During a routine well-baby clinic visit, 9-month-old Sheila Movan was diagnosed as having congenital hip dysplasia, which is presently being treated.

113. The nurse's assessment of Sheila's orthopedic status would reveal:
    ① An inability to adduct the affected leg
    ② An inability to palpate movement of the femoral head
    ③ A narrowing of the perineum with an anal stricture
    ④ An apparent shortening of one of her legs

114. Sheila's social development is best promoted by having her:
    ① Play with a large ball with a bell
    ② Manipulate soft clay
    ③ Play peek-a-boo and bye-bye
    ④ Pound on a peg board

115. A developmental assessment of 9-month-old Sheila would be expected to reveal:
    ① Closure of both anterior and posterior fontanels
    ② A two- to three-word vocabulary
    ③ The ability to sit steadily without support
    ④ The ability to feed herself with a spoon

116. If Sheila's immunization schedule is up to date for her age, the next immunization that she should receive at age 15 months is:
    ① Diphtheria
    ② Measles, mumps, rubella
    ③ Tetanus
    ④ Trivalent oral polio

Situation: Sixteen-year-old Laurie Anderson and her 1-month-old baby Elizabeth arrive via ambulance at the emergency room. Ms. Anderson states that she was holding the baby and fell down the stairs. Accompanying them is Ms. Anderson's mother, Sylvia Anderson.

117. Legally, consent for Elizabeth's medical care:
    ① Is not necessary because this is an emergency and no consent is needed
    ② Must be obtained from Mrs. Anderson, who should sign the consent
    ③ Is Ms. Anderson's responsibility, and she should sign the consent

④ Must be decided by Family Court because Ms. Anderson is a minor

118. Elizabeth has numerous abrasions, a red welt on her back, a fractured sternum, and a closed head injury. She is admitted to the pediatric intensive care unit after surgical repair of a subdural hematoma and a fractured sternum. She is intubated, on a ventilator, has one chest tube, and has a central line. When allowed to see her daughter, Ms. Anderson cries and says, "I didn't mean to do it." The nurse should:
① Notify the Child Abuse Hotline of this probable instance of abuse
② Respond by saying, "You caused your baby's injury and feel guilty."
③ Put an arm around Ms. Anderson and say, "This must be difficult for you."
④ Encourage Ms. Anderson's mother to stay with her and help comfort her

119. Ms. Anderson visits Elizabeth in the pediatric ICU. She is told that Elizabeth is no longer on the ventilator and is breathing well on her own. Ms. Anderson asks why the chest tube was not removed if Elizabeth is breathing better. The nurse should explain that the chest tube:
① Is left in to drain the extra air in the baby's chest that accumulated following the punctured lung
② Is left in to drain air from the chest because air is normally inside the lungs but not around them
③ Will not cause discomfort and is left in for emergency use
④ Will be pulled once the baby is feeding well and is afebrile

Situation: Ollie Larson, 4 years old, was diagnosed as having nephrotic syndrome at 3½ years of age. Since that time he has had two relapses that required hospitalization.

120. Ollie has been treated with prednisone for several months and thus is highly susceptible to the adverse side reactions. An important nursing assessment related to prednisone therapy would be:
① Daily checking of oral mucous membrane for ulcers
② Regular checking of urine for mucus threads
③ Daily checking of pulse for irregularities
④ Frequent checking of stools for occult blood

121. This time Ollie's admission to the hospital has been brought about by a greatly decreased urine output and weight gain resulting from massive edema. Close monitoring of his urine would be expected to reveal:
① Numerous red blood cells
② High protein levels
③ Normal specific gravity
④ Crystalline particles

122. In children with renal disease the best indicator of fluid balance is the daily measurement of:
① Body weight
② Urinary output
③ Abdominal girth
④ Urine osmolality

123. Ollie's oral fluid intake has been restricted to 600 ml for 24 hours. The nursing intervention that would be most appropriate in assisting Ollie to cope with this limitation would be:
① Dividing fluid intake equally among each shift (200 ml/each shift)
② Permitting Ollie to have 1 ounce of fluid in small 1 oz cups each hour he is awake
③ Allowing Ollie to drink fluids as desired until the 600 ml limit is reached
④ Withholding fluids from 7 PM to 7 AM and giving the entire 600 ml from 7 AM to 7 PM

124. Ollie is being kept on bedrest until he begins to diurese. The most therapeutic play activity for Ollie would be:
① Using crayons to color in a coloring book
② Fingerpainting on blank sheets of paper
③ Engaging in a checker game with his father
④ Playing dominos with an 8-year-old roommate

125. In planning self-care that would foster independence, the nurse would expect Ollie to be able to:
① Part and comb his hair appropriately
② Button his pajama shirt
③ Tie his shoes
④ Cut the meat on his dinner tray

Situation: Janet Lee is a nurse who works in the teenage clinic of a large county hospital. Ms. Lee is aware that during the adolescent period there may be sexual experimentation.

126. One day, 16-year-old Martin Starve comes to the clinic with a complaint of a thick urethral discharge. To confirm the suspected diagnosis of gonorrhea the nurse should:
① Obtain a urine specimen
② Draw blood for a VDRL
③ Get a sexual history
④ Take a urethral culture

127. Because Martin is allergic to penicillin, the physician orders tetracycline (Sumycin) to treat the infection. The nurse would know that the teaching about the administration of tetracycline was effective when Martin says he should take the drug:
① With meals or milk
② At least 1 hour before meals
③ Approximately 30 minutes after meals
④ Just before meals

128. The nurse would determine that the teaching about the side effects of tetracycline was un-

derstood when Martin says that the medication could cause:
① Constipation
② Diarrhea
③ Vertigo
④ Tinnitus

129. Another client, Abe Gold, 16 years old, comes to the clinic. He is sexually active and is worried about having syphilis. The nurse is aware that an early diagnosis of syphilis is important and its presence is often determined by:
① A discharge from the penis
② Evidence of a rash
③ Multiple gummatous lesions
④ A lesion on the penis

130. The physician diagnoses that Abe does in fact have syphilis and orders penicillin G (Pentids) and probenecid (Benemid). The nurse explains to Abe that the rationale for both drugs being used is:
① Each drug attacks the organism during different stages of cell multiplication
② Probenecid decreases the potential for an allergic reaction developing to the penicillin, which treats the syphilis
③ The penicillin treats his syphilis while the probenecid relieves his severe urethritis
④ Probenecid delays excretion of penicillin by the kidneys to maintain effective blood levels for longer periods

Situation: Kenneth Cole is born with a meningomyelocele. The meningomyelocele is repaired and an atrioventricular shunt is surgically inserted.

131. To evaluate the shunt's function, the nurse should:
① Palpate his anterior fontanel
② Note the frequency of voiding
③ Assess for periorbital edema
④ Observe for symmetrical moro reflexes

132. Kenneth develops diarrhea and metabolic acidosis with a decreased urinary output. Because of his status, the nurse anticipates the physician's orders and prepares for administration of:
① Isotonic saline
② Potassium chloride
③ Sodium lactate
④ Plasmanate

133. Kenneth recuperates and is discharged. His mother, Eileen Cole, asks the clinic nurse when Kenneth will begin immunizations. The nurse responds that immunizations will be delayed until he is 2 months of age because:
① Maternal antibodies interfere with the development of active antibodies by the infant
② The neonatal spleen is unable to produce efficient antibodies

③ Infants under 2 months are rarely exposed to infectious diseases
④ The immunization would attack the immature infant's body and produce the disease

134. Kenneth receives his first DPT immunization at 2 months. The nurse should tell Mrs. Cole to:
① Apply ice to the injection site if soreness develops; call the physician if the baby has a fever
② Apply heat to the injection site for the first day; afterwards apply ice if the arm is sore
③ Give a baby aspirin for pain; if swelling at the injection site develops, call the physician
④ Give Tylenol for fever; call the physician if marked drowsiness or convulsions occur

135. When Kenneth is 2½ years old he is readmitted for a shunt revision. Before discharge, the nurse, recognizing abnormal behavior for this age-group, tells Mrs. Cole to call the physician if Kenneth:
① When playing, frequently starts arguments by claiming all toys are "mine"
② Tries to copy all of his father's mannerisms
③ Becomes fussy when frustrated and displays a shortened attention span
④ Talks incessantly regardless of the presence of others

136. Ferrous fumarate (Feostat Drops) 30 mg is ordered for Kenneth before his discharge. The solution contains 45 mg/0.6 ml. The nurse should administer:
① 0.6 ml
② 0.9 ml
③ 6.0 minims
④ 13.0 minims

Situation: Allen Klein, 6 months old, has eczema. He is admitted to the hospital because of secondary infection of his face and head from constant scratching.

137. The nurse is aware that eczema is a nonspecific ailment that is:
① Associated with chronic respiratory infections
② Predominantly found in infants
③ Easily treated
④ Highly contagious

138. The most important nursing care for infants with eczema is:
① Prevention of secondary infections
② Identification of causative factors
③ Provision of sufficient hydration
④ Promotion of physical growth

139. Allergic reactions in eczematous clients are most often caused by:
① Woolens, house dust, and dog hairs
② Fruit, eggs, and wheat

③ Milk, eggs, and peanuts
④ Woolens, meat, and milk

140. An assessment of Allen's growth and developmental level should reveal that he can:
① Hold his bottle by himself
② Crawl forward
③ Say,"Mama"
④ Turn pages in a book

141. The nurse evaluates that Allen's mother needs more teaching regarding Allen's care when she states:
① "I will be careful not to cut Allen's nails short."
② "I am going to buy him a whole new set of cotton clothing."
③ "I will make sure not to give him any whole milk products."
④ "I have given all his woolen blankets to my nephew."

Situation: Five-year-old Norman Toll is hit by a car while riding his bicycle. He sustains a fractured femur and a supracondylar fracture of the humerus.

142. On admission the x-ray films reveal evidence of fractures of the long bones in various stages of healing. The nurse understands that Norman should be assessed for:
① Child abuse
② Osteogenesis imperfecta
③ Vitamin D deficiency
④ Inadequate calcium intake

143. The pain is intense and analgesics prn are prescribed for Norman. When administering the analgesics to Norman, the nurse should consider that:
① Pain is not as strongly felt by children as by adults, so analgesics are not needed frequently
② Even though children do not like medicines, analgesics will make them more comfortable
③ Children do not need analgesics, as they are easily distracted and quickly return to playing or sleeping
④ Children should rarely receive analgesics, because this may result in addiction or respiratory depression.

144. Once Norman is better, he begins to play with his 5-year-old roommate. The nurse should be aware that 5-year-olds engage in play that is known as:
① Parallel
② Aggressive
③ Cooperative
④ Ritualistic

Situation: Angela Wiley brings Lyman, 4 weeks old, to the emergency pediatric clinic with a history of intermittent vomiting after feeding for the past few days and frequent, very forceful, projectile vomiting after today's feeding.

145. The pediatrician examines Lyman and makes a tentative diagnosis of hypertrophic pyloric stenosis. When assessing Lyman, the nurse would expect to find:
① Visible peristaltic waves across the lower abdomen
② Tenderness over the epigastric region not relieved by heat application
③ A palpable mass in the epigastrium to the right of the umbilicus
④ Lower abdominal distention with vomiting of bile-stained gastric contents

146. Lyman is hospitalized for surgical correction of the pyloric obstruction. The nurse explains to Mr. and Mrs. Wiley that this type of procedure has a high success rate when:
① It is performed before the infant's vomiting becomes severe and projectile
② The fluid and electrolyte imbalances are corrected preoperatively
③ The infant receives small, frequent feedings of thickened formula preoperatively
④ Gastric decompression is monitored for amount and type of drainage

Situation: Larry, the newborn son of Mary and Joe West, has tetralogy of Fallot. He is being cared for at home by his parents and is receiving digoxin (Lanoxin) and spironolactone (Aldactone).

147. The public health nurse periodically reviews Larry's care and medication instructions with Mrs. West. The nurse would know that Mrs. West understood the medication instructions when she indicates:
① Vomiting should be reported to the physician
② Larry should have orange juice daily
③ Larry's activity should be carefully restricted
④ Aspirin should be avoided while the child is taking Aldactone

148. At the age of 2 months Larry is admitted to the pediatric unit with a diagnosis of congestive heart failure (CHF). The nurse is aware that in children with CHF:
① The treatment differs vastly from adult treatment
② Digoxin (Lanoxin) and furosemide (Lasix) are the most commonly used medications
③ Treatment is still experimental because infants rarely experience congestive heart failure
④ The illness is an acquired congenital anomaly

149. When planning teaching sessions with Mr. and Mrs. West, who both work full time, the nurse should:
① Insist both parents attend the teaching sessions
② Schedule a whole evening for teaching
③ Provide written and oral information in short sessions

④ Point things out to them when they are visiting Larry

150. The physician decides to perform palliative surgery for Larry's tetralogy of Fallot. The aim of the palliative surgery is to directly increase the blood flow to the:
① Lungs
② Brain
③ Myocardium
④ Right ventricle

Situation: Margo Howe, 5 years old, is admitted to the hospital with acute lymphocytic leukemia (ALL).

151. When obtaining a health history from Margo's parents, Beth and Leonard Howe, the nurse would expect them to report that the first sign they observed was:
① A paleness of the skin
② Sores in the mouth
③ A loss of appetite
④ Purplish spots on the skin

152. The physician plans to administer the alkylating agent cyclophosphamide (Cytoxan) as part of the chemotherapeutic regimen. During the administration of this drug, the nurse should assess Margo for:
① Unexpected nausea
② Extent of hydration
③ Increased irritability
④ Hyperplasia of gums

153. After the initial administration of chemotherapy, Margo is being discharged home. The nurse would know that Mr. and Mrs. Howe understood the discharge instructions when they say, "We should:
① Provide her with structured activities each day."
② Allow her to eat her food at her own pace."
③ Isolate her from other children her age."
④ Have her rinse her mouth with mouthwash."

154. To prevent the spread of the leukemia to areas of the body not affected by systemic chemotherapy, Margo is to be readmitted and given methotrexate and cranial radiation. Mrs. Howe asks the nurse if Margo should be started on multiple vitamins so that she won't be so weakened. The nurse's best response would be:
① "That is an excellent idea; I'll ask the doctor to order some for Margo."
② "Unfortunately, vitamin supplements won't make her feel any better now."
③ "Some vitamins contain folic acid, which interferes with methotrexate."
④ "Margo will benefit from vitamins and will be receiving them soon."

155. Margo needs special mouth care because of the potential for mouth lesions from the chemotherapy. The nurse would recognize that Mr. and Mrs. Howe understand the instruc-

tions about mouth care when they say, "Margo should:
① Brush her teeth with a toothbrush."
② Rinse her mouth with hydrogen peroxide."
③ Brush her teeth with a foam-tipped applicator."
④ Rinse her mouth with undiluted mouthwash."

156. Margo is readmitted to the pediatric unit for intrathecal methotrexate. Allopurinol (Zyloprim) is prescribed for Margo. She asks, "Why do I have to take that pill?" The nurse's best response would be:
① "Because your doctor ordered it. He would not order anything for you unless it was very important."
② "Because this pill helps the other medicines get rid of the things that are making you sick."
③ "To protect your body from developing other problems after your treatment has been stopped."
④ "To stop your sick white cells from going to other parts of your body where they can cause problems."

157. Margo looks very pale and feels warm to the touch. The nurse suspects a fever and checks Margo by taking an axillary and oral temperature because:
① Rectal temperatures are too upsetting for a 5-year-old child
② Axillary temperatures alone are not accurate when fever is suspected
③ Oral temperatures alone are inaccurate in children with leukemia
④ Rectal temperatures are avoided to reduce the risk of rectal trauma

158. Margo is scheduled to begin cranial radiation. The nurse is aware that this is being done to:
① Reduce the risk of systemic infection
② Improve the quality of Margo's life
③ Avoid metastasis to the lymphatic system
④ Prevent central nervous system involvement

Situation: Marguerite Colon, newly arrived from Puerto Rico, brings her daughter, Julie, 5½ years old, to the pediatric clinic for a physical examination. Julie attends kindergarten where everyone speaks English.

159. Mrs. Colon tells the nurse that Julie cries all the time, is no longer outgoing, and is very passive in the classroom. The nurse suspects that Julie:
① Is undergoing cultural shock
② Is not mature enough for kindergarten
③ Lacks adequate motivation for school
④ May be experiencing discrimination

160. The nurse begins to assess Julie. To bring about effective communication with any

child, the nurse must first take into consideration the child's:
① State of health
② Developmental level
③ Ability at self-expression
④ Fear of authoritarian figures

161. When Julie is 6 years of age, she develops rubeola. The nurse knows this is the medical name for the disease that is commonly called:
① Chickenpox
② Measles
③ German measles
④ Whooping cough

162. The nurse advises Mrs. Colon that rubeola will cause Julie to have:
① A macular rash
② A paroxysmal cough
③ Enlarged parotid glands
④ Generalized vascular lesions

Situation: Daniel and Florence Shaw's new infant daughter, Sharon, is born with a cleft lip.

163. Immediate nursing care for Sharon should be directed primarily toward:
① Preventing the occurrence of infection
② Modifying feeding methods
③ Keeping the baby from crying
④ Minimizing handling by parents

164. Mrs. Shaw bottle feeds Sharon with a special nipple. To minimize regurgitation of the feedings, the nurse instructs Mrs. Shaw to:
① Feed Sharon while sitting her up in an infant seat
② Hold and burp Sharon frequently while feeding
③ Give Sharon the thickened formula as ordered
④ Lay Sharon on her side with the bottle firmly propped

165. Mr. and Mrs. Shaw ask when Sharon's cleft lip will be repaired. The nurse responds:
① "When the baby is 8 to 12 weeks old."
② "Usually at about 18 months of age."
③ "Not until she has teeth in her mouth."
④ "As soon as she starts to lose weight."

166. Sharon's lip is repaired surgically. Postoperatively, the nurse will provide nutrition for the baby via:
① A plastic teaspoon
② Intravenous feedings
③ A rubber-tipped syringe
④ Nasogastric tube feedings

167. Following each feeding the first action by the nurse should be to:
① Cuddle Sharon for a few minutes
② Place Sharon on her abdomen
③ Burp Sharon several times
④ Clean and rinse Sharon's suture line

168. A priority nursing measure for Sharon during the postoperative period is to:
① Minimize her crying
② Restrain her at all times
③ Oxygenate her frequently
④ Handle her as little as possible

Situation: Jay Larro, 9 years old, was recently diagnosed as having insulin-dependent diabetes mellitus (IDDM). He was admitted for insulin regulation and education. During the nursing history, his parents, Jules and Harriet Larro, tell the nurse that Jay has been diagnosed as learning disabled and attends a special school for his disability.

169. When the nurse tells Mr. and Mrs. Larro that Jay will be taught about his disease, Mrs. Larro responds, "That won't be necessary. With Jay's disability we recognize that he is unable to care for himself." The best response by the nurse would be:
① "Then we will just teach you what he needs to have done."
② "Jay cannot always depend on you for his health needs."
③ "Jay seems bright enough to me, I think he can learn this."
④ "This material is not difficult; even a slow child can learn it."

170. While Jay is hospitalized for dosage regulation, he has been exhibiting some manipulative behavior. He has been observed sneaking forbidden foods and trying to talk his mother into allowing him extra sweets. One day, he comes to the nurse complaining of symptoms of hypoglycemia. Based on his behavior, the most appropriate nursing action would be to:
① Administer orange juice with sugar
② Obtain a blood sugar level
③ Test his urine for glucose
④ Ask him when he last ate anything

171. Jay has trouble correctly measuring his insulin dose. He frequently draws up 42 units of insulin instead of his prescribed 24 units. The most appropriate intervention to ensure dosage safety is to:
① Provide Jay with pre-set syringe guides originally developed for the blind
② Teach Jay to use a magnifying glass to read the numbers on the syringe
③ Allow Jay to have the number written down on paper as he fills the syringe
④ Exchange the insulin syringe Jay has been using for a tuberculin syringe

172. When Jay is 12 years old he is admitted to the hospital in acidosis. The nurse should recognize that the sequence of events that occurs in the respiratory response to acidosis is:
① Hypoventilation; increased CO_2 elimination; decreased blood H^+ ions; increased pH
② Hypoventilation; decreased blood H^+ ions; increased CO_2 elimination; decreased pH
③ Hyperventilation; decreased CO_2 elimina-

tion; decreased blood H$^+$ ions; decreased pH

④ Hyperventilation; increased CO_2 elimination; decreased blood H$^+$ ions; increased pH

173. While in the hospital Jay's insulin regimen is reevaluated. He is prescribed 15 units of regular insulin and 30 units of NPH insulin at 7:00 AM each morning. The nurse should expect that a hypoglycemic reaction from the NPH insulin is most likely to occur:
① Within 30 minutes
② In the late morning
③ In the late afternoon
④ During the night

174. One day the nurse suspects that Jay is hypoglycemic when he manifests:
① Redness of the face and deep, rapid breathing
② A change in behavior, hunger, and diaphoresis
③ Increased thirst, sleepiness, and some vomiting
④ A decreased level of consciousness and a dry mouth

175. Mrs. Larro tells the nurse that Mr. Larro has been giving Jay his insulin injections for the past 3 years. The nurse evaluates Jay and believes he can give his own injections. The nurse plans to teach Jay to give himself insulin before discharge. In learning to give his own injections Jay should:
① Draw up the NPH insulin first and then draw up the regular insulin
② Alternate the sites until he finds the best one to use
③ Administer his own injections immediately after he is taught the technique
④ Learn to use a needle and syringe on an orange first

Situation: Joan Wise, a school nurse, encounters a variety of infestations common in the school-age child.

176. A student comes to Ms. Wise complaining of intense itching behind her ears. After examination, Ms. Wise determines the student has head lice (pediculosis capitis) and advises immediate treatment to prevent the development of a secondary infection that may occur as a result of scratching. The most common secondary infection is:
① Cellulitis
② Impetigo
③ Eczema
④ Tinea capitis

177. Louise Stope, the mother of 7-year-old Bob, telephones Ms. Wise and tells her that the physician has asked her to obtain a specimen of pinworms from Bob for diagnostic evaluation. Ms. Wise instructs her to:
① Insert a cotton tipped swab into Bob's rec-

tum to collect a small amount of stool after a bowel movement
② Make an anal impression on cellophane tape before Bob uses the bathroom in the morning
③ Give Bob a tap water enema and save all returns for testing
④ Tape a 4×4 gauze tightly over Bob's anus during the night

Situation: Elaine Mariono, 4 years old, is brought to the pediatrician's office with complaints of earache, sore throat, low-grade fever, a cough, and general malaise. The nurse prepares the necessary equipment to perform an otoscopic examination, a throat examination, and a throat culture.

178. To properly visualize the canal during the otoscopic examination, the pinna of the ear must be pulled:
① Down and forward
② Up and back
③ Up and forward
④ Down and back

179. When examining Elaine's throat, the nurse should position a tongue blade to the side of the child's tongue primarily to avoid:
① Interfering with the visual examination
② Eliciting the gag reflex
③ Hurting any of the teeth
④ Obstructing the airway

180. Dorcol pediatric cough syrup ½ tsp is ordered for Elaine. Each teaspoonful contains dextromethorphan hydrobromide 7.5 mg. When administering the cough syrup the nurse should administer:
① 0.5 ml
② 2.5 ml
③ 3.75 ml
④ 7.5 ml

181. In assessing 4-year-old Elaine the nurse would expect her to:
① Have a vocabulary of 1500 words
② Use just three- or four-word sentences
③ Ask the definitions of new words
④ Name two or three different colors

182. Several weeks later Elaine is admitted with a diagnosis of rheumatic fever. She is exhibiting manifestations of carditis and polyarthritis. Penicillin, probenecid (Benemid), and aspirin are started, and she is prescribed bedrest. In examining Elaine's lab work the nurse would expect to see:
① A negative C-reactive protein
② A positive antistreptolysin titer
③ A decreased erythrocyte sedimentation rate
④ An elevated reticulocyte count

183. When Elaine is 8 years old she has a tonsillectomy under general anesthesia without any untoward sequelae. During the immediate postoperative period, a nursing intervention for Elaine would be to maintain:

① Hydration by providing cool liquids frequently
② Consciousness by encouraging interaction with her mother
③ Airway patency by positioning her on the side
④ Aeration by assisting with coughing and deep breathing

Situation: Ten days after Michael Jones, age 6, recovers from an upper respiratory infection, his mother, Lily Jones, notices puffiness around his eyes. At this time, Michael tells her that he has a stomachache, that he does not want to eat, and that his urine is dark colored, like cola. After a visit to his physician, Michael is admitted to the hospital with a probable diagnosis of acute glomerulonephritis.

184. On Michael's admission, the physician orders tests to confirm the diagnosis. The nurse is aware that the tests ordered would probably include:
① Routine urinalysis, chest x-ray films, blood sugar levels, IVP
② Upper GI series, 24-hour urine collection, complete blood chemistry, nasopharyngeal culture
③ Routine urinalysis, complete blood chemistry, nasopharyngeal culture, ASO titer
④ Electrocardiogram, heterophil antibody test, urinalysis, chest x-ray film

185. Mrs. Jones is concerned about Michael's 4-year-old sister developing acute glomerulonephritis. In explaining the etiology of the disease, the nurse should respond:
① "The cause of acute glomerulonephritis is unknown, so it is difficult to know how to prevent it."
② "Acute glomerulonephritis is inherited by an autosomal recessive trait but usually occurs only in males."
③ "Acute glomerulonephritis is caused by clot formation in the small renal tubules secondary to systemic infection."
④ "Acute glomerulonephritis is caused by an antigen-antibody response secondary to group A beta-hemolytic streptococcus."

186. When Michael is marking the dietary preference list for dinner, the nurse encourages him to choose the most appropriate combination of foods. This would include:
① Baked potato, ground beef, canned carrots, banana, buttermilk
② Canned green beans, baked ham, bread and butter, peach, milk
③ Corn on the cob, baked chicken breast, rice, applesauce, milk
④ Hot dog on a bun, potato chips, dill pickle slices, brownie, milk

187. In assessing Michael's condition and testing his urine the morning after admission, the nurse would not be surprised to note a:
① Decreased blood pressure, periorbital edema, 1+ proteinuria, and a specific gravity of 1.001
② Moderately elevated blood pressure, periorbital edema, 4+ proteinuria, and a specific gravity of 1.030
③ Normal blood pressure, anorexia, 1+ proteinuria, and a 3+ glycosuria
④ Anorexia, hematuria, 1+ proteinuria, and decreased blood pressure

188. The physician orders antibiotic therapy for Michael. Initial medications that the nurse would expect the orders to include are:
① Reserpine and hydralazine
② Digitalis and hydralazine
③ Reserpine and phenobarbital
④ Furosemide and phenobarbital

189. In caring for Michael, the nurse plans to:
① Promote rest, monitor intake and output, weigh Michael daily, and provide a regular diet with no added salt
② Maintain bed rest, use isolation techniques, force fluids, and provide meticulous skin care
③ Prevent chilling, monitor vital signs every 2 hours, provide a no-sodium diet, and get Michael up in a chair for 2 hours
④ Maintain bed rest, provide a low-sodium diet, monitor blood pressure every hour, and monitor IV therapy

190. Before Michael's discharge the nurse should plan to provide his parents with:
① A sample of a sodium-restricted diet because he will continue to be on this diet
② The nurse's phone number so that Mrs. Jones can call if she has any questions
③ Suggestions about activities that will keep Michael active for long periods of time
④ Instructions as to when Michael should return for a work-up for a kidney transplant

Situation: Karl Fredricks, a 6-year-old child with celiac disease, is brought to the pediatric clinic by his mother, Ruth Fredricks. Karl is a small, thin child whose growth curve falls below the normal for his age.

191. When taking the health history and assessing Karl, the nurse would expect to find:
① Constipation, abdominal distention, flatulence, rickets
② Constipation, abdominal distention, peripheral edema, increased clotting time
③ Diarrhea, muscle wasting, anemia, osteomalacia, steatorrhea
④ Diarrhea, malnutrition, rickets, anemia, steatorrhea

192. Karl is placed on a low-gluten diet. The nurse explains to Mrs. Fredricks that the low-gluten diet will mainly restrict:
① Milk and dairy products
② The grains of wheat, rye, oat, and barley

③ The grains of corn and rice
④ Saturated and unsaturated fats

193. The effectiveness of a gluten-restricted diet in a child with celiac disease can be assessed on the second day by having the nurse and mother evaluate the child for:
① Decreased irritability
② Maintenance of weight
③ Normal bowel movements
④ Disappearance of steatorrhea

194. Karl is anemic. The nurse suspects that the anemia is caused by:
① An inadequate amount of the intrinsic factor
② The small amount of iron included in his diet
③ The poor absorption of iron and folic acid
④ His minimal appetite and low food intake

195. When teaching Mrs. Fredricks about a diet for Karl, who is malnourished, the nurse should teach her to:
① Supplement Karl's diet with megadoses of vitamins A, D, E, and K to correct the coagulation deficiencies
② Give foods high in potassium and magnesium to correct the bone growth deficiencies
③ Provide foods high in folic acid, iron, and vitamin B_{12} to correct the blood dyscrasia
④ Encourage a high-calorie diet composed of high-protein and high-fat foods to foster weight gain

196. The nurse's plan should include helping Karl to:
① Express his feelings, while focusing on ways in which he can still be normal like his friends
② Understand the relationship of diet to disease so that he will be more willing to adhere to his diet and refrain from eating snack foods
③ Learn which snack foods can be substituted for the hot dogs and hamburgers that have wheat fillers, because occasional noncompliance is permitted
④ Select meals from those high-residue, high-carbohydrate foods that are gluten-free and permitted

197. In the management of a child with chronic celiac disease the primary nursing goal is to:
① Prevent celiac crisis and resulting complications
② Prevent complications from respiratory involvement
③ Teach the parents to control the diet to promote normal growth
④ Help the parents and child adjust to the lifelong dietary restrictions

198. Karl returns with Mrs. Jones to the clinic 6 months later. Compliance to the dietary regimen can be evaluated by assessing his:
① Knowledge of foods allowed on the diet
② Understanding of the disease process

③ Physical and emotional progress
④ Ability to handle stressful situations

199. Karl, now 7 years old, is admitted for an emergency appendectomy. The anesthetist examines Karl and leaves a preanesthesia medication order for atropine and meperidine (Demerol). The nurse should:
① Give Karl the preanesthesia medication and call the surgeon with a reminder about Karl's celiac condition
② Take Karl's vital signs, administer the preanesthesia medication, and attach a note to the front of Karl's chart noting his celiac condition
③ Withhold Karl's preanesthesia medication, note his celiac condition in the nurse's notes, and transport him to the operating room
④ Call the anesthetist, tell him of Karl's celiac condition, and question the preanesthesia order

Situation: Natalie Post, 8 years old, is admitted with Reye's syndrome.

200. When doing the nursing history the nurse would probably learn that Natalie has recently recovered from:
① Rubella
② Chickenpox
③ Bacterial meningitis
④ Rheumatic fever

201. The early symptoms that usually bring the child with Reye's syndrome to the hospital are:
① Intractable vomiting and confusion
② Low-grade fever and petechiae
③ Diarrhea and rash
④ Jaundice and oliguria

202. The nurse should expect that Natalie will be:
① Placed on strict isolation
② Admitted to the intensive care unit
③ Treated on an ambulatory basis initially
④ Taken to surgery immediately

203. Mrs. Post, who has two younger children, asks the nurse for some guidelines to possibly prevent Reye's syndrome in her other children. The nurse should respond:
① "If their temperature reaches 101° F, begin sponge bathing with alcohol."
② "Restrict their carbohydrate intake when they have symptoms of a cold."
③ "Use an antipyretic other than aspirin when they have a respiratory infection."
④ "Ask your doctor about inoculating them with a specific immunization serum."

Situation: Six-year-old Eloise Hurley has just returned from surgery, where she was placed in a spica cast.

204. When providing care for Eloise immediately after she returns from application of the cast, the nurse plans to include:
① Drying the cast with a hair dryer

② Touching the cast with the palms of the hands

③ Turning by using the crossbar

④ Logrolling every 6 hours until the cast is dry

205. Eloise had the cast applied while under general anesthesia. The priority care for her in the immediate postoperative period is:
① Teaching her to use the overhead trapeze
② Checking her peripheral circulation
③ Giving her oral fluids
④ Encouraging deep breathing

206. The nurse knows that an appropriate toy for Eloise, who is 6 years old, would be a:
① Set of building blocks
② Ball and jacks
③ Coloring book and crayons
④ Game of checkers

207. Three days after the cast application, Eloise has a temperature of 101.4° F. Suspecting an infection the nurse should first assess Eloise for:
① Any complaints of tingling in her toes
② A foul smell coming from the cast
③ The presence of itching around the top of the cast
④ Rapid irregular respirations

208. Before discharge, cast care is taught to Eloise's mother, Jane Hurley. The nurse assesses that Mrs. Hurley understands the instructions when she says, "If Eloise is itchy around the cast, I will:
① Pat the area with an alcohol swab."
② Gently scratch the itchy area."
③ Sprinkle a layer of powder around the itchy spots."
④ Ask the physician for an antihistamine."

Situation: Bonnie Kross, 13 years old, gives birth to a girl, who she names Jessica. Ms. Kross and Jessica return to live with Olive Kross, Ms. Kross' mother.

209. During a well-baby visit to the pediatric clinic when Jessica is 6 weeks old, the statement by Ms. Kross that would lead the nurse to assess Jessica for the presence of an abnormality is:
① "I seem to have a hard time getting her diaper between her legs."
② "She wants to sleep curled up on her stomach all the time."
③ "I can't get her to straighten out her legs when I try to stand her up."
④ "Her feet look very flat when I put both of her booties on her."

210. Jessica is diagnosed as having congenital hip dysplasia, and she is admitted to the hospital for immediate corrective measures because:
① The infant's hip joint is still cartilaginous, and molding of the acetabulum is possible
② Infants are easier to manage in spica casts than toddlers
③ Bryant's traction cannot be used effec-

tively after a child reaches the age of 2 years
④ Mobility will be delayed if correction is postponed until later

211. When Jessica is being admitted the nurse notes that her mother is 13 years old and that both live with Jessica's grandmother. The nurse should obtain the informed consent from the:
① 13-year-old mother
② Maternal grandmother
③ Family court, who must make the decision
④ 13-year-old mother and Jessica's legal father

Situation: Margaret O'Malley, age 7, accompanied by her parents, James and Irene O'Malley, is admitted for observation because of myoclonic seizures of the right arm and leg lasting 1 to 2 minutes. The number of seizures per day is increasing. Seizure precautions are instituted.

212. While in the playroom, Margaret has a myoclonic seizure of the right arm and leg that almost immediately progresses to a grand mal seizure with clenched jaws. The nurse's best initial action would be to:
① Take the other children to their rooms
② Put a padded tongue blade into Margaret's mouth
③ Move furniture and toys away from Margaret
④ Place a large pillow under Margaret's head

213. During the seizure Margaret becomes cyanotic. The nurse should:
① Insert an oral airway
② Continue to observe the seizure
③ Administer oxygen by mask
④ Notify the physician immediately

214. Margaret is given phenytoin (Dilantin) 75 mg po bid. The nurse teaches Mr. and Mrs. O'Malley about care pertinent to long-term Dilantin therapy. The nurse would recognize that the teaching was effective when Mr. and Mrs. O'Malley say, "We should:
① Observe her urine for a reddish brown discoloration."
② Give her the medication 2 hours after she eats breakfast and dinner."
③ Supplement her diet with high-caloric foods and force fluids."
④ Provide oral hygiene, especially gum massage and flossing of teeth."

215. After discharge, Margaret is scheduled for routine medical follow-up because of the potential for the development of status epilepticus. The nurse is aware that the most common reason for status epilepticus is that the prescribed dosage of Dilantin is:
① Toxic to the child
② At the therapeutic level

③ Probably not taken consistently

④ Insufficient to cover the child's activities

Situation: Four-year-old Candy Vernon has recently been diagnosed as having Hirschsprung's disease. Candy will be at home awaiting surgery until her malnourished condition is improved.

216. The nurse is aware that Candy's parents, Hope and Thomas Vernon, understand the care that will be required when they tell the nurse that care at home will most likely include:
① Soapsuds enemas
② A low-protein diet
③ Nasogastric feedings
④ A high-calorie diet

217. The nurse recognizes that Mr. and Mrs. Vernon need further teaching about Candy's diet when they indicate they are going to allow her to have:
① Ripe bananas
② Spaghetti
③ Ice cream
④ Apples

218. Once Candy's malnutrition is corrected, she is admitted to the hospital for a colostomy. Preparation for surgery must include consideration of Candy's age-related fear of:
① Separation from parents
② Disruption of routines
③ Intrusive procedures
④ Strangers

219. Teaching is to be provided for Mr. and Mrs. Vernon before Candy's discharge following the colostomy. The nurse plans to include the information that:
① An enterostomal therapist is available to assist with home care
② Fluids should be limited between meals, although permitted at meals
③ They should try correcting Candy's poor eating habits at mealtime
④ Candy should not take part in physical education when she begins school

Situation: Christopher Renn, 5½ months old, was admitted with the diagnosis of fever of unknown origin. His mother, Ginger Renn, reveals that he had a fever and was vomiting for 48 hours before admission.

220. In view of Christopher's responses, the assessment by the nurse that would influence his care initially is:
① Asking Mrs. Renn whether he is breastfed or bottle-fed
② Checking his neurologic status and urinary output
③ Determining his vital signs and weight
④ Inspecting his skin for poor turgor

221. According to Mrs. Renn, Christopher is fully immunized as scheduled. The nurse can assume that he has already received:

① Two doses of diphtheria, tetanus, and pertussis vaccine
② Measles, mumps, and rubella vaccines
③ A booster dose of trivalent oral poliovirus vaccine
④ The first booster dose of diphtheria, tetanus, and pertussis vaccine

222. As Christopher's temperature returns to normal, his play could be expected to consist of:
① Picking up his rattle or toys and putting them into his mouth
② Exploratory searching when his cuddly toy is hidden from view
③ Simultaneously kicking his legs and batting his hands in the air
④ Waving his clenched fists and dropping toys placed in his hands

223. The primary nurse assigned to Christopher understands that his emotional development should normally make Christopher:
① Cling furiously to his mother when the nurse tries to take him away
② Cry when the nurse approaches his crib for the first time
③ Welcome the attention that the primary nurse gives him
④ Smile socially in recognition of his primary nurse's face

224. On the evening before Christopher's discharge from the pediatric unit Mrs. Renn voices her concern about taking her son Christopher home because his 4-year-old brother Oliver has chickenpox. In replying to Mrs. Renn, the nurse should convey the concept that chickenpox is:
① Not communicable as long as the vesicles are intact and surrounded by a red areola
② No longer communicable after a high fever has subsided
③ Still communicable until all the vesicles have dried
④ Still communicable even when only dry scabs remain

225. In discussing susceptible persons who should be protected from exposure to Oliver during the acute phase of his chickenpox, the nurse should question Mrs. Renn about relatives or friends who are receiving:
① Long-term anticonvulsant therapy
② Therapeutic doses of vitamins and minerals
③ Prolonged topical antibiotic therapy
④ High doses of systemic steroid therapy

226. Mrs. Renn asks the nurse whether there is something she can do to hasten the drying of Oliver's varicella lesions and relieve the itching. The nurse suggests that Mrs. Renn should try:
① Using wet to dry saline dressings over the oozing vesicles
② Patting the lesions gently with a paste of baking soda and warm water

③ Rubbing bacitracin (Bacitin) ointment into the open lesions

④ Having Oliver wear mittens and cutting his fingernails short

227. As she leaves the hospital, Mrs. Renn carefully covers young Christopher with blankets. The nurse understands that Mrs. Renn is preventing heat loss in her young child by the principle of:
① Radiation
② Active transport
③ Conduction
④ Fluid vaporization

Situation: Baby Martin Carey was born in the thirty-second week of pregnancy after his parents, Mabel and Frank Carey, were involved in a car accident. He has hypospadias.

228. Mr. and Mrs. Carey are upset about the hypospadias and ask if it was caused by the accident. The nurse explains that it occurred during fetal development in the:
① First trimester
② Second trimester
③ Third trimester
④ Implantation phase

229. Mr. and Mrs. Carey are told by the physician that surgery will be needed to repair Martin's hypospadias. The parents ask the nurse when this surgery will be done. The nurse should reply:
① "Within the next 2 months."
② "When he is between 3 and 4 years old."
③ "When he is between 5 and 6 years old."
④ "Before discharge from the hospital."

230. The nursing care plan for a newborn with hypospadias should include:
① Carefully explaining the genetic basis for the defect to the parents
② Preparing the infant for the insertion of a cystostomy tube
③ Keeping the penis wrapped with petrolatum gauze
④ Explaining to the parents why a circumcision will not be done

231. At 2 months of age Martin is brought to the pediatric clinic. During this visit he is given his first diphtheria, tetanus, and pertussis vaccination. Before Mrs. Carey takes Martin home, the nurse discusses with her the possible reactions to this immunization because these reactions are:
① Often serious and may require hospitalization
② Sometimes responsible for deep ulceration at the site of injection
③ Often responsible for permanent neurologic damage
④ Common and may be local or systemic

Situation: Janet Long, age 7, is admitted to the hospital. On admission she is febrile and extremely pale. She has petechiae and bone and joint pain. The physician diagnoses acute lymphatic leukemia. She is receiving several antineoplastic agents, including vincristine.

232. When assessing Janet for possible side effects of vincristine, the nurse should be aware that a sign of toxicity is:
① Diarrhea
② Alopecia
③ Hemorrhagic cystitis
④ Peripheral neuropathy

233. When assessing Janet's status the nurse would know that her fluid intake should be increased when her:
① Uric acid level is elevated
② Output for the last 24 hours totaled 1700 ml
③ Temperature is 99.8° F
④ Urine's specific gravity is 1.026

234. When giving Janet morning care, the nurse notices dried blood on the pillowcase and numerous bloody tissues in the bedside bag. The nurse should check the chart for the:
① Uric acid level
② Prothrombin time
③ Red blood cell count
④ Platelet count

235. Janet is to be sent home on a protocol that includes several antineoplastics after intrathecal administration of methotrexate. The instruction to Janet's parents that should be included in the nurse's teaching before discharge is:
① Limit contact with peers because they tend to have communicable diseases
② Return weekly for bone marrow aspiration to determine the effectiveness of therapy
③ Schedule routine laboratory appointments for evaluation of response to medication
④ Withhold medications when nausea occurs to prevent additional episodes of vomiting

Situation: Denise and Otto Marks bring Steven, their 4-year-old son, to the emergency room. They tell the nurse that the child has been complaining of pain in his abdomen and is running a temperature of 102.8° F.

236. The nurse would assess a 4-year-old child's pain by:
① Asking the child to point to where the hurt is
② Asking the parents about the child's bowel movements
③ Observing the child's position at rest and when in motion
④ Auscultating the abdomen for bowel sounds

237. Steven is diagnosed as having appendicitis, and surgery is performed. After the opera-

tion, he should be positioned in a semi-Fowler's or right Sims' position because:
① The lungs can aerate fully in both of these positions
② Drainage is facilitated, preventing subdiaphragmatic abscesses
③ Splinting of the wound is accomplished by pressure on the operative site
④ Movement is easier, thus reducing complications from immobility

238. Mr. and Mrs. Marks constantly blame each other for Steven's illness. The response by the parents that would indicate that the nurse's attempts to point out reality had been successful would be:
① The father bringing the child many expensive gifts
② The mother assuming the blame for not paying attention to the child's complaints
③ The parents making an appointment with a family counselor
④ The parents promising the child a trip to Disney World

239. The nurse's charting for a child who has had an appendectomy should include, in addition to "coughing and deep breathing," documentation of:
① Teaching to prevent dumping syndrome and early ambulation
② Mouth care and frequency of dressing changes
③ Bowel sounds, intake and output, and teaching about the low-residue diet
④ Dressing changes, intake and output, and bowel sounds

240. When doing a dressing change the nurse understands that a basic principle of surgical asepsis is:
① Sterile items held below the waist are considered sterile
② Wounds with exudates are contaminated and dry wounds are sterile
③ The entire sterile field is considered sterile
④ Sterile objects in contact with clean objects are considered clean

Situation: Lenny Powel is admitted to the pediatric unit in sickle cell crisis. He is in pain and will not take any oral fluids.

241. In addition to relief of pain, the nurse should direct Lenny's care toward:
① Oxygenation and adequate hydration
② Hydration and psychologic counseling
③ Antibiotics and narcotic regulation
④ Oxygenation and Factor VIII replacement

242. Lenny, who is 16 years old, understands that his sickle cell anemia symptoms appear when he has:
① A low iron intake
② An increased WBC production
③ A breakdown of RBCs
④ A fluid and electrolyte imbalance

243. A nursing intervention for a child with sickle cell anemia is:
① Teaching the child about the prophylactic medications
② Teaching the child to prevent sickling
③ Preparing the child for occasional blood transfusions
④ Explaining how excess oxygen sickles the RBCs

244. The nurse lists all of Lenny's problems associated with his sickle cell anemia that require nursing intervention and recognizes that priority must be given to:
① The interruption of learning as a result of multiple hospitalizations
② His altered body image resulting from skeletal deformities
③ The separation from his family during periods of hospitalization
④ His restriction of movement during periods of arthralgia

Situation: Ginny Sims is an 8-month-old child who had a cast applied to her right arm. Her parents, Lola and Hyman Sims, are at her bedside.

245. When doing the assessment the nurse finds that the fingers of Ginny's right hand feel cool. The nurse should first:
① Call the physician to report Ginny's circulatory impairment
② Clip the edge of Ginny's cast to reduce pressure
③ Compare the temperature of Ginny's right and left hands
④ Elevate Ginny's right arm to reduce swelling

246. The nurse recognizes that behaviors typical of an 8-month-old include:
① Drinking from a cup, using the words "Mama" and "Dada," and standing by herself
② Smiling spontaneously, clasping her hands, and keeping her head steady when sitting
③ Removing some of her clothing, building a tower of two cubes, and stooping to pick up toys
④ Being shy with strangers, playing peek-a-boo, and standing by holding onto furniture

247. The nurse, teaching Mr. and Mrs. Sims how to care for the plaster cast, tells them that to keep Ginny's cast clean they should:
① Remove surface dirt with a damp cloth
② Cover the cast with a piece of plastic
③ Scrub the cast with a soft brush and a mild abrasive
④ Rub the dirty area with a diluted bleach solution

248. Mrs. Sims tells the nurse that Ginny will eat only mashed potatoes and pancakes, and will drink only milk. She is concerned about this

diet even though Ginny is receiving Poly Vi-Sol daily. The nurse recognizes that Ginny's diet could lead to:

① A potassium deficit
② A vitamin deficiency
③ An amino acid deficiency
④ An iron deficiency anemia

249. Mrs. Sims brings Ginny, now 20 months old, to the well-baby clinic. Mrs. Sims indicates that she is concerned that Ginny's bedtime thumbsucking will cause her teeth to protrude. The nurse's most appropriate response would be:

① "You should seek counseling; her thumbsucking may indicate that she has an emotional problem."
② "You should switch her to a pacifier in the next 2 months to avoid protrusion of the teeth."
③ "You need not be concerned about her teeth protruding unless it persists after permanent teeth appear."
④ "You should restrain her from sucking her thumb because it prematurely loosens the first teeth."

250. The nurse notes that Ginny uses two- or three-word phrases (telegraphic speech), has a vocabulary of about 200 words, and frequently uses the word "me." The nurse would interpret her language development as being:

① Advanced for her age
② Normal for her age
③ Slow for her age
④ A developmental lag

Situation: The ambulance arrives at the emergency room with Eileen and Sean Wilkes and their 4-year-old child, Donna, who was discovered face down in a drainage ditch filled with 2 feet of water. She was not breathing when found, and the paramedics initiated CPR. Her pulse is now 50 beats per minute, she has no spontaneous respirations, and her temperature is 95° F.

251. Donna is intubated and is being bagged with 100% oxygen. The most important nursing measure at this time is to:

① Suction her endotracheal tube, mouth, and nasal passages
② Start an intravenous line to provide fluid and electrolytes
③ Assist the physician in delivering intracardiac medications
④ Call the pediatric ICU to inform them of Donna's admission

252. Donna is placed on a ventilator and is transferred to the pediatric intensive care unit. Although still unconscious, she responds to pain. Her heart rate is 85 beats per minute. The nurse recognizes that even though she has survived the near-drowning episode, she still has many problems to overcome. The nurse is aware that the ultimate prognosis will depend mainly on the extent of damage resulting from the:

① Hyperthermia
② Hypoxia
③ Aspiration pneumonia
④ Emotional trauma

253. Mr. and Mrs. Wilkes are allowed to visit Donna in the pediatric ICU. After they call her name several times, Donna opens her eyes and smiles at her mother. Mr. Wilkes states, "Look, she will get better now. What a miracle." The nurse's best response would be:

① "Yes, you are right; this is a very good sign."
② "See if you can get her to hold your hand, too."
③ "God certainly must have been watching over her."
④ "We are doing everything we can to help her recover."

254. Donna is breathing on her own and is removed from the ventilator. Oxygen 30% is ordered. The nurse is aware that in routine oxygen therapy the oxygen:

① Should be labeled as flammable
② May be administered without a prescription
③ Must be humidified before administration
④ Is warmed before administration

255. A few days later the nurse notices that Donna seems distressed and is clutching her chest. It appears that Donna is having a cardiac arrest. The physician orders epinephrine as a cardiac stimulant. The nurse is aware that the one factor that would still permit administration of an epinephrine solution that is on hand would be that the reconstituted solution:

① Is no more than 72 hours old
② Contains only slight sediment
③ Has been exposed to light
④ Is slightly discolored

256. When assessing Donna after the administration of epinephrine, the nurse should monitor for toxicity, which would be indicated by:

① Decreased blood pressure
② Constricted pupils
③ Hypoglycemia
④ Tachycardia

257. Donna soon regains her strength and appears to have recovered completely. She is transferred to the pediatric unit. Mr. and Mrs. Wilkes ask what playthings they can bring in for Donna. Utilizing knowledge about a 4-year-old's developmental level, the nurse is aware that the toy that would be most appropriate for Donna would be a:

① Six-piece jigsaw puzzle
② Blunt scissor and cut-out paper dolls

③ Fuzzy stuffed animal
④ Pocketbook filled with plastic figures

Situation: David Buxton, age 12, has been complaining of a rash on his chest, chills, a fever of 102.2° F, and a headache since he returned from a 1-week camping trip near the seashore. He comes to the clinic for evaluation accompanied by his parents, Jeanne and Matthew Buxton.

258. The nurse recognizes that David's history and physical assessment should include:
① A developmental screening and history of exposure to chickenpox
② The date of his flu vaccination and history of sunburn
③ A history of allergies and duration of symptoms
④ Sports played on the trip and when he is to return to school

259. David reports that he received many insect bites and two of the insects were pulled off by his father with tweezers. These areas became swollen and reddened, and the other symptoms began 3 days later. The physician suspects Lyme disease. David asks, "What is Lyme disease?" The nurse's best response would be:
① "You sound upset, but the medicine will make you better."
② "You are concerned. Why don't you ask me what you want to know."
③ "The insect bite gave you an infection, but the medications will stop it."
④ "It's a spirochetal infection that the penicillin will treat."

260. Mr. Buxton asks the nurse what the best way is to remove ticks from the skin. The nurse's best response would be:
① "Pour ammonia over the tick and it will shrivel up."
② "Touch the tick with a lighted cigarette."
③ "Remove the tick carefully with tweezers."
④ "Spray the tick with insect repellent and it will fall off."

261. David tells the nurse that he is afraid to go camping any more because of the ticks. The nurse's best response would be:
① "Frequent checks for ticks are a defense against infection."
② "Tell me more about your fears about camping."
③ "You are afraid to go camping just because of a tick?"
④ "Oh, camping is fun. Just think of what you will be missing."

Situation: Sam Katz, a toddler, is admitted to the pediatric unit with gastroenteritis caused by *Salmonella*.

262. After Sam's admission, the priority nursing action to be initiated for a child with a diagnosis of salmonellosis should be to:

① Weigh the child
② Establish a skin care routine
③ Obtain a recent food history
④ Set up enteric isolation

263. The physician has ordered 1000 ml of Isolyte-H (a balanced electrolyte solution) to run over the next 36 hours. Sam's IV drip-chamber delivers 60 gtt/ml. To administer 1000 ml of solution in the next 36 hours, the nurse should set the IV drip rate at:
① 0.5 gtt/min
② 3.0 gtt/min
③ 27.0 gtt/min
④ 36.0 gtt/min

Situation: Kevin Croce, a 16-year-old high school student, is admitted to the hospital with a fever of 104° F, a blood pressure of 130/90, a heart rate of 90, and respirations of 25. He is coughing and complaining of a sore throat, superficial chest pain, and fatigue.

264. During the physical examination Kevin is placed in the supine position. Immediately after being positioned flat he experiences shortness of breath. The nurse is aware that the term that best describes this phenomenon is:
① Dyspnea
② Hyperpnea
③ Orthopnea
④ Apnea

265. When assessing Kevin's respiratory pattern, the nurse understands that this pattern is controlled by the:
① Medulla
② Cerebral cortex
③ Hypothalamus
④ Cerebellum

266. Kevin's breathing becomes more difficult, and blood gases are taken. Normal arterial blood gas values would be most accurately reflected by readings of:
① pH 7.25, P_{O_2} 60 mm Hg, P_{CO_2} 50 mm Hg, base excess −4
② pH 7.40, P_{O_2} 85 mm Hg, P_{CO_2} 40 mm Hg, base excess 0
③ pH 7.50, P_{O_2} 85 mm Hg, P_{CO_2} 35 mm Hg, base excess 0
④ pH 7.45, P_{O_2} 70 mm Hg, P_{CO_2} 25 mm Hg, base excess +4

267. Kevin has an order for placement of a pulse oximeter. To assure accuracy of the pulse oximeter reading the nurse should:
① Place the probe on the abdomen or upper leg
② Calibrate the oximeter at least every 8 hours
③ After application wait 30 minutes before obtaining a reading
④ Place the probe on a finger or earlobe

Situation: Kay Robinson, 5 years old, is mentally retarded. She is admitted to the pediatric unit with a diagnosis of pneumonia.

268. The nurse realizes that the concept that Kay could probably learn the fastest is:
① Love vs hate
② Right vs wrong
③ Large vs small
④ Life vs death

269. The nurse understands that the first activity of daily living that should be taught to a child who is mentally retarded is:
① Dressing
② Hair combing
③ Self-feeding
④ Toileting

Situation: Marty Jamison, 3½ years old, is admitted with a suspected tetralogy of Fallot. He had no cyanosis at birth but had some difficulty feeding. During his first year he gained weight slowly and experienced frequent distress while feeding, unless fed slowly. He has gradually developed cyanosis on exertion and has recently experienced what his parents, Diane and David Jamison, call "weak spells." Exertion also results in weakness, which seems to be relieved when he squats for brief periods.

270. When reviewing Marty's history the nurse should understand that:
① In the absence of cyanosis, poor sucking is insignificant
② Many infants retain mucus that may interfere with feeding
③ Feeding problems are fairly common in infants during the first year
④ Poor sucking and swallowing may be early indications of heart defects

271. The nurse is aware that a common adaptation of children with tetralogy of Fallot is:
① Clubbing of fingers
② Slow, irregular respirations
③ Subcutaneous hemorrhages
④ Decreased red blood cell count

272. Marty is returned to his room after a cardiac catheterization. Postprocedure nursing care should include:
① Encouraging early ambulation
② Monitoring the insertion site for bleeding
③ Restricting fluids until blood pressure is stabilized
④ Comparing blood pressure in affected and unaffected extremities

273. Marty's parents leave with the promise to return soon. Marty nods his head that he understands, but after they leave he begins to cry frantically and his cyanosis and dyspnea worsen. Remembering that he squats if fatigued while walking, the nurse attempts to achieve relief for him by placing him in the:
① Semi-Fowler's position
② Lateral Sims' position
③ Orthopneic position
④ Knee-chest position

274. Based on an understanding of normal preschool behavior during hospitalization, the nurse tells Mr. and Mrs. Jamison that Marty will probably:
① Refuse to cooperate with nurses during his parents' absence
② Demonstrate despair if his parents do not visit at least once a week
③ Cry when his parents leave and return but not during their absence
④ Be unable to relate to peers in the playroom if there are parents present

275. If death should become a concern to Marty, the nurse should understand that to a preschooler, death is thought of as:
① An end to life
② A reversible separation
③ Something that happens to old people
④ A persona who takes one away from his family

CHAPTER 5

Maternity Nursing Review Questions

Situation: Nadia Lustig has just had a baby girl. Before delivery she indicated she wished to breastfeed her infant.

1. The delivery room nurse explains to Mrs. Lustig and her husband, Ira, that an Apgar score recorded 5 minutes after birth helps to evaluate the:
   ① Effectiveness of the labor and delivery
   ② Adequacy of transition to extrauterine life
   ③ Possibility of respiratory distress syndrome
   ④ Gestational age of the infant

2. The nurse is aware that the nursing action that would best promote parent-infant attachment behaviors would be:
   ① Encouraging rooming-in, with parental infant care
   ② Keeping the new family together immediately postpartum
   ③ Restricting visitation on the postpartum unit
   ④ Supporting the parents' choice of breastfeeding

3. Mrs. Lustig is breastfeeding her infant on the delivery table. The nurse assists her by:
   ① Touching the infant's cheek adjacent to the nipple to elicit the rooting reflex
   ② Leaving them alone and allowing the infant to nurse as long as desired
   ③ Positioning the infant to grasp the nipple so as to express milk
   ④ Giving the infant a bottle first to evaluate the baby's ability to suck

4. Mr. and Mrs. Lustig note petechiae on the newborn's face and neck. The nurse informs them that this is a result of:
   ① Increased intravascular pressure during delivery
   ② Decreased vitamin K level in the newborn infant
   ③ A rash called erythema toxicum
   ④ Excessive superficial capillaries

5. A physician has just written several medication orders for Mrs. Lustig. In reviewing the physician's orders the nurse evaluates that one of the drugs is contraindicated for breastfeeding mothers. The nurse should contact the physician and question the order for:
   ① Heparin
   ② Propylthiouracil (PTU)
   ③ Gentamicin (Garamycin)
   ④ Diphenhydramine (Benadryl)

6. Mrs. Lustig asks the nurse what she can do to ease the discomfort caused by a cracked left nipple. She should be instructed to:
   ① Use a breast shield to keep the baby from direct contact with the nipple
   ② Nurse the baby on the right side first until the left side heals
   ③ Stop nursing for 2 days to allow the nipple to heal
   ④ Manually express milk and feed it to the baby from a bottle

7. Baby Lustig has a total body response to noise or movement that is distressing to her parents. It is important for the nurse to teach them that this is:
   ① A reflexive response that indicates normal development
   ② A voluntary response that indicates insecurity in a new environment
   ③ An automatic response that may indicate that the baby is hungry
   ④ An involuntary response that will remain for the first year of life

8. When changing her infant, Mrs. Lustig notices a reddened area on the infant's buttocks. The nurse should:
   ① Have staff nurses, instead of Mrs. Lustig, change the infant
   ② Use both lotion and powder to protect the involved area
   ③ Encourage Mrs. Lustig to cleanse and change the infant more often
   ④ Notify the physician and request an order for a topical ointment

9. The nurse is aware that during the taking-in phase of the postpartum period the area of health teaching that Mrs. Lustig will be most responsive to is:
   ① Family planning
   ② Infant feeding
   ③ Infant hygiene
   ④ Perineal care

Situation: Bella Otis is 42 weeks pregnant. An oxytocin challenge test is to be performed to evaluate fetal status.

10. Before this test the nurse should:
    ① Place the client in the supine position
    ② Instruct the client to take nothing by mouth
    ③ Have the client empty her bladder
    ④ Prepare the client for insertion of internal monitors

11. When direct monitoring of the fetal heart rate during the first stage of labor shows an irregular baseline with variability, a nursing priority is to:
    ① Notify the physician

② Continue to monitor the client
③ Administer oxygen
④ Change the client's position

12. The nursing action that has the highest priority for a client in the second stage of labor is to:
① Help the client push effectively
② Prepare the client to breastfeed on the delivery table
③ Check the fetal position
④ Administer medication for the pain

13. The nurse is aware that when local anesthesia is used for delivery:
① There is danger of maternal aspiration
② Reactions such as vertigo and tinnitus may occur
③ Labor is slowed after its administration
④ Maternal respirations may be depressed

14. At 1 minute after birth the nurse notes that Mrs. Otis' infant boy is crying, has a heart rate of 140, has acrocyanosis, resists the suction catheter, and keeps his arms extended. The nurse should assign him an Apgar score of:
① 4
② 6
③ 8
④ 10

15. The nurse assesses Mrs. Otis during the fourth stage of labor for:
① Level of maternal love
② Distention of the bladder
③ Ability to relax
④ Knowledge of newborn behavior

Situation: Gail Saunders, 28 years old and newly married, makes an appointment with a family planning clinic. She expresses an interest in using some form of family planning but is uncertain about which method to use.

16. Mrs. Saunders eventually decides to use oral contraceptives. When obtaining the health history, the nurse should consider that oral contraceptives are contraindicated in a client who:
① Has a family history of CVA
② Is over 30 years of age
③ Smokes a pack of cigarettes per day
④ Has a history of a multiple pregnancy

17. The physician orders progesterone oral contraceptives (minipills). The nurse instructs Mrs. Saunders to take one pill daily:
① During the first 5 days of the menstrual cycle
② During the 5 days surrounding ovulation
③ Throughout the menstrual cycle
④ Throughout the first 21 days of the menstrual cycle

18. The nurse would know that Mrs. Saunders understood the teaching about the side effects of excessive estrogen when she indicates it would cause:

① Nausea and vomiting
② Amenorrhea
③ Depression and lethargy
④ Hypomenorrhea

19. The nurse recognizes that Mrs. Saunders understands the teaching about minipills when she states that she will discontinue the oral contraceptive at once if she experiences:
① Increased leukorrhea
② Chest pain
③ Mittelschmerz
④ Menorrhagia

Situation: Agnes Busch, a 21-year-old primigravida, calls the physician's office complaining of a headache and blurred vision. The nurse notes in the chart that she is 36 weeks pregnant, and at her last prenatal visit, a week ago, her vital signs and laboratory results were within normal limits. The nurse, suspecting impending eclampsia, instructs her to come to the office.

20. Mrs. Busch arrives at the office. Her blood pressure is 170/110 and her urine is 3+ for albumin. A characteristic symptom of eclampsia for which the nurse should assess is:
① Increased blood pressure
② Anasarca
③ Excessive weight gain
④ Convulsions

21. Mrs. Busch is admitted to the high-risk prenatal unit for observation and therapy. Her blood pressure is 170/110, her pulse is 108, and her respirations are 24. Magnesium sulfate 0.5 g every 4 hours as necessary is ordered. Eight hours later, after 2 doses, her blood pressure is 150/110, her pulse is 98, and her respirations are 14. She also has an absent knee-jerk reflex. The nurse should:
① Eliminate the next dose of magnesium sulfate and notify the physician
② Administer the next dose of magnesium sulfate because the blood pressure is still high
③ Wait 1 hour, monitor the vital signs and reflexes again, and then administer the next dose
④ Administer calcium gluconate as an antidote for the magnesium sulfate

22. Mrs. Busch has an unexpected cesarean delivery. A common concern of the mother after cesarean delivery that the nurse should anticipate is the:
① Postoperative pain and scarring
② Sense of failure in the birthing process
③ Inability to assume her mothering role
④ Prolonged period of hospitalization

Situation: Shirley Ramirez, age 30, first comes to the prenatal clinic at 30 weeks gestation. At 33 weeks, after a fall, Mrs. Ramirez delivers a baby girl whose Apgar scores are 3 and 7 at 1 and 5 minutes. She is transferred to the high-risk nursery.

23. At 6 hours of age, Baby Ramirez develops respiratory distress syndrome (RDS). Assessment of the infant at this time would probably reveal:
    ① A high-pitched cry
    ② A respiratory rate of 20
    ③ A heart rate of 140
    ④ Intercostal retractions

24. Nursing care of Baby Ramirez during this crisis should be directed toward:
    ① Keeping her in oxygen concentrations of 40%
    ② Stimulating deep breathing by tapping her soles
    ③ Maintaining her in a warm environment
    ④ Turning her frequently to prevent apnea

25. Respiratory acidosis is confirmed when the nurse notes that the laboratory report of blood gases reveals:
    ① A pH of 7.35
    ② An elevated PCO_2
    ③ An arterial O_2 level of 80 mm Hg
    ④ A potassium level of 4.6 mEq/L

26. Baby Ramirez is to receive oxygen by an overhead hood. During the time Baby Ramirez is under this hood it would be appropriate for the nurse to:
    ① Put a hat on her head
    ② Keep the O_2 concentration at 100%
    ③ Remove her q 15 min for stimulation
    ④ Hydrate her q 15 min

Situation: Rose Clancy, a 32-year-old attorney, is admitted to the labor and delivery suite at 39 weeks gestation and informs the nurse that she thinks her membranes have ruptured.

27. The nurse uses phenaphthazine (nitrazine) paper to test the pH of the leaking fluid. If amniotic fluid is present, the nitrazine paper will become:
    ① Red
    ② Orange
    ③ Blue
    ④ Purple

28. Ms. Clancy's labor does not progress, and a cesarean delivery is performed. Afterward she tells the nurse that she is a "natural childbirth flunkie." The postpartal phase of adjustment that this statement most closely typifies is:
    ① Taking hold
    ② Working through
    ③ Taking in
    ④ Letting go

29. Baby boy Clancy weighs 2450 g (5.5 lb) at delivery. He would be classified as being:
    ① Average for gestational age
    ② Small for gestational age
    ③ Average for gestational age but preterm
    ④ Preterm and immature

30. After Baby Clancy is admitted to the newborn nursery, the nurse observes that he has a weak high-pitched cry, seems jittery, and has irregular respirations. The nurse should associate these symptoms with:
    ① Hypoglycemia
    ② Hypercalcemia
    ③ Hypovolemia
    ④ Hypothyroidism

31. Ms. Clancy chooses to bottle feed her newborn because this will cause the least interference with full resumption of her law practice. Before discharge the nurse should teach Ms. Clancy that if breast engorgement occurs, she should:
    ① Take 2 aspirins every 4 hours
    ② Apply hot compresses to the breasts
    ③ Wear a tightly fitted brassiere
    ④ Cease drinking milk for 2 weeks

Situation: Patricia and Neil Josephs are expecting their first baby and express an interest in childbirth classes.

32. The nurse explains to the Josephs that in childbirth classes the emphasis is on:
    ① Birth as a family experience
    ② Education, breathing, and exercise
    ③ Nutrition, relaxation, and breathing
    ④ Labor without using analgesics

33. Mrs. Josephs asks how the Lamaze method differs from the Read method. The nurse explains that the Lamaze method:
    ① Is a calm, relaxed approach based on "childbirth without pain"
    ② Forbids the use of pain-relieving drugs during labor
    ③ Requires much prenatal preparation
    ④ Is a much easier method to teach and learn

34. Mr. and Mrs. Josephs enroll in a Lamaze class. The nurse knows that Mrs. Josephs understands how to use effleurage correctly when the client is observed:
    ① Taking deep breaths before simulated contractions
    ② Rocking gently back and forth on her knees
    ③ Practicing panting to avoid pushing during labor
    ④ Massaging her abdomen gently with her fingertips

35. The need to improve pubococcygeal muscle tone is explored during one of the childbirth classes. The nurse recognizes that Mrs. Josephs understands the instructions on how to strengthen this muscle when she states she should do:
    ① Pelvic rocking
    ② Forward tilting
    ③ Kegel exercises
    ④ Tailor sitting

Situation: Sarah Jones, 33 weeks gestation, comes to the prenatal clinic because she is having contractions. An examination reveals cervical dilation of 2 cm, no bloody show, head at −2, and membranes intact. She is discharged to her home and prescribed bedrest.

36. The teaching plan for Mrs. Jones should include the information that:
    ① She should lie on her side with her head raised on a small pillow
    ② Blocks should be placed at the foot of the bed to raise it
    ③ For 10 minutes every 2 hours she should assume the knee-chest position
    ④ She should sit in an upright position with several pillows behind her back

37. After hearing that she must remain in bed Mrs. Jones starts to cry and says, "I have two small children at home who need me." The nurse's best response would be:
    ① "You are worried about how you will be able to manage."
    ② "You'll need someone to care for the children."
    ③ "You'll be able to fix light meals, and the children can go to nursery school a few hours each day."
    ④ "You can get a neighbor to help out, and your husband can do the housework in the evening."

38. The nurse should also explain to Mrs. Jones that coitus:
    ① Is safe as long as she is in the side-lying position
    ② Should be restricted because it may stimulate labor
    ③ Is permitted if penile penetration is not deep
    ④ Need not be modified in any way by either partner

39. Mrs. Jones follows the prescribed regimen. However, a few days later, Mrs. Jones' contractions increase in intensity and frequency. She is admitted to the labor room and placed on IV ritodrine (Yutopar) therapy. During the initial administration of IV ritodrine, the nurse should:
    ① Monitor Mrs. Jones' blood pressure q 10 min
    ② Insert a Foley for accurate measurement of urinary output
    ③ Check Mrs. Jones' deep knee reflexes q 2 h
    ④ Institute safety measures because of altered consciousness

Situation: Maura Williams, who is 28 years old, was diagnosed as having diabetes mellitus as a young child. She is newly married and visits the clinic because she has not been feeling well.

40. The nurse suspects that Mrs. Williams is probably pregnant when:
    ① She complains of nausea and vomiting episodes every morning
    ② Her menses are already 7 days late
    ③ She relates that urinary frequency occurs every 2 to 3 hours
    ④ Her urine immunoasssay test is positive

41. Mrs. Williams' pregnancy is confirmed. When explaining the effects of pregnancy on diabetes mellitus to the client, the nurse should inform her that to minimize fetal-neonatal complications the most important action for her to take is to:
    ① Check her blood glucose level as ordered
    ② Keep all the physician's appointments made for her
    ③ Adhere strictly to the prescribed diet to limit weight gain
    ④ Cooperate with the physician to maintain normal blood sugar

42. Mrs. Williams asks the nurse when her baby's heartbeat will first be heard. The nurse's best response would be:
    ① "With a fetoscope around 8 weeks."
    ② "With a fetoscope at 12 to 14 weeks."
    ③ "With an electronic doppler after 17 weeks."
    ④ "With an electronic doppler at 10 to 12 weeks."

43. At 36 weeks gestation a nonstress test is performed on Mrs. Williams. It is interpreted as being nonreactive. Based on this finding, the contraction stress test, or oxytocin challenge test (OCT), is performed. The OCT is also interpreted as being negative. The nurse knows that this means:
    ① The fetus at this time is likely to tolerate the stress of labor, but the test must be repeated weekly
    ② Immediate delivery should be considered because there is no fetal heart acceleration with fetal movement
    ③ A trial induction should be started because fetal heart rate acceleration with movement is indicative of a false result
    ④ The test should be repeated in 24 hours because the examination results indicate hyperstimulation

44. At 38 weeks Mrs. Williams has an amniocentesis done to determine fetal maturity. The proper L/S ratio for lung maturity is:
    ① 1:2
    ② 2:1
    ③ 1:1
    ④ 1.5:1

45. Mrs. Williams goes into active labor. She is admitted to the labor unit and is being monitored externally. When Mrs. Williams' membranes rupture, the nurse detects a deceleration in the fetal heart rate. The nurse inspects the vaginal area and notes a prolapsed cord. The nurse should immediately:
    ① Administer oxygen by face mask at 7 L/minute
    ② Instruct the client to assume a dorsal recumbent position

③ Notify the physician of the findings of the examination

④ Elevate the presenting part off the cord until delivery

46. A cesarean delivery is performed, and a male infant weighing 9 lb 4 oz is born. Because of his large for gestational age (LGA) classification and his being the baby of a diabetic mother, the nursery nurse should assess him for:
① An axillary temperature below 98° F
② Cyanotic episodes accompanied by tremors
③ Elevated bilirubin levels in the first 24 hours
④ A blood glucose level below 45

Situation: Jill South, the mother of two children, comes to the prenatal clinic for a pregnancy test. Mrs. South's pregnancy test comes back positive, and on bimanual examination the uterus feels enlarged. Mrs. South is determined to be approximately 8 weeks pregnant.

47. As she is leaving the prenatal clinic, Mrs. South states, "I just don't feel like making love to my husband. Just last night he wanted to make love and I just couldn't and he just doesn't understand." The nurse could most appropriately respond:
① "How long have you had this problem?"
② "Why don't you feel like having intercourse?"
③ "A decrease in libido is a normal occurrence in pregnant women during the first trimester."
④ "I'm sure your husband eventually will understand that your feelings are related to pregnancy."

48. Two weeks later, Mrs. South calls the prenatal clinic complaining of urinary frequency without dysuria and asks the nurse for suggestions. The nurse is aware that Mrs. South will have to:
① Decrease her fluid intake during the day
② Maintain increased fluid intake during the day
③ Contact her physician as soon as possible
④ Try to resist the urge to void as long as possible

49. In discussing dietary needs, Mrs. South tells the nurse that milk constipates her at times. The nurse should explain that it is preferable to:
① Treat constipation in some way other than omitting milk
② Substitute skimmed or buttermilk for whole milk
③ Substitute a variety of cheeses for the milk
④ Increase her prenatal capsules and omit the milk

50. Mrs. South asks if there are foods other than milk that are a good source of calcium. The nurse advises her that she should eat:
① Corn
② Lean meat
③ Liver
④ Broccoli

51. Between 12 and 24 weeks gestation, applicable prenatal teaching for Mrs. South should include information about:
① Growth of the fetus, interventions for nausea and vomiting, and expectations for care
② Growth of the fetus, personal hygiene, and nutritional guidance
③ Danger signs of preeclampsia, relaxation breathing techniques, and signs of labor
④ Preparation for the baby, travel to the hospital, and signs of labor

52. When Mrs. South is 16 weeks pregnant, the nurse assesses her fundal height. The nurse determines the fundal height to be one finger above the umbilicus. The nurse should:
① Assess for two distinct fetal heart rates
② Ascertain the birth weights of children of any siblings
③ Inform Mrs. South that she is mistaken about her dates
④ Instruct Mrs. South on appropriate weight gain during pregnancy

53. After an uncomplicated labor and delivery, Mrs. South is now 24 hours postpartum and has blood drawn for a complete blood count. The CBC reveals Mrs. South's WBC count to be 17,000/mm³. The nurse should interpret Mrs. South's WBC count as being indicative of:
① A bacterial infection of the reproductive system
② An acute sexually transmitted viral disease
③ A normal decrease in white blood cells
④ A normal response to the labor process

Situation: Theresa Evans, a 24-year-old primipara, is admitted to the hospital. She is 35 weeks pregnant and this morning began having a small amount of bright red vaginal bleeding without contractions.

54. After placing Mrs. Evans in the bed the nurse should:
① Perform a vaginal examination
② Check fetal heart tones
③ Administer a Fleet's enema
④ Obtain an amniotomy setup

55. Mrs. Evans' bleeding increases, and an emergency cesarean delivery is performed. Baby Evans is suctioned, dried, and transported to the neonatal intensive care unit (NICU). The admitting nurse assesses Baby Evans' Silverman-Anderson Index to be 3. This value reflects the baby's need for:
① Increased caloric intake and fluids

② Respiratory support and observation
③ Continuous cardiac monitoring
④ Assessment of neurologic reflexes

56. A finding of the physical assessment that may indicate that Baby Evans is preterm is:
① Many superficial veins
② A positive Babinski reflex
③ Absent femoral pulses
④ Flexion of extremities

57. Eight hours after birth Baby Evans is observed to have a respiratory rate of 68 per minute with nasal flaring and cyanosis. He is diagnosed as having respiratory distress syndrome. A finding consistent with this diagnosis is:
① Pulse rate 100
② Arterial blood pH 7.50
③ Diminished breath sounds
④ Inspiratory stridor

58. Supplemental oxygen is ordered as part of Baby Evans' treatment. To prevent retrolental fibroplasia the nurse plans to:
① Analyze O_2 concentration frequently
② Warm and humidify all oxygen flow
③ Apply eye patches to both eyes
④ Administer the oxygen by hood

59. The primary nurse in the NICU who is caring for Baby Evans suspects that he has necrotizing enterocolitis (NEC) when:
① Several severe bouts of projectile vomiting are observed
② Large amounts of residual formula are withdrawn before gavage
③ An increased number of explosive stools are noted
④ Circumoral pallor develops during gastric feeding

60. Nursing care for the infant with necrotizing enterocolitis includes:
① Measuring abdominal girth every 2 hours
② Diluting the formula mixture as ordered
③ Giving half-strength formula by gavage feeding
④ Administering oxygen before gastric feeding

61. Mrs. Evans expresses concern about her baby. To best facilitate mother-infant bonding the nurse should:
① Avoid discussing negative aspects of the baby's condition
② Encourage the mother to let the nursing staff care for the baby
③ Have the mother stroke the baby whenever possible
④ Assure Mrs. Evans that her baby will be fine

Situation: Betty Johnson is a 20-year-old term primipara with a history of phenylketonuria.

62. Baby Johnson is delivered and at 1 minute is crying vigorously with an apical pulse of 110.

The nurse notes acrocyanosis and flexion of the extremities. The baby's Apgar is:
① 10
② 9
③ 8
④ 7

63. Eight hours postpartum the nurse finds Ms. Johnson's fundus to be 3 cm above the umbilicus and displaced to the right. The statement by the client that is most significant to the nurse at this time would be:
① "I've been so thirsty the past few hours."
② "I've changed my pads once since I got to my room."
③ "I've had a lot of contractions, especially when nursing."
④ "I've been up to the bathroom but can't seem to urinate."

64. Ms. Johnson is receiving methylergonovine maleate (Methergine) postpartum. The nurse should withhold this drug if Ms. Johnson is found to have a:
① Positive Homan's sign
② Blood pressure of 160/90
③ Respiratory rate of 12 per minute
④ Negative Babinski reflex

65. On her third postpartum day Ms. Johnson asks the nurse why her baby's skin has begun to appear yellow. The nurse should plan to teach her that the change in skin tone is a result of:
① Breast milk ingestion
② An immature vascular system
③ Inadequate fluid intake
④ Breakdown of red blood cells

66. Ms. Johnson is breastfeeding her baby. Diet counseling for the client with a history of phenylketonuria should include providing a food list displaying the amount of:
① Lactose
② Amino acids
③ Glucose
④ Fatty acids

67. To best assist Ms. Johnson to understand the unique characteristics of a newborn the nurse should discuss with her the:
① Infant's response to routine feeding schedules
② Newborn's states of wakefulness and behaviors
③ Importance of reading about parent-infant bonding
④ Testing of the normal newborn's auditory acuity

Situation: Ann Murray's physician telephones the delivery room to say that Mrs. Murray is on her way to the hospital. Mrs. Murray is a primipara, 36 weeks pregnant, whose membranes have ruptured spontaneously. Her cervix is 2 cm dilated and 75% effaced.

68. When admitting Mrs. Murray, one of the first questions the nurse should ask is:

① "How frequent are your contractions and how long do they last?"

② "What time was your last meal and what did you eat?"

③ "Are you planning to breastfeed or to bottle feed?"

④ "What is your expected date of delivery?"

69. Mrs. Murray's physician arrives and examines her. The physician states that her cervix is completely effaced, dilation is 4 cm, and station is 0. On the basis of this information, the nurse should:

① Check the fetal heart rate every 5 minutes and record it on her chart

② Continue to help Mr. Murray coach her in the use of breathing techniques

③ Call the anesthesia department and alert them to an imminent delivery

④ Ask Mrs. Murray how bad her pain is and whether she wants medication

70. The teaching plan for Mr. Murray should include the information that it would be best for him to:

① Leave Mrs. Murray alone periodically so that she can rest between contractions

② See that Mrs. Murray remains supine so that the monitoring equipment is not disturbed

③ Keep the conversation in the labor room to a minimum so that Mrs. Murray can concentrate

④ Let Mrs. Murray know the progress she is making and that she is doing a good job

71. During labor Mrs. Murray says, "We're so worried about our baby because I'm a whole month early." The nurse's best response would be:

① "Don't worry; the care of preterm babies has greatly improved."

② "I can understand why you and your husband are worried."

③ "Your physician is very good; try not to worry about it now."

④ "I don't blame you for worrying; there is some danger."

72. Later in labor an internal cardiac monitor is attached to the fetal scalp. The nurse should be concerned about a fetal heart rate that:

① Varied from 130 to 140 beats per minute

② Dropped to 110 beats during Mrs. Murray's contractions

③ Occasionally dropped to 90 beats unrelated to contractions

④ Did not drop during Mrs. Murray's contractions

73. When the obstetrician hands the infant to the nurse after delivery, the nurse's first action should be to:

① Dry the infant and place him in a warm environment

② Cut the umbilical cord and attach a Hesseltine clamp

③ Perform an abbreviated systematic physical assessment

④ Administer oxygen by face mask until cyanosis clears

74. Mrs. Murray calls to the nurse, "I'm so cold, and I can't stop shaking." The nurse should say:

① "Let me check your fundus to see whether it is firm."

② "Please turn on your side so I can check the amount of lochia."

③ "I am going to take your blood pressure and pulse."

④ "I will put some warm blankets on you; the chill will subside soon."

75. In estimating the infant's gestational age the nurse should take into consideration the:

① Weight and length at birth

② Presence of a tonic neck reflex

③ Condition of skin on the extremities

④ Size of breast tissue and genitalia

76. Infant Murray weighs 1800 g, and his Apgar scores are 6 and 8 at 1 and 5 minutes. The parents are shown the infant after his birth, but then he is moved to neonatal intensive care. The nurse should plan to:

① Take Mrs. Murray to the NICU to see her infant as soon as feasible

② Find out the condition of the infant and take Mrs. Murray to see him if he is doing well

③ Ask the physician's permission to have Mrs. Murray see the infant

④ Discourage Mrs. Murray's involvement with the infant until the prognosis is favorable

77. While watching her infant, Mrs. Murray exclaims, "He is so little. How will I ever learn to care for him?" The nurse should explain to Mrs. Murray that she:

① Can watch his care to assist her in becoming familiar with the specific routines

② Will be encouraged to participate in his care as much as possible from the beginning

③ Will be able to care for him in a special nursery for a few days before his discharge

④ Should find someone with training in preterm care to help her at home the first week

Situation: Pierre and Alice Andre have been married for 2 years and are expecting their first child.

78. Mr. and Mrs. Andre attend prepared childbirth classes. The nurse discusses the importance of the "spurt of energy" that occurs prior to labor. The nurse teaches the women in the class to conserve this energy because:

① Fatigue may influence the need for pain medication

② Energy helps to increase the woman's progesterone level

③ This energy decreases the intensity of uterine contractions

④ Extra energy is needed to push during the first stage of labor

79. Mr. and Mrs. Andre ask the nurse about the cause of low back pain in labor. The nurse replies, "This occurs most often when the position of the baby is:
    ① Occiput posterior."
    ② Mentum anterior."
    ③ Transverse."
    ④ Breech."

80. The position Mrs. Andre should be taught to avoid when she experiences back pain during labor is the:
    ① Side-lying position
    ② Knee-chest position
    ③ Supine position
    ④ Sitting position

81. Mrs. Andre begins labor and is admitted to the hospital. She is experiencing back pain. The nurse might suggest that Mr. Andre try to comfort her by:
    ① Encouraging her to do Kegel exercises between contractions
    ② Applying pressure to the sacrum during contractions
    ③ Having her perform a panting breathing pattern
    ④ Positioning her with her legs elevated

82. While doing her shallow breathing during transition, Mrs. Andre experiences tingling and numbness of her fingertips. Mr. Andre should suggest that she breathe into:
    ① An oxygen mask
    ② A paper bag
    ③ A trichloroethylene (Trilene) mask
    ④ Room atmosphere

83. The nurse is aware that the management of a client in transition is primarily directed toward:
    ① Reducing the client's discomfort with medication
    ② Helping the client maintain control
    ③ Decreasing the client's intravenous fluid intake
    ④ Having the client breathe simple patterns

84. The nurse would know that the childbirth preparation classes were effective when during the transition phase the couple uses the breathing pattern of:
    ① Shallow chest
    ② Pant-blow
    ③ Slow chest
    ④ Accelerated-decelerated

Situation: Barbara and Bill James, both 39 years old, are having their first child. They tell the nurse in the prenatal clinic that because of their ages they are concerned about having a normal child and want to have an amniocentesis procedure.

85. The nurse tells them that this procedure can be done:
    ① Immediately after conception
    ② After the fourteenth week of pregnancy
    ③ As soon as Mrs. James feels life
    ④ In the last trimester only

86. After an amniocentesis the nursing care should include:
    ① Observing for signs of labor
    ② Giving perineal care
    ③ Forcing fluids every hour
    ④ Changing the abdominal dressing

87. Mrs. James vaginally delivers a baby girl. The baby develops jaundice 72 hours after birth. The nurse explains to Mrs. James that the jaundice is probably due to:
    ① Some Rh negative blood that is still present in the baby's bloodstream
    ② Normal physiologic destruction of immature RBCs
    ③ An obstruction in the bile duct, which is common in newborns
    ④ An allergic response to her feedings

88. Rho (D antigen) immune globulin (RhoGAM) has been ordered for Mrs. James, who is Rh negative. Before giving the medication, the nurse must verify that the baby is:
    ① Rh positive, negative Coombs'
    ② Rh negative, positive Coombs'
    ③ Rh positive, positive Coombs'
    ④ Rh negative, negative Coombs'

89. Mrs. James is breastfeeding her infant. The baby sucks very vigorously, and as a result, Mrs. James' nipples have become sore and tender. The best nursing action would be to:
    ① Remove the baby from the breasts for a few days
    ② Expose the nipples to air several times a day
    ③ Give analgesic medication as ordered
    ④ Apply continuous ice packs

Situation: Colleen Reilly, age 32, delivers a baby girl who is admitted to the newborn nursery.

90. Later, while inspecting her baby, Mrs. Reilly asks the nurse if her newborn has flat feet. The nurse recalls that:
    ① Flat feet are common in children and infants
    ② This is difficult to assess because the feet are so small
    ③ The arch of the newborn's foot is covered with a fat pad, giving the appearance of being flat
    ④ Flat feet are associated with major deformities of the bones of the feet such as clubfoot

91. The nurse palpates the femoral pulses of Baby Reilly. This procedure is done to detect the presence of:
    ① Ventricular septal defect
    ② Coarctation of the aorta

③ Patent ductus arteriosus
④ Atrial septal defect

92. The nurse also assesses Baby Reilly for central cyanosis. Central cyanosis is indicative of congenital heart defects that affect cardiac circulation by:
① Shunting blood right to left
② Shunting blood left to right
③ Obstructing the flow of blood from the left side of the heart
④ Preventing shunting of blood between the left and right sides of the heart

93. The nurse understands that congestive heart failure is the usual sequela to congenital cardiac defects that result from left-to-right shunting of blood in the heart. With this knowledge, the nurse would be aware that a sign that would be most indicative of early onset of congestive heart failure in the infant would be:
① Decreased heart rate
② Increased respiratory rate
③ Liver 2 cm below the costal margin
④ Cyanosis of skin

Situation: Sonia Martin is a 32-year-old primigravida who uses cocaine and narcotics. Following a 2½ hour second stage of labor she delivers a 9 lb 3 oz male with the aid of low-outlet forceps. She develops periurethral tears and has a second-degree episiotomy.

94. In light of Ms. Martin's history of narcotic abuse the nurse's initial plans for providing pain relief measures should include:
① Scheduling pain medication at regular intervals
② Administering the medication just when the pain is severe
③ Avoiding the administration of medication unless it is requested
④ Recognizing that she will not need as much pain medication as others

95. The nurse is aware that the best initial intervention that should help to limit perineal edema would be:
① Aspirin 10 grains po q 4 h
② Ice packs to the perineum
③ Hot sitz baths tid
④ Elevation of hips on a pillow

96. In the postpartum period the nurse anticipates that Ms. Martin is most likely to develop:
① Difficulty voiding spontaneously
② Delayed onset of milk production
③ Maladaptive bonding and attachment
④ Posterior vaginal varicosities

97. The nurse should be aware that Ms. Martin may be experiencing drug withdrawal if she develops:
① Depression and tearfulness
② Extreme hunger and thirst
③ Irritability and muscle tremors
④ Paranoia and evasiveness

98. To help prevent postpartum infection the most important discharge instruction given by the nurse would be:
① "Wash your hands before and after changing your sanitary napkins."
② "Don't take tub baths for at least 6 weeks after delivery."
③ "Tampons are better than napkins for inhibiting bacteria in the postpartum period."
④ "Douche gently with Betadine solution twice a day for a week or more after delivery."

99. Ms. Martin's baby develops feeding problems. He is very irritable and cries in a high shrill voice. It is suspected that he has cytomegalovirus disease. The nurse recognizes that his mother probably contracted this disease from:
① Eating improperly cooked meat
② Handling a cat litter box
③ Drinking contaminated water
④ Having sex with many partners

Situation: Baby Thomas Marks is brought to the nursery directly from the delivery room. On assessment he is noted to be pale pink with mottling. His pulse is 160 beats per minute and his respirations are 80 breaths per minute without retractions. His birth weight is 1000 g. The gestational examination estimates the age at 34 weeks.

100. Based on the assessment of 34 weeks gestation and 1000 g birth weight, the nurse considers this infant to be:
① Term, average for gestational age (AGA)
② Preterm, large for gestational age (LGA)
③ Term, small for gestational age (SGA)
④ Preterm, small for gestational age (SGA)

101. It is most important for the nurse to know the infant's gestational age and how it compares with the birth weight because:
① This information will help identify potential newborn problems
② The infant will lose 10% of birth weight the first few days of life
③ Evaluation and classification records are necessary for health insurance
④ This information must be documented on the admission record

102. After assessing the infant and determining that he is experiencing temperature instability, the nurse should:
① Assess him for signs of hyperglycemia and begin temperature stabilization
② Rapidly rewarm him over the next hour until his temperature is stabilized
③ Slowly rewarm him over the next several hours while closely observing the infant
④ Assess and record his skin temperature every hour until his temperature is stable

103. When Mrs. Marks sees the baby for the first time, she asks, "When will I be able to

breastfeed my baby?" The nurse's most appropriate response would be:
① "He is preterm and sucks weakly, so it will be several weeks before you may breastfeed."
② "Even though he is preterm, he is stable. You may try now if you would like."
③ "Preterm infants should not breastfeed. It takes more calories than bottle feeding."
④ "Pump your breasts now and then feed him the milk by bottle to conserve his energy."

Situation: Edith Jayce is a single 16-year-old high school dropout who is in the fourth month of pregnancy. She lives with her divorced mother and a younger sister. She works part time at a fast food restaurant and is underweight. She has been sexually active since age 15. The health department is providing prenatal care.

104. The nurse explains to Ms. Jayce that hormones play an important role in all phases of the reproductive process, from the production of the sperm and ova to the nourishment of the newborn. The nurse is aware that the corpus luteum secretes:
① Prolactin
② Oxytocin
③ Progesterone
④ Cortisol

105. Folic acid supplements are prescribed for Ms. Jayce. The nurse is aware that these are necessary to:
① Promote normal erythropoiesis
② Treat pernicious anemia
③ Prevent anaphylactic shock
④ Prevent erythroblastosis fetalis

106. Ms. Jayce complains of a foamy white discharge and painful intercourse, and is treated for *Trichomonas* vaginitis. The statement that best indicates to the nurse that Ms. Jayce has learned measures to prevent recurrence is, "I will:
① Douche immediately after sexual intercourse."
② Persuade my sexual partner to be treated."
③ Insert a vaginal suppository after intercourse."
④ Void immediately after intercourse."

107. Ms. Jayce comes to the hospital in active labor at 40 weeks gestation. A baby boy is delivered and given to his mother. After repair of the episiotomy the nurse notes a continuous trickle of blood from Ms. Jayce's vagina. Her fundus is firm and even with the umbilicus. The best nursing action is to:
① Massage the uterus
② Have Ms. Jayce void
③ Notify Ms. Jayce's physician
④ Monitor vital signs q 30 min

108. Ms. Jayce is now 12 hours postpartum. Before the nurse administers the prescribed drugs to Ms. Jayce, the client states that she is allergic to penicillin. Until the physician is contacted about Ms. Jayce's stated allergy, the nurse should hold her prescribed:
① Cephradine (Velosef)
② Casanthranol and docusate sodium (Peri-Colace)
③ Bromocriptine mesylate (Parlodel)
④ Methylergonovine maleate (Methergine)

109. Ms. Joyce confides that she hopes her baby will be good and sleep all night without crying. The nurse should plan to teach Ms. Jayce to:
① Cuddle the baby and talk softly when crying occurs
② Add cereal to the bedtime bottle to ensure deep sleep
③ Keep the baby awake for longer periods during the day
④ Put a soft cuddly toy next to the baby at bedtime

110. Ms. Jayce indicates correct understanding of postpartum discharge instructions when she states she will take her iron supplement with:
① Water
② Orange juice
③ Milk
④ Each meal

Situation: Arlene Charl is a 38-year-old primipara who successfully achieved pregnancy with Clomid therapy after 8 years of infertility. She is carrying twins and will deliver via elective cesarean under epidural anesthesia.

111. Mrs. Charl's preoperative teaching should include instructions that after cesarean delivery she can generally expect to:
① Be discharged between 7 and 10 days postpartum
② Be ambulating whenever she wants the day after surgery
③ Take sponge baths until the incision is completely healed
④ Need an enema to have an effective bowel movement

112. A statement by Mrs. Charl that indicates the nurse's teaching about stimulating the breastfeeding let-down reflex has been successful is, "I will:
① Apply warm moist packs and massage my breasts before each feeding."
② Wear a snug-fitting breast binder 24 hours a day."
③ Take a cool shower before each breastfeeding."
④ Drink at least 2 quarts of low-fat milk a day."

113. The best indication that a baby has correctly attached to the breast is when the:

① Baby sucks each breast vigorously for 5 minutes before falling asleep
② Baby's mouth covers most of the areolar surface
③ Baby's tongue is securely on top of the nipple
④ Baby makes frequent loud clucking sounds while nursing at each breast

114. The nurse tells Mrs. Charl that the best indication that her milk supply is adequate for the babies' growth and development is when the babies gain weight and:
① Awaken to feed every 4 hours
② Void six or more times a day
③ Have several hard stools daily
④ Rarely suck on a pacifier

115. The comment by Mrs. Charl on her fourth postpartum day that indicates a need for further assessment by the nurse is:
① "My lochia is bright red with small brown clots the size of my thumb."
② "I've been urinating large amounts ever since I delivered."
③ "My breasts feel full, heavy, and tingly before I feed the babies."
④ "I hope I'll be a good mother to these sweet babies."

Situation: Clint Shaw brings his pregnant wife Rose to the hospital because she had a sudden gush of vaginal bleeding. The physician diagnoses placenta previa. Mrs. Shaw is 35 weeks pregnant and is apprehensive about her baby. The physician's orders include nothing by mouth and complete bed rest.

116. The nurse knows that placenta previa occurs when:
① The placenta is not implanted securely in place on the uterine wall
② There is premature separation of a normally implanted placenta
③ There is premature aging of a placenta implanted in the uterine fundus
④ The placenta is implanted in the lower uterine segment covering part of the os

117. The nurse gently performs Leopold's maneuvers on Mrs. Shaw's abdomen. From the data, the nurse expects to find the:
① Fetal head firmly engaged
② Uterus hard and tetanically contracted
③ Fetal presenting part high and floating
④ Fetal small parts difficult to palpate

118. The nursing diagnosis that the nurse should consider in planning Mrs. Shaw's care is:
① Pain related to bleeding from placental tears
② Potential for infection related to placental location
③ Impaired skin integrity related to placental damage
④ Anticipatory grieving related to possible genetic birth defects

119. The best way for the nurse to assess the blood loss of a client with placenta previa is to:
① Monitor the pulse and blood pressure
② Check hemoglobin and hematocrit levels
③ Measure the height of the fundus
④ Count or weigh perineal pads

120. Mrs. Shaw is scheduled for an amniocentesis to determine fetal maturity. Both Mr. and Mrs. Shaw express nervousness about the baby's safety during the test. The nursing intervention that would best promote the parents' ability to cope is:
① Reassuring them that the procedure is safe
② Arranging for Mr. Shaw to be present during the test
③ Informing them about the procedure step by step
④ Initiating a parent-physician conference

121. Mrs. Shaw is to have an ultrasonogram to determine the location of the placenta. When preparing her for this procedure the nurse should:
① Insert an indwelling urinary catheter
② Cleanse her abdomen with a germicidal soap
③ Instruct her to drink two large glasses of water
④ Give a cleansing enema of 500 ml normal saline

122. The painless, bright red bleeding continues, and a vaginal examination is to be done by the physician. In preparation for this examination the nurse plans to:
① Attach the client to an internal monitor to closely watch the fetus' response
② Prepare a supply of ritodrine (Yutopar) in case early labor begins
③ Prepare for a double setup that includes equipment for a cesarean delivery
④ Have equipment ready for a fetal scalp pH after the examination

123. When the physician examines Mrs. Shaw vaginally, the nurse should have available:
① Two units of typed and cross-matched blood
② Vitamin K for intramuscular injection
③ One unit of freeze-dried plasma
④ Heparin sodium for intravenous injection

Situation: Violet Brow, a primigravida who is 11 weeks pregnant, comes to the prenatal clinic for her obstetric workup. Mrs. Brow's prepregnant weight falls within the range designated as appropriate for her height, body build, and age.

124. Mrs. Brow is to receive a tuberculin test as part of her obstetric workup. Before administering the tuberculin test, the most important information for the nurse to collect is whether or not Mrs. Brow has:
① Previously had a tuberculin test

② Ever had a positive tuberculin test

③ Had any serious respiratory diseases

④ A history of tuberculosis in the family

125. Before answering Mrs. Brow's questions about immunity, the nurse recalls that active immunity occurs when:

① Blood antigens are aided by phagocytes in defending the body against pathogens

② Protein antigens are formed in the blood to fight invading antibodies

③ Protein substances are formed by the body to destroy or neutralize antigens

④ Sensitized lymphocytes from an immune donor act as antibodies against invading pathogens

126. Mrs. Brow, now 42 weeks pregnant, comes to the emergency room complaining of back pain radiating to her abdomen and leaking of fluid for the last 4 hours. On physical assessment the nurse notes the following findings: contractions approximately every 3 to 4 minutes of moderate intensity with a 30 to 45 second duration; fetal heart tones 140 beats per minute in the right lower quadrant (RLQ); cervix 2 cm dilated and 70% effaced; presenting part floating; streaks of blood from the vagina; nitrazine test positive. The nurse is aware that the finding that indicates that a problem with delivery may occur is the:

① Fetal heart tones of 140 beats per minute in the RLQ

② Streaks of blood from the vagina

③ Presenting part is floating

④ Nitrazine test is positive

127. Twelve hours after Mrs. Brow is admitted to the hospital, she delivers a baby boy with Apgar scores of 8 and 9. On the baby's admission to the nursery, the nurse transporting him from the delivery room states, "It was a difficult delivery; he has wide shoulders." Based on this information, the nursery nurse's priority assessment would be to check for a normal:

① Moro reflex

② Stepping reflex

③ Babinski reflex

④ Plantar grasp

Situation: Myra Ames, 36 weeks pregnant, has been admitted to the antepartum unit with a diagnosis of pregnancy-induced hypertension. She is prescribed bed rest for 3 days.

128. The nurse should encourage the pregnant client prescribed bed rest to assume the:

① Supine position

② Semi-Fowler's position

③ Side-lying position

④ Slight Trendelenburg position

129. A nonstress test is scheduled for Mrs. Ames. The nurse explains that the nonstress test is a way of evaluating the condition of the fetus by comparing the fetal heart rate with:

① Maternal blood pressure

② Fetal gestational age

③ Maternal uterine contractions

④ Fetal physical activity

130. During the nonstress test the nurse should be aware that if nonperiodic accelerations of the fetal heart rate occur with fetal movement it most likely indicates:

① Head compression

② Uteroplacental insufficiency

③ Umbilical cord compression

④ Fetal well-being

131. Mrs. Ames' nonstress test is inconclusive, so an oxytocin challenge test (stress test) is scheduled. This test result is positive, indicating potential fetal distress. The nurse knows that this means that during uterine contractions the fetal heart rate showed:

① Normal baseline

② Early decelerations

③ Variable decelerations

④ Late decelerations

Situation: Mary Cook is admitted in early labor. She has had a normal prenatal course and is presently at 34 weeks gestation.

132. Mrs. Cook's labor progresses and she begins to experience severe back discomfort. She asks the nurse, "Can't I have a hypo for the pain?" The nurse's response is best guided by understanding that the use of analgesic medications during preterm labor is:

① Contraindicated at any time

② Reduced to a minimum

③ Based on the client's comfort level

④ Not influenced by fetal age

133. Mrs. Cook delivers a baby boy weighing 2300 g. His Apgar scores were 3 and 8 at 1 and 5 minutes respectively. These scores indicate that:

① Resuscitation was necessary and measures used were appropriate

② Oxygen under pressure would be necessary if the Apgar drops below 8

③ The preterm newborn was responding according to his gestational age

④ Respiratory stimulation will be needed for the first 24 hours

134. Baby Cook develops severe respiratory distress, and a diagnosis of respiratory distress syndrome (RDS) is made. Continuous positive-pressure ventilation therapy is initiated via an endotracheal tube. The nurse notes that Baby Boy Cook's breath sounds on the right side are diminished. He seems restless, and the point of maximum impulse (PMI) of his heartbeat is in the left axillary line. Interpretation of this assessment data should lead the nurse to understand that:

① These are normal findings because infants

with this disorder frequently have some degree of atelectasis

② The endotracheal tube has probably slipped into the left main stem bronchus and needs to be pulled back to ventilate both lungs

③ The inspiratory pressure on the ventilator is probably too low and needs to be increased for adequate ventilation

④ He may have a pneumothorax, and the physician should be contacted immediately so that treatment can be instituted

135. During Mrs. Cook's first visit to the neonatal intensive care nursery the nurse notes that she stands about 2 feet away from her son and does not touch him. Mrs. Cook's only comment to the nurse is, "He looks so fragile. Do you think he'll make it?" The most appropriate comment for the nurse to make would be:

① "The staff is confident, because all preterm babies look like this at first."

② "He is very small, but many babies born as small as he is have done just fine."

③ "I can understand that he looks fragile to you. What did the doctor tell you about his condition?"

④ "He's not as fragile as he might appear. You just need to get used to him, and then it won't be so frightening."

136. Mrs. Cook is visiting the neonatal intensive care unit when it is time for her baby's nasogastric feeding. As the nurse prepares to start the feeding, Mrs. Cook asks, "Would it hurt him to suck a pacifier during the feeding?" The nurse's most appropriate response would be:

① "It might tire him out because he's still so small. We don't want him to use up all his energy."

② "If he sucks on a pacifier a lot now he may have problems learning how to suck from a bottle later."

③ "There's no real benefit in using a pacifier, and there is a relationship between the use of a pacifier and buck teeth."

④ "Sucking on a pacifier during tube feedings may help him associate sucking with food so that he'll adjust better to bottle feedings."

Situation: At 40 weeks gestation, Bertha Horn is admitted to the labor room in active labor. She is complaining of severe pain with each contraction.

137. The physician orders meperidine hydrochloride (Demerol) and promethazine (Phenergan) prn for pain. Mrs. Horn asks why she is getting Phenergan. The nurse explains that this drug:

① Reverses the analgesic effects of Demerol

② Decreases the analgesic effects of Demerol

③ Potentiates the analgesic effects of Demerol

④ Initiates the analgesic effects of Demerol

138. Mrs. Horn delivered a baby girl and is now 6 hours postpartum. Before giving the ordered medications, the nurse assesses Mrs. Horn and notes the following findings: BP 178/110; TPR 98/60/18; fundus firm, one fingerbreadth below umbilicus; episiotomy edematous, red, and approximated; one Peri-pad saturated with lochia rubra in 6 hours. In light of the assessment findings, the nurse should contact the physician before administering:

① Cephradine (Velosef)

② Hydrocortisone acetate (Epifoam)

③ Methylergonovine maleate (Methergine)

④ Casanthranol and docusate sodium (Peri-Colace)

Situation: A nurse works with a group of teenage girls from 13 to 17 years of age in a community center. The nurse encourages the girls to ask questions that concern them.

139. Lisa Baker, 13 years old, has been menstruating for about 2 years and complains of having some mild upper abdominal pain between each period. The nurse understands that this:

① Requires immediate medical attention

② Usually occurs when menses first begins

③ Will disappear when ovulation is well established

④ Is a common occurrence known as mittelschmerz

140. Diane Stull, age 16, has a steady boyfriend and is having sexual relations with him. She is seeking advice as to how she can protect herself from contracting AIDS. The nurse advises her to:

① Make certain their relationship is monogamous

② Have her partner withdraw before ejaculating

③ Have her partner use a condom during sexual activity

④ Seek counseling about various contraceptive methods

141. Carmela Uzzo tells the nurse that her sister had a tubal pregnancy about 3 months ago and she had to have a tube removed. The nurse knows that Carmela needs further explanation about this when Carmela states:

① "I guess I'll have to wait a while to become an aunt."

② "This kind of thing can happen to my sister again."

③ "This kind of thing can happen after a pelvic infection."

④ "My sister is lucky because she'll never have a period again."

142. Margaret Wilson tells the group that her mother complains about having dysmenor-

rhea and asks the nurse what this means. The nurse should describe dysmenorrhea as:
① Spotting between menstrual periods
② Uterine pain with menstruation
③ Abnormal vaginal bleeding
④ Cessation of menstruation

143. The nurse would know that one of the students did not understand the teaching about fetal growth and development when she states:
① "The fetus gets food from the amniotic fluid."
② "There are two umbilical arteries and one vein."
③ "The mother must observe proper nutrition."
④ "The baby's oxygen needs are provided for by the mother."

Situation: Sigrid Sens has come to the prenatal clinic in her second month of pregnancy for her first visit.

144. Mrs. Sens tells the nurse that her mother told her she should not take tub baths during pregnancy because she will get an infection. The nurse should tell Mrs. Sens that tub bathing:
① Is permitted through late pregnancy
② Is not recommended during pregnancy
③ Makes the pregnant woman prone to infections
④ Is permitted only during the first trimester

145. An ultrasound examination is ordered for Mrs. Sens. This test is used primarily to:
① Rule out congenital defects
② Estimate fetal age
③ Detect mental retardation
④ Approximate fetal linear growth

146. Mrs. Sens, now 34 weeks pregnant, begins to experience contractions. To halt the preterm labor, Mrs. Sens is started on a ritodrine hydrochloride (Yutopar) infusion. The nurse is aware that an expected side effect of this drug is:
① Hypotension
② Bradycardia
③ Hypertonic uterine contractions
④ Difficulty falling asleep

147. Mrs. Sens has indicated to the physician that she desires anesthesia but wants to participate in her delivery. The nurse is aware that a type of anesthetic block that will provide perineal anesthesia but allow her to feel her contractions and push during the delivery is a:
① Pudendal block
② Paracervical block
③ Saddle block
④ Epidural block

148. At 38 weeks Mrs. Sens comes to the hospital in labor. During the transition phase the nurse should be concerned primarily with:

① Monitoring uterine contractions
② Assessing the client's vital signs
③ Monitoring intake and output
④ Helping the client maintain control

149. Mrs. Sens delivers a healthy infant. She is bottle feeding the baby. During postpartal care, the nurse discusses breast care with Mrs. Sens. The nurse plans further teaching when Mrs. Sens states:
① "How should I apply heat to my breast to help my milk dry up?"
② "I must call my husband and ask him to bring my new brassiere."
③ "The discomfort I am feeling will go away in a couple of days."
④ "May I have my medication for this discomfort in my breasts?"

150. Mrs. Sens asks the nurse how human milk compares with cow's milk. The information given to Mrs. Sens should include the following:
① Lactose content is significantly higher in cow's milk
② Protein content of human milk is higher than that of cow's milk
③ Fat in human milk is easier to digest and absorb than that in cow's milk
④ Immunologic and antiallergic factors are now found in cow's milk

Situation: Ann Morales is an 18-year-old gravida I, para I single mother with a history of alcohol abuse during her pregnancy. She begins labor at 30 weeks gestation and is admitted to the labor and delivery unit. She is immediately moved to the delivery room where she spontaneously delivers a baby girl.

151. The nurse notes that baby Morales' heart rate is 86 beats per minute, and she has slow, irregular respirations. She grimaces in response to suctioning, is cyanotic, and has flaccid muscle tone. The nurse should assign the infant an Apgar score of:
① 2
② 3
③ 4
④ 5

152. When assessing Baby Morales the nurse notes the following findings: arms and legs slightly flexed; skin smooth and transparent; abundant lanugo on the back; slow recoil of pinna; few sole creases. In light of these findings, the care plan for Baby Morales should include nursing orders to monitor her for:
① Polycythemia
② Hyperglycemia
③ Postmaturity syndrome
④ Respiratory distress syndrome

153. The nurse caring for a 30 week appropriate for gestational age (AGA) neonate such as Baby Morales establishes the following list of potential interventions for the baby. The one that should receive the highest priority is:
① Supporting body temperature

② Maintaining respirations
③ Preventing infection
④ Promoting bonding

154. The nurse recognizes that survival in the neonatal period is largely related to:
① Parental health habits and social class
② Gestational age and birth weight
③ Timing and adequacy of prenatal care
④ Reproductive history of the mother

155. During the first week of life, Baby Morales experiences several episodes of periodic apnea. An apnea monitor is used and sounds an alarm 10 seconds after cessation of respirations. The nurse should respond first by:
① Assessing skin color and respirations
② Using tactile stimuli on the chest or extremities
③ Checking the device for signs of malfunction
④ Resuscitating with a face mask and Ambu-bag

156. Baby Morales is started on digoxin (Lanoxin) and furosemide (Lasix) for persistant patent ductus arteriosus. The nursing assessment that would provide the best indication that the Lasix is effective is that:
① The fontanels are depressed
② The pedal edema is reduced
③ Urine output exceeds intake
④ There are no signs of digitalis toxicity

157. Ms. Morales has been participating in her daughter's care for several days in preparation for the baby's discharge. On the last hospital day, Ms. Morales comes to the unit with alcohol on her breath and her speech is slurred. The nurse's most appropriate action would be to:
① Talk with Ms. Morales about her condition and assess her willingness to participate in an alternate plan for discharge
② Avoid confrontation by asking Ms. Morales to wait in the hospital lobby and calling the physician to cancel the discharge order
③ Continue with the discharge procedure, alerting the home health nurse that immediate follow up is needed for Ms. Morales
④ Speak openly to Ms. Morales about her condition and have her see a social worker about discharge to a foster home

Situation: Krista Hanover, 4 months pregnant, complains of fatigue and anorexia. Her hemoglobin indicates iron-deficiency anemia, and ferrous sulfate 300 mg daily is prescribed.

158. To increase iron absorption, the nurse should suggest that Mrs. Hanover eat foods high in:
① Vitamin B complex
② Vitamin C
③ Water content
④ Fat content

159. The nurse is aware that absorption of drugs taken orally during pregnancy may be decreased as the result of:
① Decreased glomerular filtration rate
② Delayed emptying of gastric contents
③ Developing fetal-placental circulation
④ Increased secretion of hydrochloric acid

160. An ultrasound is ordered for Mrs. Hanover. In addition to measuring fetal age, the ultrasound of the fetus can identify:
① Mental retardation
② Biliary atresia
③ Spina bifida
④ Cleft palate

161. Mrs. Hanover is now 32 weeks pregnant. During an antepartal visit, she reveals that a recent sexual contact has gonorrhea. Probenecid (Benemid) is added to therapy with penicillin. The nurse knows that Mrs. Hanover understands the instructions when she states that the probenecid will:
① "Activate my immune defense mechanisms."
② "Minimize any allergy to penicillin."
③ "Increase the penicillin in my blood."
④ "Reduce the side effects of the disease."

162. Mrs. Hanover tells the nurse that she has taken tetracycline (Achromycin) on other occasions and would prefer to take it now. The nurse should tell Mrs. Hanover that tetracycline is avoided in the treatment of infections in pregnant women because it:
① Increases the baby's tolerance to the drug
② Produces allergies to the drug in the baby
③ Permanently stains the baby's teeth
④ Adversely affects breastfeeding

Situation: Accompanied by her husband, Joan Carey—gravida II, para I—is admitted in early labor.

163. As the nurse inspects her perineum, Mrs. Carey suddenly turns pale and says that she feels as if she is going to faint, although she is lying flat on her back. The nurse should:
① Elevate her head
② Elevate her feet
③ Start oxygen and IV fluids
④ Turn her on her left side

164. During labor Mrs. Carey begins to experience dizziness and tingling of her hands. The nurse tells Mr. Carey to instruct his wife to:
① Hold her breath with the next contraction
② Breathe into her cupped hands or a paper bag
③ Use a fast deep-breathing pattern
④ Pant during the next three contractions

165. Mrs. Carey has been in labor for 4 hours and her cervix is 5 cm dilated. She had been having good contractions until the past 30 minutes, when her contractions gradually became irregular and of fair quality. In caring for her the nurse should first check her for:
① Uterine dysfunction
② False labor

③ A full bladder

④ A breech presentation

166. In assessing Mrs. Carey for signs that the transitional phase is beginning, the nurse would expect her to have:
    ① Bulging of the perineum
    ② Crowning of the fetal head
    ③ Pinkish vaginal discharge
    ④ Rectal pressure during contractions

167. After delivering a baby boy, Mrs. Carey, who is not nursing, is taught how to care for her engorged breasts. The nurse realizes Mrs. Carey does not understand the teaching when she states:
    ① "I'm expressing milk from my breasts every 3 to 4 hours."
    ② "I'm wearing a well-fitting, tight brassiere."
    ③ "I do not let warm water run over my breasts when showering."
    ④ "I am drinking 2 quarts of fluid every 24 hours."

Situation: Sheila Elkind is 8 weeks pregnant and has many questions about her nutritional needs during pregnancy. She is 5 feet 3 inches tall and weighs 125 pounds.

168. The nurse is aware that, to fall within the recommended weight gain during pregnancy, at term, Mrs. Elkind should weigh about:
    ① 130 pounds
    ② 135 pounds
    ③ 140 pounds
    ④ 150 pounds

169. The nurse instructs Mrs. Elkind to increase her protein intake by at least:
    ① 15 grams
    ② 30 grams
    ③ 60 grams
    ④ 90 grams

170. Mrs. Elkind is curious about when the fetus gains the most weight. She is told by the nurse that fetal weight gain is:
    ① Greatest during the first trimester
    ② Equally distributed throughout pregnancy
    ③ Begun in the second trimester
    ④ Most marked in the third trimester

Situation: Florence Scott is admitted to the labor room at 39 weeks gestation. The nurse assesses that the baby is in the left breech position.

171. The nurse places the fetal heart transducer on Mrs. Scott's abdomen in the:
    ① Left upper quadrant
    ② Midline of the lower quadrant
    ③ Right lower quadrant
    ④ Left lower quadrant

172. Mrs. Scott is in the transitional phase of labor (8 cm dilation). Mr. Scott, who is coaching his wife, demonstrates understanding of this stage when with each contraction he instructs his wife to:
    ① Take cleansing breaths and push
    ② Take quick shallow breaths and blow
    ③ Use slow, rhythmic diaphragmatic breathing
    ④ Switch from accelerated to decelerated breathing

173. Mrs. Scott's membranes rupture spontaneously. The nurse notes fresh meconium in the vaginal introitus and realizes that this:
    ① Is a normal occurrence in breech presentations
    ② Requires immediate notification of the physician
    ③ Indicates that the cord will prolapse
    ④ Is evidence of impending fetal distress

174. Baby Scott is delivered without the aid of forceps. He is active and crying lustily, but the bottoms of his feet have a marked bluish tinge. His Apgar score at 1 minute will probably be:
    ① 3
    ② 5
    ③ 7
    ④ 9

Situation: Yvonne Bradshaw, age 34, who has a history of two spontaneous abortions, comes to the prenatal clinic with a history of amenorrhea for the past 3 months, enlarged breasts, and nausea every morning. Her blood work reveals that she is Rh negative.

175. During a prenatal visit the nurse explains to Mrs. Bradshaw that RhoGAM will be administered:
    ① Within 72 hours after delivery if her infant is found to be Rh positive
    ② To her infant immediately after delivery if the Coombs' test is positive
    ③ Weekly during the ninth month because this is her third pregnancy
    ④ During the second trimester if an amniocentesis indicates a problem

176. An article about toxoplasmosis in the local newspaper prompts Mrs. Bradshaw to ask the nurse for more information about this problem in pregnancy. The nurse teaches her that:
    ① Toxoplasmosis is a disease that is prevalent just in foreign countries
    ② Pork and beef should be properly cooked before eating
    ③ Raw shellfish are intermediary hosts and should be avoided during pregnancy
    ④ Eating salads with mayonnaise should be avoided during the summer

177. Because of her high-risk status, Mrs. Bradshaw has a nonstress test. When the test is nonreactive, an oxytocin challenge test (OCT) is ordered. The nurse understands that this test, which uses Pitocin, would not be done if Mrs. Bradshaw had:

① Vaginal bleeding
② Sickling of the red cells
③ Blurred vision
④ Increasing hypertension

178. Mrs. Bradshaw delivers a full-term healthy male child. Before her discharge Mrs. Bradshaw asks the nurse for contraceptive information. The nurse, as part of the teaching plan on contraception, tells Mrs. Bradshaw that:
① No sperm can reach the ovum if the man uses coitus interruptus and withdraws before ejaculation
② Individuals using periodic abstinence should have intercourse on days when the woman has a rise in temperature
③ The rim of the condom must be held in place during removal of the penis from the vagina
④ Diaphragms are equally effective whether or not the partners choose to use spermicidal creams

Situation: Arlene Dannon is 17 years old and is 36 weeks pregnant. When she comes to the prenatal clinic she is found to have mild pregnancy-induced hypertension. The physician plans to treat her on an outpatient basis.

179. Although the exact cause of pregnancy-induced hypertension is unknown, the nurse knows that it is often associated with:
① A limited amount of calories
② A vitamin deficiency
③ An inadequate intake of protein
④ An inability to absorb minerals

180. When providing health teaching concerning pregnancy-induced hypertension, a therapeutic instruction that the nurse should give Mrs. Dannon is:
① Rest frequently in the side-lying position
② Eat a sodium-free diet
③ Limit fluid intake to 1000 ml a day
④ Walk at least a mile a day

181. Mrs. Dannon's physical status gets progressively worse and she is admitted to the high-risk prenatal unit at the local community hospital. During the admitting history and physical assessment the nurse should expect to find:
① Difficulty in breathing
② Vaginal spotting
③ Blood pressure of 130/80
④ Proteinuria of 3+

182. The physician orders large doses of magnesium sulfate. To evaluate the therapeutic effectiveness of this therapy, the nurse should assess for:
① Excessive urinary output
② Absent deep tendon reflexes
③ A decreased respiratory rate
④ An increase in blood pressure

183. The nurse encourages Mrs. Dannon to lie in the left lateral recumbent position because it maximizes:
① Uterine and kidney perfusion and relieves compression of the major vessels
② Intraabdominal pressure on the iliac veins and increases blood in the pelvic area
③ Hemoconcentration, reduces blood volume and cardiac output, and increases placental perfusion
④ Aortic compression, decreases uterine arterial pressure, and increases uterine blood flow

Situation: After missing two periods, Natalie Greene, a Class B diabetic who is pregnant for the first time, comes to the high-risk OB clinic.

184. The nurse knows that diabetic women who become pregnant:
① Require intensive and thorough prenatal care
② Have decreased insulin requirements
③ Have 30% or higher fetal mortality
④ Should have their babies by cesarean delivery

185. A primary long-term goal for the pregnant diabetic client such as Mrs. Greene is to:
① Minimize the amount of insulin given
② Keep blood sugar levels stable
③ Minimize dietary fluctuations
④ Deliver an optimally healthy baby

186. In the thirty-seventh week of gestation, an L/S ratio done on Mrs. Greene's amniotic fluid indicates adequate fetal lung maturity. Based on this information the nurse assesses that:
① The baby will have to be delivered immediately
② The baby should be free from major respiratory problems
③ Labor will probably be induced very shortly
④ There will be no need for further fetal monitoring

187. Mrs. Greene is now in late active labor and is experiencing severe back pain. The best nursing intervention at this time is:
① Instructing her to increase her effleurage and relaxation exercises
② Placing her in a supine position, using pillows for sacral support
③ Assisting her to walk about the room until her membranes rupture
④ Applying external pressure manually in the area of the lower back

188. It is the first day postpartum for Mrs. Greene, and her baby is rooming in. She asks the nurse to take the baby to the nursery and only bring the baby back for feedings. The best response by the nurse would be:
① "All right Mrs. Greene, I'll inform the nursery nurses."

② "Oh, you must be tired; I'll bring her back at feeding time."

③ "It seems like you have changed your mind about rooming in."

④ "I think you are having difficulties caring for the baby."

189. Mrs. Greene asks the nurse about birth-control methods. When counseling the diabetic client who requests contraceptive information, it would be most therapeutic for the nurse to focus on:
① Oral contraceptives
② The IUD
③ Rhythm
④ A diaphragm

Situation: Ann David is admitted to the labor room in active labor with her second child. On inspection of the perineum, the umbilical cord is observed outside the vagina.

190. After observing the prolapsed cord, the first action of the nurse should be to:
① Start oxygen at 2 L per minute via a face mask
② Check the fetal heart rate every 15 minutes
③ Cover the cord with a sterile moist dressing
④ Gently replace the cord in the vaginal vault

191. A 6 lb 10 oz baby girl is born by cesarean delivery. When the nurse brings her to be breastfed, Mrs. David asks if she may drink a small glass of wine to help her relax. The nurse's best response would be:
① "I'm sure that drinking one glass of wine would not cause any harm."
② "You seem a little tense. Tell me about your past breastfeeding experiences."
③ "I'm sure a glass of wine would be okay, but you had better check with your doctor."
④ "Yes, it's relaxing, but I do think you should find another, better way to relax."

192. A few weeks after discharge Mrs. David develops mastitis and telephones for advice concerning breastfeeding. The nurse should tell her to:
① Pump her breast and wear a tight-fitting bra to suppress milk production
② Start to wean the baby from the breast because it will reduce the pain
③ Breastfeed often because this will keep the breasts empty and reduce pain
④ Get an antibiotic from the physician and start the baby on bottle feedings

Situation: Ruth and Bart Trent have just completed a Lamaze course in preparation for the birth of their first child. They arrive at the hospital with Mrs. Trent in active labor. Mr. Trent will be assisting his wife during the birth.

193. The nurse realizes Mr. Trent has successfully learned his role when during the early phase of labor he is observed assisting his wife to:
① Pant-blow breathe
② Accelerate-decelerate breathe
③ Shallow chest breathe
④ Slow chest breathe

194. Leopold's maneuvers are performed to determine the position of Mrs. Trent's baby. In assessing Mrs. Trent the nurse notes the presence of a firm round prominence over the pubic symphysis, a smooth convex structure down her right side, irregular lumps down her left side, and a soft roundness in the fundus. The nurse should conclude that the fetal position is:
① RSA
② LOA
③ LOP
④ ROA

195. When Mrs. Trent experiences the urge to push at 9 cm dilation, the breathing pattern the nurse should remind the Trents to use is:
① Panting or blowing
② Slow chest
③ Accelerated-decelerated
④ Expulsion

196. Mrs. Trent's membranes rupture spontaneously. The nurse observes the umbilical cord protruding from the vagina. The nursing action that receives the highest priority in this situation is:
① Administering oxygen by mask
② Auscultating the fetal heart tones
③ Raising the foot of the bed
④ Preparing for a cesarean delivery

197. Mrs. Trent delivers a healthy baby girl. Twelve hours after delivery Mrs. Trent's temperature is 100.4° F. This elevation is most likely an indication of:
① Mastitis
② Dehydration
③ Puerperal infection
④ Urinary tract infection

Situation: Millie Borg, 16 years old, comes to the adolescent clinic concerned that she has missed a menstrual period. She is 7 days overdue. She has been sexually active for the past year with several partners, some of whom she has known only casually. She also gives a history of smoking and drug and alcohol use on a regular basis. Her health history reveals that she was maintained on a low-phenylalanine diet until she was 9 years old.

198. The nurse is aware that babies born to very young mothers are at risk for neglect or abuse because adolescents characteristically:
① Do not plan for their pregnancies
② Resent having to give constant care to the baby
③ Cannot anticipate the baby's needs
④ Are involved in seeking their own identity

199. Ms. Borg is pregnant. Considering Ms. Borg's history of phenylketonuria, the nurse teaches her that:
① The baby will probably be mentally retarded because of her history of PKU
② Reinstitution of the low-phenylalanine diet will protect her baby from PKU
③ The fetus is at no risk prenatally but will require immediate care at birth to prevent PKU
④ She should avoid phenylalanine even when not pregnant so that her body is able to support a pregnancy

200. Ms. Borg's baby girl is tested for phenylketonuria immediately after birth. This is done primarily to prevent:
① Growth retardation
② Failure to thrive
③ Mental retardation
④ Spread of the disease

201. The child with PKU has a characteristic urinary odor best described as:
① Mousy or musty
② Aromatic or pungent
③ Fishy
④ Ammoniacal

202. The effect PKU has on development will depend on:
① Diagnosis within the first 3 days after birth
② The level of phenylalanine in the blood at birth
③ Compliance with a corrective diet and how early it is instituted
④ The presence of phenylpyruvic acid in the urine at 1 week of age

Situation: Baby Tommy Jones was delivered at term by a cesarean delivery because of cephalopelvic disproportion. In the nursery Tommy is assessed as a healthy newborn.

203. While observing Tommy during sleep, the nurse notes periods of irregular breathing and occasional twitching movements of his arms and legs. His heart rate is 150 per minute and his respiratory rate is 50 per minute. The glucose test strip reading 1 hour ago was 60 mg/100 ml. The most appropriate assessment would be:
① The baby requires no intervention; all findings are normal.
② The baby's blood sugar is low; twitching movements suggest hypoglycemia
③ The rapid respiratory rate and irregular breathing suggest respiratory distress
④ The twitching movements suggest the baby may be having seizures

204. When Tommy is 2 days old his parents ask the nurse whether they should have him circumcised. The nurse's most appropriate response would be:
① "It would probably be a good idea because circumcision is known to prevent penile cancer."
② "That's something you both will have to decide after you discuss it thoroughly with your doctor."
③ "I'm sure you have discussed this with your doctor, but let's discuss the benefits and risks of circumcision."
④ "The Academy of Pediatrics recommends that circumcision not be done routinely because of the risks associated with the procedure."

Situation: Lenore Carr, 40 weeks pregnant, is admitted to the labor room with ruptured membranes for 12 hours and a few irregular contractions. An oxytocin (Pitocin) induction is started and she is placed on a fetal monitor.

205. The physician's order states: add 10 units of Pitocin to 1000 ml of D5W and administer 0.01 units per minute. The IV setup has a drop factor of 60 gtt/ml. To administer the correct amount of medication the nurse should set the flow rate at:
① 20 gtt/min
② 40 gtt/min
③ 60 gtt/min
④ 80 gtt/min

206. Aware of the adverse effects of the oxytocin drug, the nurse should observe Mrs. Carr for:
① Contractions occurring more frequently than every 2 minutes
② A fetal heart rate of 120 to 150 beats per minute
③ Contractions with a duration of 30 seconds
④ Intrauterine pressure of 60 mm Hg

207. It is important for the nurse to assess the character of Mrs. Carr's amniotic fluid to prepare for potential:
① Prolapsed cord
② Abruptio placentae
③ Placenta previa
④ Maternal sepsis

208. On observing a deceleration in the fetal heart rate, the nurse should first:
① Administer oxygen
② Place the mother on her left side
③ Check the blood pressure
④ Discontinue the oxytocin infusion

209. Mrs. Carr has a paracervical block for delivery. Aware of the risk most often associated with administration of paracervical block, the nurse should observe for:
① Aspiration of stomach contents
② Maternal hypertension
③ Fetal bradycardia
④ Maternal respiratory paralysis

210. Twelve hours after delivery Mrs. Carr's blood pressure is 160/90 and she is prescribed magnesium sulfate. Before administering magne-

sium sulfate the nurse should assess her:
① Clinitest, Acetest, and specific gravity
② Temperature, blood pressure, and respirations
③ Urinary output, respirations, and patellar reflexes
④ Level of consciousness, funduscopic appearance, and knee reflex

Situation: Molly Davis is pregnant for the second time. Mrs. Davis' first infant died of sudden infant death syndrome (SIDS) at 2 months of age. Mrs. Davis expresses concern that the same thing may happen to the child she is now carrying.

211. Mrs. Davis asks the nurse if the risk of having another infant die from SIDS is increased because her first child died of SIDS. The nurse should inform Mrs. Davis that a subsequent sibling of a SIDS infant is at:
① Greater risk for SIDS than is the general population
② Lower risk for SIDS than is the general population
③ No particular risk for the development of SIDS
④ The same risk for SIDS as is the general population

212. After an uncomplicated labor, Mrs. Davis delivers a baby boy under epidural anesthesia. Baby Davis, who is 12 hours old, is experiencing respiratory distress and is to be transferred to a regional neonatal intensive care unit. The nursing action that would best promote parent-infant attachment would be:
① Encouraging Mr. and Mrs. Davis to call their infant by name
② Allowing Mr. and Mrs. Davis to hold their infant before departure
③ Helping Mr. and Mrs. Davis to phone the neonatal intensive care unit daily
④ Giving Mr. and Mrs. Davis a picture of their infant in the intensive care unit

213. Baby Davis improves and is to be discharged. On the day of his discharge, the nurse enters the nursery dressing room and finds Mrs. Davis crying. Before the nurse can say anything, Mrs. Davis states, "I know I should not be crying but I have to work. I know my baby will suffer in a day-care center without me." The best response by the nurse would be:
① "No ill effects have been noted when children are placed in high-quality day-care centers."
② "Only a few children suffer mentally from being placed in a high-quality day-care center."
③ "Motor development is advanced in children attending day-care centers."
④ "Children fare better when taken to a sitter's home for care."

Situation: Catherine Martinez, an active and healthy 23-year-old, is in her first pregnancy. She and her husband are both concerned that she have the necessary nutritional support.

214. The nurse knows that Mrs. Martinez understands the need to increase her intake of complete proteins of high biologic value during her pregnancy when she reports she is eating more:
① Milk, eggs, and cheese
② Whole grains and breads
③ Beans, peas, and lentils
④ Nuts and seeds

215. Mrs. Martinez' increased need for vitamin A to meet rapid tissue growth during pregnancy may be met by using increased amounts of such foods as:
① Nonfat milk
② Extra egg whites
③ Carrots
④ Citrus fruits

216. Following an uneventful pregnancy, Mrs. Martinez delivers a 9 lb 9 oz, male infant. Thirty minutes after her admission to the recovery room, her uterus is relaxed and her lochia is excessive. The first action by the nurse, after discovering Mrs. Martinez' excessive bleeding, should be to:
① Elevate the foot of her bed
② Check her vital signs
③ Massage her uterus and expel any clots
④ Immediately notify her physician

217. Mrs. Martinez has decided to breastfeed her baby and asks the nurse about her diet needs. The nurse can best respond:
① "Just eat as you have been doing during your pregnancy."
② "You'll need greater amounts of the same foods you've been eating and more fluids."
③ "Just drink a lot of milk; you need the calcium to make your own milk."
④ "Don't worry about it, your body will produce the amount of milk your baby needs."

218. Mrs. Martinez' nipples become sore and cracked. The best intervention for Mrs. Martinez would be to:
① Remove the baby from the breast for a few days
② Expose her nipples to air several times a day
③ Give her an analgesic medication as ordered
④ Apply continuous ice packs to her nipples

Situation: Sylvia Drewer, a 37-year-old college professor, comes to the gynecology clinic. She has been unable to conceive after 4 years of unprotected intercourse. Mrs. Drewer says she has generally enjoyed good health; however, lately she has been experiencing headaches with pain radiating down the back of the neck. The physical examination reveals a blood pressure of 172/110.

219. Mrs. Drewer is requested to monitor her basal temperature for 5 months and is told to limit salt intake. The health professionals are:
    ① Encouraging self-responsibility
    ② Overlooking the hypertension
    ③ Not helping Mrs. Drewer
    ④ Avoiding the major problem

220. Five months after the first visit Mrs. Drewer returns to the clinic. Her blood pressure is 150/100. The nurse tells Mrs. Drewer to prepare for a Papanicolaou test. Mrs. Drewer replies, "I don't want to be examined today. I want to talk with the doctor." The nurse should:
    ① Encourage Mrs. Drewer to comply with clinic procedures
    ② Recognize that Mrs. Drewer is uncooperative
    ③ Inform the gynecologist of Mrs. Drewer's request
    ④ Remind Mrs. Drewer of the importance of cancer detection

221. Mrs. Drewer's temperature charts indicate that she is ovulating. Her menstrual cycle is normal. The client again requests fertility drugs. The nurse should recognize that:
    ① Mrs. Drewer has a right to receive this drug
    ② Mr. Drewer's semen should be examined first
    ③ Mrs. Drewer will require an endometrial biopsy
    ④ Mrs. Drewer will need to have a culdoscopy

222. At the next visit, Mrs. Drewer's blood pressure is 154/98. During the past month she has lost 8 pounds. The client states that she is using self-control strategies to reduce her blood pressure and weight. The nurse should:
    ① Acknowledge Mrs. Drewer's achievement and encourage the continuation of the client's action program
    ② Point out to Mrs. Drewer that her action program is inadequate, because her blood pressure remains abnormal
    ③ Encourage Mrs. Drewer to take antihypertensive drugs until her blood pressure is reduced to normal limits
    ④ Emphasize the importance of Mrs. Drewer's exercising in addition to the reduction of sodium and calories

Situation: Cindi Waxe, gravida II, para I, gave birth to a preterm infant 14 hours ago via cesarean delivery.

223. On the first postpartum day, a major goal of nursing intervention for Mrs. Waxe would be:
    ① Relieving gaseous distention
    ② Promoting dietary intake
    ③ Relieving postoperative pain
    ④ Promoting bowel function

224. After the Foley catheter is removed, Mrs. Waxe has difficulty voiding. The nurse can best evaluate if Mrs. Waxe has emptied her bladder by:
    ① Asking her if she still feels the urge to void
    ② Catheterizing her for residual urine
    ③ Measuring the amount of urine she has voided
    ④ Palpating her bladder for distention

225. Infant Waxe has respiratory distress syndrome. A nursing intervention for infants with this diagnosis is to:
    ① Observe carefully for possible congenital birth defects
    ② Set Isolette temperature at 85° F to prevent shivering
    ③ Promote respiratory efforts with careful positioning
    ④ Avoid handling to minimize overstimulation and conserve O_2

226. Mrs. Waxe is told by her pediatrician that her baby also has a maternal-fetal blood group incompatibility. Mrs. Waxe asks the nurse what blood types would result in this condition. The nurse informs Mrs. Waxe that an ABO incompatibility most commonly arises when the mother is:
    ① Type A
    ② Type B
    ③ Type O
    ④ Type AB

Situation: Ellen Woods, 39 weeks pregnant, awakens with heavy, bright red painless vaginal bleeding. Her physician advises her to go to the hospital. She is admitted with a diagnosis of possible placenta previa.

227. The nurse is aware that the client most likely to be predisposed to placenta previa would be a:
    ① 19-year-old, gravida 1, para 0
    ② 25-year-old, gravida 2, para 1
    ③ 40-year-old, gravida 2, para 1
    ④ 30-year-old, gravida 6, para 5

228. The labor room nurse instructs and coaches Mrs. Woods about the importance of:
    ① Keeping all movement to a minimum to diminish bleeding
    ② Remaining on her back to minimize pressure on the cervix
    ③ Lying on her side to avoid putting pressure on the vena cava
    ④ Breathing deeply to ensure that the fetus gets oxygen

229. An important nursing action in the care of Mrs. Woods during labor is:

① Evaluation of external blood loss by pad count
② Frequent vaginal and rectal examinations
③ Assessment of fetal heart tones by fetoscope
④ Monitoring of the height of the fundus

230. To allay some of the concerns that Mrs. Woods has about placenta previa and the baby, the nurse should tell her that:
① With a very aggressive approach the infant morbidity is almost nonexistent
② Infant mortality from placenta previa is less than maternal mortality
③ There is little danger to mother or child as long as the physician's orders are followed
④ With conservative therapy, the dangers to mother and infant are greatly decreased

231. After birth, Baby Woods' Apgar score is 4, and 5 minutes later it is 6. The nurse should be aware that:
① The infant is probably hypoglycemic
② The infant is in immediate danger
③ There is a chance the infant may be neurologically impaired
④ There is an immediate need to resuscitate the infant

Situation: Dena Makowitz, age 36, is pregnant with her second child. Her first child has Down's syndrome and is now 4 years old. She is scheduled for a sonogram and amniocentesis in the physician's office.

232. When Mrs. Makowitz arrives for her scheduled visit she is extremely nervous. While undressing she anxiously says, "I don't know what I'll do if this baby has Down's too. Do you think abortion is the same as killing?" The nurse's best response would be:
① "No, I don't think so, but it's your decision to make."
② "Some people think this is what an abortion is."
③ "I really can't answer that question. You seem ambivalent about abortion."
④ "I don't want to answer that question at this time. How do you feel about it?"

233. Mrs. Makowitz is to have a sonogram followed by an amniocentesis. The nurse should direct Mrs. Makowitz to void:
① Just before each procedure is begun
② After the first sonogram tracing is obtained
③ At least 1 hour before the procedures are scheduled to begin
④ After the sonogram is completed and before the amniocentesis is begun

234. Before the amniocentesis the nurse should:
① Obtain an informed consent from Mrs. Makowitz
② Perform a vaginal examination to assess cervical dilation

③ Initiate the intravenous therapy as ordered by the physician
④ Inform Mrs. Makowitz that the procedure could precipitate an infection

Situation: Rebecca Ewing is 28 weeks pregnant and has gained 13 pounds. She tells the nurse in the antepartum clinic that she's glad that she has not gained as much weight as her sister did during her pregnancy.

235. An appropriate response by the nurse to Mrs. Ewing's comment would be:
① "Are you trying to watch your figure?"
② "Tell me what you have been eating lately."
③ "You have to eat right during pregnancy."
④ "Do you think you are getting fat?"

236. An iron deficiency is identified. In counseling Mrs. Ewing, the nurse teaches her that iron use is more efficient when she takes her iron supplement:
① At bedtime
② At mealtime
③ With orange juice
④ With a milkshake

237. Mrs. Ewing is admitted to the labor room in her thirty-ninth week of pregnancy with 2 to 3 minutes between contractions that last from 70 to 90 seconds. She complains of rectal pressure. The nurse should:
① Attach an external fetal heart monitor
② Inspect the perineum for bulging
③ Ask if her membranes have ruptured
④ Determine when labor began

238. Baby Ewing is born with an Apgar score of 3 at 1 minute. The nurse is aware that this score necessitates:
① Oxygen by mask
② Immediate resuscitation
③ Additional warming measures
④ Stimulation to the soles of the feet

239. Baby Ewing is admitted to the neonatal intensive care unit and placed in an Isolette with a temperature setting of 89° F to increase his body temperature. In the well neonate, heat production is accomplished by:
① Shivering vigorously
② Breaking down brown fat
③ Increasing muscular activity
④ Oxidizing fatty acids

240. In preparing Mrs. Ewing to breastfeed the nurse teaches her that:
① Suckling stimulates the pituitary gland to release oxytocin, which initiates lactation
② Milk secretion is under the control of hormones and starts immediately after delivery
③ High levels of estrogen stimulate secretions of lactogenic hormones
④ High levels of progesterone stimulate the secretion of oxytocin

Situation: Ellen Mills, in labor for 8 hours, has been receiving oxytocin (Pitocin) for a prolonged period of time.

241. An adverse reaction from prolonged Pitocin administration for which Mrs. Mills must be closely monitored is:
    ① A change in affect
    ② An elevated temperature
    ③ Hyperventilation
    ④ Water intoxication

242. Mrs. Mills delivers a baby girl and is taken to the recovery room. The nurse is aware that Mrs. Mills could be at increased risk for post-partal hemorrhage if she:
    ① Breastfed in the delivery room
    ② Delivered a baby who weighed 9 lbs 8 ozs
    ③ Received a pudendal block for delivery
    ④ Had a third stage that lasted 10 minutes

243. Aware of the signs of an impending postpartal hemorrhage, the nurse assesses Mrs. Mills for:
    ① A decrease in pulse rate
    ② An increase in blood pressure
    ③ Persistent muscular twitching
    ④ Continuous trickling of blood

Situation: Angelica and Alvin Ross devoted the early years of their marriage to their careers and travel. At 35 years of age Mrs. Ross became pregnant.

244. During the 6-month prenatal office visit Mrs. Ross states that she is getting fat all over and that she even needs bigger shoes because her old ones are too tight. The nurse should:
    ① Teach her about the basic four food groups
    ② Obtain her weight, blood pressure, and fundal height
    ③ Encourage her to use a comfortable walking shoe
    ④ Reassure her that weight gain is expected

245. Mrs. Ross shows signs of developing mild pregnancy-induced hypertension (PIH). A home-care regimen is outlined for her use. When assessing the effectiveness of the teaching plan about self-care and conservative management of PIH the nurse would know that Mrs. Ross understood when she recognized the importance of:
    ① Joining a weight reduction program
    ② Eating a low-protein diet
    ③ Maintaining a normal sodium intake
    ④ Following the diuretic regimen as ordered

246. Mrs. Ross asks how she can relieve her occasional heartburn. As part of the teaching plan the nurse should warn against taking antacids containing:
    ① Aluminum
    ② Calcium
    ③ Sodium
    ④ Magnesium

247. Mrs. Ross' condition worsens, and she is hospitalized. The physician's order states, "Provide a neutral environment." The nurse knows this is important because a nonstimulating environment for a client with increased cerebral irritability:
    ① Increases the duration of hypotensive medications
    ② Reduces the probability of grand mal seizures
    ③ Improves intracellular fluid reabsorption
    ④ Reduces the severity of frontal headaches

248. Mrs. Ross complains of a severe headache. Her BP is 170/120 and she has hyperactive reflexes. Magnesium sulfate ($MgSO_4$) intravenously is ordered. High magnesium blood levels from $MgSO_4$ therapy can be reversed by administration of:
    ① Edetate disodium (EDTA)
    ② Sodium polystyrene sulfonate (Kayexalate)
    ③ Hydralazine hydrochloride (Apresoline)
    ④ Calcium gluconate (Kalcinate)

Situation: Bridget Lums, a 36-year-old gravida III, para II, is approximately 16 weeks pregnant. Her second child, a son, was born with congenital defects. Mrs. Lums is admitted for an amniocentesis.

249. To obtain informed consent from Mrs. Lums for the amniocentesis, it is unnecessary for the nurse to give her:
    ① A copy of the Patient's Bill of Rights
    ② A complete description of possible dangers and discomforts
    ③ An offer to answer questions about the procedure
    ④ An explanation of usable alternative procedures

250. To detect possible complications immediately after the amniocentesis, the nurse caring for Mrs. Lums should first:
    ① Check her for vaginal bleeding or discharge
    ② Assess the fetal heart rate (FHR)
    ③ Position her on her left side
    ④ Apply pressure for 5 minutes at the puncture site

251. After Mrs. Lums delivers a healthy baby girl, Mr. and Mrs. Lums decide they do not want any more children. Because of their religious beliefs they decide to use the rhythm method of birth control. Mrs. Lums tells the nurse that she menstruates every 32 days for 2 days. The nurse should teach Mrs. Lums that based on this cycle, ovulation probably occurs:
    ① On the fourteenthth day of the cycle
    ② 10 days after the first day of bleeding
    ③ 14 days before the start of the next menses
    ④ 2 to 3 days after the last day of menstrual bleeding

Situation: Kimberly Abrams, 32 years old, develops severe pain in her left leg during her twenty-ninth week of pregnancy. Thrombophlebitis is diagnosed, and she is admitted to the hospital, prescribed bed rest, and started on anticoagulant therapy.

252. The nurse should be aware that the only anticoagulant that Mrs. Abrams can safely receive is:
    ① Heparin sodium
    ② Warfarin sodium
    ③ Dicumarol
    ④ Embolex

253. Mrs. Abrams has blood drawn for activated partial thromboplastin time (APTT). One day her APTT is reported to be 98 seconds. The nurse notifies the physician because the anticoagulant should be:
    ① Increased for better clotting results
    ② Omitted for today and the APTT rechecked tomorrow
    ③ Changed to one of the other effective anticoagulants
    ④ Discontinued because the APTT is normal

254. In her thirty-second week of pregnancy, Mrs. Abrams is scheduled for ultrasonography. The ultrasonography demonstrates a low-lying placenta. The nurse is aware that as the pregnancy concludes and labor begins, Mrs. Abrams may first experience:
    ① Sharp abdominal pain
    ② Early rupture of membranes
    ③ Increased lower back pain
    ④ Painless vaginal bleeding

Situation: Gladys and Hugh Williams, who have been married for 5 years and have used no contraception at all, come to the infertility clinic.

255. At the first interview, Mr. Williams tells the nurse that his parents are impatient about having a grandchild. He says, "They promised me a down payment on a house if Gladys gets pregnant this year." The nurse's best response to Mr. Williams' comment is:
    ① "Five years without a pregnancy is a long time. Do you think there is something wrong with both of you?"
    ② "You're lucky; I wish someone would give me a down payment for a house."
    ③ "How do the two of you feel about having a baby?"
    ④ "You know, you don't have to worry about satisfying your parents. Having a child should be a decision you make."

256. Mr. and Mrs. Williams are to undergo infertility testing, and in preparation for one test the nurse teaches Mrs. Williams to examine her cervical mucus. After listening to the explanation Mrs. Williams says, "That sounds gross. I don't think I can do it." The nurse is aware that:

① Some women are uncomfortable touching their genitals and discharges
② It is possible that Mrs. Williams is being unduly fastidious
③ Having a baby is not that important to Mrs. Williams
④ Mrs. Williams is afraid of finding out that the problem is her fault

257. Mrs. Williams comes in for a carbon dioxide insufflation test to determine if her tubes are patent. As part of the teaching before the test the nurse tells Mrs. Williams:
    ① "You will have to rest in bed for 8 hours after the test is completed."
    ② "There is a strong possibility that you will become nauseated during the test."
    ③ "You will receive a local anesthetic to lessen the pain of the test."
    ④ "You may have some persistent shoulder pain for 24 hours after the test."

258. Because an infertility workup involves both partners, Mr. Williams is to have a semen analysis; as part of his instructions he is told to:
    ① Use a condom to collect the semen specimen
    ② Refrigerate the specimen until it can be delivered to the laboratory
    ③ Ejaculate 2 to 3 days before collection to ensure a pure specimen
    ④ Make sure that the specimen is collected as soon as he awakens

259. Mr. and Mrs. Williams attend the prenatal clinic to confirm a pregnancy. When preparing Mrs. Williams for the pelvic examination, the nurse notes that Mrs. Williams is very anxious. The best nursing intervention at this time would be to:
    ① Maintain eye contact, touch gently, and thoroughly explain the procedure
    ② Distract her by asking her preference as to the sex of the child
    ③ Assist the physician so that the examination can be finished quickly
    ④ Encourage her to close her eyes and hold her breath during the examination

260. Mrs. Williams tells the nurse that she is a vegetarian. To ensure proper nutrition the nurse should:
    ① Advise her to include meat in her diet at least once daily
    ② Discontinue the vegetarian practice entirely until she delivers
    ③ Help her plan meals that use foods that she is willing to eat
    ④ Encourage her to join a diet group to teach her good nutrition

261. During the discussion on nutrition, the nurse explains to Mrs. Williams that she will need additional calcium during pregnancy and that the best source is milk. Mrs. Williams

states, "I never drink milk or eat milk products. They turn my stomach." The best reply by the nurse would be:
① "How unfortunate; this may cause your teeth to loosen."
② "Just make sure the rest of your diet is nutritionally sound."
③ "You will have to try and drink some milk so that the baby will have strong bones."
④ "There are mineral and vitamin supplements that the physician can order for you."

Situation: Mrs. Jones' labor was precipitated by an automobile accident, and at 32 weeks' gestation she has just delivered a preterm infant with an Apgar score of 8.

262. When discussing gestational age with Mrs. Jones, the nurse points out that in an infant of 32-weeks' gestation the:
① Areola and nipple are barely visible
② Palms have clearly defined creases
③ Ear pinna springs back when folded
④ Square window sign shows a 0-degree angle

263. Understanding that preterm infants are prone to respiratory distress, the nurse should observe Baby Jones for:
① Flaring nares
② Acrocyanosis
③ Respirations of 40 per minute
④ Abdominal breathing

264. The nurse is aware that a preterm infant may have a potential nutritional problem because of:
① A decreased metabolic rate
② A poor sucking reflex
③ Increased absorption of nutrients
④ Decreased caloric requirements

265. Mrs. Jones expresses the desire to breastfeed her infant. The nurse should:
① Discourage her because of the time and effort it will take to pump her breasts
② Tell her this is not possible because the infant is being fed by gavage
③ Instruct her that breast milk is inadequate for a preterm infant because it does not contain all the necessary nutrients
④ Support her decision and explain that the infant will initially lose weight because of the energy expended when breastfeeding

266. The nurse observes Mrs. Jones' behavior but cannot decide whether Mrs. Jones is anxious about her baby or experiencing postpartal depression. The client's behaviors that would clarify this confusion for the nurse would be:
① Decreased appetite, crying, and insomnia
② Ambivalence, lethargy, and increased appetite
③ Increased appetite, insomnia, and ambivalence

④ Long periods of sleep, lethargy, and anorexia

Situation: Baby Boy Lewis, 45 minutes old, has just been admitted to the newborn nursery after a cesarean delivery.

267. In doing the newborn assessment, the nurse notes that the infant's head circumference is 1½ inches smaller than his chest. The nurse is aware that this finding:
① Is normal in male newborns regardless of mode of birth
② Could indicate microcephaly
③ Is indicative of anencephaly
④ Commonly occurs in babies born by cesarean delivery

268. Baby Lewis develops physiologic jaundice, and phototherapy is ordered to:
① Activate the liver to dispose of the bilirubin
② Break down the bilirubin into a conjugated form
③ Activate vitamin K to facilitate excretion of bilirubin
④ Dissolve the bilirubin and allow it to be excreted from the skin

269. Baby Lewis is circumcised. Additional teaching of Mrs. Lewis regarding care of her son after his circumcision would be indicated if she plans to:
① Give the baby a tub bath the day after he is discharged
② Change the baby's diapers very frequently
③ Place petrolatum gauze or A & D ointment on his penis
④ Call the physician if there is excessive bleeding

Situation: Crystal Collins, a 28-year-old primigravida, is brought to the labor unit by her husband. She is having contractions every 4 minutes, and her membranes are intact. Mrs. Collins is in her fortieth week of the pregnancy, which has progressed without problems.

270. On Mrs. Collins' admission, the nurse notes the fetal heartbeat is loudest in the upper left quadrant. The nurse should be aware that the position of the fetus is probably:
① Left occipital anterior
② Left sacral anterior
③ Left mentum anterior
④ Left occipital transverse

271. The nurse should use the data from the assessment of this fetal position to observe for:
① Symptoms of primary uterine inertia, such as cessation of contractions
② Signs of precipitate labor, such as rapid dilation of the cervix
③ Symptoms of fetal distress, such as a prolapse of the cord

④ Signs that normal labor is progressing, such as increased contractions

Situation: In the thirty-ninth week of gestation, Jodi Flax is admitted to the labor unit in active labor, and a pelvic examination is performed.

272. The examination reveals a 6 to 7 cm dilation. Based on this finding the nurse should expect that Mrs. Flax would:
    ① Have a profuse bloody show
    ② Appear unable to control her shaking legs
    ③ Be uncomfortable because of nausea and vomiting
    ④ Have contractions every 5 to 7 minutes of 45-second duration

273. The nurse is aware that Mrs. Flax is beginning the second stage of labor when:
    ① The bloody show appears to lessen
    ② Beads of perspiration appear on her upper lip
    ③ About a "dime's worth" of caput is showing

④ A gush of watery fluid bursts from the vagina

274. Mrs. Flax delivers a baby girl. Five minutes later the nurse assesses that the placenta is separating when:
    ① The client complains of unbearable abdominal pain
    ② Bright red blood continually seeps out of the vagina
    ③ The fundus becomes completely relaxed
    ④ There is a lengthening of the umbilical cord

275. Mrs. Flax required an extensive episiotomy because her baby was large. A priority nursing intervention that will minimize edema and lessen discomfort at the incision site would be:
    ① Applying some form of cold to the perineum
    ② Giving her an oral analgesic immediately
    ③ Spraying the area with a local anesthetic
    ④ Positioning the client on her side, off the area

Comprehensive Examinations

Comprehensive Examination One

Test 1

Situation: During Johnny Cole's 6-month health care visit to a clinic, a diagnosis of spastic cerebral palsy was confirmed.

1. The clinic nurse was especially observant for signs of cerebral palsy in Johnny because he:
   ① Was born by elective cesarean delivery
   ② Weighed less than 1500 g at birth
   ③ Was born to a mother over 35 years old
   ④ Had a positive Moro reflex at birth

2. The hypertonicity of Johnny's muscles causes scissoring of his legs. The nurse should suggest to Mrs. Cole that the best way to carry him in a sitting position is:
   ① Wrapped tightly in a blanket
   ② Strapped in an infant seat
   ③ Astride one of her hips
   ④ Under the arm using a football hold

3. On a later clinic visit Mrs. Cole asks why she was not told that Johnny had cerebral palsy when he was a newborn. The nurse should reply:
   ① "The joint deformities of cerebral palsy appear only after 6 months of age."
   ② "The health care personnel in the clinic did not want to alarm you until it was necessary."
   ③ "The neurologic lesions responsible for Johnny's condition may have changed as he matured."
   ④ "Early diagnosis of cerebral palsy is difficult in infants until they develop control of voluntary movements."

4. When Johnny is older, he is admitted to the hospital for orthopedic surgery. During the admission interview the nurse should:
   ① Ask Mrs. Cole about the therapy program used by the family at home
   ② Explain to Mrs. Cole that the hospital will provide a pureed diet
   ③ Tell Mrs. Cole that Johnny will be put in a private room
   ④ Let Mrs. Cole know at what hours she will be permitted to visit Johnny

Situation: Sam Traver, a 52-year-old engineer, is admitted to the hospital with a history of alcohol abuse, Laënnec's cirrhosis, and chronic pancreatitis.

5. Bile salts are ordered for Mr. Traver, and he asks why he needs to take them. The nurse tells him that they:
   ① Aid absorption of vitamins A, D, and K
   ② Stimulate prothrombin production
   ③ Promote bilirubin secretion in the urine
   ④ Stimulate contraction of the common bile duct

6. Mr. Traver develops portal hypertension. He has an elevated serum aldosterone level. The nurse caring for Mr. Traver observes him carefully for:
   ① Chloride depletion and hypovolemia
   ② Potassium retention and arrhythmias
   ③ Sodium retention and fluid accumulation
   ④ Calcium depletion and pathologic fractures

7. Mr. Traver fails to respond to chlorothiazide, and spironolactone (Aldactone) is prescribed in addition to the chlorothiazide. The advantage of Aldactone is that it:
   ① Reduces arterial blood pressure
   ② Stimulates H_2O excretion
   ③ Stimulates sodium excretion
   ④ Helps prevent potassium loss

8. Mr. Traver is malnourished and nauseated. He has ascites and gastrointestinal bleeding. The nurse recognizes that his ascites is largely due to his malnourished state, especially his lack of adequate:
   ① Sodium to maintain its proper concentration in tissue fluid
   ② Vitamins to maintain cell coenzyme functions
   ③ Iron to prevent proper hemoglobin synthesis
   ④ Plasma protein to maintain proper capillary-tissue circulation

9. Mr. Traver is given 2 units of salt-poor albumin IV. The purpose of salt-poor albumin is to:
   ① Increase the client's protein stores
   ② Provide parenteral nutrients
   ③ Increase the client's circulating blood volume
   ④ Temporarily divert blood flow away from the liver

10. Mr. Traver improves and is to be discharged. In planning his discharge with family members, the nurse tells them about:
    ① The need for a high-protein diet
    ② The use of chlorpromazine for relaxation
    ③ The importance of reporting personality changes to the physician
    ④ The need for increased fluids to increase kidney output

Situation: Eighteen-year-old Helen Roles, a primigravida who is 36 weeks pregnant, is admitted to the antepartum unit with a diagnosis of pregnancy-induced hypertension.

11. The nurse who admits Ms. Roles is aware that nursing care measures for this client will be directed chiefly toward reducing:
① Bleeding
② Blood pressure
③ Anxiety
④ Vasospasms

12. A major complication of hypertensive disease that the nurse should anticipate is:
① Placenta previa
② Abruptio placentae
③ Oligohydramnios
④ Isoimmunization

13. Ms. Roles is placed on a fetal monitor, as well as a blood pressure monitor. The continuous monitoring of blood pressure is essential to reduce the potential for:
① Premature delivery
② Hemorrhage
③ Convulsions
④ Fetal death

14. The nurse should expect the physician's orders for Ms. Roles to include:
① Diuretics, low-salt diet, intake and output monitoring
② Daily weights, intake and output monitoring, high-protein diet
③ Bed rest, intake and output monitoring, diuretics
④ Daily weights, fractional urines, bed rest

15. Ms. Roles' condition warrants therapy with intravenous magnesium sulfate. The nurse caring for Ms. Roles should immediately notify the physician if the client's:
① Respirations are 18 per minute
② Output is less than 100 ml in 4 hours
③ Patellar reflexes can be elicited
④ Blood pressure begins to decrease

16. The nurse should have available at Ms. Roles' bedside:
① Calcium gluconate
② Adrenalin
③ Neo-Cortef
④ Calcium chloride

Situation: Rose Shawn, 36 years of age, has just been admitted to the psychiatric unit. She appears seclusive and mistrustful of everyone. Ms. Zarr is assigned to work with this client.

17. Ms. Zarr can help Ms. Shawn to develop trust by:
① Handing her medication and not watching to see whether she swallows it
② Listening attentively to her positive feelings and ignoring her negative feelings
③ Attempting to be prompt for their scheduled meetings
④ Telling her simply and sincerely that she cares about her feelings

18. The most important aspect of a therapeutic contract is:
① Determining time and place of meeting with the client
② Planning frequency and duration of meetings with the client
③ Discussing and defining the client's goals for treatment
④ Understanding the professional responsibilities of the nurse

19. Each time the physician or head nurse visits Ms. Shawn, Ms. Zarr notices that she becomes extremely anxious. Today after visiting with her physician Ms. Shawn sits wringing her hands. The best initial response by Ms. Zarr would be:
① "How do you handle your anxiety?"
② "I notice that you are wringing your hands."
③ "Tell me why you are afraid of authority figures."
④ "Do you realize why you are wringing your hands?"

20. Ms. Zarr can best initially prepare Ms. Shawn for termination of their relationship by:
① Telling her how long she will be working with her during their first meeting
② Waiting until the termination phase, then reminding her periodically of the duration of their meetings
③ Periodically summarizing Ms. Shawn's progress during the working phase
④ Reminding Ms. Shawn that, if she feels it is necessary, their meetings could be extended

21. One morning during the working phase of the relationship, Ms. Shawn suddenly becomes very hostile. The most appropriate interpretation of this behavior is that:
① Flare-ups often occur when the nurse and client have a good working relationship
② This behavior is a form of regression and implies deterioration in the client's condition
③ Hostility is being used as a defense because the nurse has come too close
④ The client is exercising assertiveness, which implies improvement in her condition

22. During the termination phase of the relationship Ms. Shawn misses a series of appointments without any explanation. Ms. Zarr should:
① Attend the remaining designated meetings and wait
② Terminate the relationship immediately
③ Contact the client to encourage another session
④ Explore her personal reactions with her supervisor

Situation: Nancy Woodwood is admitted for a right modified radical mastectomy.

23. Before Mrs. Woodwood signs the informed consent, the nurse should be certain that she knows her surgery includes the removal of:
    ① Axillary lymph nodes on the affected side
    ② Pectoral muscles
    ③ Skin overlying the breast tissue
    ④ The involved half of the breast and nodes

24. Mrs. Woodwood returns from surgery with a portable suction unit in place and a dry sterile dressing covering the site of the incision. When observing Mrs. Woodwood for signs of bleeding, the nurse should:
    ① Turn her on the affected side to inspect for blood that may flow backward
    ② Empty and measure the output in the portable suction unit hourly
    ③ Reinforce the operative site with a pressure dressing if any drainage appears on the dressing
    ④ Inspect the bedclothes under the axillary area for signs of drainage

25. The nurse empties the portable suction unit when it is only half full because:
    ① It is easier and safer to empty the unit when it is only half full
    ② As fluid collects in the unit it exerts positive pressure, forcing drainage back up the tubing and into the wound
    ③ This facilitates a more accurate measurement of drainage output
    ④ The negative pressure in the unit lessens as fluid accumulates in it, interfering with further drainage

26. After emptying the portable suction unit, the nurse creates negative pressure by:
    ① Attaching it to a wall suction unit
    ② Compressing the device and then closing the air plug
    ③ Keeping it in a position lower than the site of insertion
    ④ Periodically milking the tubing toward the suction unit

27. On the first postoperative day the nurse encourages exercises such as flexion and extention of fingers and pronation and supination of the forearm. These interventions are done primarily to:
    ① Assess extent of lymphedema
    ② Stimulate circulation
    ③ Prevent contractures
    ④ Preserve muscle tone

28. The nurse would know that Mrs. Woodwood understands the discharge teaching when she states she will report to the physician any:
    ① Slightly irregular-appearing skin around the incision
    ② Persistent itching around the incision
    ③ Decreased sensations in the area around the incision
    ④ Swelling and erythema around the incision

Situation: Five-month-old Felix Heinz was probably exposed to an adolescent sibling who contracted measles.

29. The clinic nurse is asked by a very anxious Mrs. Heinz whether the baby can be vaccinated against measles at his age. The nurse's reply should take into consideration the history of:
    ① Immunization of this baby
    ② Maternal diseases and immunizations
    ③ Preexisting tuberculosis of the mother
    ④ Previous viral illnesses of this baby

30. It is later determined that vaccination is indicated for this baby. The nurse should help Mrs. Heinz understand that to ensure continued protection against measles, Felix should be revaccinated when he is approximately:
    ① 8 months old
    ② 10 months old
    ③ 12 months old
    ④ 15 months old

Situation: Elsie Simpson comes to the prenatal clinic for the first time. She tells the nurse that her last menstrual cycle began on January 11. She also states that she had 1 day of light bleeding on February 7.

31. Mrs. Simpson's due date is calculated to be:
    ① October 14
    ② October 18
    ③ November 14
    ④ November 18

32. In the fortieth week of gestation Mrs. Simpson is admitted in active labor. As she is relaxing between contractions, the nurse performs Leopold's maneuvers to determine the position of the fetus. The examination reveals a soft rounded mass at the fundus, smooth irregular curvature on the right side of the abdomen, and bumpy projections on the left. The fetal position is:
    ① RScA
    ② LSP
    ③ ROA
    ④ LOP

33. During labor Mrs. Simpson states, "I feel all wet. I think I urinated." The nurse should first:
    ① Auscultate the fetal heart rate
    ② Inspect the perineal area
    ③ Give her the bedpan
    ④ Change the bed linens

34. A few hours after admission, Mr. Simpson asks, "How much longer will this take? She's complaining of back pain and is so uncomfortable." The nurse responds:
    ① "It shouldn't be much longer now."

② "Everything is progressing nicely as expected."

③ "Let me show you how to provide back pressure."

④ "I think you should take a break for a while."

Situation: Saul Glass, who is 56 years old, comes to the emergency room with complaints of chest pain.

35. The doctor orders an electrocardiogram (ECG). Mr. Glass asks the nurse, "What is the purpose of this test?" The nurse replies, "This test will:
   ① Enable us to detect heart sounds."
   ② Enable us to detect heart damage."
   ③ Help us to change your heart rhythm."
   ④ Tell us how much stress your heart can endure."

36. Mr. Glass is admitted to the CCU. After attaching him to the monitor the nurse notes six premature ventricular contractions (PVCs) per minute. The nurse, following established protocols, should first:
   ① Initiate cardiopulmonary resuscitation on Mr. Glass
   ② Encourage him to cough and deep breathe
   ③ Administer a bolus of cardiac xylocaine
   ④ Obtain an orthostatic blood pressure reading

37. Mr. Glass receives 15 mg of morphine sulfate for chest pain. Fifteen minutes later, he complains of feeling dizzy. The nurse should:
   ① Tell him this is a normal sensation after receiving morphine
   ② Ask him if he is having an allergic reaction
   ③ Elevate his head and keep his extremities warm
   ④ Place him in a supine position and take his vital signs

38. Before discharge Mr. Glass asks the nurse how long he should wait before having sexual relations with his wife. The nurse's best reply would be:
   ① "It depends on how you are feeling."
   ② "Two weeks is the usual waiting time."
   ③ "Have you discussed this with your physician?"
   ④ "You should wait until your heart feels stronger."

Situation: Helen Jackson, 57 years old, has been admitted to the psychiatric unit with a diagnosis of schizophrenia, paranoid type.

39. On entering the unit, Mrs. Jackson says, "They all are trying to kill me. They all are." The nurse's best response would be:
   ① "No, Mrs. Jackson. No one wants to hurt you."
   ② "Mrs. Jackson, we are here to protect you."

③ "Mrs. Jackson, you are having very frightening thoughts."

④ "Tell me more about their wanting to kill you, Mrs. Jackson."

40. Mrs. Jackson says to the nurse, "I know they're spying on me in here too. I'm not safe anywhere!" The most therapeutic response by the nurse would be:
   ① "You don't feel safe anywhere, not even in the hospital."
   ② "Why do you feel they'd want to follow you here, Mrs. Jackson?"
   ③ "Mrs. Jackson, nobody's spying on you in here."
   ④ "You are safe in the hospital; nothing can happen to you here."

41. Mrs. Jackson appears very suspicious of the nurse. The most effective approach to this problem would be for the nurse to:
   ① Engage Mrs. Jackson in a discussion about her thoughts
   ② Make brief, frequent contacts with Mrs. Jackson
   ③ Allow Mrs. Jackson to stay in her room without interruption
   ④ Assign various caregivers to Mrs. Jackson

42. Mrs. Jackson continues to have delusions. The nurse understands that delusions are:
   ① The result of paleological thinking
   ② A defense against anxiety
   ③ Precipitated by external stimuli
   ④ Subconscious expressions of anger

43. Mrs. Jackson and the nurse are standing next to each other in the dayroom when Mrs. Jackson gets down on her hands and knees and says, "I am a table." It would be most effective for the nurse to:
   ① Offer a hand to help her up while saying, "You are not a table; you are a person."
   ② State, "You were never a table before and you are not a table now."
   ③ Touch her arm while saying, "You must be very frightened to feel this way."
   ④ State, "You are safe here in the hospital. You do not need to be a table."

Situation: Larry Gaines, 6 years old, is admitted to the pediatric unit with a diagnosis of acute glomerulonephritis.

44. A nursing diagnosis of fluid volume excess would be correct if the assessment data includes:
   ① Dysuria, pruritus, weight loss
   ② Periorbital edema, smoky urine, headaches
   ③ Diarrhea, polyuria, weight gain
   ④ Hypotension, tachycardia, hematuria

45. When doing the nursing history, the nurse would expect Mrs. Gaines to report that:
   ① Larry had just gotten over the measles
   ② Larry had a sore throat 3 weeks ago

③ Larry's father has a history of urinary infections
④ Larry's immunizations for camp were completed last week

46. Nursing care for Larry should be directed toward:
① Enforcing strict bed rest
② Promoting diuresis
③ Forcing fluids
④ Eliminating sodium from his diet

Situation: Ken Madison is a 30-year-old steamfitter who weighs 143 pounds and has 40% of his body surface area burned.

47. The physician orders fluid replacement of 7200 ml during the first 24 hours. The hourly IV fluid intake will be approximately:
① 125 ml/hr
② 200 ml/hr
③ 300 ml/hr
④ 425 ml/hr

48. To best help manage Mr. Madison's pain during dressing changes, the nurse can teach the client:
① Deep-breathing exercises
② Active range-of-motion exercises
③ To alternately contract and relax his muscles
④ The importance of wound care

49. Two weeks after the burn, the nurse notes that Mr. Madison is losing 2 pounds of weight per day. The nurse's best action would be to adjust his diet by adding:
① High-protein drinks
② Fruit juices low in potassium
③ Low-sodium milk
④ 10% more calories in the form of fats

50. The best approach to wound care for Mr. Madison, who is receiving hydrotherapy, is to:
① Prepare equipment while doing the procedure and explain interventions to the client
② Use a consistent approach to care and encourage the client's participation
③ Change staff every 4 to 5 days and have the client select the time for the procedure to be done
④ Heat the water to 102° F to prevent loss of body temperature and prepare the equipment before starting

51. Mr. Madison receives an autograft. One week after the graft Mr. Madison, while changing his own dressing, notices the edges of the graft curling up and asks the nurse about it. The nurse's best response would be:
① "It's time for another graft."
② "Let me see if it is infected."
③ "May I take a look at it?"
④ "Is there any sign of redness?"

Situation: Jeri Marin, 24 years old, has been in control of her diabetes with daily insulin, diet, and exercise since its onset 6 years ago. She and her husband have decided they would like to start a family.

52. Mrs. Marin is concerned about how a pregnancy is going to affect the diabetes, especially her diet and insulin needs. The nurse should inform Mrs. Marin that pregnancy:
① Is a normal state, and that a revised diet and her usual insulin regimen will meet her and the fetus' needs
② Increases the need for protein, and adjustments have to be made to meet the need for increasing doses of insulin
③ Will vary her diet and insulin needs, and she will have to monitor her blood sugar more often to make appropriate adjustments
④ Decreases the need for insulin because the excess glucose will be used by the fetus for growth

53. Mrs. Marin is pregnant and is now in the thirty-fourth week. The doctor tells her that her baby may have to be delivered at about 38 weeks gestation instead of the usual 40 weeks. She asks the nurse why early delivery is necessary. The best initial reply is:
① "After 36 weeks the placenta may not be as efficient in providing for the fetus' needs."
② "You need to be delivered early before the fetus gets too big to fit through the birth canal."
③ "You need to be delivered early so you don't develop toxemia of pregnancy."
④ "Early delivery will reduce the chance of your infant developing hyperglycemia."

54. Mrs. Marin delivers an 8 lb baby boy who is given an injection of vitamin K on his admission to the nursery. The nurse knows that this is done to:
① Promote liver formation of clotting factors
② Replace necessary bacteria in the intestine
③ Prolong the prothrombin time of the infant
④ Improve the absorption of biliary salts

55. During discharge instructions Mrs. Marin states that she does not want another baby for at least 3 years. The nurse knows that Mrs. Marin understood the family planning teaching when she states, "The best type of contraception for a woman with diabetes is:
① An oral contraceptive."
② A diaphragm with foam."
③ The intrauterine device."
④ Tying the fallopian tubes."

Situation: John Swift, 8 years old, has a history of severe asthma since 3 years of age and is admitted to the hospital after an attack at home.

56. John is extremely short of breath. To facilitate breathing and to promote respiratory drainage, the nurse should place him in a:
① Supine position
② High-Fowler's position
③ Left lateral position
④ Trendelenburg position

57. After the administration of epinephrine, the nurse carefully monitors John for the common side effect of:
① Hypotension
② Tachycardia
③ Flushing
④ Dyspnea

58. John is being discharged from the hospital on oral theophylline. The nurse recognizes that the parents understand the discharge teaching when they tell the nurse they will observe John for the side effect of:
① Nausea and vomiting
② Apneic episodes
③ Frequent urination
④ Spasmodic hiccoughs

59. Long-range management for children with asthma includes exercise. The nurse should teach the parents to encourage John to participate in the sport of:
① Baseball
② Basketball
③ Soccer
④ Wrestling

Situation: Hattie Breaker, 19 years of age, is admitted to the psychiatric unit for treatment of her drug addiction. Her mother accompanies her and tells the nurse that Hattie has been taking all sorts of drugs. The initial urine analysis for drugs shows traces of heroin, barbiturates, amphetamines, and methadone.

60. In caring for individuals with a history of abuse of multiple drugs, the nurse is aware that the most serious life-threatening symptoms during withdrawal usually result from:
① Heroin
② Barbiturates
③ Amphetamines
④ Methadone

61. In planning care for Ms. Breaker after the withdrawal period the nurse should take into consideration that the client is probably:
① Unconcerned with reality
② Unable to give up drugs
③ Unable to delay gratification
④ Unaware of the dangers of drug addiction

Situation: Harry Charles, 23 years of age, is admitted to the surgical unit with superficial wounds of both wrists as the result of an abortive suicide attempt. His father accompanies him to the unit and states to the nurse, "I really think I caused this; I told him I was calling the police to have him arrested for stealing our silver set. He should have known I didn't mean it." The client has a history of psychiatric problems and has been diagnosed as having an antisocial personality disorder.

62. When the nurse enters Mr. Charles' room, he states, "I suppose you're going to ask me about my suicide attempt!" The nurse's best response would be:
① "Do you want to talk about it, Mr. Charles?"
② "Why do you think I'd ask you about it, Mr. Charles?"
③ "It's best not to dwell on it, Mr. Charles."
④ "Tell me how you feel about it, Mr. Charles."

63. The nurse should recognize that Mr. Charles has probably had a long history of:
① Stringent parental discipline
② Interpersonal difficulties
③ Sexual aberrations
④ Diminished contact with reality

64. Mr. Charles is very hostile and threatening to the staff and other clients. He refuses to turn off his television set at bedtime and is continually found in other clients' rooms. One client on the unit states that his watch is missing, and another has lost his wallet. The nurse's best response to this situation would be to:
① Have Mr. Charles transferred to the psychiatric unit or discharged
② Call the hospital security and tell them Mr. Charles is stealing
③ Search Mr. Charles' belongings for the missing articles without telling him
④ Tell Mr. Charles that the staff knows he took the articles in question

65. The primary difficulty in establishing long-range goals for clients like Mr. Charles is related to the fact that such clients are usually:
① Unable to deal with their feelings of guilt
② Unwilling to accept their need for help
③ Reluctant to change their life-style
④ Resistant to any demonstration of feeling

66. Mr. Charles is being discharged and is to continue psychotherapy on an outpatient basis. In evaluating his chances for improvement, the nurse recognizes that:
① Mr. Charles requires intensive psychotherapy combined with tranquilizers to produce a remission
② Mr. Charles' prognosis for adjusting to a limited life-style is excellent
③ Mr. Charles will not change unless he is ready to accept the pain associated with change
④ Mr. Charles will not change unless his parents are willing to set and keep firm limits

Situation: Lilly Justice, 34 years old, is admitted to the medical unit with a diagnosis of insulin dependent diabetes mellitus.

67. Insulin dependent diabetes is classified as:
    ① Gestational diabetes
    ② Impaired glucose tolerance diabetes
    ③ Type I diabetes mellitus
    ④ Type II diabetes mellitus

68. The factor, learned during the nursing history, that probably predisposed Mrs. Justice to diabetes mellitus is:
    ① Drinking a daily alcoholic drink
    ② Eating low-cholesterol foods
    ③ Being 20 pounds overweight
    ④ Having diabetes insipidus

69. The nurse should expect Mrs. Justice's fasting blood sugar to be:
    ① 30 mg/100 ml
    ② 60 mg/100 ml
    ③ 110 mg/100 ml
    ④ 160 mg/100 ml

70. The physician prescribes regular insulin each morning for Mrs. Justice. After administering the insulin at 8:00 AM, the nurse should observe Mrs. Justice for a potential insulin reaction:
    ① At breakfast
    ② Before lunch
    ③ In the early afternoon
    ④ Before dinner

71. Mrs. Justice is taught the symptoms associated with hypoglycemia. The nurse would know that Mrs. Justice understands the teaching when she states she will notify the nursing staff if she experiences:
    ① Abdominal pain, nausea, fruity odor to breath
    ② Thirst, excessive urination, blurred vision
    ③ Confusion, vomiting, rapid deep breathing
    ④ Generalized nervousness, headache, perspiration

72. During the teaching about insulin injections, Mrs. Justice asks the nurse, "Why can't I take the insulin in pills instead of taking shots?" The nurse should respond:
    ① "Insulin cannot be manufactured in pill form."
    ② "The route of administration is decided on by the physician."
    ③ "Insulin is destroyed by gastric juices, rendering it ineffective."
    ④ "Your doctor will order pills when you are ready."

73. Mrs. Justice is placed on a 1500 calorie ADA diet. She should be taught that 1 gram of carbohydrate contains:
    ① 2 calories
    ② 4 calories
    ③ 9 calories
    ④ 12 calories

74. When making rounds the next afternoon the nurse finds Mrs. Justice unconscious. She has Kussmaul respirations; an acetone odor to her breath; and dry, hot, flushed skin. The nurse suspects that Mrs. Justice is experiencing:
    ① Hyperosmolar, non-ketotic coma
    ② The Somogyi effect
    ③ Diabetic ketoacidosis
    ④ A hypoglycemic reaction

Situation: Sam Flowers has a bronchoscopy and biopsy, which confirms cancer of the lung. A pneumonectomy is performed.

75. Mr. Flowers has an IV running postoperatively. In light of his particular surgery, he is most vulnerable to the complication of:
    ① Air embolism
    ② Phlebitis
    ③ Infiltration
    ④ Pulmonary edema

76. In a three-chamber underwater drainage system, the main purpose of the third chamber is to:
    ① Act as a drainage container
    ② Control the amount of suction
    ③ Provide an air-tight water seal
    ④ Allow for escape of air bubbles

77. Mr. Flowers has had a tremendous weight loss. He is told by his physician that he must eat more protein foods to get the essential amino acids that he needs. He asks the nurse why these substances in protein foods are "essential." The nurse should respond:
    ① "They contain the necessary nitrogen you need for healing."
    ② "They are essential for rebuilding your body tissue protein."
    ③ "They will give you the added energy you need."
    ④ "Your body can't make them, so you must get them in your food."

Situation: Nancy Elwood, 32 years old, has had rheumatic heart disease since childhood and is now pregnant. She has been classified as having Class I heart disease.

78. Although Mrs. Elwood will experience some symptoms during her pregnancy that are related to her cardiac pathology, she will also experience some normal symptoms of pregnancy such as:
    ① Dyspnea at rest
    ② Tachycardia
    ③ Shortness of breath on exertion
    ④ Progressive dependent edema

79. Mrs. Elwood expresses concern about her delivery and asks the nurse what she should expect. The nurse should be aware that the physician will probably:
    ① Induce her labor with oxytocin
    ② Perform an elective cesarean delivery
    ③ Use prophylactic forceps after a pudendal block
    ④ Prematurely rupture her membranes

80. Mr. and Mrs. Elwood arrive in the delivery suite. The nurse explains to the couple that Mrs. Elwood should avoid lying on her back during labor. The nurse has based this statement on the knowledge that the supine position can:
    ① Unduly prolong labor
    ② Cause decreased placental perfusion
    ③ Interfere with free movement of the coccyx
    ④ Lead to transient episodes of hypertension

81. Mrs. Elwood delivers a healthy baby boy. The nurse should plan Mrs. Elwood's postpartum care based on the knowledge that:
    ① The first 48 hours postpartum are the most stressful on the cardiopulmonary system
    ② Mrs. Elwood is out of immediate danger because the stress of pregnancy is over
    ③ Clients with cardiac problems should maintain bed rest for a minimum of 7 days
    ④ Mrs. Elwood should increase her fluid intake, particularly if she is breastfeeding.

82. Mrs. Elwood and her baby, who is 3 weeks old, are being seen by the visiting nurse at home. When the nurse arrives, Mrs. Elwood appears exhausted and the baby is crying. The most appropriate question by the nurse would be:
    ① "Is everything OK? You look exhausted."
    ② "When did the baby have his last feeding?"
    ③ "Tell me a little about your daily routine."
    ④ "Oh, you're having a terrible day."

Situation: Carmen Trindale brings her 5-year-old son, Tony, to the pediatric clinic because he has had a cold for a month. He is pale, irritable, and has a poor appetite. Preliminary blood work reveals abnormal results, and Tony is admitted to the hospital to rule out a leukemic process.

83. On admission, the most important nursing assessment is to determine:
    ① What Tony has been told about his diagnosis
    ② The parents' ability to cope in stressful situations
    ③ Tony's previous experience with illness and hospitalization
    ④ Tony's growth percentile and developmental abilities

84. In assessing Tony, the nurse recalls that some of the most common early signs of leukemia that he may present are:
    ① Fatigue, mouth lesions, hepatomegaly
    ② Pallor, joint pain, anorexia, fever
    ③ Fatigue, pallor, alopecia, hemorrhage
    ④ Lethargy, petechiae, splenomegaly

85. Before a bone marrow aspiration, the nurse prepares Tony for the procedure by telling him that:
    ① He will be put to sleep and will not feel anything
    ② After the test is over he will have to stay in bed until supper
    ③ He will feel a little pressure, and when it's over a Band-Aid will be applied
    ④ He will have a few stitches at the site, but he can get up and go to the playroom

86. Methotrexate is to be administered IV. The appropriate amount has been dissolved in 500 ml of D5W. The IV drip delivers 45 gtt/ml. The 500 ml are to be absorbed in 4 hours. The nurse should set the flow rate at:
    ① 22 gtt/minute
    ② 45 gtt/minute
    ③ 90 gtt/minute
    ④ 125 gtt/minute

87. Vincristine is added to Tony's medication regimen. Once this medication is begun, the nurse adds to his nursing care plan: check bowel sounds bid, and record. This action is necessary because a side effect of this drug is:
    ① Increased antigen-antibody reactions, which cause edematous bowels
    ② Decreased innervation to the GI tract
    ③ Hyperactivity of the bowel from diarrhea
    ④ Nausea that decreases fluid intake and produces constipation

88. In planning Tony's care, the nurse must keep in mind that the prognosis of the child with acute lymphocytic leukemia who is receiving therapy is:
    ① Very positive, with a probable cure in 90% of the children affected
    ② Very poor, but the therapy keeps them pain free
    ③ Limited to a few months in 70% of the children affected
    ④ Extended to at least 5 years in 60% of the children treated

Situation: Cathy Adams, a 19-year-old college student with a history of regional enteritis (Crohn's disease), is admitted to the hospital with a possible small bowel obstruction.

89. Ms. Adams is to have an intestinal tube inserted. Before assisting the physician with this procedure, the nurse should:
    ① Reassure the client that the procedure will not cause discomfort
    ② Place the client flat in bed, lying on her right side
    ③ Instruct the client in techniques of mouth breathing
    ④ Spray the client's oropharynx with a local anesthetic solution

90. After insertion of the intestinal tube, nursing care should include:

① Securing the tube by taping it to the nose
② Keeping the client on absolute bed rest
③ Allowing the client frequent sips of water
④ Confirming tube position by testing the pH of the drainage

91. A subclavian catheter is inserted and Ms. Adams is started on total parenteral nutrition (TPN). In order to prevent the most common complication of TPN the nurse should plan to teach the client to:
① Keep her head as still as possible whenever moving
② Weigh herself daily at the same time, wearing the same clothing
③ Regulate the flow rate on the infusion pump as necessary
④ Avoid touching the dressing as much as possible

92. Ms. Adams is scheduled for an ileostomy. When teaching her before the ileostomy, the nurse plans to include a statement that:
① Regular bowel habits can be established within a few weeks postoperatively
② Skin irritation at the stoma site will occur easily
③ Effluent discharge from the stoma will be formed fecal matter if the diet is regulated
④ A continent ileostomy will be the procedure of choice

93. The nurse expects drainage from the ileostomy in the first 24 to 48 postoperative hours to be:
① Clear with mucoid shreds
② Bloody with clots
③ Fecal with flatus
④ Mucoid and serosanguinous

Test 2

Situation: Sally Crane, 44 years old, has been attending the community mental health day treatment center for the past 6 weeks. She has been diagnosed as having an obsessive-compulsive personality disorder and although her symptoms have decreased, she still demonstrates ritualistic behavior, anxiety, and difficulty with decision making.

94. Care in a day treatment center is often indicated early in the treatment program for clients with incapacitating symptoms resulting from obsessive-compulsive personality disorders because it:
① Provides a neutral environment in which the client can work through conflicts
② Limits the client's time to carry out the symptomatic rituals
③ Resolves the client's anxiety, since opportunities requiring decision making are reduced
④ Allows the therapeutic staff to exert control over the client's activities

95. In developing a plan of care for Mrs. Crane the nurse should be aware that her anxiety level would be increased if the staff:
① Helped her to understand the nature of her anxiety
② Involved her in establishing and implementing the therapeutic plan
③ Provided a nonjudgmental and accepting environment
④ Permitted her ritualistic behaviors to be carried out at three set times during the day

96. Mrs. Crane's ritual focuses on her checking her pocketbook for her keys and other belongings every 4 minutes. If prevented from doing this, she gets quite upset. The nurse should:
① Lock her pocketbook in a safe place in the morning, thereby relieving her of the necessity to check it
② Allow her to continue to check her pocketbook for as long as she wants and wait for her to get tired
③ Keep her actively involved in projects to distract her so she will forget about checking her pocketbook
④ Allow the behavior, but with the client's agreement, set limits on the amount of time and the frequency of the checks

97. The treatment team decides it would be therapeutic for Mrs. Crane to get a part-time job and she eagerly begins her search for employment. On the day of her job interview, she comes to the center very anxious and displays an increase in compulsive behaviors. The nurse could best respond to these behavioral changes by stating:
① "If going to an interview makes you this anxious, it seems to me that you're not ready to work."
② "It must be that you really don't want that job after all. I think you should think more about it."
③ "Going for your interview triggered some feelings in you. Describe what you're feeling at this time."
④ "I know you're anxious, but make yourself go to the interview and try to conquer your fear."

Situation: Mark Goode, age 73, is admitted to the hospital for severe malnutrition and dehydration. He is being treated with intravenous fluids, a well-balanced diet, and between-meal dietary supplements. During the diagnostic workup the physician also diagnoses Parkinson's disease.

98. While setting up Mr. Goode's dinner tray, the nurse notices that he has a tremor of the right hand when it is lying in his lap but the tremor disappears when he reaches for his fork. The nurse recognizes that this is a:
① Resting tremor

② Intention tremor
③ Voluntary tremor
④ Idiopathic tremor

99. To relieve the symptoms of parkinsonism the nurse should expect the physician to order:
① Dopamine
② Vitamin B$_6$
③ Levodopa
④ Isocarboxazid

100. When Mr. Goode begins drug therapy a nursing priority would be to:
① Perform a physical assessment daily
② Monitor the intake and output every 8 hours
③ Assess the vital signs every 4 hours
④ Observe his sleeping patterns weekly

101. Mr. Goode experiences orthostatic hypotension, a side effect of drug therapy. To help limit this adaptation the nurse should:
① Initiate gait training
② Apply elastic stockings
③ Withhold the next dose
④ Increase the fluid intake

102. When removing Mr. Goode's tray the nurse notices that he did not eat his chicken. When asked why he did not eat his chicken he states, "I only eat meat once a week because old people don't need protein every day." Based on this statement the nurse knows that Mr. Goode should be taught about the:
① Need for home-delivered meals
② Continued need for the basic four
③ Effect of aging on the need for some foods
④ Need for meat at least once per day throughout life

Situation: Dan Bello, a married 65-year-old retiree, has a history of an enlarged prostate gland. He has been unable to urinate for 2 days and is experiencing suprapubic pressure and discomfort when he comes to the emergency room for assistance. After decompression of the bladder, Mr. Bello is scheduled for outpatient diagnostic studies, and prostatic carcinoma is identified.

103. Mr. Bello is scheduled for a transurethral prostatectomy. As he is being admitted to the surgical unit, he tells the nurse he is concerned that his operation will result in impotence. The nurse's best reply would be:
① "You may be impotent for a while, but normal functioning will probably return within 5 months."
② "I can understand why you are worried; it is a very real possibility."
③ "Most men worry about their ability to function. Why don't you speak with your physician?"
④ "I can understand that you are concerned, but this operation rarely causes impotence."

104. During preoperative teaching, the nurse tells Mr. Bello that following the surgery:
① Oral fluids should be avoided because of continuous urinary irrigation
② He can expect spasms of the bladder during the first 24 to 48 hours
③ His urine will be bright red for at least 24 to 48 hours
④ He should use the Valsalva maneuver to decrease bladder contractions

105. Following the transurethral prostatectomy, Mr. Bello returns to the recovery room with a three-way Foley catheter. An initial nursing priority in his care plan would be to:
① Observe the suprapubic dressing for drainage
② Maintain Mr. Bello in a semi-Fowler's position
③ Observe for signs of confusion and agitation
④ Force fluids by mouth as soon as the gag reflex returns

106. The physician has ordered alternate liters of D5W and D5RL at the rate of 175 ml/hour. The drop factor of the IV set is 15 gtt/ml. The nurse should adjust the flow to provide:
① 40 gtt/min
② 42 gtt/min
③ 44 gtt/min
④ 46 gtt/min

107. The nurse is preparing Mr. and Mrs. Bello for Mr. Bello's discharge. The nurse is aware that Mr. Bello understands the teaching when he states:
① "I am so glad this is over. Now I don't have to keep going to the doctor."
② "I was so worried and now I can hardly wait to get home and have sex with my wife."
③ "I will use stool softeners regularly for 1 to 2 months after I get home."
④ "I will drink 8 cups of fluid daily, but none after 9 PM."

Situation: Ellen Roy, 20 years old, comes to the OB clinic for her first prenatal visit.

108. The nurse tells Mrs. Roy that the most common emotional reaction to pregnancy, experienced in the first trimester, is:
① Depression
② Rejection
③ Ambivalence
④ Narcissism

109. For Mrs. Roy's complaint of "morning sickness" the nurse should plan to teach her to:
① Increase fluid intake
② Increase calcium in the diet
③ Eat three small meals a day
④ Avoid long periods without food

110. Mrs. Roy questions all the changes in her body. The nurse, when explaining these

changes to her, knows that the most profound change of all occurs in the:
① Cardiovascular system
② Urinary system
③ Endocrine system
④ Gastrointestinal system

111. The nurse is also aware that in a normal pregnancy another adaptation that occurs is:
① Decreased gastrointestinal motility
② Increased ovarian activity
③ Decreased glomerulofiltration rate
④ Increased pulmonary capacity

112. The nurse schedules Mrs. Roy for an ultrasound to confirm the expected date of delivery. When preparing her for the sonography, the nurse should tell her to:
① Avoid eating for 8 hours before the test
② Empty her bladder before the ultrasound
③ Force fluids for 1 hour before the ultrasound
④ Take a laxative the night before the sonogram

113. In the fortieth week Mrs. Roy delivers a 7 lb 13 oz baby boy by cesarean delivery because of fetal distress. When doing postoperative coughing and deep-breathing she complains of localized pain in the incision site, which subsides in a few moments. The nurse should:
① Call her physician immediately and then check for wound dehiscense
② Instruct her to splint the wound with a pillow when coughing
③ Place her in the supine position and inspect the wound site
④ Assess the intensity of the pain and give her the ordered analgesic

Situation: Leah Spencer delivers a baby boy and names him Thomas.

114. The nurse recognizes that Thomas has a left talipes equinovarus (club foot) when on physical examination his toes are:
① Higher than his heel, and his foot points inward
② Lower than his heel, and his foot points inward
③ Higher than his heel, and his foot points outward
④ Lower than his heel, and his foot points outward

115. Thomas is examined by a pediatric orthopedist who confirms the diagnosis of talipes equinovarus. The physician applies a cast to Thomas' left lower extremity. Mrs. Spencer should expect to bring Thomas back to the physician's office for a cast change:
① Each week
② Once a month
③ When the cast is soiled
④ Every other day

116. After the cast is removed the nurse teaches Mrs. Spencer how to exercise Thomas' foot. The nurse would know that Mrs. Spencer understood the instructions when she says that she will exercise the foot:
① Once a day, after his nap
② Twice a day, in the AM and PM
③ Every 4 hours without fail
④ With each diaper change

117. Mrs. Spencer would like to have more children but she is afraid that another child would have the same problem. The best intervention by the nurse would be to:
① Reassure her that this is unlikely to happen again in the same family
② Explore with her the environmental and hereditary factors involved
③ Discuss the certainty of the defect occurring in later children
④ Explain that future children will have a 1 in 4 chance of having the deformity

Situation: Sherri Decker, age 55, returns from surgery following a cholecystectomy. She has IV fluids, a T-tube attached to gravity drainage, a nasogastric tube attached to suction, and an abdominal dressing.

118. The location of Mrs. Decker's surgical site high in the abdominal cavity places her at high risk for the postoperative complication of:
① Hemorrhage
② Wound infection
③ Paralytic ileus
④ Atelectasis

119. The nurse encourages Mrs. Decker to perform deep breathing and coughing every hour. Mrs. Decker resists doing these exercises primarily because the:
① Nasogastric tube is irritating
② Pain at the incision site increases
③ Bandage on the abdomen is constricting
④ T-tube moves and causes cramps

120. Mrs. Decker's total bile drainage from the T-tube 24 hours after surgery is 150 ml. The nurse should:
① Notify the physician immediately of the excessive amount of bile drainage
② Empty the drainage bag and record amount on the I and O record
③ Check the tube for kinks because the drainage is less than expected
④ Clamp the T-tube and drain small amounts of bile every 4 hours

121. Before irrigating Mrs. Decker's nasogastric tube, the nurse must first:
① Check the tube for placement
② Auscultate for bowel sounds
③ Assess breath sounds
④ Instill 15 ml of normal saline

122. An intravenous solution of Lactated Ringer's is ordered to replace Mrs. Decker's T-tube

output. To evaluate whether the solution was therapeutically effective, the nurse should observe Mrs. Decker for symptoms associated with:
① Urinary stasis
② Metabolic acidosis
③ An increased potassium
④ A paralytic ileus

123. Mrs. Decker asks if she can keep her own intake and output record. The nurse should:
① Explain that this job is the responsibility of the nurse
② Assess her ability to measure her intake and output
③ Identify her reason for wanting to do this task
④ Determine her willingness to really help

124. Dehiscence is a complication with gastrointestional surgery. A factor that would further predispose Mrs. Decker to wound dehiscence would be:
① Weight 25% above recommended level
② Presence of a T-tube
③ The age of the client
④ The presence of excessive flatus

Situation: Jim Verset has a history of chronic obstructive pulmonary disease (COPD). He is admitted to the respiratory care unit in acute respiratory failure. On his admission the clinical observations include listlessness, cyanosis of the nailbeds, respirations 30, and pulse 122. Arterial blood gases (ABGs) are pH 7.25, PO_2 50 mm Hg, and PCO_2 60mm Hg.

125. After Mr. Verset has received low-flow oxygen by nasal cannula for 4 hours, the nurse notes that he has increased restlessness and confusion. This is followed by a decreased respiratory rate and lethargy. The nurse should:
① Percuss and vibrate the chest wall
② Quietly ask him about his confusion
③ Increase the oxygen by 2% increments
④ Decrease or discontinue the oxygen flow

126. Mr. Verset's status stabilizes. One evening he tells the nurse that he recently restarted smoking but limits it to a cigarette or two a day. He also tells the nurse that he has been lax in doing the prescribed respiratory hygiene exercises because they are too tiring. The nurse should respond:
① "Tell me more about your typical day before you changed your routine."
② "Your being so sick is probably because of your smoking and not exercising."
③ "Smoking is probably a primary cause of the increased severity of your disease."
④ "I can't make you stop doing what you are doing. It's your choice to be sick or well."

127. Following Mr. Verset's comments, the nurse revises the nursing care plan. The nursing diagnosis that is most indicated for Mr. Verset as a result of this discussion is:

① Knowledge deficit related to causal relationship of smoking to lung disease
② Noncompliance with therapeutic regimen related to nonacceptance
③ Altered thought processes related to cerebral anoxia
④ Bathing/hygiene self-care deficit related to fatigue

128. Mr. Verset is receiving intravenous aminophylline. The adverse reaction for which the nurse should observe is:
① Oliguria
② Hypotension
③ Bradycardia
④ Hypoventilation

129. Because Mr. Verset has been getting little relief after using his nebulizer, the nurse observes him during therapy. The observation by the nurse that would indicate Mr. Verset is not using the nebulizer correctly and needs additional instruction is that he:
① Positions the tip of the nebulizer beyond the lips
② Holds the inspired breath for at least 3 seconds
③ Exhales slowly through the mouth with lips pursed slightly
④ Inhales with his lips tightly sealed around the mouthpiece

130. In helping to break the vicious cycle of fear, dyspnea, and avoidance of activities commonly found in clients with COPD, the nurse should place primary emphasis in the teaching program on:
① Education about the disease and breathing exercises
② Judicious use of aerosol therapy, especially nebulizers
③ Teaching about priorities in carrying out daily activities
④ Learning to control or prevent respiratory infections

Situation: Jane French, a 42-year-old social worker, is admitted to the psychiatric unit after acting wild in her office and threatening to hit a co-worker with a chair. She has a history of three previous hospitalizations with a diagnosis of mood disorder, manic episode.

131. During the admission interview, the nurse would expect Ms. French to demonstrate:
① Delusions of persecution
② Flight of ideas
③ Associative looseness
④ Ritualistic behaviors

132. Ms. French answers the nurse's questions rapidly. Her speech is pressured and punctuated with profanity. It would be most therapeutic for the nurse to deal with Ms. French's behavior by:
① Allowing her to express her hostility in a safe manner without being judgmental

② Quietly telling her that the use of profanity is unbecoming and will not be tolerated

③ Thoroughly explaining to her the behavior that is allowed in the facility

④ Assisting her to interact with another client who is exhibiting similar behavior

133. The physician starts Ms. French on a regimen of chlorpromazine and lithium carbonate. The nurse is aware that the rationale behind this regimen is that the chlorpromazine:
① Potentiates the action of lithium for more effective results
② Helps decrease the incidence of lithium toxicity in the first week of therapy
③ Acts with the lithium to prevent progression to the depressive phase
④ Acts to quiet the client while allowing time for lithium to take effect

134. An initial priority in planning care for Ms. French would be:
① Planning to encourage her to participate in a daily discussion group
② Varying the staff assigned to care for her to reduce the opportunity for manipulation
③ Reducing the number of people interacting with her during any given day
④ Encouraging frequent close contact with staff and a few selected clients

135. The supervised activity that would be most therapeutic for Ms. French during the early phase of her hospitalization would be:
① Joining a brief swimming competition
② Walking around the hospital grounds with one of the nurses
③ Writing letters and doing needlepoint
④ Playing a board game with another client

136. During the third week of therapy with lithium, the nurse would be aware that it is effective when Ms. French is:
① Able to laugh off criticism
② More high-spirited
③ Able to spend the morning alone in her room
④ More appropriately groomed

Situation: Daniel James, 3 years old, has been diagnosed as having chronic lead poisoning and is admitted to the hospital for chelation therapy.

137. Mrs. James asks the nurse how Daniel got lead poisoning. The nurse bases the response on the knowledge that this problem in children is:
① Clearly related to the child's ingestion of nonfood substances
② Unknown, but high-risk groups include those with pica and those exposed to environmental hazards
③ Attributed to an indigent and passive mother who fails to supervise them

④ Considered to be caused by an environment with lead available for oral exploration by unsupervised children

138. The nurse takes Daniel's health history from Mrs. James. The nurse knows that an early sign of chronic lead poisoning (plumbism) is:
① Mental retardation
② Convulsions
③ Oliguria
④ Anemia

139. Lead poisoning affects various organ systems, but its irreversible side effects are exerted mainly on the:
① Hematologic system
② Urinary system
③ Central nervous system
④ Skeletal system

140. Chelation therapy with Ca EDTA is started. The nurse can evaluate the success of this therapy by monitoring for:
① Increased urinary excretion of lead
② Elevated blood lead levels
③ Increased fecal excretion of lead
④ Decreased deposition of lead in the bones

141. Daniel will have 60 injections before the lead is chelated and removed from his system. The nurse should prepare Daniel for this painful treatment by:
① Allowing Daniel to play with a syringe and a doll before the therapy is initiated and after receiving each injection
② Carefully explaining the rationale for the injections so that Daniel does not feel he is being punished for eating paint chips
③ Rotating the injection sites and adding procaine to the chelating agents to lessen the discomfort
④ Role playing with puppets dressed as physicians and nurses to minimize Daniel's fear of unfamiliar adults

142. The nurse's projected goal for Daniel would be to relieve the local discomfort from the painful injections required by his therapy. The nurse plans to accomplish this by:
① Assisting Daniel to ambulate immediately after each injection
② Applying warm soaks to the affected area
③ Vigorously massaging the affected injection site with a sponge
④ Giving Daniel a cool tub bath after each injection

143. A condition that can be attributed both to lead toxicity and to the side effects of the chelating agent, Ca EDTA, is:
① Hypocalcemia
② Bone marrow depression
③ Increased intracranial pressure
④ Nephrotoxicity

Situation: Betsy Ames, 32 weeks pregnant, delivers a 3 pound male child whose Apgar scores are 4 and

7. The infant is immediately transferred to the neonatal intensive care unit.

144. The nurse should plan to take Mrs. Ames to visit her baby in intensive care:
① As soon as Mrs. Ames feels up to it
② When the infant is out of immediate danger
③ After the physician writes an order permitting it
④ When the infant's condition has stabilized

145. The nurse is aware that Mrs. Ames has still not begun the normal bonding process when Mrs. Ames says:
① "Do you think he will make it?"
② "Why does he need to be in an incubator?"
③ "He looks so much like my husband."
④ "It looks like such a tiny baby."

146. To aid Mrs. Ames in the bonding process, the nurse should say to her:
① "It must be hard to let yourself love a baby when you're not sure he'll make it."
② "He'll gain weight gradually and look better."
③ "Many mothers are shocked when they first see their babies; you'll see him grow."
④ "I will give you instructions on how to care for him."

147. Mrs. Ames names the baby Dennis. Because Dennis is at risk for respiratory distress syndrome, immediate nursing intervention is required when he develops:
① Tachycardia of 160 per minute
② A respiratory rate of 50 per minute
③ An expiratory grunt
④ Substernal retractions

148. Dennis experiences occasional periods of apnea and is placed on an apnea monitor. If the apnea monitor sounds, the nurse's initial action should be to:
① Provide oxygen by hood
② Suction his nasopharynx
③ Institute resuscitative measures
④ Provide light tactile stimulation

149. Baby Dennis develops hyperbilirubinemia, and phototherapy is begun. The nursing care plan for Dennis during therapy should include:
① Taking vital signs q 1 h
② Dressing him in a light shirt and diaper
③ Giving additional fluids q 2 h
④ Drawing blood for a Guthrie test qid

150. When an infant is receiving phototherapy the nurse should plan to:
① Discontinue the therapy and hold him during feedings
② Cover his head with a cap to minimize heat loss
③ Use mineral oil on his skin to prevent skin excoriation
④ Regulate radiant heat to keep the skin at 99° F

Situation: Bob Sant, age 29, is admitted to the hospital because of a suspected pituitary tumor, which is causing Cushing's syndrome.

151. Clinical manifestations of this syndrome that the nurse might observe in Mr. Sant may include:
① Hypotension and a rapid, thready pulse
② Increased fatty deposition in the extremities
③ Hypoglycemic episodes in the early morning
④ Retention of sodium and water

152. Mr. Sant's mother expresses anxiety about her son's condition. To help Mrs. Sant better understand his illness, the nurse should inform her that:
① His physical changes are permanent but will improve with time
② He will need to take exogenous steroids for several months
③ He may have mood swings or depression as a result of his disease
④ His condition is improving, as demonstrated by his weight gain

153. Mr. Sant undergoes removal of his pituitary tumor through a transsphenoidal approach. Postoperatively, the nurse should plan to:
① Raise the head of the bed to a 30 degree angle at all times
② Provide vigorous oral hygiene, including brushing the teeth
③ Encourage the client to deep breathe and cough frequently
④ Keep the client NPO until nasal packing is removed

154. The nurse should assess Mr. Sant for increasing intracranial pressure by monitoring his pulse pressure. The nurse understands that a client's pulse pressure is actually the:
① Difference between the apical and radial rates
② Force exerted against an arterial wall
③ Degree of ventricular contraction in relation to output
④ Difference between systolic and diastolic readings

155. Dexamethasone (Decadron) is ordered. While Mr. Sant is receiving the Decadron the nurse should plan nursing care considering his predisposition to:
① Urinary stasis
② Infection
③ Hypotension
④ Weight gain

Situation: A 72-year-old widower, Donald Rose, is admitted to the rehabilitative psychiatric unit for an evaluation related to his behavior. The nurse notes that he seems quite anxious, frequently paces about, has a short attention span, and is very forgetful. He relates at length the activities of his youth and early married years. His conformance to social norms, hygiene, and dress requirements have deteriorated over the last 3 months.

156. While Mr. Rose remains on the psychiatric unit, the nurse can best cope with the behaviors associated with dementia by:
① Consistently having all staff members reinforce reality with each client contact
② Providing a restrictive environment, including restraints, to prevent self-injury
③ Ignoring instances when denial is used, as well as the client's memory lapses
④ Focusing on the client's coping skills, to avoid making him feel more inadequate

157. The nurse develops a care plan related to Mr. Rose's altered mental status. In planning care for Mr. Rose the nurse should remember that confusion in the elderly:
① Is a common finding and is to be expected with aging
② Follows transfer to new surroundings
③ Results from brain pathology and cannot be cured or stopped
④ Is always progressive and will get worse

158. At night Mr. Rose becomes more disoriented and sleeps very little. Confusion caused by sleep deprivation can often be decreased by:
① Administering prescribed sedative medications
② Giving him a back rub and shutting his door tightly
③ Leaving a subdued light on in his room all night long
④ Restraining him so he will remain in his bed

159. Mr. Rose becomes progressively confused and tries to climb out of bed. The physician orders Mr. Rose to be restrained at night while in bed. The nurse should apply:
① Arm restraints secured to the headboard
② A jacket restraint secured to the underbed frame
③ Leg restraints secured to the footboard
④ Mitt restraints secured under the bed

160. One evening Mr. Rose chokes on his food and becomes panicky and cyanotic. The nurse performs the abdominal thrust maneuver and a wad of food pops out of his mouth. After several deep respirations his cyanosis disappears. It would be most appropriate at this time for the nurse to:
① Inform the client that everything is fine
② Provide psychologic support to the client
③ Teach the client how to prevent future problems
④ Stand the client up and check his pulse

Situation: Gino Testani, 28 months old, is admitted to the pediatric unit at 1 AM with a tentative diagnosis of meningitis. Physician's orders include: isolation; NPO; IV D5 ⅓NS at 45 ml/hour; chloramphenicol 100 mg IVPB q 6 h; and vs q 1 h.

161. Based on the physician's order for isolation the nurse should place Gino on:
① Syringe and needle precautions
② Enteric precautions
③ Respiratory isolation
④ Reverse isolation

162. All of the following beds are available on the pediatric unit. The night nurse should plan to put Gino in:
① A corner of a four-bed room next to the nurses' station
② An isolation room away from activity at the far end of the hall
③ A private room two doors away from the nurses' station
④ A semiprivate room in the middle of the hall

163. At 3 AM, after Gino is settled down, his mother tells the night nurse, "I have to leave now, but whenever I try to go, Gino gets so upset and then I start to cry." The nurse should:
① Encourage Gino's mother to spend the night
② Stay with Gino while his mother leaves
③ Tell her to wait until Gino falls asleep
④ Walk Gino's mother to the elevator

164. By 5 AM, Gino has assumed an opisthotonic position. At this time the nurse should place Gino in a:
① Side-lying position
② Trendelenberg position
③ Knee-chest position
④ High-Fowler's position

165. Gino has a pediatric microdrip set up. A 500 ml bottle of D5 ⅓NS was hung at 1 AM. At 6 AM, the night nurse notes that Gino's IV bottle has 125 ml left. The nurse correctly evaluates that the:
① IV has infused at the prescribed rate through the night
② Total amount of fluid infused is more than Gino should have received
③ Total amount of fluid infused is less than ordered for him
④ Amount of fluid infused should be calculated at the change of shift or 7 AM

166. At 7 AM, the physician orders the IV rate for Gino increased to 55 ml/hour. The night nurse should change the flow rate to:
① 9 to10 gtt/minute
② 13 to14 gtt/minute
③ 55 gtt/minute
④ 60 gtt/minute

167. Gino is receiving Chloramphenicol q 6 h. The nurse should be sure to monitor Gino's blood tests for side effects, which include:
① Hyperuricemia
② Polycythemia

③ Hypoalbuminemia
④ Aplastic anemia

Situation: Judy Carson, 58 years old, is admitted to the emergency room with a blood pressure of 240/150. She is complaining of a severe headache, blurred vision, and swelling of the ankles.

168. At this time it would be most appropriate for the nurse to:
① Place her in the supine position
② Obtain urine and blood samples
③ Obtain a glucometer reading
④ Assess other vital signs

169. Ms. Carson is admitted to the hospital. The physician orders furosemide (Lasix) 20 mg IV, and a Nipride infusion is begun. When administering the Lasix, the nurse should tell Ms. Carson that she:
① Will need to void in 5 to 10 minutes
② Should drink 240 ml of orange juice
③ May have problems with her hearing
④ Will feel some burning at the IV site

170. Later, the nurse enters Ms. Carson's room and finds her having a seizure. The nurse should:
① Attempt to place a tongue blade between her teeth
② Restrain her head and limb movements
③ Return to the nurses' station for help
④ Turn her to the side and hyperextend her neck

171. Ms. Carson's blood pressure is lowered with therapy and the physician orders a low-fat, 2 gram sodium diet. The nurse understands that a low-sodium diet will:
① Cause fluid to move toward the interstitial compartment
② Prevent reabsorption of water in the distal tubules
③ Chemically stimulate the loop of Henle
④ Diminish the thirst response of the client

172. The nurse schedules time to teach Ms. Carson about her diet. The nurse should instruct her to:
① Drink carbonated beverages instead of decaffeinated coffee
② Restrict her intake of green vegetables
③ Use lemon juice to season her meat
④ Refrain from eating canned fruits

173. Ms. Carson asks why her ankles are swollen. To respond, the nurse must understand that in the human body, where a semipermeable membrane divides two solutions, the solution with the greatest number of particles:
① Gives up water to the side with fewer particles
② Draws water in its direction
③ Does not contribute particles to the other side
④ Draws particles in its direction

Situation: Mabel Collier, age 74, fell off a stepstool, sustaining an injury to her left hip. She is transported to the hospital by ambulance.

174. X-rays reveal that Mrs. Collier has an intracapsular fracture of her left hip and she is temporarily placed in Buck's traction. When caring for Mrs. Collier the nurse should:
① Turn her from side to side every 2 hours
② Put each extremity through passive range of motion
③ Raise the head of the bed to semi-Fowler's position
④ Monitor her for tenderness in the left calf

175. An open reduction is performed. The nurse plans Mrs. Collier's postoperative care knowing that she:
① Cannot bear weight on the affected leg for 3 months
② Can be ambulated for short distances 1 to 2 days after surgery
③ Will not be permitted to lie on her affected side
④ Should be positioned with the legs in adduction

176. Mrs. Collier develops a thrombophlebitis in her left leg. She is prescribed bed rest, and heparin sodium IV is started. When describing the purpose of this drug to Mrs. Collier, the nurse should explain that it:
① Dissolves the blood clot in the vein
② Reduces the size of the thrombus
③ Promotes absorption of red blood cells
④ Prevents extension of the blood clot

177. While caring for Mrs. Collier, the nurse encourages active leg and foot exercises of her right leg every 2 hours. This activity will specifically help to:
① Maintain muscle strength
② Prevent additional clots
③ Reduce leg discomfort
④ Limit venous inflammation

Situation: Joseph Coe, a 30-year-old high school dropout who is employed as a dishwasher, and Linda, his 37-year-old wife of 9 years, have five children between the ages of 2 months and 8 years. Mr. Coe drinks heavily, especially on weekends. When he drinks, it takes little or no provocation to send him into a rage, yelling obscenities, throwing and breaking furniture, and occasionally hitting his wife and the older children.

178. The nurse recognizes that Mr. Coe's abusive behavior is probably related to his:
① Living in the culture of poverty
② Long-standing problem with alcohol
③ Feeling trapped in a marriage
④ Low socioeconomic background

179. Because Mrs. Coe appears to be a victim of abuse, it would be most therapeutic for the nurse to:
① Discuss birth control with her

② Report her experiences to the police

③ Let her talk about her family problems

④ Discuss the possibility of her leaving him

180. The Coes bring their 5-year-old daughter, Ann, to the emergency room with a broken arm and contusions. It is decided that Ann is a victim of child abuse. Through conversation with Mr. and Mrs. Coe and the child, the nurse is unsure who is responsible for the abuse. The nurse suspects it may be Mrs. Coe because of her:

① Effective use of defense mechanisms

② Isolation and lack of emotional support

③ Assertive and dominating personality

④ Lack of knowledge about child development

181. Focusing attention on individuals who may be at high risk for child abuse is an example of:

① Legal prevention

② Primary prevention

③ Secondary prevention

④ Tertiary prevention

Situation: Rene Heyt, who is at 43 weeks' gestation, is taken to the delivery room where she delivers a baby boy.

182. The obstetrician hands the baby to the nurse. The nurse's first action should be to:

① Dry the infant and place him in a warm environment

② Perform a physical assessment and instill eye drops

③ Stimulate the baby to cry

④ Administer oxygen by mask

183. Baby Boy Heyt is classified as postmature. This classification is based on the assessment finding of:

① Testicles undescended with few rugae over the scrotum

② Abundant lanugo and vernix caseosa

③ Skin thick with desquamation over most of the body

④ Sole creases over the anterior two thirds of each foot

184. Two hours after delivery, Mrs. Heyt is transferred to the postpartum unit. In planning Mrs. Heyt's care for the morning, the nurse's highest priority is:

① Planning activities so that Mrs. Heyt has time to rest and offering mild analgesics as ordered and other comfort measures to facilitate rest

② Arranging an individual session during which Mrs. Heyt can learn all that is necessary about successful breastfeeding

③ Anticipating the probability of postpartum hemorrhage and assessing Mrs. Heyt's uterus every 15 minutes for firmness and position

④ Anticipating possible safety needs and instructing Mrs. Heyt to remain in bed and call for assistance before attempting to ambulate

185. On the day after delivery, Mrs. Heyt mentions that her nipples are becoming sore from breastfeeding. The nurse should:

① Provide a breast shield for her to keep the infant's mouth off the nipples

② Assess her breastfeeding and hygiene techniques to identify possible causes

③ Instruct her to limit breastfeeding to 5 minutes per side until the soreness subsides

④ Instruct her to apply warm compresses before she begins to breastfeed

186. In assessing the rate of involution of Mrs. Heyt's uterus on the second postpartum day, the nurse palpating the fundus would expect it to be:

① One fingerbreadth above the umbilicus

② At the level of the umbilicus

③ One to two fingerbreadths below the umbilicus

④ Three to four fingerbreadths below the umbilicus

187. On the fourth postpartum day, Mrs. Heyt's vaginal discharge is a pinkish color and does not contain clots. This discharge is called:

① Lochia pinkosa

② Lochia alba

③ Lochia rubra

④ Lochia serosa

Test 3

Situation: Andrew Smith, who has angina pectoris, is instructed by the physician to take one nitroglycerin tablet sublingually when an angina attack occurs.

188. The nurse should teach Mr. Smith that he will know the nitroglycerin is effective when his:

① Sublingual area tingles because sensory nerves are being triggered

② Pulse rate increases because the cardiac output is stimulated

③ Pain subsides because his arterioles and venules dilate

④ Capacity for activity escalates because of increased collateral circulation

189. Mr. Smith's angina is usually very intense. To hasten the absorption of the nitroglycerin tablet, the nurse should instruct Mr. Smith to:

① Break up the tablet before placing it under the tongue

② Take the tablet with a glass of warm water

③ Swallow saliva before placing the tablet under the tongue

④ Move the tablet around with the tip of the tongue

190. Mrs. Smith visits her husband during visiting hours. As she is leaving the unit, Mrs. Smith says to the nurse, "He looks so pale." The nurse should reply:
① "Paleness is expected with heart problems."
② "You both must be terribly frightened by this."
③ "I can understand why you are worried, but he will be all right."
④ "Other clients get pale and recover without any complications."

191. Mr. Smith is diagnosed as having had a myocardial infarction. Two days after admission Mr. Smith has a temperature of 100.2°F. The nurse should:
① Notify the physician immediately about the temperature
② Encourage deep breathing and coughing every 2 hours
③ Record the temperature and monitor vital signs at routine intervals
④ Auscultate the chest for diminished breath sounds

192. Mr. Smith is on a low-sodium, weight-reducing diet. The nurse knows that the dietary teaching was effective when Mr. Smith chooses:
① Baked chicken and mashed potatoes
② Stir-fried Chinese vegetables and rice
③ Tuna fish salad with celery sticks
④ Lean steak and carrots

193. Mr. Smith begins a supervised progressive jogging regimen and asks the nurse how he will know it is helping. The nurse should reply:
① "When you perspire less when you run, because you'll use less energy."
② "When the intermittent claudication is reduced."
③ "When your breathing becomes regular and shallow."
④ "When you can run progressively longer distances before tiring."

Situation: Peter Goldner, 56 years old, seeks medical attention for hoarseness and frequent bouts of laryngitis. After a laryngoscopy and biopsy of a lesion on the vocal cords, cancer of the larynx is diagnosed and a total laryngectomy with a radical neck dissection is planned. The physician carefully explains all the ramifications of surgery to Mr. Goldner.

194. When reinforcing the physician's statements, the nurse should review with the client what the surgery entails and what abilities will be lost. The discussion should also focus on what abilities Mr. Goldner will retain, such as the ability to:
① Smell and differentiate odors
② Sip through a straw

③ Blow his nose
④ Chew and swallow food

195. Mr. Goldner returns from the operating room with a laryngectomy tube in the permanent stoma, an intravenous infusion running, and a portable suction unit draining the surgical site. To facilitate respirations and promote comfort, Mr. Goldner should be placed in the:
① Side-lying position
② Semi-Fowler's position
③ Orthopneic position
④ High-Fowler's position

196. During the immediate postoperative period a priority nursing goal for Mr. Goldner should be to:
① Observe for signs of infection
② Provide emotional support
③ Keep the trachea free of secretions
④ Promote a means of communication

197. Two days after surgery the physician orders a progressive diet as tolerated for Mr. Goldner. The nurse should:
① Administer pain medication as ordered 30 minutes before meals to limit discomfort
② Encourage intake of pureed foods because they promote the swallowing reflex
③ Keep a suction apparatus readily available in case aspiration occurs
④ Administer the diet through a nasogastric tube until the suture line heals

198. Mr. Goldner is using a pad and pencil to communicate. He becomes very frustrated and writes, "When can I learn how to speak again?" The nurse's best response would be:
① "Every client is different. It's difficult to say just how long it will be."
② "You have to give the incision time to heal before going to speech therapy."
③ "Perhaps I can arrange for a member of the Laryngectomy Club to speak with you."
④ "It must be difficult for you, but be patient. These things take time."

Situation: Susan White is admitted to the psychiatric unit. She appears dejected, barely responds to questions, and walks very slowly about the unit.

199. Ms. White tells the nurse in a barely audible voice that life is no longer worth living. The nurse's most therapeutic response to this statement would be:
① "Have you been thinking about suicide?"
② "Let's talk about something pleasant, and you'll feel better."
③ "What could be so bad to make you feel that way?"
④ "We'll talk about your feelings after you have rested."

200. In caring for clients who are at risk for suicide, the nurse should be aware that:
① A client who talks about suicide never

commits suicide; it is just a way to get attention

② It is best not to talk to clients about suicide because it may give them the idea

③ A client who fails in a suicide attempt will probably not try again

④ The more formalized the plan, the greater the possibility that the client will attempt suicide

201. In talking with Ms. White, her statement that would give the nurse a clue that she may be going to attempt suicide would be:
① "I don't feel too good today."
② "I feel a little better, but it probably will not last."
③ "I'm very tired today, and I'd like to be alone."
④ "I feel much better; today is a lovely day."

202. Ms. White is to start electroconvulsive therapy (ECT) in the morning and asks how the treatment will help. The nurse should reply:
① "The important thing is it will help you."
② "It works on chemical substances in the brain, and it does help."
③ "Why don't you ask the physician? He can explain it better."
④ "It changes your usual behavior patterns."

203. Succinylcholine chloride (Anectine) is administered to Ms. White before she receives ECT. The nurse should observe her for:
① Nausea and vomiting
② Convulsions
③ Respiratory difficulties
④ Loss of memory

204. When Ms. White returns from ECT, she complains that she has lost her memory. The nurse should reply:
① "This is only temporary; your memory will return after the therapy is completed."
② "It is better if you forget what happened before you became ill."
③ "The fact that you are getting well is the most important thing for you right now."
④ "I will help you try to remember when the treatments are over."

Situation: Timmy Loomis is born with a cleft lip.

205. Timmy's nursing care, unlike that of other newborns, includes:
① Using modified techniques of feeding
② Keeping him on strict intake and output
③ Changing his position frequently
④ Keeping his head elevated at all times

206. Timmy is going to have surgery for the repair of his lip when he is about 10 weeks old. In preparation for the postoperative period the nurse should instruct Mrs. Loomis to:
① Teach him to drink from a cup
② Keep his arms in restraints at all times

③ Place him on his back for long periods
④ Burp him as little as possible after feeding

207. Timmy, now 10 weeks old, is recovering from reparative surgery. His mother is with him constantly and participates actively in his nursing care. Mrs. Loomis demonstrates that she has a good understanding of Timmy's postoperative needs when she:
① Gives Timmy his feeding while he lies on his side
② Cleanses his suture line after each feeding
③ Allows him to cry for short periods of time
④ Offers Timmy a pacifier when he becomes restless

208. For a few days after the repair of his lip Timmy should be fed via:
① Intravenous infusion
② Nasogastric tube
③ A bottle with a premie nipple
④ A rubber-tipped syringe

209. Mrs. Loomis questions the nurse about the elbow restraints on Timmy's arms. The nurse's best response regarding the use of the restraints would be:
① "They are used routinely on all children with lip surgery."
② "Keeping his arms straight makes it difficult for him to touch his mouth."
③ "The surgeon insists that all his clients have them on."
④ "We can't be with him all the time to watch that he doesn't touch his mouth."

Situation: Kevin and Laura Kett are both attending graduate school and plan to wait a few years to start a family. The Ketts attend a family planning clinic to determine which contraceptive method would be most appropriate for them.

210. When discussing intrauterine devices, Mrs. Kett asks the nurse during which phase of the menstrual cycle should the IUD be inserted. The nurse responds that the insertion is usually done on the:
① First to fourth day
② Fifth to tenth day
③ Fourteenth to sixteenth day
④ Twenty-fifth to twenty-eighth day

211. The Ketts also ask about the cervical mucus method of family planning. The nurse explains that if they use this method, they must avoid intercourse when the cervical mucus is:
① Yellow and thin
② Clear and thick
③ Cloudy and viscid
④ Clear and stretchable

212. The nurse knows that Mrs. Kett understands the discussion about the use of a diaphragm when she states, "After intercourse, a diaphragm must be left in place for:
① 1 to 2 hours."
② 6 to 8 hours."

③ 10 to 12 hours."

④ 16 to 20 hours."

213. Mr. and Mrs. Kett discuss the various methods of family planning. Together, they decide to use the basal body temperature method. Before they begin using this method they should understand that the fertility period surrounding ovulation usually extends from:
① 12 hours before to 24 hours after ovulation
② 72 hours before to 24 hours after ovulation
③ 24-48 hours before to 48 hours after ovulation
④ 72-80 hours before to 72 hours after ovulation

Situation: Glendal Gray, a primigravida, calls the nurse midwife in the antepartum clinic to complain of a sharp shooting pain in the lower quadrant of her abdomen. She also has vaginal spotting. Mrs. Gray is told to go to the hospital so that she can be examined. A diagnosis of a ruptured tubal pregnancy is made.

214. When the nurse in the hospital questions Mrs. Gray about the initial appearance of her symptoms, she should expect Mrs. Gray's answer to indicate that her symptoms started:
① Immediately after implantation occurred
② About the sixth week of pregnancy
③ Midway through the second trimester
④ At the beginning of the last trimester

215. The nurse prepares Mrs. Gray for immediate surgery. In view of her symptoms, the nurse will probably be preparing Mrs. Gray for a:
① Dilation and curettage
② Hysterectomy
③ Salpingectomy
④ Myomectomy

216. While Mrs. Gray is being prepared for surgery, she complains of feeling light-headed. Her pulse is very rapid, and her color is pale. The nurse assesses that Mrs. Gray may be:
① Hyperventilating
② Going into shock
③ Extremely anxious
④ Developing an infection

217. Nursing care plans for Mrs. Gray after surgery should include:
① Counseling for an intrauterine device (IUD) so as to prevent another tubal pregnancy
② Administering Rho (D) immune globulin (RhoGAM) to prevent isoimmunization
③ Assuring her that she is still capable of becoming pregnant
④ Telling her not to douche after intercourse because this may dislodge a fertilized egg

Situation: Aaron Jacobs, 67 years old, is widowed suddenly when his wife is killed in a car accident.

218. The first action by the nurse in the emergency room to best help Mr. Jacobs at this time would be:
① Referring him to a support group that meets near his home
② Asking the clergyman of his faith to visit him
③ Assuring him that everything possible was done for his wife
④ Having the physician order a tranquilizer for him

219. A potential nursing diagnosis for Mr. Jacobs related to the death of his wife would be:
① Ineffective individual coping
② Defensive coping
③ Altered family processes
④ Personal identity disturbance

220. Eight months later Mr. Jacobs comes to the mental health clinic. He reports that he has been very depressed since the death of his wife and he has not been seeing any of his friends or attending any of the activities he previously enjoyed. His married children live in another state and he rarely has any contact with them. The most accurate nursing diagnosis for Mr. Jacobs would be:
① Impaired verbal communication related to social isolation
② Dysfunctional grieving related to difficulty reestablishing life-style following the death of his wife
③ Ineffective individual coping related to low motivation to resume activities of daily living
④ Ineffective family coping related to separation from children

221. Studies have shown that the grieving process may last longer for people who have:
① Feelings of guilt
② Ambivalent feelings about the death
③ Failed to remarry within 3 years
④ A close relationship with their family

222. Formulating a nursing diagnosis for Mr. Jacobs occurs during the stage of the nursing process known as:
① Assessment
② Analysis
③ Planning
④ Evaluation

223. The nursing diagnosis made for Mr. Jacobs could be defined as a statement:
① Made to explain his present needs
② That describes his health status and related factors
③ Of his responses that are within the scope of nursing
④ That rewords his medical diagnosis in nursing terminology

224. A long-term goal for Mr. Jacobs would be that he will be able to:
① Relocate to the state in which his children reside

② Eat at least two meals a day with another person
③ Decrease his negative thinking about himself and others
④ Resume the activities he previously enjoyed

Situation: Carol Jones, a 47-year-old teacher, went to her Health Maintenance Organization for a routine examination. She was found to have an enlarged thyroid gland. It is suspected that she has hyperthyroidism.

225. On assessment of Ms. Jones, the nurse should expect to find:
① Thickened and coarse skin
② Menstrual disturbances and loss of libido
③ Tachycardia and palpitations
④ Apathetic attitude and masklike facies

226. Ms. Jones is referred to the laboratory for a radioactive iodine (RAI) uptake test. In teaching about this test, the nurse should explain that:
① Her urine will not contain any radioactive particles
② This test is one of several needed for an accurate diagnosis
③ Test results will not be influenced by any medications
④ An accurate measure of thyroid hormone levels will be obtained

227. Hyperthyroidism is confirmed. Ms. Jones is treated with propylthiouracil, an antithyroid drug, along with potassium iodide. The nurse teaches her about these medications with the knowledge that:
① The drugs will be discontinued as soon as the client's temperature and pulse rate return to normal
② The client should carefully observe for signs of infection or bleeding while on this therapy
③ Iodide solutions such as these must be taken on an empty stomach and diluted in water
④ Use of these drugs before thyroidectomy will increase the risk of postoperative hemorrhage

228. If the medication is not effective, an additional health problem may develop as a result of her continued tachycardia. The nurse should tell Ms. Jones to immediately report the development of:
① Nervousness and irritability
② Weight gain or pedal edema
③ Changes in appetite or bowel habits
④ Flushed skin and diaphoresis

229. One week later, Ms. Jones reports that she has diarrhea, abdominal pain, and fever. Ms. Jones is admitted for thyrotoxicosis. The most important goal of immediate treatment for this condition is:

① Rapid reduction of body temperature and heart rate
② Prevention of fluid overload by limiting the client's intake
③ Observation for an exaggerated response to sedatives
④ Treatment of associated hyperglycemia and ketoacidosis

Situation: James Nide, with a history of chronic obstructive pulmonary disease, is admitted to the hospital with pneumonia. He is placed on bed rest with the head elevated and is receiving humidified oxygen at 2 L. An IV antibiotic and Bronkosol, a bronchodilator, via ultrasonic nebulizer are ordered.

230. When teaching Mr. Nide how to use the nebulizer the nurse instructs him to:
① Seal his lips around the mouthpiece, taking rapid, shallow breaths through the nose
② Hold his breath while spraying the medication carefully into each nostril
③ Instill the medication from the nebulizer while exhaling through the nose
④ Loosely place his lips around the mouthpiece taking a slow, deep breath through the mouth

231. On the third day of Mr. Nide's hospitalization, he complains of a sharp pain on the right side of his chest. The nurse suspects a right pneumothorax. In assessing breath sounds on the affected side, the nurse should expect to hear:
① Wheezing sounds
② Crackling sounds
③ Adventitious sounds
④ Decreased breath sounds

232. The physician assesses the client and diagnoses right pneumothorax, and a chest tube is inserted. The primary purpose of the chest tube for Mr. Nide is to:
① Drain accumulated fluid from the pleural cavity
② Lessen Mr. Nide's chest pain and discomfort
③ Prevent subcutaneous emphysema in the chest wall
④ Restore negative pressure in the pleural space

233. While Mr. Nide's chest tube is in place, the nurse plans to:
① Encourage coughing, deep breathing, and ROM to the right arm
② Administer cough suppressants at appropriate intervals as ordered
③ Empty and measure the drainage in the collection chamber each shift
④ Apply clamps below the insertion site whenever he gets out of bed

234. Mr. Nide is to be taken to the Radiology Department via stretcher. When transporting him, the nurse should keep the:

① Chest tube clamped between the water seal chamber and the client
② End of the chest tube covered with sterile 4X4s securely taped
③ Collection device below the level of the client's chest
④ Collection device attached to mechanical suction

Situation: Eric Mason, 4 months old, is admitted to the pediatric unit with the diagnosis of nonorganic failure to thrive (NFTT). Eric is the first child of adolescent parents

235. When assessing a young infant, inspection, palpation, percussion, and auscultation are used. The technique the nurse should perform last is:
① Auscultation of his heart and breath sounds
② Inspection of his general condition
③ Percussion of his lung fields
④ Palpation of his abdominal organs

236. Considering Eric's medical diagnosis and family situation the priority nursing diagnosis for this family would be:
① Altered nutrition: less than body requirements related to child abuse
② Sensory/perceptual alterations (gustatory) related to infant deprivation
③ Potential for injury related to mothering failure
④ Altered parenting related to knowledge deficit

237. Considering Eric's age, his mother should be encouraged to provide him with:
① Push-pull type toys
② Nesting blocks and cups
③ Snap beads and strings
④ Soft squeeze toys with squeakers

238. With therapy, Eric improves and begins to meet the developmental milestones appropriate for his age. At his 18-month checkup the nurse recognizes that Eric's growth and development is within the normal range when he:
① Builds a tower of eight blocks
② Climbs up the stairs
③ Says 150 different words
④ Pedals a tricycle easily

239. During the health history, the nurse learns that Eric recently had a fever, runny nose, cough, and white spots in his mouth for 3 days. He then developed a rash that started on his face and spread to his whole body. The nurse should suspect that Eric probably had:
① Varicella
② Rubeola
③ Rubella
④ Scarlet fever

Situation: Michael Hazlitt, 3 years of age, has had swollen cervical lymph nodes and a prolonged high fever that has not responded to antibiotics. When he develops erythema of the extremities, he is admitted to the pediatric unit for further evaluation.

240. A diagnosis of Kawasaki disease is made based on:
① An elevated ASO titer
② A combination of symptoms
③ An elevated sedimentation rate
④ A decreased serum protein level

241. Aspirin is prescribed along with intravenous gamma globulin. When administering the aspirin to Michael the nurse should:
① Disguise the medication in his favorite food
② Offer Michael a reward for taking his prescribed medication
③ Not respond to questions about the taste of the drug to avoid lying
④ Let him decide how he will take his medication

Situation: Steve Farmer's diagnostic findings reveal adenocarcinoma of the descending colon with a partial obstruction. Chemotherapy is initiated to reduce the tumor mass, after which a hemicolectomy is planned.

242. Mr. Farmer is receiving Adriamycin IV. The nurse should assess for signs of toxicity which include:
① An alteration in cardiac rhythm
② A minor skin rash
③ A blue tinge to the urine
④ An increased feeling of nervousness

243. While undergoing chemotherapy, it is most essential for Mr. Farmer to immediately report to the nurse any:
① Loss of hair
② Nausea
③ Sore throat
④ Constipation

244. When receiving chemotherapy Mr. Farmer states, "I get so sick to my stomach. The medication is useless." The response by the nurse that employs the technique of paraphrasing is:
① "You don't think the medication is helping you?"
② "I'll get an order for an antiemetic."
③ "You get sick to your stomach?"
④ "Tell me more about how you feel."

245. Mr. Farmer is scheduled for the hemicolectomy. The nurse's primary role in informed consent for surgery is one of client advocate. The nurse should recognize that in regard to informed consent:
① As a witness, the nurse must be present to see the client actually sign the form
② Either a nurse or a physician can give the client the necessary information to obtain informed consent for surgery
③ Clients need to know about the procedure;

they need not be frightened with information about potential risks

④ A consent is only valid for 7 days; if a longer time passes a new form must be signed

246. One of the medical orders the nurse would expect for Mr. Farmer preoperatively would be:
① Administer Neomycin 1 gram q 6 h orally for 2 days preoperatively
② Have a Sengstaken-Blakemore tube at the bedside preoperatively
③ Oil retention enemas daily for 2 days preoperatively
④ Give a high-protein, high-carbohydrate regular diet for 2 days preoperatively

247. Mr. Farmer returns from the operating room with a nasogastric tube in place. The nurse understands that the purpose of this tube is to:
① Remove fluids and gas from the upper gastrointestinal tract
② Provide a route for liquid tube feeding when possible
③ Monitor the acidity of the gastric secretions
④ Permit continuous decompression of the large bowel

248. Mr. Farmer's condition improves, and he is placed on a regular diet. The food he will most likely be able to tolerate with little discomfort is:
① Whole milk
② Bran cereal
③ Baked fish
④ Fresh fruit

Situation: Beth Stern is pregnant with her first child.

249. About the eighth or ninth week, an assessment of Mrs. Stern's adaptations to pregnancy would reveal:
① Lightening
② Goodell's sign
③ Braxton Hicks contractions
④ Quickening

250. Mrs. Stern's last menstrual period was February 11. On July 18 a physical assessment of Mrs. Stern should indicate that the top of her fundus is:
① Even with the umbilicus
② Half way between the symphysis and umbilicus
③ Two fingerbreadths above the umbilicus
④ Just above the symphysis pubis

251. At 39 weeks, Mrs. Stern begins having uterine contractions. When her cervix is 3 to 4 cm dilated and 60% effaced, and the vertex is at −1 station, Mrs. Stern has a sudden spurt of dark blood from the vagina. Her uterus is irritable on palpation and does not relax well between contractions. The nurse should immediately:

① Transport her to the delivery room without delay
② Perform a vaginal examination to determine dilation
③ Check her BP and FHR and monitor her uterine activity
④ Change Mrs. Stern's underpad and position her on her back

252. Mrs. Stern delivers a baby girl by cesarean delivery. The nursery nurse suspects that Baby Stern has Down's syndrome when the initial assessment reveals:
① High-pitched catlike cry, microcephaly, and low-set ears
② Low-set ears, micrognathia, and rocker bottom feet
③ Lymphedema of dorsa of hands and feet, webbed neck, and widely spaced nipples
④ Hypotonia, low-set ears, simian crease, and epicanthal folds

253. The physician tells Mr. and Mrs. Stern that their daughter may have Down's syndrome and additional diagnostic studies should be performed. In the plan of care, the nurse should prepare for:
① Aminocentesis
② Karyotyping
③ A buccal smear
④ Enzyme assay

254. Mrs. Stern tells the nurse that she could not possibly take a retarded child home and asks if she should plan to place her daughter in an institution. An appropriate statement by the nurse at this time would be:
① "You should not make such a hasty decision; your baby is like any other baby right now."
② "At this young age no one is able to predict the baby's ultimate level of functioning."
③ "Give yourself time to get acquainted with your baby, and see that she isn't retarded yet."
④ "I understand how you feel, and I will notify the nursery personnel of your decision."

Situation: The Salk children, 2, 4, and 6 years old, are termed accident prone because of several accidents. The community health nurse involves the parents in a teaching program to avoid accidents.

255. The nurse instructs Mr. and Mrs. Salk to lower the risk of accidents with discipline that stresses:
① Rational consistency
② Realistic rigidity
③ Guarded indifference
④ Serious overprotection

256. Two-year-old Billy Salk should be closely supervised for potential accidents at this age because he is learning primarily from:
① His mother and father

② Trial and error
③ His playmates
④ Older siblings

Situation: Four-year-old Ann Russo is diagnosed with Wilms' tumor and is admitted to the hospital for surgery.

257. When preparing a preschooler for a surgical procedure, the best time to tell the child what will happen is:
   ① Just before it happens
   ② 1 month in advance
   ③ 2 weeks before
   ④ 3 to 4 days before

258. On admission to the pediatric unit the nurse should place a sign on Ann's crib that says:
   ① No IV medications
   ② Do not use diapers
   ③ Strain all urine
   ④ Do not palpate abdomen

259. The nurse knows that the most important aspect of the preoperative care of the child with Wilms' tumor is to:
   ① Monitor the blood pressure
   ② Maintain the child in a prone position
   ③ Check the size of the liver
   ④ Obtain urine for culture and sensitivity

260. A preschool child views death:
   ① As permanent and irreversible
   ② As a departure from which the person returns
   ③ Without comprehending its meaning in any way
   ④ In a frightening and horrible way

261. Before Ann's discharge the nurse explains to her parents that because Ann has only one kidney, precautions will have to be taken to preserve the remaining kidney. The nurse is aware they understand the teaching when they say:
   ① "We will limit Ann's fluid intake to 3 glasses daily."
   ② "We will not prevent Ann from taking part in sports when she is older."
   ③ "We will teach Ann to wipe from front to back after going to the bathroom."
   ④ "We will keep Ann away from those individuals with infections."

Situation: Arnie Smothers, 50 years old, is admitted with chronic hypertension, syncope, right hemiparesis, and expressive aphasia.

262. Mr. Smothers has difficulty communicating because of the aphasia. When the nurse asks him how he is feeling, Mrs. Smothers answers for her husband. The nurse should:
   ① Instruct Mrs. Smothers to let Mr. Smothers speak for himself
   ② Acknowledge her but look at Mr. Smothers for a response
   ③ Ask Mrs. Smothers how she knows how he feels

④ Return later after Mrs. Smothers has gone home

263. The nurse assists Mr. Smothers with lunch. The nurse suspects that Mr. Smothers may have left-side hemianopsia when he:
   ① Ignores the food on the left side of his tray when eating
   ② Asks to have all food moved to the left side of the tray
   ③ Drops the coffee cup when trying to use his right hand
   ④ Complains he cannot use his left arm to help eat

264. The physician orders a stationary (nonrolling) walker for Mr. Smothers to aid his ambulation. The nurse plans to teach Mr. Smothers to:
   ① Place the walker flat on the floor about 12 inches in front of his feet, shift his body weight to the walker, and step forward
   ② Move the walker about 8 inches forward while stepping forward to the walker with his body weight on the walker and his legs
   ③ Place the back legs of the walker about 10 inches in front of his feet, shift his body weight to the walker, and step forward
   ④ Move the walker about 10 inches in front of his feet with only the front legs of the walker on the floor, then step forward and put the walker flat

265. The nurse begins planning for Mr. Smothers' discharge. Information the nurse should include in the education program is the:
   ① Importance of bed rest at home
   ② Need to decrease protein in the diet
   ③ Importance of a safe environment
   ④ Use of oxygen therapy at home

Situation: Mark Payer, 6 years old, is admitted to an inpatient child psychiatric unit with a diagnosis of attention-deficit hyperactivity disorder. He exhibits a short attention span and demonstrates excessive motor activity with intermittent head banging.

266. The nurse is aware that a 6-year-old with normal psychosocial development would have achieved Erikson's developmental tasks of trust, autonomy, and:
   ① Identity
   ② Intimacy
   ③ Initiative
   ④ Belonging

267. The most important nursing diagnosis for Mark at this time would be:
   ① Anxiety related to shortened attention span
   ② Potential for violence: self-directed, related to self-destructive behavior
   ③ Altered parenting related to inability to set limits on child's behavior
   ④ Sleep pattern disturbance related to hyperactivity

268. The most important nursing objective when planning care for Mark would be to:
① Prevent Mark from causing any self-injury
② Assist Mark to develop an ability to test reality
③ Help Mark to formulate realistic ego boundaries
④ Provide Mark with opportunities to discharge energy

269. It has been decided that Mark is ready for discharge. The behavior that would indicate that nursing interventions have been effective for Mark would be that he:
① Is no longer enuretic during the nighttime
② Has an increased attention span in school
③ Is not inhibited by rules or routines
④ Enjoys playing with his cars by himself

Situation: Rick Ronson is a 36-year-old supermarket manager who is married and has two children. Whenever he attempts to ride in an elevator, he experiences extreme terror. He is also very uneasy in large crowds. He feels uncomfortable about his fears and is beginning to experience difficulty concentrating at work. He makes an appointment to see the nurse at a mental hygiene clinic.

270. In assessing the situation, the nurse should understand that Mr. Ronson's symptoms are probably associated with:
① Depression about life events, which frequently leads to unreasonable fears
② Generalized anxiety about conflicts, which has been displaced into specific unreasonable fears
③ The development of an obsession as a result of his conflicts with society
④ A terrifying incident in an elevator in Mr. Ronson's past that has been repressed but unresolved

271. A suitable short-term goal for Mr. Ronson would be that he will:
① Ride an elevator without anxiety, accompanied by the nurse
② Experience relief from his depression and an elevation of mood
③ Describe the thoughts and feelings he experiences in terrifying situations
④ Identify the early childhood conflicts leading to his fears

Situation: Diane Worth, a primigravida, is admitted in active labor. The baby is in a breech position.

272. During labor the nurse should expect to note:
① Deceleration at the end of a contraction
② Irregularity of the fetal heart rate
③ Heavy bleeding from the vagina
④ Meconium staining of the amniotic fluid

273. Mrs. Worth is scheduled for a cesarean delivery. An important nursing intervention during labor to prevent postoperative complications should include:

① Frequent monitoring of maternal vital signs
② Maintenance of adequate hydration
③ Notification of the neonatal intensive care unit
④ Provision of scrupulous skin care

274. A cesarean delivery is performed, and Mrs. Worth is transferred to the recovery room. A nursing diagnosis of altered tissue perfusion is made related to the:
① Inability of Mrs. Worth to turn from side to side
② Increased risk for hemorrhage following cesarean delivery
③ Unfavorable position of the fetus during labor
④ Use of regional anesthesia during the delivery

Situation: Marion Jay, a primigravida in the thirteenth week of gestation, is admitted to the labor and delivery suite via stretcher. She is unaccompanied and is crying. On assessment, the nurse, Ms. Swep, determines that Ms. Jay is having uterine cramping and moderate bleeding and is aborting the pregnancy.

275. It is important for the nurse to first deal with her own feelings about abortion, death, and loss so that she can:
① Maintain complete control of the situation
② Allow the client to express her grief fully
③ Share her personal grief with the client
④ Teach the client to cope more effectively

276. Ms. Jay's anxiety is displayed in her question, "Could this have happened because I had the flu?" Ms. Swep's best response would be:
① "The doctor will be here soon and at that time will tell you what is causing the bleeding. Wait until then."
② "I'm sure that there is absolutely nothing you could have done to cause this. You need not worry about that."
③ "We know that maternal infections sometimes result in miscarriages. Perhaps the flu did cause it."
④ "You feel that you did something to cause the bleeding? Tell me more about what you think."

Situation: Harriet Jakes, a 50-year-old librarian, is admitted to the hospital with a suspected brain tumor. She has been experiencing morning headaches, loss of equilibrium and coordination, and occasional mental clouding.

277. Based on the history of loss of equilibrium and coordination, the nurse suspects the tumor is located in the:
① Basal ganglia
② Parietal lobe
③ Occipital lobe
④ Cerebellum

278. The diagnostic test the nurse would expect Ms. Jakes to have soon after admission is:
① Myelography
② Electromyography
③ Lumbar puncture
④ Computerized tomography

279. A brain tumor is confirmed, and surgery is scheduled. Part of Ms. Jakes' preoperative preparation should include:
① Gently shampooing the hair
② Administering morphine sulfate
③ Forcing nutrient fluids
④ Administering cleansing enemas

280. Dexamethasone (Decadron) is ordered for Ms. Jakes following surgery. The nurse recognizes that the expected response should be:
① Reduced cell proliferation
② Reduced cerebral edema
③ Increased renal reabsorption
④ Increased response to sedation

281. Ms. Jakes' condition deteriorates. She repeatedly expresses that she does not want to be a burden and wants to die. She asks the nurse for help. Before responding, the nurse recognizes that a nurse actively or passively aiding a client with euthanasia is:
① Liable to be tried for a crime
② Acting within the law in most states
③ Practicing medicine without a license
④ Negligent in performing nursing duties

Test 4

Situation: Sally Ochs is pregnant for the first time. In the sixteenth week she develops vaginitis for which the physician prescribes daily douches.

282. The nurse provides Mrs. Ochs with instructions for douching. The most important aspect of the instruction is that Mrs. Ochs should:
① Use a sterilized bulb syringe
② Recline with head and shoulders elevated slightly
③ Hold the labia together while instilling the solution
④ Insert the douche tip 5 to 6 inches

283. Mrs. Ochs was 20 pounds overweight when she became pregnant. She has already gained another 20 pounds during this pregnancy. The nurse understands that treating Mrs. Ochs' obesity during pregnancy is not advisable because:
① Additional calories are needed for her increased activity
② Weight loss can best be achieved after pregnancy
③ Protein is utilized for energy when carbohydrates are decreased
④ Calcium utililzation varies proportionately with calorie intake

284. Mrs. Ochs is now 42 weeks pregnant. She is admitted for a nonstress test. The nurse is aware that this is being scheduled because a prolonged pregnancy can:
① Result in a baby that is LGA
② Lead to placental insufficiency
③ Predispose the mother to postpartal infection
④ Indicate subclinical gestational diabetes

285. Fifteen days after Mrs. Ochs' due date, a healthy baby boy is born. When assessing this newborn, the nurse will most likely find:
① Large amounts of lanugo over his shoulders
② Ample fatty tissue distributed over his entire body
③ That he seems to want to sleep for long periods
④ That he is constantly putting his fists in his mouth

286. During Baby Ochs' bath, the nurse teaches Mrs. Ochs to disinfect the base of his umbilical cord and tells her, "It's important to do this since the cord stump is a potential site for infection because:
① It is touched by blankets and clothing."
② Wharton's jelly is no longer present."
③ It contains necrotic tissue and blood."
④ Newborns have no resistance to infection."

287. By the third day of life, Baby Ochs weighs 5% less than he did at birth. His weight loss most likely results from:
① The development of sepsis
② Generalized muscle response to stimulation
③ An obstructive gastrointestinal anomaly
④ An imbalance between nutrient intake and elimination

288. Later that day, Mrs. Ochs tells the nurse that her breasts feel warm, firm, and tender. The skin appears shiny and taut. The nurse suspects that the cause of Mrs. Ochs' discomfort is:
① Inadequate emptying of the breast during each feeding
② Stasis of milk in the mammary ducts
③ Overdistention of the acini with milk
④ Increased lymphatic and venous circulation in the breasts

Situation: Irene Daily, a 65-year-old widow, has been admitted to the hospital for an acute episode of rheumatoid arthritis. She complains that lately she has lost weight, has been tired, and has had migratory pain in her joints.

289. Mrs. Daily asks why her roommate Mrs. Tane, who also has arthritis, goes to physical therapy every day and she does not. The most appropriate response by the nurse would be:
① "Her condition is much more advanced than yours."

② "Physical therapy is an important aspect of rheumatology care."

③ "It usually depends on who your physician is."

④ "Your joints are still inflamed and it would be harmful."

290. The physician orders aspirin therapy to be continued at home. In teaching Mrs. Daily regarding aspirin intake, the nurse should emphasize that she should:
① Switch to Tylenol if tinnitus occurs
② Take the medicine on a full stomach or with meals
③ See her dentist if she develops gum bleeding
④ Avoid spicy foods during the time she is taking the medication

291. Mrs. Daily progresses to the stage where she can no longer care for herself, and she is admitted to a health-related facility. According to Erikson the major developmental conflict for Mrs. Daily is:
① Ego integrity vs despair
② Generativity vs stagnation
③ Identity vs role diffusion
④ Intimacy vs isolation

292. Mrs. Daily is in severe pain and tells the nurse that the only time she is pain free is when she lies perfectly still. The nurse should explain that she needs to exercise every day to prevent:
① Shortening of the muscles
② Loss of muscular coordination
③ Paresthesias of the feet
④ Osteoblastic development

293. When discussing with Mrs. Daily the frequency of her tub baths, the prime factor that should be considered is:
① Her ability to assist
② The condition of her skin
③ Her degree of orientation
④ The history of allergic reactions

294. Mrs. Daily develops a small decubitus ulcer on the sacral area. The nurse should plan to deal with this problem by:
① Keeping the area dry
② Providing a low-calorie diet
③ Applying moist dressings
④ Keeping her on her right side

Situation: The local voluntary hospital is instituting various outreach programs for the community. One of the programs will be for scoliosis screening.

295. In the designing of the program, the most appropriate site to implement the actual screening would be in a:
① Well-baby clinic
② Senior high school
③ Preschool day care center
④ Junior high school

296. Tammy Mitchell is examined by the nurse practitioner, and scoliosis is suspected. A note is sent to her parents suggesting that she be seen by her pediatrician for evaluation. Tammy's mother calls the school nurse to ask what scoliosis actually is. To answer the question, the nurse must understand that it is:
① A pathologic process involving the vertebrae
② Concave lumbar curvature that is very exaggerated
③ Curvature of the thoracic spine that has an increased convex angulation
④ Lateral curvature of the spine with a rotary deformity

297. Mrs. Mitchell takes Tammy to the pediatrician, and she is diagnosed as having idiopathic scoliosis with a mild structural curve. Mrs. Mitchell asks the nurse if the problem can be corrected with exercise. The nurse should reply that an exercise program will be:
① The only intervention needed to correct the curvature
② Used in conjunction with a Milwaukee brace
③ Avoided because it can exaggerate the curvature
④ Employed if Tammy appears highly motivated.

298. Tammy is very upset about the treatment regimen and is worried that she will be different from her friends. To help Tammy develop a positive self-image during treatment the nurse should:
① Refer Tammy for psychologic counseling until the treatment program is over
② Assist Tammy in the selection of appropriate clothing to minimize her condition
③ Remind Tammy how crooked her back would be if she did not get treatment
④ Exaggerate Tammy's positive attributes and avoid focusing on negative attributes

Situation: Mary Court, a fourth-grader, is sent home from school because the school nurse identifies that Mary has pediculosis capitis (head lice). Mary's mother takes her to the pediatrician, who orders 1% gamma benzene hexachloride (Kwell) shampoo.

299. When teaching Mary's mother about the treatment for head lice, the nurse should tell her that:
① Clothing and personal belongings must be boiled or discarded
② Other children should be kept away from Mary for 1 week
③ The shampoo must be repeated within 7 to 10 days
④ The medicated shampoo has no known side effects

300. When Mary returns to school, her mother asks the school nurse how she could have

gotten the head lice. When replying the school nurse should remember that:

① Infestation is most common where crowded conditions exist
② Transmission occurs through direct personal contact
③ Infestation is more widespread among lower socioeconomic groups
④ Transmission occurs through household pets

301. Mary tells the school nurse, "My mother said I got the lice because I don't keep clean." The nurse's best reply would be:

① "Lice are more common if you have poor personal hygiene."
② "You have problems getting along with your mother?"
③ "There is no relationship between cleanliness and lice."
④ "You feel that your mother is putting you down?"

Situation: Marsha Banes brings her 2-year-old daughter Nancy to the pediatric clinic for her yearly physical. The clinic nurse observes Nancy in the waiting room. Nancy is not socializing with the other children but sits in the corner rocking and staring at a small shiny top she is spinning around.

302. During the interview, Mrs. Banes related to the nurse her concern about Nancy, stating, "When I go near her, she pushes me away. She really does not speak and only shows feelings when I take her top away. Is it something I've done?" It would be most therapeutic for the nurse to respond to Mrs. Banes by:

① Telling her not to be concerned, that she will outgrow this phase of development
② Asking her how she held Nancy when she was an infant
③ Asking her about her relationship with Mr. Banes
④ Telling her that it's nothing she has done and sharing observations of Nancy

303. The nurse can be most therapeutic in approaching Nancy by:

① Waiting for Nancy to make the initial contact before moving close
② Gently stroking Nancy's arm to gain her attention
③ Holding Nancy to provide a sense of support and security
④ Bending down and staring at the spinning top with Nancy

304. While walking to the examination room with the nurse, Nancy suddenly runs over and begins to bang her head on the wall. The nurse's initial action should be to:

① Ask Nancy to stop this behavior
② Tell Nancy her behavior is not acceptable
③ Restrain Nancy to prevent injury
④ Allow Nancy to act out her feelings

Situation: Ann Knox, a 22-year-old college senior with a history of binge eating and purging, is admitted to the eating disorder unit with a diagnosis of bulimia nervosa.

305. The nurse is aware that bulimia can best be defined as the:

① Uncontrollable ingestion of large quantities of food in a short period of time
② Mood swings, ranging from euphoria to depression, associated with meals
③ Uncontrollable pilfering and hoarding of food for later consumption
④ Refusal to eat in public and engaging in private excessive overeating

306. The nurse should assess Ms. Knox for the psychologic characteristics commonly demonstrated by clients with bulimia nervosa, which include:

① Unmet dependency needs
② An unwillingness to discuss problems
③ Rigidity of character and inflexibility
④ A flattened affect

307. For lunch on the second day of hospitalization Ms. Knox eats two sandwiches, two salads, and four desserts. After the meal the nurse would expect to observe her:

① Hoarding more food for a later binge
② Performing excessive exercises
③ Withdrawing from the group to the bathroom
④ Actively socializing with small groups of clients

308. Considering her diagnosis, the nurse should observe Ms. Knox for symptoms of:

① Hyperglycemia
② Dehydration
③ Hyperactivity
④ Weight gain

309. A primary component of the nursing care plan for a client with bulimia would be:

① Intake and output
② Daily weighing before eating
③ Careful observation after meals
④ Daily room search for hoarded food

Situation: Lili Chong, 57 years old, has severe angina pectoris. She is admitted for a cardiac catheterization, which is to be done via the femoral approach.

310. In planning preoperative preparation for Mrs. Chong, the nurse should include information that:

① A general anesthetic will be given, and she will not be awake during the procedure
② She will be on bed rest, supine, with the affected leg extended for about 8 hours
③ She will be permitted to get up and walk around as soon as she returns to her room
④ Her physician will immediately tell her about the results of the procedure

311. Following her cardiac catheterization, Mrs. Chong is discharged and is scheduled to re-

turn for coronary bypass surgery. Mr. Chong asks, "When my wife gets chest pain at home, how will we know if we should call the doctor?" The nurse should teach the family to call the physician if the pain:
① Is not relieved by rest or by nitroglycerine
② Radiates to the arms, neck, or jaw
③ Is accompanied by mild diaphoresis
④ Repeatedly occurs after mild exercise

312. Before obtaining informed consent for surgery from Mrs. Chong the nurse should:
① Explain to Mrs. Chong the risks involved in the surgery
② Evaluate whether Mrs. Chong's knowledge level is sufficient to give consent
③ Witness the signature, since this is what the nurse's signature documents
④ Explain to Mrs. Chong that obtaining the signature is routine for surgery

313. Mr. Chong is present when the surgical consent is being obtained from his wife and asks how the coronary bypass surgery will help Mrs. Chong. The nurse bases the response on the knowledge that:
① Studies have consistently shown that this surgery increases an individual's life span
② Evidence substantiates that surgery can prevent progression of coronary artery disease
③ The bypass will permit the client to return to gainful employment after healing occurs
④ This surgery significantly decreases symptoms in a large percentage of clients

314. Before Mrs. Chong's open heart surgery the nurse should plan to include in the teaching plan a:
① Visit by recovery room and/or ICU nursing staff
② Detailed description of the surgical procedure
③ Thorough discussion of discharge plans
④ Discussion of the specific areas of the body that will be shaved

315. In the postoperative period immediately following coronary bypass surgery the nurse should be particularly alert for the common complications of:
① Postpericardotomy syndrome, with fever and audible friction rub
② Graft closure, with recurrence of angina-like chest pain
③ Supraventricular arrhythmias, especially atrial fibrillation
④ Elevation of hemoglobin and hematocrit levels, with risk of embolization

316. Mrs. Chong is to be discharged. The nurse prepares her for discharge by teaching her that there will be:
① No further drainage from the incisions after hospitalization
② Increased edema in the leg used for the donor graft when she is more active
③ Little incisional pain and tenderness after 3 to 4 weeks following surgery
④ A mild fever and extreme fatigue for several weeks following surgery

317. The physician prescribes propranolol (Inderal) 20 mg po qid to be taken after discharge. The teaching plan should include telling Mrs. Chong that she:
① May drink alcoholic beverages in moderation
② Should report a pulse rate below 70 beats per minute
③ Should not abruptly discontinue her medication
④ May increase the medication if chest pain occurs

Situation: Blossom Tyler, gravida VI, Para V, planned to have her baby at the birthing center. However, her labor has progressed so rapidly that she is afraid to go by car. She calls her neighbor, who is a nurse, for help.

318. The nurse assesses Mrs. Tyler's perineum and notes that it is bulging. The priority action is to:
① Encourage her to pant during the contraction
② Place a clean drape under the perineal area
③ Accurately time the length of each contraction
④ Contact the physician by phone for instructions

319. As the fetal head begins to crown, the nurse should:
① Press firmly on the fundus
② Encourage Mrs. Tyler to take prolonged deep breaths
③ Apply gentle perineal pressure
④ Suggest that she push down vigorously

320. During the delivery the nurse remembers that the most common complication associated with a too rapid expulsion of the fetus in a precipitate labor is:
① Dural or subdural tears in fetal brain tissue
② Premature separation of the placenta during the delivery
③ Pitting edema of the fetal scalp
④ Prolonged retention of the placenta

321. Immediately after delivery, the nurse should:
① Control maternal bleeding
② Cut the umbilical cord
③ Expel the placenta
④ Keep the infant warm

322. To facilitate the expulsion of the placenta the nurse should plan to:
① Push down vigorously on the fundus
② Have the mother breastfeed the baby

③ Place gentle continuous tension on the cord

④ Encourage the mother to vigorously bear down

323. Mrs. Tyler and her newborn are transported to the local hospital after the delivery. After a thorough physical assessment Baby Tyler is suspected of having toxoplasmosis. Toxoplasmosis, one of the TORCH diseases, may have been transmitted to the baby through:
① A blood transfusion given to the mother
② Breastfeeding
③ Contact with the maternal genitals
④ The placenta

324. One of the adaptations associated with toxoplasmosis that the nurse might observe when assessing Baby Tyler is:
① A head circumference of 34 cm (13.5 inches)
② Irregular respirations when he is awake
③ Small size for his gestational age
④ Pigmentation spots on his buttocks

Situation: As part of the sex education program, the school nurse is scheduled to speak to the junior and senior classes about herpes genitalis.

325. The nurse should tell the students that:
① Herpes genitalis is curable with penicillin
② The disease generally is painless in women
③ Herpes genitalis causes both local and systemic reactions
④ The disease is not transmitted via fomites such as toilet seats

326. When one of the students asks if recurrent infection is possible with herpes genitalis, the nurse should reply that:
① Unfortunately, recurrent attacks do occur but are not as severe as the initial infection
② Good health practices, such as getting adequate rest and nutrition, will prevent recurrences
③ Once herpes genitalis has been adequately treated, recurrence is rare
④ The only sure way to prevent recurrent attacks is to abstain from sexual activity

Situation: Lila Bray, a sexually active female, has been experiencing frequency and burning on urination for 24 hours. She comes to the walk-in clinic, and a diagnosis of cystitis is made.

327. The physician prescribes sulfisoxazole with phenazopyridine (Azo Gantrisin). The nurse knows Ms. Bray understands the teaching about taking this medication when Ms. Bray says she will:
① Report any changes in color of urine
② Drink 10 glasses of water daily
③ Take it with antacids to avoid GI upset
④ Strain all urine for calculi

328. Outcome criteria on discharge from the clinic should include a statement that Ms. Bray will:
① Understand the need for 7 to 8 liters of fluid per day
② Have relief of symptoms and show no further loss of kidney function
③ Be able to plan menus to include any dietary restrictions
④ Be able to state activities to be avoided because of possible bleeding

329. Ms. Bray mentions she has heard cranberry juice prevents infection. The nurse replies that cranberry juice is helpful because it:
① Increases the acidity of the urine
② Improves the glomerular filtration rate
③ Destroys microorganisms in the urinary tract
④ Soothes the irritated bladder walls

330. Ms. Bray asks if there is anything she can do to prevent cystitis in the future. The nurse tells her to plan to:
① Increase her intake of orange juice
② Void immediately after intercourse
③ Cleanse from vaginal orifice to urethra
④ Avoid the regular use of tampons

331. Ms. Bray has repeated episodes of cystitis. A cystoscopy is scheduled to determine the possibility of urinary abnormalities. In answer to Ms. Bray's questions the nurse describes the procedure as:
① The visualization of the urinary tract through ureteral catheterization using a radiopaque material
② The visualization of the inside of the bladder with an instrument connected to an illuminating source
③ A computerized scan that clearly outlines the bladder and surrounding tissue
④ An x-ray film of the abdomen, kidneys, ureters, and bladder after administration of dye

Situation: Irene Sharpe, a 19-year-old college sophomore, is admitted to the psychiatric unit of the community hospital. Her behavior on the unit is quite bizarre. She sits in a corner for long periods of time rocking and responds to voices using words that the staff cannot understand. The admitting diagnosis is schizophrenia, undifferentiated type.

332. In developing the plan of care for Ms. Sharpe, the nurse should:
① Include her in a discussion group on the unit
② Encourage her to talk to other clients during the day
③ Plan to spend short periods of time with her
④ Allow her to be by herself, but observe her from a distance

333. Ms. Sharpe's communication contains many words that sound like she is speaking a dif-

ferent language. The nurse recognizes that this is an example of:
① Clanging
② Echolalia
③ Echophrasia
④ Neologisms

334. When Ms. Sharpe is actively hallucinating, it would be most therapeutic for the nurse to:
① Involve her in a simple game of cards
② Request her to lower her voice
③ Ask her to whom she is talking
④ Allow her to continue without interrupting

335. Ms. Sharpe is started on chlorpromazine hydrochloride (Thorazine). The nurse is aware that this antipsychotic drug is used primarily to:
① Keep the client quiet and relaxed
② Reduce the need for restraints
③ Control the client's behavior and reduce stress
④ Make the client more receptive to psychotherapy

336. One morning Ms. Sharpe tells the nurse that she is Joan of Arc and is going to be burned at the stake. The most therapeutic response by the nurse would be:
① "It seems like the world is a pretty scary place for you."
② "Tell me more about being Joan of Arc."
③ "You are safe here, we won't let you be burned."
④ "You are not Joan of Arc. You are Irene Sharpe."

Situation: Brian Monroe, 2½ years old, is admitted to the pediatric unit with a severe upper respiratory tract infection. He has cystic fibrosis, which was diagnosed when he was 6 months old.

337. An early symptom that the nurse commonly observes in newborns who are later diagnosed as having cystic fibrosis is:
① Elevated bilirubin level
② Rapid respiratory rate
③ Meconium ileus
④ Imperforate anus

338. Brian is very small for his age. His slowed growth is probably related to:
① The absence of pancreatic enzymes
② The retention of CO_2
③ An atrial ventricular defect
④ Increased salt retention

339. The nurse plans to include scheduled times for postural drainage in Brian's care plan. This therapy should be scheduled:
① Tid, halfway between meals
② Tid, before meals
③ Bid, on awakening and at bedtime
④ Qd, after breakfast

340. In view of the adaptations of cystic fibrosis, the diet the nurse should provide for Brian should be:

① Low in salt and high in carbohydrate
② High in fat and high in protein
③ Low in fat and high in carbohydrate
④ Low in fat and low in salt

341. The play teacher gives Brian's nurse the key to the play room so that an appropriate toy can be chosen for Brian. The best choice would be a:
① Colorful hanging mobile
② Plastic mirror
③ Wooden puzzle with large pieces
④ Set of nesting blocks

342. The nurse reviews Brian's care after discharge with Mr. and Mrs. Monroe. The nurse realizes that further explanation is needed about the problems caused by cystic fibrosis when Brian's parents state, "We will:
① Keep Brian in an air-conditioned room."
② Give Brian his pancreatic enzymes with his meals."
③ Give Brian skin care after each bowel movement."
④ Take Brian to Florida this summer to visit his grandparents."

Situation: After exposure to a nephrotoxic substance, John Sullivan is admitted to the hospital in the oliguric phase of acute renal failure. His urine output for the last 12 hours is estimated by his wife to be less than 1 cup. His BUN level is 96.

343. Mr. Sullivan's fluid order is for 900 ml of water by mouth during the next 24 hours. In carrying out this order, the nurse realizes that the rationale for the order is that 900 ml of fluid will:
① Equal the expected urinary output for the next 24 hours
② Prevent the development of complicating hypostatic pneumonia
③ Compensate for both insensible and measured fluid losses over the next 24 hours
④ Prevent hyperkalemia, which could result in his having serious cardiac arrhythmias

344. When reviewing the laboratory slips the nurse notes that Mr. Sullivan's serum potassium level is 6.2 mEq. The nurse should first:
① Call the cardiac arrest team to alert them
② Obtain an ECG strip and have lidocaine available
③ Take Mr. Sullivan's vital signs and notify the physician
④ Call the laboratory to schedule a repeat test

345. When the nurse is administering care to Mr. Sullivan, he says, "My doctor said he is going to give me some insulin. Do I also have diabetes?" The response by the nurse that best demonstrates an understanding of the use of insulin in acute renal failure would be:
① "No, but insulin will reduce the toxins in your blood by lowering your metabolic rate."

② "Why don't you ask your physician that question when he comes to see you to-day?"

③ "You probably had an elevated blood sugar level and your physician is cautious."

④ "No, the insulin will help your body handle a chemical element called potassium."

346. Mr. Sullivan is scheduled for peritoneal dialysis. When explaining this procedure to him, the nurse should review that its purpose is to:
① Help do some of the work usually done by his kidneys
② Remove bad chemicals from his body so that his condition will not worsen
③ Prevent him from developing complicating heart problems
④ Speed his recovery, since his kidneys are not responding to other therapy

347. During the dialyzing procedure the nurse observes that drainage of dialysate from the peritoneal cavity has ceased before the required amount has drained out. The nurse should assist Mr. Sullivan to:
① Drink 8 ounces of water
② Deep breathe and cough
③ Turn from side to side
④ Periodically rotate the catheter

348. The nurse is aware that one reason the dialysis solution is warmed to body temperature before its instillation into the peritoneal cavity is to:
① Encourage removal of serum urea by dilating the peritoneal blood vessels
② Force potassium back into the cells, thereby decreasing serum levels
③ Add extra warmth to the body because metabolic processes are diturbed
④ Help prevent cardiac arrhythmias by speeding removal of excess serum potassium

349. After 1 week Mr. Sullivan moves into the diuretic phase of acute renal failure. During this phase the client must be carefully assessed for signs of:
① Hyperkalemia
② Metabolic acidosis
③ Hypovolemia
④ Renal failure

Situation: Margaret Knight, 36 weeks pregnant, comes to the clinic because she is having painless intermittent periods of bleeding. She is admitted with a tentative diagnosis of placenta previa.

350. The diagnosis of placenta previa is usually confirmed by:
① Amniocentesis
② Laparoscopy
③ Ultrasonography
④ Amnioscopy

351. The diagnosis of placenta previa indicates to the nurse that the placenta is:

① Separating prematurely
② Immaturely developed
③ Low lying
④ Infarcted

352. Mrs. Knight is concerned that she may have done something to cause the bleeding. Recognizing that the client is worried, it would be most therapeutic for the nurse to say:
① "It's not your fault; these things happen."
② "The placenta is lying low and separates when you dilate."
③ "Don't worry; it's just a sign of beginning labor."
④ "You probably have a weak uterus."

353. The nurse is aware that Mrs. Knight's labor has started when assessment demonstrates:
① Increased vaginal bleeding
② Decreased fetal heart rate
③ Decreased vaginal bleeding
④ Rhythmic uterine contractions

Situation: Mary Monica, 16 years old, is admitted to a medical unit with malaise, fever, and a persistent cough. Her history shows she has continually run away from home and has been remanded to a juvenile detention center by the court. Ms. Monica demonstrates little emotion, and it does not seem to bother her that her running away from home and her behavior have caused emotional distress to others. She has been diagnosed as having an antisocial personality disorder.

354. Ms. Monica's lack of remorse and behavior is probably related to an underdeveloped:
① Id
② Ego
③ Limbic system
④ Superego

355. Some of the staff are having difficulty handling Ms. Monica's manipulative behavior. The nurse should explain to them that Ms. Monica's behavior can best be controlled by having the staff:
① Designate one staff member to approach her about her behavior
② Avoid focusing on her behavior
③ Develop and use a unified approach
④ Assign members who are not easily manipulated to care for her

Situation: Jane Conklin was admitted to the hospital because she could not walk. After a physiologic basis for the problem was ruled out, a diagnosis of somatoform disorder, conversion type was made.

356. The nurse realizes that Mrs. Conklin's paralysis is:
① A way of getting attention
② The result of intrapsychic conflict
③ A loss of contact with reality
④ A nondisabling illness

357. The nurse would expect Mrs. Conklin to display an affect that is:
① Frightened and upset

② Happy and cheerful
③ Sad and depressed
④ Calm and matter-of-fact

358. When caring for Mrs. Conklin, the nurse should:
① Avoid discussing the paralysis
② Ask her how she feels about being paralyzed
③ Encourage her to get up, pointing out that she can walk
④ Explain the reason for her paralysis

359. In formulating a plan of care for Mrs. Conklin, the nurse must realize that:
① There is no physiologic basis for the illness; therefore only emotional care is needed
② Although the client believes she has the illness, there is no cause to be concerned
③ The client really believes she is ill and needs good nursing care
④ Good nursing care is needed even though the nurse recognizes that the client is not ill

Situation: Victor Jamison, 65 years old, has had NIDDM for the past 15 years. He is admitted to the hospital in a coma. On inspection it is noted that he has gangrene of the right foot and ulcerations of the ankle. A pedal pulse is not found on the right and is barely perceptible on the left.

360. Individuals like Mr. Jamison with adult onset diabetes mellitus:
① Have a lower incidence of chronic complications
② Seldom develop ketoacidosis
③ Have a sudden and dramatic onset of symptoms
④ Secrete no endogenous insulin

361. On physical examination of Mr. Jamison, in addition to the lesions on the lower extremities, the nurse might expect to find:
① Arthritic changes in the hands
② Increased vascularization of the retina
③ Dependent pallor of the lower legs and feet
④ Hyperactive knee- and ankle-jerk reflexes

362. In a comatose client such as Mr. Jamison, the laboratory value that would support a diagnosis of diabetic ketoacidosis would be:
① Normal BUN
② Elevated serum lipids
③ Low serum calcium
④ Decreased hematocrit

363. Warm saline soaks tid are ordered for Mr. Jamison's ulcers. A staff nurse has placed a clean basin, wash cloth, and protective pad at the bedside in preparation for the soak but is unable to continue the procedure. The nurse assigned to complete the soak should:
① Continue the procedure as started
② Collect new supplies before starting
③ Report the first nurse to the supervisor

④ Discuss the type of soak with the physician

364. Two weeks after Mr. Jamison's admission a below-the-knee amputation of the right leg is performed. The nurse should understand that after this type of surgery:
① The stump dressing is usually changed daily by the physician
② Strict bed rest is usually maintained for at least several days
③ Hemorrhage rarely occurs during the early postoperative period
④ The client is usually positioned with the stump elevated for the first 24 hours

365. Mr. Jamison is now being given regular insulin even though he was taking an oral hypoglycemic before being admitted to the hospital. The nurse recognizes that regular insulin is now needed because:
① He will need a higher serum glucose level as long as he is on bed rest
② The dosage can be adjusted to his changing needs during recovery from surgery
③ The possibility of recurrence of acidosis is greater when a client is taking oral hypoglycemics
④ Regular insulin is readily available in the event of complications following surgery

366. One week after surgery Mr. Jamison refuses to go to physical therapy and tells the nurse, "I'll never be a whole person again!" The nurse's best response would be:
① "You must go to physical therapy every day or you will develop muscle contractures."
② "You may feel that way, but I'm sure your family considers you a whole person."
③ "Relax, Mr. Jamison, you're still the same person you've always been."
④ "You've lost a part of yourself. That must be very difficult for you."

Situation: Jason Mack has just had surgery for pyloric stenosis.

367. An immediate postoperative nursing care priority for Jason would be:
① Reporting any vomiting to the physician
② Giving the oral feedings very slowly
③ Observing for signs of infection at the incision site
④ Checking the patency of the nasogastric tube

368. Mrs. Mack is reluctant to resume feeding him but is readily in favor of assisting with the other aspects of his care. The care plan 24 hours after surgery includes encouraging Mrs. Mack to participate in the oral feedings. The rationale for the focus of nursing care is that Mrs. Mack is:
① Uncertain of how the thickened oral feedings are administered

② Reluctant to feed Jason because of his present need to use a special nipple
③ Probably afraid to resume feedings because of the frequent vomiting before surgery
④ Unaware that family involvement in care is permitted

Situation: Tommy Brown, 8 years old, has sickle cell anemia and comes to the pediatric clinic monthly for checkups. Tommy's parents are both free of the disease.

369. The nurse is aware that the genotypic makeup of Tommy's parents is:
① Father-normal homozygous   Mother-heterozygous
       ↓   ↓
(no sickle trait)   *(sickle trait)*

② Father-heterozygous   Mother-homozygous
       ↓   ↓
(sickle trait)   *(no sickle trait)*

③ Mother-homozygous   Father-homozygous
       ↓   ↓
(has sickle cell disease)   *(normal)*

④ Mother-heterozygous   Father-heterozygous
       ↓   ↓
(sickle trait)   *(sickle trait)*

370. Tommy is admitted in sickle cell crisis. Appropriate nursing care during this period includes:
① Active range-of-motion exercises to all joints
② Administration of oxygen
③ Restricted fluids until the crisis is over
④ Cold compresses to painful joints

371. After Tommy recovers from the crisis, the nurse teaches the parents all the "do's and don'ts" concerning Tommy's care. The nurse knows that the parents understand the basic principles of care when they state that they are:
① Getting Tommy a private tutor for his schoolwork
② Not permitting Tommy to play soccer or go backpacking with the Boy Scouts
③ Keeping Tommy's fluid intake restricted at night
④ Not allowing Tommy to play with other children

372. Long-term care for Tommy's parents includes periodic conferences with groups of parents whose children have sickle cell disease to:
① Air their feelings regarding the transmission of the disease to the child
② Choose a means of birth control to avoid future pregnancies
③ Find special schooling facilities for the child
④ Make plans for moving to a more therapeutic climate

Situation: Rita Owen is admitted with a rigid and painful abdomen. The diagnosis of ruptured peptic ulcer is made. A nasogastric tube is inserted to decompress the stomach, and intravenous fluids with antibiotics are administered. The client is scheduled to have a partial gastrectomy in 4 hours.

373. Before surgery the nurse should place Mrs. Owen in the:
① Sims' position
② Dorsal recumbent position
③ Semi-Fowler's position
④ Supine position

374. After surgery the nurse can determine that peristalsis has returned when:
① Mrs. Owen has a bowel movement
② The abdomen is no longer rigid and tender
③ The feeling of nausea passes
④ Borborygmi are auscultated

375. After a gastric resection the nurse should expect to observe:
① Bloody drainage for the first 12 hours
② Gastric distention
③ Vomiting
④ Intermittent periods of diarrhea

Comprehensive Examination Two
Test 1

Situation: Mary and Frank Pulman are expecting their first child. Because of a family history of congenital defects, the physician informs them that an alpha fetoprotein test of amniotic fluid should be performed to detect the presence of neural tube defects.

1. Mrs. Pulman asks the nurse when this test will have to be performed. The nurse replies that the physician will schedule it sometime during the:
   ① Eighth to tenth week
   ② Fourteenth to sixteenth week
   ③ Twentieth to twenty-fourth week
   ④ Thirty-second to thirty-sixth week

2. A neural tube defect is suspected based on the elevated alpha fetoprotein. Following an otherwise uneventful pregnancy and labor, a baby girl is born with a meningomyelocele. The baby has an Apgar score of 9/10. An immediate priority of nursing care should be:
   ① Placing a name bracelet on her ankle and taking foot prints
   ② Administering O_2 by nasal catheter
   ③ Protecting the sac with sterile moist gauze
   ④ Transferring the infant to the intensive care nursery

3. The physician orders intravenous fluids. The intravenous is placed in the scalp vein, and Mr. Pulman asks why the intravenous is not started in the hand like for an adult. The nurse responds:
   ① "Putting the IV in the scalp improves the absorption rate of the IV."
   ② "Veins are closer to the surface of the scalp, making it easier to insert the IV."
   ③ "Inserting the IV in the scalp decreases the need to restrain the baby."
   ④ "The IV solution is too irritating to be introduced through a vein in the hand."

4. Two days after her delivery, Baby Pulman's head circumference is 16 inches (40.6 cm) and her chest circumference is 13 inches (33 cm). These measurements:
   ① Are both normal parameters at birth
   ② Indicate that the baby's head is enlarged
   ③ Suggest the presence of microcephaly
   ④ Demonstrate a smaller than normal chest

5. Baby Pulman is scheduled for surgery. The priority preoperative nursing goal is to make certain that Baby Pulman:
   ① Gains 1 ounce per day
   ② Develops a strong sucking reflex
   ③ Remains infection free
   ④ Remains sedated

6. Postoperatively Baby Pulman is being fed by gavage feedings. When checking placement of the tube the nurse is unable to hear the air injected because of noisy breath sounds. The nurse should:

① Advance the tube 1 to 2 cm
② Notify the physician
③ Carefully insert 1 ml of formula
④ Attempt to aspirate stomach contents

Situation: Eli Stepp, 56 years old, is brought to the emergency room after experiencing a sudden onset of retrosternal chest pain while shoveling snow. The pain stopped before he arrived at the hospital, but admission is recommended because of past myocardial infarctions.

7. The nurse explains to Mr. Stepp that the physician will diagnose his pain on the basis of the findings from:
   ① Physical examination
   ② A stress test
   ③ A detailed history
   ④ X-ray films of the heart

8. The physician orders an electrocardiogram (ECG). Mr. Stepp asks the nurse, "Why are they doing this test?" The best reply by the nurse would be, "This test will:
   ① Enable us to detect heart sounds."
   ② Enable us to detect heart damage."
   ③ Help us to change your heart rhythm."
   ④ Tell how much stress you can tolerate."

9. Mr. Stepp is admitted to the coronary care unit. After attaching Mr. Stepp to the cardiac monitor, the nurse notes six premature ventricular contractions (PVCs) in a row. Using the protocol generally established in most CCUs, the nurse should first:
   ① Initiate cardiopulmonary resuscitation on Mr. Stepp
   ② Encourage Mr. Stepp to cough and deep breathe
   ③ Administer a 50 to 100 mg bolus of cardiac xylocaine
   ④ Notify Mr. Stepp's physician of the findings immediately

10. Mr. Stepp is placed on digoxin (Lanoxin) and procainamide hydrochloride (Pronestyl). Because of the combined effect of Lanoxin and Pronestyl, the nurse should monitor Mr. Stepp for signs of increased:
    ① Respiratory stimulation
    ② CNS depression
    ③ Myocardial depression
    ④ Reflex stimulation

11. A calcium deficit is suspected, and the nurse checks for hypocalcemia by placing a blood pressure cuff on Mr. Stepp's arm and inflating it. After about 3 minutes he develops carpopedal spasm. The nurse records this finding as a positive:
    ① Chvostek's sign
    ② Trousseau's sign
    ③ Homan's sign
    ④ Romberg sign

12. The physician orders 10 ml of a 10% solution of calcium gluconate for Mr. Stepp's severely

depressed serum calcium. The nurse should be aware that calcium gluconate:
① Cannot be added to the IV of 1000 ml D5W
② Is nonirritating to surrounding tissues
③ Is compatible with all IV solutions
④ Potentiates the action of digitalis preparations

13. Before discharge Mr. Stepp is placed on the "Prudent Diet" advocated by the American Heart Association and designed to control saturated fats and cholesterol. To best explain the dietary nature of these two food substances the nurse should teach him that:
① Polyunsaturated fats come from animal foods such as meat and cheese
② The more saturated fats come from plant foods such as seeds and grains
③ Cholesterol is a necessary body constituent that cannot be eliminated
④ Plant sources of cholesterol must also be controlled in the diet every day

14. Mrs. Stepp says to the nurse, "I guess with this 'Prudent Diet' I'm going to have to cook two meals, one for my husband and one for my daughter and myself." The most appropriate response by the nurse would be:
① "The diet that has been prescribed for your husband is a healthy diet that is recommended for all of us to follow."
② "You're right, and be careful not to cook his favorite meals because he will probably not want to adhere to the diet."
③ "I wouldn't bother. This diet is really easy to follow; just cut down the salt you use and fry foods in peanut oil."
④ "This is a very difficult diet to follow. I would recommend that you shop daily for food so that there are no temptations in the kitchen."

Situation: Hilda Townes, 51 years old, paces back and forth across the floor and speaks very rapidly, loudly, and incoherently. Mrs. Townes spends most of her time talking to persons who are not present, and it often appears as if she is verbally fighting with these persons.

15. The initial therapeutic intervention by the nurse should be directed toward:
① Engaging Mrs. Townes in a structured, reality-oriented activity
② Setting limits on Mrs. Townes' verbal aggression
③ Establishing a relationship to reduce Mrs. Townes' loneliness
④ Isolating Mrs. Townes to decrease her aggression

16. When Mrs. Townes mumbles incoherently, the most appropriate intervention would be for the nurse to:
① Consistently ask Mrs. Townes to repeat what she said, so that she will learn to recognize she is mumbling
② Ignore Mrs. Townes because she is using this pathologic manner of speech to get attention
③ Set limits on her behavior by refusing to talk with her unless she stops mumbling
④ Indicate to her that she needs to slow down because what she says is important and cannot be understood

17. Mrs. Townes becomes increasingly agitated. She screams at, curses at, fights with, and bites other clients. The physician orders a stat injection of hydroxyzine hydrochloride (Vistaril). The nurse should carry out the order to administer the Vistaril:
① Quickly, with an attitude of concern
② Before Mrs. Townes suspects she is being sedated
③ Quietly, without any explanation about the reason for it
④ After Mrs. Townes agrees

18. The nurse should monitor Mrs. Townes for the common side effects of Vistaril, which include:
① Ataxia and confusion
② Slurred speech and headache
③ Drowsiness and dry mouth
④ Vertigo and impaired vision

19. Lithium therapy is instituted. In regard to lithium therapy, the nurse should teach Mrs. Townes to maintain a normal daily intake of:
① Magnesium
② Sodium
③ Potassium
④ Iron

20. During lithium administration the nurse should assess Mrs. Townes':
① Potassium level
② Bowel sounds
③ Visual acuity
④ Weight

21. After Mrs. Townes has been receiving lithium for 10 days, the laboratory calls to report her lithium level is 1.9 mEq/liter. The nurse should:
① Monitor the client closely because the level of lithium in the blood is slightly elevated
② Report the findings to the physician so that the dosage can be increased because the level is below therapeutic range
③ Continue to administer the medication as ordered because the level is within the therapeutic range
④ Immediately report the finding to the physician because the level is dangerously high

Situation: Sandra Nash has been losing weight despite a ravenous appetite. She has been irritable and cries easily. She visits her physician, who suspects hyperthyroidism and prescribes propylthiouracil.

22. Two months after being started on the antithyroid medication Mrs. Nash calls the

physician because she is feeling tired, and her family says she looks pale. The nurse should:

① Schedule an appointment for her
② Advise her to get more rest
③ Tell her to increase her medication
④ Instruct her to skip one dose daily

23. Several months later Mrs. Nash has a thyroidectomy. After the surgery, the nurse should position Mrs. Nash in the:
    ① Supine position
    ② Prone position
    ③ Left Sims' position
    ④ Semi-Fowler's position

24. To check for wound hemorrhage after a thyroidectomy the nurse should:
    ① Outline the blood as it appears on the dressing to observe any progression
    ② Press gently around the incision to express accumulated blood from the wound
    ③ Observe the dressing at the back of the neck for the presence of blood
    ④ Loosen an edge of the dressing and lift it to visualize the wound

25. The nurse is aware that after the thyroidectomy Mrs. Nash should be observed carefully for symptoms indicating:
    ① Laceration of the esophagus
    ② Perforation of the lung
    ③ Fracture of the laryngeal cartilage
    ④ Accidental removal of the parathyroids

26. Hyperextension of the neck for the first few postoperative days may cause:
    ① Cervical trauma
    ② Laryngeal spasm
    ③ Laryngeal edema
    ④ Wound dehiscence

Situation: Barbara Swensen, a 16-year-old primipara, is admitted to the delivery room accompanied by her mother. Ms. Swensen states she is in labor.

27. To verify that Ms. Swensen is experiencing true labor the nurse should:
    ① Obtain slides for a fern test
    ② Time any uterine contractions
    ③ Prepare her for a pelvic examination
    ④ Place nitrazine paper at the cervical mouth

28. Ms. Swensen requests that her mother remain at the bedside but refuses her mother's assistance with comfort measures, stating, "I can do this myself." Ms. Swensen's conflicting behavior is representative of the adolescent's attempt to achieve the developmental task of:
    ① Integrity
    ② Identity
    ③ Industry
    ④ Intimacy

29. The laboratory finding that reflects a major problem commonly found in pregnant teenagers is:

① Urine glucose 2+
② White blood cells 12,000
③ Platelets 75,000
④ Hemoglobin 9.1g

30. When checking Ms. Swensen's cervical dilatation, the nurse notices that the umbilical cord has prolapsed. The nurse's first action should be to:
    ① Cover the cord with sterile saline soaks
    ② Take the fetal heart rate
    ③ Turn Ms. Swensen on her side
    ④ Put Ms. Swensen in a modified Trendelenburg position

31. The nurse anticipates that Ms. Swensen's delivery will be:
    ① Augmented with oxytocin
    ② Via a cesarean delivery
    ③ Postponed as long as possible
    ④ A low-forceps vaginal delivery

32. A 7 lb baby boy is delivered and admitted to the normal newborn nursery with an order for phytonadione (AquaMEPHYTON, vitamin K) 1 mg IM. The nurse is aware that this treatment is administered to:
    ① Increase liver glycogen stores
    ② Facilitate bilirubin excretion
    ③ Promote normal blood clotting
    ④ Stimulate normal bowel flora

33. Baby Swensen is being fed by bottle. Ms. Swensen's breasts become engorged. The measure most appropriate to relieve the engorgement would be:
    ① Restriction of oral fluid intake to less than 1000 ml daily
    ② Application of ice packs and a binder to her breasts
    ③ Expression of breast milk to relieve pressure
    ④ Use of hot moist towels as compresses on her breasts

Situation: Melissa Baines, 4 years old, is admitted for a diagnostic workup for pulmonic stenosis.

34. The nurse understands that pulmonic stenosis is a:
    ① Hardening of the lining of the pulmonary artery at a point close to the lungs
    ② Narrowing of the valve between the left atrium and left ventricle
    ③ Narrowing of the valve between the right ventricle and the pulmonary artery
    ④ Hardening of the valve between the right atrium and right ventricle

35. A cardiac catheterization is performed on Melissa. The nurse is aware that children with pulmonic stenosis have increased pressure:
    ① On the left side of the heart
    ② On the right side of the heart
    ③ In the pulmonary vein
    ④ In the pulmonary artery

36. A pulmonary valvotomy is performed. When Melissa is in the intensive care unit after her

operation, she is told that she can have medicine to keep her comfortable. The nurse should tell her that when she feels uncomfortable:

① The nurses will give her injections to make her feel better

② She will be given a pill to "make the hurt better."

③ The nurses will put medicine in her IV to make her more comfortable

④ She will be given medicines that will take all the hurt away

37. Several months after surgery Melissa develops iron deficiency anemia, and the physician orders supplemental iron orally. With proper administration of iron to a child, Mr. and Mrs. Baines should be informed to expect Melissa to develop:

① Orange-colored urine

② Positive stool guiac

③ Staining of the teeth

④ Greenish-black stools

38. After 3 months of supplemental oral iron therapy there is no significant rise in Melissa's hemoglobin level. The physician orders iron dextran (Imferon). When administering this medication, the nurse should:

① Use a 25-gauge ⅝ inch needle

② Avoid aspiration before injection

③ Use the Z-track method

④ Massage the injection site

Situation: Ben Collins, 60 years old, is brought to the emergency room by his wife at 11 PM with severe pain in the upper right quadrant. He is overweight, and his skin appears jaundiced. Acute cholecystitis is diagnosed, and a cholecystectomy is scheduled in 2 weeks.

39. Mr. Collins is placed on a low-fat, high-protein diet to help prepare him for the surgery. The nurse should teach Mr. Collins that his diet can include:

① Poached eggs

② Skimmed milk

③ Boiled beef

④ Steamed broccoli

40. Two weeks later a cholecystectomy is performed and Mr. Collins returns to his room with a nasogastric tube to low continuous suction, a T-tube, and a Foley catheter. The nurse should first:

① Check drainage tubes and collection devices

② Fasten each tubing to the bed sheets

③ Irrigate each tube with normal saline

④ Empty drainage from the collection devices

41. A nursing goal is to have Mr. Collins achieve alveolar expansion. This goal would be most effectively achieved by:

① Blow bottles

② Postural drainage

③ Prolonged exhalation

④ Sustained inspirations

42. During the first 48 hours after surgery the nurse should:

① Prevent the client from turning onto the right side

② Connect and maintain the T-tube to low intermittent suction

③ Maintain T-tube patency via gravity drainage

④ Irrigate the T-tube with 30 ml of normal saline q 2 h

43. The nurse is aware that the bile flow into the duodenum has been reestablished after surgery when:

① Serum bilirubin returns to normal

② The liver is no longer tender

③ Stools are normal brown in color

④ Colic is absent after ingestion of fats

44. In teaching Mr. Collins about his diet, the priority intervention on discharge should be:

① Teaching him the importance of a low-calorie diet to promote weight reduction

② Listing those fatty foods he may include in his diet until he sees his physician

③ Explaining that he may not be able to tolerate fatty foods for several weeks

④ Encouraging him to join a weight reduction program in his local community

Situation: Joanne Christe has just lost her first job in a city about 100 miles away from her home town. Ms. Christe comes to the Mental Health Clinic very upset. On being questioned, she states, "Without warning, I just start crying without any reason."

45. The nurse's initial response should be:

① "Do you know what makes you cry?"

② "Most of us need to cry from time to time."

③ "Crying unexpectedly must be very upsetting."

④ "Are you having any other problems at this time?"

46. As Ms. Christe is talking, she starts crying again. She appears to be upset that she cannot control her crying. The most appropriate response by the nurse would be:

① "Sometimes it helps to get it out of your system."

② "Is talking about your problem upsetting you?"

③ "You look upset; let's talk about why you are crying."

④ "It is OK to cry; we can talk when you're ready."

47. An appropriate nursing diagnosis for Ms. Christie would probably be:

① Social isolation related to absence of satisfying personal relationships

② Altered thought processes related to impaired judgment

③ Potential for violence, self-directed, related to panic state

④ Personal identity disturbance related to inability to distinguish self from nonself

48. A continuing goal of care appropriate for Ms. Christie would be:
   ① Limiting tearfulness
   ② Increasing self-esteem
   ③ Promoting acceptance by others
   ④ Controlling feelings of sadness

Situation: Betty Wells is admitted to the hospital in active labor at 40 weeks gestation.

49. The nurse should avoid placing Mrs. Wells in a supine position during labor, primarily because it can:
   ① Prolong labor because of the influence of gravity
   ② Cause decreased perfusion of the placenta
   ③ Impede free movement of the symphysis pubis
   ④ Lead to transient episodes of hypertension

50. When Mrs. Wells begins to experience contractions q 2 minutes that last 50 to 70 seconds, she complains of a severe backache and becomes very irritable. The nurse determines that Mrs. Wells is in the stage of labor known as:
   ① Early first
   ② Transition
   ③ Late second
   ④ Early third

51. An important nursing intervention during the fourth stage of labor is to:
   ① Vigorously massage the fundus
   ② Monitor the vital signs q 1 h
   ③ Turn the client on her side to check lochia
   ④ Assist the client to the bathroom to void

52. About 6 hours after delivery the nurse notes that Mrs. Wells' fundus is two fingerbreadths above the umbilicus and is deviated to the right of the midline. The nurse suspects that Mrs. Wells has:
   ① Retained placental fragments
   ② Bladder distention
   ③ Begun involution
   ④ Second-degree uterine atony

53. The nurse is preparing Mrs. Wells for discharge. Mrs. Wells says, "I don't think I'll be able to take care of the baby when I go home." The nurse's best response would be:
   ① "It will come naturally. Give yourself time."
   ② "I know it can be frightening, but you'll do just fine."
   ③ "What is it that makes you think that?"
   ④ "Is there anything specific that concerns you?"

Situation: Letitia Barnes, age 9, is admitted with a diagnosis of possible infratentorial brain tumor.

54. The nurse identifies the common presenting symptoms of an infratentorial tumor when Letitia demonstrates:
   ① Cranial enlargement
   ② Ataxia
   ③ Seizures
   ④ Papilledema

55. The diagnosis is confirmed. The nurse is aware that 60% of brain tumors in children result in symptoms of increased intracranial pressure and are most commonly found in the:
   ① Cerebellum
   ② Temporal lobe
   ③ Cortex
   ④ Subarachnoid space

56. Surgery is scheduled and the nurse initiates preparation of Letitia for the infratentorial craniotomy. The nurse plans to:
   ① Provide a minutely detailed explanation of her anatomy and the surgery to be performed
   ② Encourage doll play with blunt tools and dressings
   ③ Have the child draw her concept of the brain and briefly clarify any misconceptions
   ④ Schedule role playing with others who are having similar surgery

57. The tumor has been surgically removed. The nurse notes an area of serosanguinous drainage on Letitia's head dressing about the size of a quarter. The nurse should:
   ① Notify the physician immediately
   ② Mark the area with nonabsorbable ink
   ③ Remove the dressing and check the sutures
   ④ Reinforce the dressing with gauze pads

58. Biopsy reveals the excised tumor is a cerebellar astrocytoma. Mrs. Barnes is crying softly in her daughter's room. When the nurse enters Mrs. Barnes says, "Do you think my Letitia will make it? I can't bear the thought of losing her." The nurse bases a response on the fact that this tumor is:
   ① Fast growing and highly malignant
   ② Close to vital centers, and only partial excision is possible
   ③ Benign and associated with a high rate of cure
   ④ The cause of pituitary malfunction as the child grows

59. During the postoperative period, Letitia develops a sudden right pupillary dilation. The nurse recognizes this as a sign of:
   ① Severe pain
   ② Uncal herniation
   ③ Reduced intracranial pressure
   ④ Intense fear

Situation: Frank Rudolf, age 40, is suspected of having Hodgkin's disease. He is admitted to the hospital for confirmation of the diagnosis.

60. Mr. Rudolf and his wife are concerned that he may have cancer. Mrs. Rudolf states, "Wouldn't it be unlikely for someone like Frank to have cancer?" Before responding to

the emotional aspects of the question, the nurse should recall that:

① Cancer is typically a disease of older, rather than younger, adults
② Hodgkin's disease is more common among women than men
③ Hodgkin's disease occurs most often in males ages 20 to 40
④ It is impossible to predict who will develop cancer or when

61. Mr. Rudolf asks how the surgeon will know he definitely has Hodgkin's disease. The nurse tells him the diagnosis is routinely confirmed by:

① Lymph node biopsy
② Bone scan
③ Radioactive iodine (^{131}I) uptake studies
④ Computerized axial tomography (CAT) scan

62. The physician diagnoses Hodgkin's disease, Stage III. Mr. Rudolf is started on a MOPP regimen of nitrogen mustard, vincristine (Oncovin), procarbazine, and prednisone. Mr. Rudolf wonders why so many drugs have to be used at once. The nurse's best response would be to explain that:

① The drugs are used to destroy cells that are not susceptible to radiation therapy
② Using groups of drugs reduces the likelihood of serious side effects
③ Each drug destroys the cancer cell at a different time in the cell cycle
④ Because there are stages of Hodgkin's disease, if one drug is ineffective another will work

63. Mr. Rudolf wants to know how the drugs in the protocol work. The nurse tells him that the cyclic antineoplastic vincristine (Oncovin) helps destroy the malignant cells by:

① Inhibiting the synthesis of pyrimidine
② Arresting mitosis in metaphase
③ Inactivating DNA and inhibiting RNA synthesis
④ Alkylating nucleic acids needed for mitosis

64. The nurse should also tell him that the nitrogen mustard is believed to act by:

① Binding the DNA strands and interfering with cell replication
② Interfering with cellular protein synthesis
③ Inhibiting the synthesis of purine and pyrimidine
④ Binding the DNA to interfere with RNA production

65. Mr. Rudolf is treated on an outpatient basis. About halfway through the first 6-month course of treatment, he complains of burning and tingling in his feet. The nurse should recognize that these complaints are symptoms of:

① Electrolyte imbalances caused by anorexia and vomiting

② Neurotoxicity caused by vincristine
③ Peripheral vasoconstriction caused by nitrogen mustard
④ Side effects of prednisone therapy

66. Nine months after treatment with MOPP is completed, Mr. Rudolf has a relapse. An ABVD combination chemotherapeutic treatment regimen is begun. This protocol includes doxorubicin HCl (Adriamycin), bleomycin sulfate (Blenoxane), vinblastine (Velban), and dacarbazine (DTIC). Because Adriamycin is part of this therapy, the nurse teaches Mr. Rudolf to:

① Expect urine to turn red for 1 to 2 days after taking this drug
② Cease taking any medication that contains vitamin D
③ Keep Adriamycin in a dark area, protected from light
④ Take Adriamycin on an empty stomach with plenty of fluids

Situation: Milton August is admitted to the hospital for an elective prostatectomy. When taking the nursing history the nurse notes that Mr. August is extremely anxious and has hand tremors. Mr. August states, "I often get very tense and I find that having a few drinks before bedtime calms my nerves and soothes my stomach." Later Mrs. August informs the nurse that Mr. August has been drinking heavily for the last 5 years.

67. When Mr. August is unpacking his suitcase, the nurse notices him hiding a bottle of whiskey in the rear of the drawer. The nurse's responsibility in relation to the alcohol includes:

① Asking Mr. August how much alcohol he really drinks
② Waiting for Mr. August to bring up the subject of drinking
③ Trying to catch Mr. August drinking the alcohol
④ Confiscating the alcohol when Mr. August is not looking

68. During the night, Mr. August demonstrates signs of acute alcohol withdrawal, and surgery is cancelled. When caring for Mr. August during the acute withdrawal period the nurse should:

① Keep his room dimly lit to counter the visual distortions he probably will experience
② Encourage Mr. August to relate hallucinations and delusions in detail
③ Apply restraints to provide security and keep Mr. August calm
④ Continually reassure him that his symptoms are part of the withdrawal syndrome

69. In the late afternoon on the day after admission the nurse finds Mr. August standing in the corner of his room. He appears frightened

and points toward his bed and says, "Bugs are crawling all over my bed and on me." The most therapeutic response by the nurse would be:
① "Do you want me to brush them away for you?"
② "Those are not bugs; it is just the design on the bedspread."
③ "I do not see any bugs on your bed."
④ "The bugs will go away when you feel better."

70. In planning for Mr. August's care during the detoxification phase, the nurse should anticipate the need to:
① Restrain Mr. August when he is upset
② Speak to him in a loud, clear voice
③ Keep his room lights dim
④ Supervise Mr. August at all times

71. As part of his treatment plan, Mr. August has agreed to attend Alcoholics Anonymous meetings at the hospital. One day Mr. August says he cannot attend his second AA meeting because he is expecting an important phone call. The nurse's most therapeutic response would be:
① "You can wait for the call and skip the meeting."
② "You can go to the meeting after the call."
③ "You are expected to go to the meeting."
④ "Is your phone call really that important?"

Situation: Link and Rhoda Dee bring their 1-year-old son Ken to the emergency room with a possible fracture of the right femur. Mrs. Dee, a prominent community leader, vaguely reports that Ken fell off the dressing table while she was changing his diaper. Ken has a number of bruises in various stages of healing. The nurse suspects child abuse.

72. The nurse's primary responsibility must be to:
① Treat the child's traumatic injuries
② Have the child examined by the physician
③ Protect the child from future abuse
④ Confirm the suspected child abuse

73. To therapeutically relate to the abusing parent the nurse must first:
① Identify personal feelings about child abusers
② Gather information about the child's home environment
③ Call authorities to report the suspected incident
④ Recognize the emotional needs of the parent

74. The nurse is aware that group therapy with abusing parents should be designed to help these parents to:
① Share information about their parenting techniques and skills
② Admit publicly and to themselves that they are child abusers

③ Confront their own rage at being abused as children
④ Recognize the long-range psychologic effects of child abuse

Situation: Joel Isaacs, a 50-year-old professor, visits the college health office because of persistent pyrexia, abdominal pain, and neuritis, symptoms that the physician feels are suggestive of polyarteritis nodosa.

75. When assessing Professor Isaacs the nurse should expect to find:
① An unexplained excessive gain in weight
② An elevation in blood pressure
③ Enlarged cervical lymph nodes
④ A hypersensitivity of the fifth cranial nerve

76. The physician advises a muscle biopsy to confirm the diagnosis of polyarteritis. Professor Isaacs tells the nurse, "They'd better give me a general anesthetic. I don't want to feel anything." The most therapeutic response by the nurse would be:
① "Tell them when you have pain, and they'll take care of it."
② "This test is always done under local anesthesia."
③ "Try not to think about it; you won't feel a thing."
④ "You seem to be worried about the test."

77. After the muscle biopsy, the nurse advises Professor Isaacs that once home, he should:
① Bathe or shower according to preference
② Change the dressing as needed
③ Resume his usual diet as soon as he feels able
④ Expect a rise in body temperature for 48 hours

78. In response to Professor Isaacs' question concerning the etiology of polyarteritis nodosa, the nurse should respond that:
① The disease affects both males and females in equal numbers
② Arteriolar pathology of the disease affects only the kidneys and the retina of the eye
③ With current therapy, clients with this disease have an excellent prognosis
④ The disease is considered one of hypersensitivity, but the exact cause is not known

79. The biopsy confirms the diagnosis of polyarteritis, and steroid therapy is started. One day Professor Isaacs meets the college nurse in the hall and states, "I have had difficulty controlling my temper, which is so unlike me, and I don't know why this is happening." The nurse's best response would be to:
① Tell Professor Isaacs it is nothing to worry about
② Encourage Professor Isaacs to talk further about these findings
③ Tell Professor Isaacs to attempt to avoid situations he knows will irritate him

④ Try to determine if Professor Isaacs has been experiencing mood swings

80. Later in the semester, Professor Isaacs calls the health office to complain that he is thirsty continually and urinates so frequently that it interferes with his classes. The best initial action is to have Professor Isaacs stop at the office so that the nurse can:
① Assess the lower extremities for presence of pitting edema
② Perform a finger stick to test for the blood glucose level
③ Have the physician assess for an enlarged prostate
④ Obtain a urine specimen for screening purposes

Situation: Geraldine Glasser is 70 years old and has osteoporosis. When lifting a bag of groceries she fell and fractured the head of the left femur.

81. Mrs. Glasser's left leg is placed in Buck's extension to reduce pain from muscle spasms until she can be scheduled for surgery the next afternoon. Buck's traction is a type of:
① Skeletal traction
② Skin traction
③ Balanced suspension
④ Transfixation

82. Mrs. Glasser is restless and appears anxious. When the nurse and nurse's aide enter the room to provide evening care, Mrs. Glasser becomes upset. The nurse should:
① Reassure her that she will be handled carefully
② Explain that hip fractures are not life threatening
③ Describe the need for various personnel at this time
④ Suggest that she turn on the television for diversion

83. The nurse recognizes that the increased incidence of fractures with osteoporosis in the United States occurs because of the:
① Dietary use of skim milk
② Increased number of hysterectomies
③ Immobility associated with early retirement
④ Aging of the American population

84. After surgery, Mrs. Glasser is encouraged to drink milk. She refuses the milk because she says it causes gasiness and bloating. A food rich in calcium that may be easily digested by those clients who do not tolerate milk is:
① Yogurt
② Eggs
③ Potatoes
④ Bananas

85. Mrs. Glasser has an internal fixation to reduce the fractured head of the femur. In the recovery room Mrs. Glasser's vital signs remained stable for an hour at BP 130/78, P 68, R 16. An hour after returning to her room her

vital signs are BP 100/60, P 74, R 22, and she is restless. The nurse should:
① Increase her IV flow rate
② Check her dressing
③ Raise the head of her bed
④ Monitor her again in 1 hour

86. Mrs. Glasser is to be transferred to a chair on the second postoperative day for a half hour. Before the transfer the nurse should:
① Instruct her to bear weight evenly on both legs
② Assess the strength of the affected leg
③ Explain how the transfer will be accomplished
④ Encourage her to keep the affected leg elevated

Situation: Bertha West, age 27, is admitted to the labor and delivery suite in active labor.

87. When Mrs. West has a contraction the nurse notes a 15 beat per minute acceleration of the fetal heart rate above the baseline rate. The nurse should:
① Prepare for immediate delivery
② Turn Mrs. West on her left side
③ Call the physician immediately
④ Record this normal fetal response

88. Mrs. West's contractions are now 2 to 3 minutes apart and last approximately 45 seconds. The fetal heart rate between contractions is about 100 beats per minute. The nurse should:
① Record this normal fetal response
② Notify the physician immediately
③ Obtain the mother's vital signs
④ Continue to monitor the fetal heart rate

89. An episiotomy is performed to facilitate delivery and prevent tearing of maternal tissues. The physician orders sitz baths three times a day. The nurse should include in the teaching plan that sitz baths promote healing by:
① Softening the incision site
② Promoting vasodilation
③ Cleansing the perineal area
④ Tightening the rectal sphincter

90. The nurse teaches Mrs. West how to care for her episiotomy at home. The nurse would know that the client understood the priority instruction when Mrs. West states:
① "I should continue the sitz baths three times a day if they provide comfort."
② "I must not climb up or down stairs for at least 3 days after discharge."
③ "I should discontinue the sitz baths once I am in my own home."
④ "I must continue perineal care after I go to the bathroom, until healing occurs."

Situation: John Owens, 5 months old, is brought to the pediatric clinic after several episodes of abdominal pain and vomiting. The physician suspects intussusception, and John is admitted to the hospital for intravenous fluid therapy and observation.

91. To assist in confirming the diagnosis, the priority assessment should be:
    ① Noting frequency of crying
    ② Measuring fluid intake and output
    ③ Observing characteristics of stools
    ④ Listening for bowel sounds

92. John is scheduled for surgery, and the physician plans to order a vagolytic agent preoperatively. An example of this type of drug is:
    ① Atropine
    ② Morphine
    ③ Phenergan
    ④ Secobarbital

93. One month after surgery, John, now 6 months old, is brought to the pediatric clinic for a follow-up visit. The nurse observes him performing all of the following tasks. The task that would be most unusual for his age is:
    ① Putting clothespins in a plastic bottle
    ② Showing stranger-anxiety when the nurse approaches
    ③ Sitting alone for brief periods in a crib
    ④ Playing with his toes during examination

Test 2

Situation: Brina Oshin, a class A diabetic, has just become pregnant for the first time. She is 31 years of age and attends the high-risk clinic.

94. When assessing an individual with class A diabetes, the nurse would probably find that the client has:
    ① A history of diabetes for at least 15 years
    ② Retinal changes seen on eye examination
    ③ No demonstrable vascular disease
    ④ Vascular changes in the eyes

95. The nurse is aware that diabetes can affect pregnancy by:
    ① Increasing the appetite and causing excessive weight gain
    ② Decreasing the amount of amniotic fluid present at term
    ③ Predisposing the client to hypertensive states
    ④ Promoting abnormal placental implantation

96. Mrs. Oshin is admitted to the hospital in her thirty-seventh week of pregnancy for an amniocentesis. This is being done primarily to determine the:
    ① Glucose level of the amniotic fluid
    ② Exact gestational age
    ③ Lung maturity of the fetus
    ④ Presence of genetic disorders

97. Nursing care for Mrs. Oshin before amniocentesis includes:
    ① Giving the ordered sedation to minimize fetal movement
    ② Reminding her to empty her bladder

③ Administering a Fleet enema to prevent contamination
④ Restricting her to nothing by mouth

98. Mrs. Oshin has a cesarean delivery in her thirty-eighth week and delivers a 9 pound, 2 ounce male infant. The baby is admitted to the neonatal intensive care unit. Priority care for the baby of a diabetic mother on admission to the nursery is:
    ① Starting an IV with 10% glucose in water
    ② Double clamping the cord immediately
    ③ Instilling prophylactic opthalmic medication
    ④ Doing a Dextrostix test on heel blood

Situation: Michael Josephs, a 30-month-old with a history of croup, is brought to the emergency clinic in acute respiratory distress. He has a temperature of 103.2° F, inflamed pharyngeal membranes, respiratory stridor, retractions, and a bark-like cough. A diagnosis of lower respiratory tract infection with croup (acute spasmodic laryngitis) is made, and Michael is admitted to the pediatric unit.

99. Based on Michael's condition, before he is admitted the nurse should anticipate the need for a:
    ① Tracheotomy setup at the bedside
    ② Cot so that a parent can stay
    ③ Quiet, cool room to facilitate breathing
    ④ Pad for the side rails of the Croupette

100. When providing care for Michael, the priority nursing responsibility should be to:
    ① Deliver 40% humidified oxygen
    ② Constantly assess respiratory status
    ③ Initiate measures to reduce fever
    ④ Provide support to reduce apprehension

101. Several hours after Michael's admission the nurse notes tachypnea and tachycardia, accompanied by intercostal and substernal retractions and increased restlessness. The nurse should immediately:
    ① Increase the level of oxygen being delivered
    ② Remove secretions with a suction apparatus
    ③ Dislodge mucus by striking Michael on the back
    ④ Report Michael's respiratory status to the pediatrician

102. An emergency tracheotomy is performed. In addition to routine suction of the tracheotomy, the nurse should also suction if Michael:
    ① Becomes restless or pale or his pulse increases
    ② Tells the nurse he is having difficulty breathing
    ③ Becomes restless, diaphoretic, and cyanotic
    ④ Has severe substernal retractions and stridor

Situation: Brian Coles is admitted for acute gastritis and ascites secondary to alcoholism and cirrhosis.

103. It is important for the nurse to routinely assess Mr. Coles for:
① Obstipation
② Complaints of nausea
③ Blood in the stool
④ Food intolerances

104. The nurse understands that Mr. Coles' ascites is most likely the result of:
① Decreased interstitial osmotic pressure
② Excess production of serum albumin
③ Inadequate secretion of bile salts
④ Impaired portal venous return

105. The physician plans a paracentesis. Immediately before the paracentesis the nurse should:
① Instruct Mr. Coles to void
② Have Mr. Coles drink a glass of water
③ Position Mr. Coles on his side
④ Measure Mr. Coles' abdominal girth

106. The physician removes 1500 ml of fluid. It is most essential that the nurse observe Mr. Coles for:
① An increased pulse rate
② Abdominal distention
③ A hypertensive crisis
④ Dry mucous membranes

Situation: Libby Kane has had a variety of gastrointestinal irregularities and discomfort for 4 months. After performing an extensive diagnostic workup, the physician suspects a mass in the liver. Mrs. Kane is admitted to outpatient surgery at the local hospital for a liver biopsy.

107. When preparing Mrs. Kane for the liver biopsy the nurse should instruct her to:
① Breathe normally throughout the procedure
② Hold her breath at the moment of the actual biopsy
③ Bear down (Valsalva maneuver) during the insertion of the biopsy needle
④ Turn on the left side after the procedure

108. The results of the biopsy indicate malignant sarcoma, and chemotherapy via regional perfusion is the treatment of choice. This method of drug administration probably was selected for Mrs. Kane because:
① The toxic effects of the chemotherapeutic drugs will be confined to the area of the tumor
② Larger doses of drugs can be delivered to the actual site of the tumor
③ The drug therapy can be continued at home with little difficulty
④ Combinations of drugs can be used to attack neoplastic cells at various stages of the cell cycle

109. Mrs. Kane's condition deteriorates despite therapy, and the physician indicates to her that her situation is serious. Her family is concerned because she appears to be accepting less and less responsibility for her own care. To help the family plan for her care, the nurse should:
① Explain that her anger is normal and identify ways for the family to deal with it
② Point out that denial is a normal response and will be temporary
③ Encourage them to accept her regression until she can cope more effectively
④ Assist them to identify methods for giving her more control over the situation

110. Mrs. Kane is experiencing severe pain, and she is admitted to the hospice unit. The physician orders Brompton's cocktail for pain management. The nurse should explain to Mrs. Kane that when Brompton's cocktail is prescribed:
① She must request the medication before the pain becomes severe
② The potential for dependency or addiction is decreased
③ A heparin lock will be inserted for intermittent IV administration
④ It is given automatically at regular intervals around the clock

111. Mrs. Kane is at high risk for developing ascites. To assess for this condition the nurse should:
① Percuss the abdomen, listening for dull sounds
② Auscultate the abdomen, listening for decreased or absent bowel sounds
③ Palpate the lower extremities over the tibia and observe for edema
④ Observe for signs of respiratory distress

Situation: Susan Bray, 24 years old, is admitted to the psychiatric unit of a general hospital for the third time in the past year. She was brought to the hospital by the police, who were called when she barricaded herself in the ladies' room at one of the shopping malls. She is about 8 months pregnant.

112. During the admission, Ms. Bray shouts, "Don't come near me. My stomach is filled with bombs and I'll blow up this place if anyone comes near me." This is an example of:
① Delusional thinking
② Tactile hallucinations
③ Loose associations
④ Ideas of reference

113. When the nurse approaches, Ms. Bray yells, "You're the one that made my boyfriend leave me." The nurse should recognize that Ms. Bray:
① Is actively hallucinating at this time
② Is confused and disoriented
③ Feels a great sense of vulnerability
④ Needs to have limits set after she has calmed down

114. One morning the nurse finds Ms. Bray staring at the television set, which is on. She sud-

denly rises and shouts, "Stop saying that. Who do you think you are?" It would be most therapeutic for the nurse to:
① Attempt to distract Ms. Bray by taking her for a walk
② Take Ms. Bray to her room so that they can have a quiet place to talk
③ Point out the inappropriateness of her behavior to her
④ Tell her that the voices she hears are coming from the television set

115. Ms. Bray refuses to eat, saying, "They want to kill my baby." The most therapeutic response by the nurse would be:
① "That's not true, Ms. Bray. It's the same food everyone else is eating."
② "You feel someone is attempting to poison your food."
③ "No one is trying to harm you or your baby, Ms. Bray."
④ "If you want, Ms. Bray, I'll taste it before you do so you'll know it's okay."

116. After 3 weeks of therapy, Ms. Bray tells the nurse that she feels she is ready for discharge. The nurse can best evaluate her readiness for discharge by:
① Requiring Ms. Bray to identify specific behaviors she sees as examples of wellness
② Exchanging views with Ms. Bray about her prognosis
③ Testing Ms. Bray's level of trust of herself and the staff
④ Asking Ms. Bray to explain how her behavior has changed since she was admitted.

117. Ms. Bray tells the nurse she is fearful about her upcoming delivery and the health of her baby. The most supportive approach by the nurse would be to:
① Commend Ms. Bray on her ability to express her fears and concerns
② Share with Ms. Bray the staff's concerns about how she will handle the infant
③ Reassure Ms. Bray that she will have plenty of help with the delivery
④ Provide Ms. Bray with a detailed explanation of what occurs during labor and delivery

Situation: Agnes Anderson, a grand multipara, is brought to the emergency room by her husband because she is experiencing vaginal bleeding.

118. The nurse should suspect that Mrs. Anderson has placenta previa if the bleeding is:
① Painful vaginal bleeding in the first trimester
② Painless vaginal bleeding in the first trimester
③ Painful vaginal bleeding in the third trimester
④ Painless vaginal bleeding in the third trimester

119. The nurse asks Mrs. Anderson to approximate how much she is bleeding. The best gauge for Mrs. Anderson to use is:
① Relation to her menstrual flow
② How weak she has become
③ The presence of clots
④ Change in her fetus' activity

120. During examination of Mrs. Anderson, the nurse uses Leopold's maneuvers to palpate her abdomen to assess the:
① Strength and duration of contractions
② Rate of uterine involution
③ Station of the fetus
④ Position of the fetus in utero

121. In planning for Mrs. Anderson's care, the nurse's primary goal is to:
① Provide a calm, quiet environment
② Prevent further episodes of bleeding
③ Prepare for a possible cesarean delivery
④ Arrange periods of diversional activity and rest

122. The nurse's primary nursing goal for Mrs. Anderson, in the event a cesarean delivery is performed, is:
① Assistance with mother-infant bonding
② Avoidance of wound dehiscence
③ Prevention of hemorrhage
④ Prevention of perineal infection

123. In childbirth preparation classes a nurse taught Mrs. Anderson some exercises that could be performed on the first day after a cesarean delivery. Further teaching would be necessary if Mrs. Anderson believes that one of the exercises is:
① Foot circles
② Leg bends
③ Pelvic rocking
④ Shoulder circles

Situation: Marie Carie brings her son, Anton, to the physician because he is constantly scratching his anus.

124. In caring for Anton, who is suspected of having pinworm infestation, the initial nursing responsibility is to:
① Identify the organism
② Collect a stool specimen
③ Prevent reinfection
④ Notify the Health Department

125. The nurse teaches Mrs. Carie how to collect a Scotch tape specimen from Anton. It is recommended that she collect the specimen:
① At night after the child has had a bath
② At night after the child has had a bowel movement
③ In the late morning after the child has had a bowel movement
④ In the morning before the child has had a bowel movement or a bath

126. Mrs. Carie, exceedingly upset about her child being diagnosed as having pinworm infestation, calls the public health nurse. Several

times during the conversation she tells the nurse that she keeps a very clean home. The nurse can best evaluate the effectiveness of the explanation of the transmission of the infestation when Mrs. Carie states:

① "I'll be sure to disinfect the toilet seat after every bowel movement for the next few days."
② "My child contracted this infestation from the dirty school toilets, and I'll report that to the school nurse."
③ "I'll have to reinforce my son's handwashing before he eats or handles food."
④ "I'll need to be sure the cat stays off my son's bed at night."

Situation: Six-year-old Peggy Sims is being discharged after diagnostic studies and treatment for frequent urinary tract infections.

127. The statement by Peggy's mother that indicates that she needs further teaching would be:
① "I guess I should not use the bubble bath I got Peggy for her birthday."
② "I hope Peggy can remember to always wipe from the front to the back."
③ "When it doesn't hurt Peggy to urinate I can stop giving her these pills."
④ "I will tell Peggy's teacher to let her go to the toilet as soon as she needs to."

128. Later that year Peggy is admitted with nephrotic syndrome. The nurse should be aware that the changes in body fluid distribution that occur with Peggy's disorder are due to the fact that:
① The basement membrane of the glomerulus becomes selectively impermeable to water so that fluid is retained in the tissues
② The loss of body protein reduces oncotic pressure so that fluid moves from the intravascular to the interstitial space
③ Hyperproteinemia results in increased oncotic pressure, which causes fluid to move from the intravascular to the interstitial space
④ The loss of sodium and water from impairment of the basement membrane of the glomerulus results in hypovolemia

129. Nursing care for the child in the acute phase of nephrotic syndrome should include:
① Providing time for active play periods
② Forcing fluids every hour
③ Feeding low-protein, high-carbohydrate, and low-salt foods
④ Encouraging frequent change of position

130. The adaptation in nephrotic syndrome that would necessitate that the nurse check vital signs, especially pulse quality and rate and blood pressure, is:

① Congestive heart failure
② Pulmonary emboli
③ Hypovolemia
④ Hyperkalemia

131. Mrs. Sims asked the nurse what she should bring Peggy to play with during her hospitalization. On the basis of Peggy's age, the nurse suggests:
① Stuffed animals, large puzzles, and large blocks
② Action toys such as a hula hoop
③ Table games, checkers, simple card games, and crayons
④ A record player, transistor radio, and children's magazines

132. Peggy is discharged from the hospital and is well for several months. One day Mrs. Sims calls the clinic nurse to report that for the past week Peggy's skin has had a muddy pale appearance, her appetite has been poor, and she has been unusually tired after school. The nurse suspects that Peggy:
① May be experiencing impending renal failure
② Is developing a viral infection
③ Is not taking her medications
④ May be overextending herself at school

Situation: John Chester, 54 years old, is admitted to the hospital witih acute bronchitis and chronic obstructive pulmonary disease.

133. The nurse observes Mr. Chester sitting up in bed, appearing very anxious and dyspneic. The nurse should:
① Administer the prescribed sedative
② Administer oxygen at 2 L per minute
③ Regulate carbon dioxide at 4 L per minute
④ Encourage coughing and deep breathing

134. Mr. Chester's laboratory values show that he has an elevated hemoglobin and hematocrit. The nurse should recognize that this is due to the fact that chronic:
① Hypercapnia stimulates red blood cell production
② Hypoxia stimulates red blood cell production
③ Infection stimulates white blood cell production
④ Infection promotes loss of extracellular fluid volume

135. On assessment of Mr. Chester's thorax, the nurse would expect to find:
① A decrease in the A-P diameter
② Atrophic accessory muscles
③ A shortened expiratory phase
④ Decreased breath sounds

136. The primary goal of therapy for Mr. Chester is to:
① Limit hydration
② Improve ventilation

③ Increase oxygenation

④ Correct bicarbonate deficit

137. Mr. Chester develops bronchopneumonia. To help determine the effectiveness of therapy, the nurse should refer to the results of Mr. Chester's:

① Pulmonary function study

② Culture and sensitivity test of sputum

③ Bronchoscopy

④ Lung scan

138. Mr. Chester develops acute respiratory distress, and a tracheostomy is performed. An important intervention that should be included in his care plan is:

① Cleansing the stoma with peroxide and cotton balls

② Suctioning via the tracheostomy every hour

③ Encouraging a fluid intake of 3000 ml daily

④ Applying an occlusive dressing over the site

139. Cor pulmonale is a frequent complication of COPD. The sign that would lead the nurse to suspect that Mr. Chester is developing cor pulmonale would be:

① Twitching of extremities

② Lethargy progressing to coma

③ Productive cough

④ Peripheral edema

Situation: Bob Tucker, a 35-year-old salesman, is admitted to the emergency room with multiple injuries suffered in an automobile accident, including a crushed chest, abdominal trauma, probable head injury, and multiple fractures.

140. In order of priority, the initial emergency care interventions for Mr. Tucker are to:

① Assess vital signs, obtain a history, arrange for emergency x-ray films

② Assess vital signs, control accessible bleeding, determine presence of critical injuries

③ Conduct a thorough physical assessment, assess vital signs, cover open wounds

④ Start an IV, get blood for typing and crossmatching, obtain a history

141. Mr. Tucker is oriented as to person and place but is confused as to time. His pupils are equal and reactive. He cannot recall how the accident occurred, complains of a headache, and becomes increasingly drowsy. A significant nursing intervention should be to:

① Prevent unnecessary movement

② Keep Mr. Tucker alert and responsive

③ Monitor Mr. Tucker for symptoms of increased intracranial pressure

④ Prepare Mr. Tucker for administration of mannitol

142. The obvious right-sided paradoxical motion of Mr. Tucker's chest indicates he suffered multiple rib fractures, resulting in a flail chest. The complication the nurse should carefully observe for is:

① Mediastinal shift

② Pericardial tamponade

③ Open pneumothorax

④ Tracheal laceration

143. Chest tubes are inserted to treat hemopneumothorax resulting from Mr. Tucker's crushing chest injury. In connecting the two-chamber water-seal drainage system ordered, the nurse must understand that the chamber attached to the chest tube provides the:

① Water seal

② Suction

③ Drainage receptacle

④ Seal and suction

144. To facilitate chest drainage, Mr. Tucker should be encouraged to lie:

① On his left (unaffected) side

② On his back

③ As if he were immobilized

④ On his right (affected) side

145. X-ray films reveal that Mr. Tucker has closed fractures of the right femur and tibia. Multiple soft-tissue contusions are also present. An important short-term intervention is to:

① Reassure him that these injuries are not that serious

② Assess the circulatory, motor, and sensory status of the injured extremity

③ Prepare him for operative reduction of the injured extremity

④ Prepare him for application of skeletal traction

146. In the evaluation of Mr. Tucker's responses to the emergency room treatment of his multiple trauma, the assessments that indicate he can safely be transferred to a critical care unit are:

① Alert but restless, stable vital signs, cyanosis

② Drowsy but easily roused, improving tissue perfusion, fluctuating vital signs

③ Elevated temperature, slowing pulse rate and respiration, pain in injured extremity

④ Stable vital signs, apprehension, complaints of pain

147. Mr. Tucker's progress is slow but steady, and his chest tube is removed. He is transferred to a postoperative surgical unit. It is planned that he will be discharged with a right leg cast and crutches. In addition to teaching him the technical aspects of crutch walking, the nurse plans to advise him to:

① Avoid taking showers until the cast is removed

② Remove loose rugs and rearrange furniture as necessary

③ Increase his intake of vitamin C to enhance healing

④ Gradually increase weight bearing on the injured leg

Situation: Norma Salomon, 16 years of age, is admitted to the adolescent psychiatric unit with a diagnosis of anorexia nervosa. Norma has lost 40 pounds during the last 6 months; her current weight is 75 pounds. She appears quite emaciated and cachectic.

148. In approaching Norma, the nurse should initially:
① Refrain from discussing her appearance
② Point out how bad she looks
③ Recognize that she is deliberately trying to kill herself
④ State the rules about eating in a matter-of-fact manner

149. Norma refuses to eat, stating, "I'll get too fat." The nurse can best respond to this behavior initially by:
① Telling her she will be tube fed if she does not eat
② Not talking about the fact that Norma is not eating
③ Stopping all her privileges until she eats
④ Pointing out that she can die of malnutrition

150. The nurse should plan to involve Norma in activities that will:
① Focus on her sexual attractiveness
② Force her to make decisions
③ Save her depleted energy
④ Involve her with her peer group

Situation: Ida Brown, 28 years of age, is admitted to the psychiatric unit with the diagnosis of obsessive-compulsive disorder. Her history demonstrates an increasing, consuming obsession with dirt. She reports feeling that her hands are dirty and that she needs to wash them about 70 to 80 times a day. She uses paper towels to open doors so she does not need to touch the doorknobs. Mrs. Brown's hands are red and raw with some bleeding.

151. An immediate nursing goal for Mrs. Brown would be to get her to:
① Stop washing her hands so that the skin will heal
② Understand that her hands are not dirty
③ Limit the number of times she washes her hands
④ Develop insight into her emotional problems

152. Mrs. Brown continues to use paper towels to turn doorknobs. The nurse's best response to this would be to:
① Ignore her behavior for the present time
② Quietly remove the paper towels from the area
③ Point out that the towels may be dirty
④ Prevent Mrs. Brown from using the towels

153. Mrs. Brown tearfully tells the nurse, "I know my hands are not dirty, but I just can't stop washing them." The nurse's best response would be:
① "I think you're getting better; you're beginning to understand your problem, Mrs. Brown."
② "Don't worry about it, Mrs. Brown; these actions are part of your illness, and these feelings will pass."
③ "Let's talk about why you feel you must wash your hands, Mrs. Brown."
④ "I understand that, Mrs. Brown, but maybe we can work to limit the number of times you wash them."

154. The nurse should plan to assist Mrs. Brown by:
① Getting her involved with activities that will keep her distracted
② Allowing her to perform menial tasks to expiate her feelings of guilt
③ Attempting to reduce or limit situations that increase anxiety
④ Providing her with repetitive activities that require little thought

Situation: Louisa Alcetti, age 2½, is brought to the emergency room with a fever of 103° F, stiffness of the neck, and generalized malaise. A diagnosis of acute bacterial meningitis is made, and Louisa is admitted to the pediatric unit.

155. Priority nursing care for Louisa would include:
① Placing her in isolation
② Hydrating her
③ Giving her a tepid sponge bath
④ Administering oxygen

156. Immediately after Louisa's admission the nurse should plan to:
① Assess her vital signs once per shift
② Administer oral antibiotic medications as ordered
③ Restrict parental visiting until isolation is discontinued
④ Check her level of consciousness every hour

157. An IV of 800 ml/24 hours is ordered for Louisa. It is set up via a pediatric administration set. The solution should be regulated to run at:
① 3 drops/minute
② 6 drops/minute
③ 33 drops/minute
④ 60 drops/minute

Situation: Edwin Torres, a 9-year-old who arrived recently from Cuba, is brought to the emergency room for treatment of a badly infected wound of the right big toe. The aunt with whom Edwin is living gives an uncertain history of tetanus immunization. An immunizing dose of tetanus immune globulin (Hyper-Tet) is administered.

158. Tetanus immune globulin is prescribed because it:
① Induces longer-lasting active protection
② Confers lifelong passive immunity
③ Immediately stimulates increased production of antibodies
④ Confers immediate passive protection of short duration

159. The chief reason for using tetanus immune globulin instead of tetanus antitoxin for Edwin is that it:
① Is more convenient to administer
② Is not likely to cause anaphylaxis
③ Is as effective as the antitoxin
④ Can be safely given to everyone who needs it

160. Edwin is admitted for surgical incision and drainage of his wound and intravenous penicillin therapy. When he is discharged 10 days later, the nurse administers tetanus toxoid immunization. The rationale for this is that, unlike tetanus immune globulin, the toxoid confers:
① Longer-lasting active immunity
② Temporary passive natural immunity
③ Lifelong passive immunity
④ Lifelong active natural immunity

Situation: Michelle Brule, a college freshman, is undergoing a hearing evaluation in the ear clinic because she has been complaining that her teachers mumble when they talk in class. The physician makes a tentative diagnosis of otosclerosis.

161. Not long after her diagnosis is established, Ms. Brule undergoes a stapedectomy with insertion of a middle ear prosthesis to help restore her hearing. A few days after her operation Ms. Brule is discouraged because her hearing has not improved. The nurse should bear in mind that this is most likely due to:
① Swelling within the ear canal
② Damage to the organ of Corti
③ Perforation of the tympanic membrane
④ The graft having slipped out of position

162. After the stapedectomy the early response by Ms. Brule that may be associated with possible damage to the motor branch of the facial nerve is:
① Dryness of the mouth
② A sensation of pain behind the ear
③ A bitter metallic taste
④ Inability to wrinkle the forehead

Situation: Franklin Dellano, age 67, visits his physician with complaints of frequency, dysuria, nocturia, and difficulty starting his urinary stream. He is admitted to the hospital, and a cystoscopy and biopsy of the prostate gland are done.

163. Mr. Dellano complains that he is unable to void after the cystoscopy. The nurse should:
① Assure him that this is normal
② Limit oral fluids until he voids
③ Insert a urinary retention catheter
④ Palpate above the pubic symphysis

164. Mr. Dellano is diagnosed as having prostatic cancer and is scheduled to have a suprapubic prostatectomy. He returns from the operating room with a suprapubic tube and a three-way Foley catheter with a continuous drip of 1 liter of a GU irrigant q 8 h. The nurse realizes that the purpose of this therapy is to:
① Prevent the formation of clots in the bladder
② Promote continuous formation of urine
③ Facilitate the measurement of urinary output
④ Provide continuous pressure on the prostatic fossa

165. Mr. Dellano complains that he needs to void. The nurse should first:
① Check the tubing connected to the client's collection bag to see whether it is draining
② Assess the client's total intake and output for the day
③ Explain to the client that the balloon inflated in the bladder gives him this feeling
④ Obtain the client's vital signs and notify the physician

166. Mr. Dellano complains of painful bladder spasms. To limit these spasms the nurse should:
① Administer a narcotic every 4 hours
② Encourage Mr. Dellano not to contract his muscles as if he were voiding
③ Irrigate the Foley catheter with 60 ml of normal saline
④ Advance the catheter to relieve the pressure against the prostatic fossa

167. Mr. Dellano's serum alkaline phosphatase level is extremely elevated. This finding should prompt the nurse to plan to:
① Measure his intake and output
② Institute seizure precautions
③ Monitor his plasma pH for acidosis
④ Handle him gently when turning him

Situation: Jane Quinn, a 40-year-old school teacher, tells the school nurse she is experiencing visual changes and sometimes has blurred or double vision. She also states she has muscular weakness and is becoming clumsy.

168. When Mrs. Quinn returns to work after her visit to her physician, she tells the school nurse that he told her she has multiple sclerosis. The nurse could best respond:
① "Don't worry; early treatment often alleviates symptoms of the disease."
② "See another physician. I've heard of several treatments that aid recovery."
③ "You should see a psychiatrist who will help you cope with this shocking news."
④ "That must have really floored you. Tell me what the physician told you about it."

169. Mrs. Quinn returns to the nurse the next day with a sudden loss of vision and asks what has caused it. The nurse explains that the blindness in her case is probably caused by:
    ① Optic nerve inflammation
    ② Intracranial pressure
    ③ Closed-angle glaucoma
    ④ Virus-induced iritis

170. Mrs. Quinn develops increased visual problems and progressive muscular weakness. In addition, she experiences frequent emotional lability, which is very distressing to her. During a visit to the nurse's office she bursts into tears for no apparent reason. The nurse should:
    ① Ascertain why she is upset
    ② Tell her there is no reason to cry
    ③ Let her cry; then resume the discussion
    ④ Tell her it is perfectly normal to be upset

171. Steroid therapy is ordered for Mrs. Quinn. The change that the nurse would expect to observe is decreased:
    ① Pain in the extremities
    ② Episodes of vision loss
    ③ Muscular contractions
    ④ Emotional lability

172. Several months later Mrs. Quinn mentions that she has developed tremors in her hands. In responding to Mrs. Quinn the nurse should take into consideration that the tremors associated with multiple sclerosis usually occur when the client:
    ① Is inactive
    ② Is asleep
    ③ Attempts to do someting
    ④ Gets nervous or upset

Situation: Max and Bella Kupper, aged 82 and 80 respectively, live alone. On a home visit, a nurse finds that Mr. Kupper has a prostate condition and at times is incontinent of urine. He is alert and cooperative but forgetful. Mrs. Kupper has diabetes that is controlled by oral medication and diet. She is severely arthritic and walks with difficulty. They both need some help with dressing, bathing, and meal preparation.

173. The plan that would appear most suitable for Mr. and Mrs. Kupper is to:
    ① Place them together in a skilled nursing faciliity
    ② Place them together in a health-related facility
    ③ Move them in with one of their children but allow them to choose which one
    ④ Keep them in their home with a long-term health care program

174. The condition that would rule out care in the home as an alternative for the Kuppers is:
    ① The home being located in a rural area
    ② The need for part-time multidisciplinary services

③ The need for part-time assistance for all personal care activities
④ The need for skilled nursing care on a 24-hour basis

Situation: Grace Peal, a 79-year-old widow living alone in an apartment, has been admitted to the hospital for medical observation. She was brought in by her daughter after a neighbor found Mrs. Peal looking confused at a nearby park late one rainy afternoon. Mrs. Peal cannot remember going to the park. A tentative diagnosis of organic mental syndrome with senile dementia is made.

175. During the admission procedures the initial approach by the nurse that would be most helpful to Mrs. Peal is:
    ① "Mrs. Peal, let me introduce you and your daughter to the staff here before you get acquainted with our ward policy and routine."
    ② "Grace, you are somewhat disoriented now, but do not worry. You will be all right in a few days."
    ③ "Mrs. Peal, do not be frightened. I am the nurse, and everyone here in the hospital will help you get well."
    ④ "Mrs. Peal, I am Miss Nee, the nurse tonight. You are at the hospital. Your daughter can stay with you for a while."

176. Considering Mrs. Peal's diagnosis the behavior that the nurse would most likely observe in Mrs. Peal is:
    ① Increased capacity for adaptation to the environment based on past life experiences
    ② Increased attention span and perceptual disturbances
    ③ Inability to learn new things and disturbance in thinking
    ④ Acceptance of personality and social changes due to declining years

177. Mrs. Peal's daughter tearfully tells the nurse, "I should never have allowed Mother to live alone as she wanted to do. But she has not been this bad. I am to blame. She did not even recognize me immediately." The response by the nurse that would be the most helpful to Mrs. Peal's daughter would be:
    ① "Why do you think your mother's condition has deteriorated? Her forgetfulness is temporary. You'll help if you don't cry."
    ② "This must be a difficult time for both of you. Would you like to share your other observations to help us plan for her care?"
    ③ "I realize that you are upset now. You can visit again when she is more responsive. I am sure you'll see a change."
    ④ "I do not think that anybody could blame you. You did what she wanted. Your being here tells us that you care."

178. When developing a plan of care for Mrs. Peal, the nurse should:
① Provide consistency in carrying out nursing activities for Mrs. Peal
② Be considerate of Mrs. Peal's various likes and dislikes
③ Be firm in dealing with Mrs. Peal's attitudes and behaviors
④ Explain to Mrs. Peal the details of the therapeutic regimen

179. After lunch one afternoon the nurse notes that Mrs. Peal is alone in the dayroom away from other clients. When the nurse approaches her, Mrs. Peal says, "I am all alone; no one has any use for me." The response by the nurse that would be most appropriate at this time would be:
① "You seem upset, Mrs. Peal. Would you like to tell me what is bothering you?"
② "We need to be alone sometimes. It helps us get to know ourselves better."
③ "You should focus on ways to change this, Mrs. Peal. Let's play some games to improve your morale."
④ "Have you done anything to avoid feeling lonely? I think you should socialize more with others."

Situation: Ann Singleton, age 18, is admitted to the labor room complaining of intense colic-like abdominal pain. She is at 35 weeks gestation and is diagnosed as having abruptio placentae.

180. When assessing Mrs. Singleton, the nurse expects to observe:
① Painless bleeding
② Flaccid uterus
③ A boardlike abdomen
④ Bright red bleeding

181. The nursing care plan for Mrs. Singleton should include careful assessment for signs and symptoms of:
① Jaundice
② Hypovolemic shock
③ Impending convulsions
④ Hypertension

182. When examining Mrs. Singleton after delivery, the nurse suspects that coagulopathy (DIC) has occurred when observations demonstrate:
① A boggy uterus
② Multiple vaginal clots
③ Bleeding from the venipuncture site
④ Hypertension and tachycardia

Situation: Myrtle Price, para I gravida III, is admitted to the labor room. She is having moderate contractions every 3 to 4 minutes, which last about 35 seconds. Vaginal examination reveals that her cervix is 50% effaced and 6 cm dilated. The head is at zero station, and the fetus is in an ROA position.

183. Gravida III means that Mrs. Price:
① Has three living children at home
② Is pregnant for the third time
③ Had one premature baby
④ Has had an induced abortion

184. From the results of the vaginal examination the nurse is aware that Mrs. Price is:
① Early in the first stage of labor
② Midway through the first stage of labor
③ In the transitional phase of labor
④ Beginning the second stage of labor

185. Mrs. Price's membranes rupture spontaneously. The observation by the nurse that necessitates immediate notification of the physician would be:
① Clear fluid with specks of mucus
② Bloody show
③ Shortened intervals between contractions
④ Greenish fluid

186. In the second stage of Mrs. Price's labor, the nurse should:
① Catheterize the client so that the head can be delivered
② Teach the client how to pant with each contraction
③ Watch for bulging of the client's perineum
④ Give the client pain medication as ordered

187. Immediately after the second stage of labor the nurse administers 10 units of oxytocin (Pitocin) as ordered by the physician. The desired response from this medication will:
① Stimulate the client's breasts so that breast-feeding can be started
② Relax the uterus so that it can be emptied
③ Lessen the discomfort of the episiotomy
④ Aid in the separation of the placenta from the uterine wall

Test 3

Situation: Alice South, a 59-year-old diabetic client, is admitted in diabetic ketoacidosis. According to her physician's order, she has been adjusting her own insulin based on blood glucose levels measured at home.

188. Of the statements made by Mrs. South during the history, the nurse realizes that the one that may best explain the etiology of Mrs. South's present state of ketoacidosis is that she:
① Has been taking steroids for a rash
② Is planning to retire next year
③ Is going to turn 60 next week
④ Has a chronic postnasal drip

189. In making the initial assessment of Mrs. South the nurse notes:
① Nervousness and cool pale skin
② Erythematoxicum rash and pruritus
③ Diaphoresis and instability as with intoxication

④ Deep respirations and fruity odor to the breath

190. The physician's order states: add 500 units regular insulin to 500 ml Ringer's lactate IV and run to administer 60 units of insulin in the next 30 minutes. The IV setup has a drop factor of 10 gtt/ml. To administer the correct amount of medication, the nurse should set the flow rate at:
① 20 gtt/min
② 30 gtt/min
③ 60 gtt/min
④ 90 gtt/min

191. Mrs. South's blood sugar level eventually returns to her usual range of 120 to 140 mg/100 ml. She receives 36 units of moderate-acting insulin before breakfast. The nurse should be alert to the symptoms of insulin reaction, which include:
① Excessive thirst, anorexia, and malaise
② Headache, nervousness, and diaphoresis
③ Dry skin, drowsiness, and tachycardia
④ Ataxia, dilated pupils, and Kussmaul respirations

192. Mrs. South develops persistent glycosuria despite increased amounts of insulin daily. Mrs. South experiences frequent hypoglycemic reactions followed by more glycosuria. This Somogyi effect is caused by:
① Insufficient amounts of insulin to lower blood sugar
② Excessive insulin that causes glycogenolysis
③ Increased glycogen formation in the liver
④ Excessive glucose intake that causes gluconeogenesis

193. Mrs. South has been diagnosed as having peripheral vascular disease. She tells the nurse that before hospitalization she had been experiencing severe cramplike pain in both legs after exercise. The nurse should include in the teaching plan specific measures Mrs. South can use to increase arterial blood flow to the extremities. These measures should include:
① Elevation of the legs above the level of the heart
② Daily cleansing of the feet by soaking in hot water
③ Exercises that promote muscular activity
④ Meticulous care of minor skin breakdown

Situation: Melvin Berk, age 43, fell asleep in his chair with a lighted cigarette in his hand. He sustained second- and third-degree burns to his chest, right arm, and upper legs.

194. Emergency treatment for Mr. Berk before bringing him to the hospital should include:
① Standing him under a gentle-spray shower
② Removing clothing from the burned areas

③ Wrapping him in a clean dry sheet
④ Applying sterile dressings to burned areas

195. Twelve hours after the burn, Mr. Berk is complaining of severe thirst. His urinary output has been 60 ml/hr for the past 10 hours. No bowel sounds are heard. The nurse should:
① Give him 4 oz of water by mouth
② Increase his IV flow rate
③ Give him orange juice by mouth
④ Moisten his lips with wet gauze

196. The nursing diagnosis that takes priority in planning Mr. Berk's care is:
① Potential fluid volume deficit related to decreased intake
② Impaired gas exchange related to smoke inhalation
③ Potential for infection related to burn trauma
④ Impaired physical mobility related to bed rest

197. Mr. Berk has a skin graft to the most severe third-degree burn on his chest. During the first 24 hours after a skin graft, care of the donor site includes immediately reporting:
① A moderate area of serosanguinous oozing
② A small amount of yellowish-green oozing
③ Separation of the edges of the non-adherent dressing
④ Epithelialization under the non-adherent dressing

198. When Mr. Berk begins to recover from his burns, he is permitted to eat. The most beneficial between-meal snack for him would be:
① A chicken salad sandwich and soft drink
② A bacon and tomato sandwich and tea
③ A piece of blueberry pie and milk
④ A cheeseburger and malted milk

Situation: Darlene Arnold, 78 years old, is found on the bathroom floor by her daughter. Mrs. Arnold complains of severe pain in her right hip. Her daughter calls the local police to take her mother to the hospital by ambulance.

199. On Mrs. Arnold's admission, the nurse assesses her condition. To assess for a fracture of the hip the nurse should:
① Move the affected leg to feel and hear crepitus
② Observe for shortening of the affected leg
③ Move the affected leg to see if it causes pain
④ Observe for bruising over the affected hip

200. X-ray films confirm a fractured right head of the femur and osteoporosis. Mrs. Arnold is placed in Buck's traction before surgical repair. Until surgery is performed the nurse should plan to:
① Turn her from side to side every 4 hours to prevent pressure on the coccyx
② Raise and maintain the knee gatch on the bed to limit the shearing force of traction

③ Inspect the skin and circulation of the affected leg hourly to prevent trauma

④ Remove the weights from the traction every 2 hours to promote comfort

201. After surgery the physician orders gentamicin sulfate (Garamycin) 75 mg IVPB q 6 hr and daily "peak" and "trough" levels. This is done primarily so that:
① Any allergy that the client might have to the drug would be detected early
② The blood culture can be obtained when gentamicin is at its lowest level
③ A drop in the client's fever may be correlated with "peak" level
④ Presence of an adequate therapeutic level of the drug can be determined

202. The next dose of gentamicin sulfate 75 mg is to be administered in 1 hour. The drug is to be diluted in 50 ml of D5W and infused over a period of 30 minutes. The drop factor of the tubing is 10 gtt/ml. The nurse should set the flow to provide:
① 3 gtt/min
② 4 gtt/min
③ 12 gtt/min
④ 17 gtt/min

203. After an open reduction and fixation of a hip fracture the assessment that would require immediate nursing intervention would be:
① An inability to cough productively 2 days postoperatively
② A rectal temperature of 100.2° F 3 days postoperatively
③ Fatigue in the leg on the unaffected side 5 days postoperatively
④ Complaints of pain in the chest 6 days postoperatively

Situation: Nineteen-month-old Stanley Slade has had large, frothy, foul-smelling stools since the introduction of cow's milk and table food. His behavior has changed from pleasant and outgoing to apathetic and irritable. He is diagnosed as having celiac disease.

204. In preparing a teaching plan for Mr. and Mrs. Slade, the nurse recalls that the basic problem in celiac disease is the:
① Presence of meconium stool
② Absence of the enzyme peptidase
③ Clumping of the intestinal villi
④ Susceptibility to profound dehydration

205. Stanley is placed on a gluten-free diet. A teaching program about the diet is instituted with Stanley's parents. The nurse knows that Mr. and Mrs. Slade understand the teaching about forbidden food substances when they state that Stanley cannot have:
① Fresh applesauce
② Steamed rice
③ Mashed corn
④ Grilled frankfurter

206. While the nurse is teaching the parents about celiac disease, Mrs. Slade sighs and states, "My neighbor said Stanley would only need to watch his diet until he's about 8 years old. I'm so relieved; you know how kids are about eating!" The nurse's response should be based on the fact that:
① The basic defect of celiac disease is lifelong
② Susceptibility to celiac crisis lessens with age
③ These children can tolerate small amounts of gluten by age 5
④ Though difficult at first, the diet is fairly easy to follow

207. In evaluating Stanley's response to the gluten-free diet after 2 days, the nurse anticipates the first change will be:
① An improved personality
② A return of appetite
③ A cessation of diarrhea
④ An increase in weight

208. When preparing Stanley for discharge, the nurse should caution the Slades that the toddler characteristic that would make Stanley most susceptible to a celiac crisis is:
① Negativism
② Invention
③ Autonomy
④ Narcissism

Situation: Iona Jeffrey has just delivered a full-term male infant.

209. The best nursing action to prevent heat loss in the neonate would be to:
① Dress the baby in a shirt and gown immediately
② Bathe the infant in warm water as soon as possible after birth
③ Maintain skin-to-skin contact between mother and baby under a cover
④ Administer oxygen to prevent shivering

210. The nurse does the Apgar test on Baby Jeffrey. A value of 2 should be assigned to:
① Heart rate of 90
② Strong cry
③ Arms and legs slightly flexed
④ Body pink, extremities blue

211. The nurse in the newborn nursery admits Baby Jeffrey. As part of the physical examination the nurse palpates his abdomen. The organ the nurse would normally expect to palpate is the:
① Liver
② Stomach
③ Pancreas
④ Gallbladder

212. The nurse further examines Baby Jeffrey and assesses his hips for dislocation. Dislocation would be indicated by:
① Ability to abduct each hip 90 degrees
② Limitation in abduction of either hip

③ Legs of equal length
④ Limitation in flexion of the hips

213. In assessing the head of Baby Jeffrey, now 2 hours old, the nurse would normally expect to find:
   ① Closed suture lines
   ② Open anterior and posterior fontanels
   ③ A soft fluctuant mass that outlines a bone
   ④ A sunken anterior fontanel

214. Failure of Baby Jeffrey to make the appropriate adaptations to extrauterine life would be indicated by:
   ① Respiratory rate of 40
   ② Liver 2 cm below the right costal margin
   ③ Cyanotic lips and face
   ④ Cyanotic feet and hands

Situation: June Simon, a 43-year-old housewife and mother of four teenage children, comes to the local community hospital mental health clinic accompanied by her husband, John Simon, a college professor. Mr. Simon reports that his wife has lost about 20 pounds over the last 2 months, cries easily, sleeps poorly, and refuses to participate in any family or social activities that she previously enjoyed. Mrs. Simon is admitted to the psychiatric unit.

215. In caring for Mrs. Simon at this time, it is very important for the nurse to:
   ① Assure her that she will regain her usual function in a short time
   ② Set firm consistent limits to reduce her crying episodes
   ③ Provide her with a high-calorie, high-protein diet
   ④ Allow her to externalize her feelings, especially anger, in a safe manner

216. In talking with the nurse, Mrs. Simon states, "I feel rotten and useless. I cannot think straight. I feel overwhelmed by everything. I don't know if I can go on." In recording this encounter in the client's record, the most objective description of the client's mood would be:
   ① Client stated, "I feel rotten and useless. I feel overwhelmed by everything. I don't know if I can go on."
   ② Client appeared to be very depressed for most of the morning. Little interest in self or environment
   ③ Client expressed suicidal thoughts about not being able to go on and has decreased ability to think clearly
   ④ Client is not able to cope with her problems and this hospitalization; states, "I cannot think straight."

217. Mrs. Simon frequently repeats her doubts about going on and admits to thinking about suicide although she denies that she has developed a plan. During this period it is essential that the nurse:
   ① Have a staff member stay with Mrs. Simon at all times

② Explain in detail to Mrs. Simon how the staff will protect her from herself
③ Use frequent unobtrusive observations of Mrs. Simon's moods and activities
④ Plan to involve Mrs. Simon in activities that are interesting and absorbing

218. A tricyclic antidepressant is prescribed for Mrs. Simon. After 1 week, Mr. Simon comes to speak with the nurse and expresses concern that his wife does not seem to show much improvement after taking the medication. In responding to Mr. Simon the nurse explains that:
   ① The tricyclics are slow-acting drugs and it may take 3 to 4 weeks until therapeutic effectiveness is achieved
   ② Mrs. Simon may require other drugs in addition to the antidepressants before her behavior changes
   ③ For clients who have been depressed for a prolonged period the drug takes additional time to be effective
   ④ As Mrs. Simon's physical condition improves, the antidepressant medication will act more effectively

219. On entering Mrs. Simon's room one morning, the nurse finds her still in bed. Mrs. Simon tells the nurse she is unable to get dressed and go to breakfast. The nurse's best response would be:
   ① "I'll get you dressed. I recognize that you have difficulty helping yourself."
   ② "Take your time. It is not necessary to hurry. I'll help you if you need me to."
   ③ "You cannot just lie in bed. You must get up now and go to breakfast."
   ④ "You can lie there for a while if you promise me you'll get dressed for lunch."

220. The next day the nurse notices that Mrs. Simon is neatly dressed and well-groomed. She smiles at the nurse and states, "Things sure look better today." Based on evaluation of Mrs. Simon's behavior the nurse should:
   ① Increase Mrs. Simon's privileges as a reward
   ② Compliment her on her appearance and her smile
   ③ Begin preparing Mrs. Simon for discharge
   ④ Assign a staff member to provide constant surveillance

Situation: Ted Cohen, age 3, is seen in the emergency department. He has not been feeling well, his temperature has been 103° F for 1 week, and he has lost weight. His mother notices a whitish film in his mouth. Ted was born prematurely, had numerous blood transfusions while in the neonatal ICU, and his HIV test is positive.

221. When doing the health history, the nurse determines that Ted is at high risk for developing AIDS because of:

① The multiple blood transfusions he received
② An immature reticuloendothelial system
③ A positive HIV antibody screening test
④ The presence of an opportunistic infection

222. Ted is placed on bed rest and is being given O_2 via a tent. Mrs. Cohen has just been informed that her son has AIDS and is found visibly upset at his bedside. The nurse's most therapeutic statement would be:
① "He'll get the best care possible at this hospital."
② "It is a shame he needed so many blood transfusions."
③ "You must really feel like screaming."
④ "Let me give you a referral for social service."

223. The nurse answers Mrs. Cohen's questions about AIDS and how it is transmitted via a blood transfusion. The nurse knows Mrs. Cohen needs further teaching when she states:
① "Once tested for antibodies, negatively tested blood cannot transmit the virus."
② "The process of donor screening has been improved since the AIDS virus was discovered."
③ "Blood that has tested negative for the AIDS virus can develop antibodies at a later time."
④ "Blood obtained from individuals in high-risk groups is discarded."

224. The nurse explains to Mrs. Cohen that Ted will be placed on appropriate isolation precautions. These precautions include:
① Gloves should be worn whenever approaching the bedside
② Limited physical contact should be made when care is administered
③ Gloves should be worn when in contact with blood and body fluids
④ Gowns, masks, and gloves should be worn when providing direct care

Situation: Anita and Hal Long have been married for 4 years. Mrs. Long, 28 years old, has been on birth control pills because they had decided to postpone having children for a while.

225. The nurse is aware that an assessment finding that would indicate a potential risk with continuing use of birth control pills is:
① A BP of 140/90
② Dysmenorrhea
③ Mid-cycle bleeding
④ The lack of ovulation

226. Mr. and Mrs. Long decide to start their family, and Mrs. Long stops taking the birth control pills. After 18 months of unsuccessful attempts at conception, Mrs. Long is diagnosed as having primary infertility related to anovulatory cycles. After consultation, she decides to use Clomid for 6 months. The nurse knows Mrs. Long understands the correct time to take the Clomid when she states, "I will begin the pills on the:
① First day I start my period."
② Fifth day of my cycle."
③ Fourteenth day of my cycle."
④ Last day of my period."

227. After taking Clomid for 3 months, Mrs. Long complains of difficulty with penetration during intercourse because of vaginal dryness. An appropriate response by the nurse would be:
① "This is a common side effect; use a water-soluble lubricant to ease penetration."
② "Stop the Clomid immediately; the physician will have to prescribe another drug."
③ "I know you are concerned about it, but this is only temporary."
④ "Good; this means you are probably beginning to ovulate."

228. Mrs. Long thinks she is now pregnant. The nurse is aware that a positive sign of pregnancy is:
① Hegar's sign
② Uterine enlargement
③ A positive pregnancy test
④ Fetal movements felt by the examiner

Situation: Loretta Anton, a 52-year-old housewife, is seen in the outpatient clinic for routine health screening. The nurse obtains a blood pressure reading of 190/100.

229. After a diagnostic workup the physician informs Mrs. Anton that she has atherosclerosis and hypertension. Later while talking with the nurse Mrs. Anton wants to know more about atherosclerosis. The nurse bases the response on the fact that atherosclerosis is characterized by:
① Development of atheromas within the myocardium
② Mobilization of free fatty acid from adipose tissue
③ Lipid plaque formation within the arterial vessels
④ Gradual decrease in arterial pressure as a result of renin

230. When discussing follow-up care with Mrs. Anton, the nurse provides her with a list of foods to avoid on her low-sodium diet. This list includes:
① Luncheon meat
② Fresh salmon
③ Cooked broccoli
④ Ground beef

231. Because of Mrs. Anton's hypertension, the nurse teaches her to reduce her dietary sodium. The nurse should emphasize that:
① The taste for salt is inherent, but it can be overcome with practice
② Salt-free natural seasonings can be used and taste the same as salt
③ Salt substitutes with potassium chloride

bases can be used freely with foods to provide the same taste

④ The taste for table salt is learned and increases over time, but it is not a biologic necessity

232. Because Mrs. Anton has always been an active individual, she is interested in measures that would help maintain her health. The nurse explains to her that maintenance of vessel patency can be promoted by:
① Increasing saturated fats in the diet
② Practicing relaxation techniques
③ Decreasing the amount of exercise
④ Leading a more sedentary life-style

Situation: Nick Falk, a 22-year-old department store clerk, is admitted to the psychiatric unit with a diagnosis of schizophrenia, paranoid type. He is accompanied by his family, who are concerned with his safety and well-being because he said the voices are telling him to kill himself.

233. After doing an initial assessment on Mr. Falk, the nursing diagnosis that should have first priority is:
① Disturbed self-concept
② Sensory-perceptual alterations (auditory)
③ Impaired verbal communication
④ Potential for violence: self-directed

234. Mr. Falk is started on haloperidol (Haldol). When the nurse gives Mr. Falk the medication, he asks, "What's this for?" The nurse could best respond, "This medication:
① Will help you to relax and think more clearly."
② Maintains an even mood while keeping your temper under control."
③ Fights 'the blues' and keeps your thoughts together."
④ Will raise your seizure threshold, letting you think more clearly."

235. The nurse evaluates that Mr. Falk has understood the teaching about the side effects and precautions associated with the neuroleptics when he states:
① "I'll maintain an adequate fluid intake, since I may urinate more than usual."
② "I'll avoid direct sunlight and use sunburn preventatives when I go outdoors."
③ "I will not eat any tyramine-containing foods while I'm on Haldol."
④ "I will immediately report any diarrhea or vomiting to my doctor."

236. One day Mr. Falk's mother confides to the nurse that she is very troubled by her son's illness. The nurse's most therapeutic initial response would be:
① "Getting together with others who are coping with this problem can be quite helpful."
② "I recognize it's hard to deal with this. Try to remember that this too shall pass."
③ "You must lessen your feelings of guilt and loneliness by seeing a psychiatrist."

④ "It is very important that you become involved in volunteer work at this time."

237. Mr. Falk's physician tells the nurse that he is concerned that Mr. Falk may be developing neuroleptic malignant syndrome. The nurse should carefully assess Mr. Falk for symptoms that would include:
① Jaundice, malaise, and pruritus
② Loss of visual acuity, dry skin, and hyperbilirubinemia
③ Diaphoresis, muscle rigidity, and hyperpyrexia
④ Sore throat, seizures, and tremors

238. Neuroleptic malignant syndrome is ruled out. The nurse begins terminating the consistent one-to-one relationship with Mr. Falk because he is soon to be discharged. The nurse might expect him to respond to termination by manifesting symptoms of:
① Splitting
② Testing
③ Manipulation
④ Grief

Situation: Betty Field is a thin, unmarried, pregnant teenager living in a poor section of the city. During her second trimester her friend brings her to the clinic. Over the next few visits her blood pressure averages 92/64.

239. For a client whose blood pressure has been averaging 92/64, pregnancy-induced hypertension should be suspected when the blood pressure first rises to:
① 110/80
② 114/80
③ 124/80
④ 140/90

240. In her third trimester Ms. Fields develops extensive edema, hypertension, low serum albumin level, and albuminuria. The nutritional therapy that requires primary emphasis is the:
① Inclusion of protein to restore normal circulation of tissue fluids
② Elimination of all salt to reduce the edema and hypertension
③ Control of kilocalories to limit weight gain during this period
④ Use of iron supplements to help restore circulating blood volume

241. Ms. Fields is admitted to the hospital at 37 weeks' gestation with the diagnosis of pregnancy-induced hypertension (PIH). Assessment of Ms. Fields reveals a nutritional deficit. A physical finding that would be related to inadequate protein intake is:
① Bradycardia
② Peripheral edema
③ Bleeding gums
④ Petechiae

242. The next day Ms. Fields is anorexic and appears depressed. The nurse plans to further

explore the client's emotional status when Ms. Fields comments:

① "I was really happy before I got pregnant."
② "I'll be glad when I can sleep all night."
③ "I'm tired of feeling so clumsy."
④ "I dreamed my baby had only one arm."

243. Ms. Fields is treated with magnesium sulfate. Before administering the second injection of magnesium sulfate, it is essential for the nurse to monitor Ms. Fields' deep tendon reflexes to:
① Evaluate the mobility of the extremities
② Determine her level of consciousness
③ Avoid development of respiratory depression
④ Determine her response to painful stimuli

244. In her thirty-eighth week Ms. Fields delivers a 4 lb 3 oz baby girl. A finding in the newborn that may indicate magnesium sulfate toxicity is:
① Pallor
② Respirations of 16
③ Tremors
④ A pulse of 200

245. Baby Fields appears mottled during transfer to the nursery. The nursery nurse should first:
① Encourage an oral feeding
② Check the baby's temperature
③ Notify the physician
④ Administer oxygen

246. Baby Fields is determined to be small for her gestational age (SGA). A priority intervention for this infant would be to:
① Measure her head circumference every shift
② Place her in the Trendelenberg position
③ Test her stools for occult blood
④ Monitor her blood glucose levels

247. Ms. Fields is to be discharged and is upset that her baby has to remain hospitalized because of a rising reticulocyte count. Ms. Fields asks the nurse why the baby must stay. The nurse's response is based on an understanding that the infant needs to be observed for:
① Adequate oxygenation
② Bleeding tendencies
③ A bacterial infection
④ Significant jaundice

Situation: Gail Agar, 23 years old, comes to the emergency room stating that she has been raped. She is disheveled, pale, and staring blankly.

248. Taking what has occurred into consideration, the nurse on duty asks Ms. Agar to describe in detail what happened because:
① It helps the victim put the event in better perspective and helps begin the resolution process
② Talking about what led to the rape will

help her see what may have precipitated it
③ It will help the nursing staff in giving legal advice and providing counseling
④ Discussing details will keep the victim from covering up the intimate happenings in the rape situation

249. Ms. Agar continues to talk about the rape. The primary nursing intervention should be directed toward:
① Exploring her feelings about men to promote future relationships
② Getting her involved with a rape therapy group
③ Helping her restore emotional control to expiate feelings of shame
④ Remaining available and supportive to limit destructive anger

250. Ms. Agar, aware of the possible legal implications, decides to prosecute the rapist. The nurse carefully listens and documents all observations. This is done because with a charge of rape the burden of proof:
① Is on the defendant to prove his innocence
② Rests with the medical team
③ Rests with the rape victim
④ Must be established before the case will be heard

251. The nurse makes notes on Ms. Agar's record during the interview and examination, because the record may go to court as evidence. It is most important when charting that the nurse include:
① A summarized statement about Ms. Agar's description of the rape and the rapist
② Ms. Agar's verbatim statements about the rape and the rapist
③ Observations about Ms. Agar's reaction to male staff members
④ General statements about Ms. Agar's previous knowledge of the rapist

Situation: Tricia Volt, age 5, is admitted to the hospital with a diagnosis of acute glomerulonephritis. Her history reveals a 5 pound weight gain during the preceding week and periorbital edema. Mrs. Volt indicates that Tricia had impetigo several weeks ago.

252. Acute glomerulonephritis may occur secondary to impetigo. The treatment most beneficial in the prevention of this sequela is the:
① Removal of crust with pHisoHex and water
② Application of antibiotic ointment to the lesions
③ Administration of systemic antibiotics
④ Use of oil-based soap for bathing

253. For the most accurate information on the status of Tricia's edema, nursing intervention should include:
① Measuring intake and output
② Obtaining a daily weight measurement
③ Doing a visual inspection
④ Monitoring electrolyte values

254. After several days on bed rest, Tricia becomes demanding and will not listen to the nurses. She was found in the playroom twice on the previous shift. To best meet the needs of the hospitalized preschool child, the nurse should:
① Explain to Tricia the reason for bed rest and ask her not to get up again
② Move Tricia into a room with another 5-year-old who has a fractured femur
③ Place soft restraints on Tricia when family members cannot be present
④ Have a color television set moved into Tricia's room as soon as possible

255. Mrs. Volt asks the nurse if Tricia will have to stay in bed. The nurse should tell Mrs. Volt that bed rest:
① Will be necessary for 3 to 4 weeks regardless of response to therapy
② Is not part of the usual treatment unless the child is seriously ill
③ Is limited to 72 hours after the institution of antihypertensive drug therapy
④ Will be necessary until the blood pressure is normal and the urine clear

Situation: Bernice Sands is admitted with a diagnosis of laryngeal cancer. A laryngectomy is to be performed the next day.

256. A common early sign of laryngeal cancer for which the nurse should assess Mrs. Sands is:
① Aphasia
② Dysphagia
③ Hoarseness
④ Dyspnea

257. The physician's preoperative order states: scopolamine 0.3 mg by injection at 7:30 A.M. Available is an ampule of scopolamine labeled 0.4 mg = 0.5 ml. The nurse should administer:
① 8 minims
② 6 minims
③ 4 minims
④ 2 minims

258. Mrs. Sands has a partial laryngectomy and tracheostomy. Postoperatively, to facilitate communication, the nurse should:
① Face the client and speak slowly and distinctly
② Allow more time for the client to articulate
③ Use visual clues such as gestures and objects
④ Provide a pad and pencil for writing

259. The physician orders IV Ringer's lactate for Mrs. Sands at the rate of 150 ml/hr. The nurse calculates that a liter bottle of this solution will infuse in:
① 6 hours and 40 minutes
② 6 hours and 50 minutes
③ 7 hours
④ 7 hours and 10 minutes

260. Mrs. Sands develops subcutaneous emphysema. This is most readily detected by:
① Palpating the neck or face
② Auscultating the lung fields
③ Evaluating the blood gases
④ Reviewing the chest x-ray film

Situation: Gloria Howard, 53 years old, is admitted to the psychiatric unit after several days of increasing incapacitation at home. She complains of memory loss, nervousness, insomnia, and is afraid to go out of her house.

261. Considering her history, an initial priority in caring for Mrs. Howard should be directed toward:
① Evaluating her adjustment to the unit
② Assessing the precipitating factors for hospitalization
③ Providing her with a sense of security
④ Exploring her fear of going out and her memory loss

262. When planning the development of a nurse-client relationship, the nurse is aware that the most important aspect of this relationship during the early phase of its development is:
① Open communication
② Personal rapport
③ Trust
④ Empathy

263. The nurse is aware that the major defense mechanism used by an individual with a phobic disorder is:
① Projection
② Regression
③ Repression
④ Avoidance

Situation: Donald Lewin, a 45-year-old bank president, complains of pain in the upper epigastric area. He indicates he has found relief by taking antacids. On endoscopy a gastric ulcer is diagnosed.

264. The diet regimen that would be appropriate for Mr. Lewin would be:
① Hourly feedings of cream and milk
② A mechanical soft diet
③ A low-fat, high-protein liquid diet
④ Regular meals that can be tolerated

265. The physician orders the drug ranitidine (Zantac) to help treat Mr. Lewin's ulcer. The nurse realizes the drug will help Mr. Lewin's condition by:
① Inhibiting the Histamine H_2 receptors
② Regenerating the gastric mucosa
③ Lowering the gastric pH
④ Promoting the release of gastrin

266. The nurse recognizes that Mr. Lewin understands how to appropriately take his antacids when he states, "I will take my antacids:
① Every time I have anything to eat."
② 30 minutes after meals."

③ Every 4 hours around the clock."
④ With the onset of pain."

267. Medical treatment of Mr. Lewin's ulcer is unsuccessful. He is scheduled for a gastroduodenostomy. Dumping syndrome is a possible postoperative complication. Nursing interventions directed toward minimizing this syndrome include teaching Mr. Lewin to:
① Increase his fluid intake with meals
② Eat in a semirecumbent position
③ Remain on a diet low in fat
④ Ambulate after every meal

268. After surgery, Mr. Lewin has a nasogastric tube in place. The nurse should plan to:
① Assess placement by injecting 10 ml of water into the tube
② Connect the nasogastric tube to high continuous suction
③ Monitor for signs of electrolyte imbalance
④ Change the tube at least every 48 hours

Situation: Emily Hale, a 24-year-old computer programer, is admitted for an emergency appendectomy.

269. Ms. Hale's respiratory status may be affected after surgery. In planning care to meet this need, the behavioral objective for Ms. Hale should be:
① She demonstrates the techniques of coughing and deep breathing
② She will cough and deep breathe five or six times every hour while awake
③ Coughing and deep breathing facilitate output of secretions
④ Respirations will improve with coughing and deep breathing

270. Ms. Hale develops hyperpyrexia, and peritonitis is suspected. When caring for her the nurse should use:
① Protective isolation
② Surgical asepsis
③ Enteric precautions
④ Wound precautions

Situation: Jenny DeBeers, 9 years old, was recently diagnosed as having insulin-dependent diabetes mellitus. She and her parents attend the outpatient clinic for diabetic teaching.

271. The nurse suspects that Jenny's concerns about her illness will center on:
① Whether having diabetes means that she cannot have children when she grows up
② How her parents will react to her
③ Whether or not her physician will be successful in controlling her diabetes
④ How much school she might miss

272. When teaching Mr. and Mrs. DeBeers about Jenny's illness, it is important to differentiate between insulin-dependent and non-insulin-dependent diabetes. The nurse should tell them that with insulin-dependent diabetes it is more common to develop:
① Resistance to treatment
② Obesity
③ Hypersensitivity to other drugs
④ Ketoacidosis

273. The nurse teaches Jenny and her parents about insulin-dependent diabetes and the occurrence of hyperglycemia. The nurse would be aware that they understand the teaching when they state that ketoacidosis is most often precipitated by:
① An infection
② An insulin overdose
③ Decreased fluid intake
④ Excessive physical exercise

274. Jenny is started on insulin therapy, and she and her family are taught how to give injections. Jenny dislikes the injections and asks the nurse why she cannot take the insulin by mouth. The nurse explains that insulin:
① Is a protein and would be inactivated by digestion
② Is alkaline and would be neutralized by gastric hydrochloric acid
③ Has a carbohydrate portion that would add to the blood sugar
④ Would irritate the stomach lining and lose its potency

275. In her discussions with health team members, Jenny learns that the insulin she takes acts by:
① Helping to carry sugar into cells where it is burned for energy
② Preventing the sugar from being stored in the liver
③ Helping to break down protein and fat to provide needed glucose
④ Preventing the wasting of blood sugar by converting it to glycogen

276. Jenny likes candy and wonders if she can ever have any. She asks about sugar and sugar substitutes in her diet. The nurse and the dietician tell her that she:
① Can use sugar substitutes such as saccharin or aspartame if she wishes
② Can use honey as a natural sugar substitute
③ Should avoid using any simple sugars such as sucrose or fructose
④ Should break her sweet taste habit by eliminating sweets altogether

Situation: Dennis Moran, 50 years old, comes to the clinic complaining of a productive cough with copious yellow sputum, fever, and chills for the past 2 days.

277. The first thing the nurse should do when caring for Mr. Moran is to:
① Collect a sputum specimen
② Take his temperature
③ Begin to push fluids
④ Administer oxygen

278. During the assessment of Mr. Moran the nurse percusses an area of dullness over the right posterior lower lobe. Considering the presenting signs and symptoms, this finding may be indicative of:
① Pleurisy
② Pneumonia
③ Emphysema
④ Bronchitis

Situation: Paul Miller, age 19, was brought to the emergency room after having had a grand mal seizure during his physical education class at college. He has a 2-year history of a seizure disorder. His seizures have been well controlled by phenytoin (Dilantin) for the last 6 months. He is admitted to the hospital for observation.

279. When being admitted to the hospital he says to the nurse, "I am so upset. I didn't think I was going to have more seizures." The nurse's best response would be:
① "You must be under a lot of stress at school right now."
② "Did you forget to take your medication?"
③ "You are worried about having more seizures?"
④ "Don't be too concerned. Your medication needs to be increased."

280. In planning care for Mr. Miller, the nurse should plan to:
① Teach that anticonvulsant medications should be taken on an empty stomach
② Outline ways to prevent physical trauma from occurring during a seizure
③ Explain that he need not tell others of his illness because the medication will be increased
④ Teach him that the symptoms and treatment of seizure disorders are similar, regardless of cause

281. Before Mr. Miller's discharge the nurse should reinforce previous teaching related to the anticonvulsant phenytoin (Dilantin). The nurse should instruct Mr. Miller to:
① Immediately report any unsteadiness of gait
② Avoid massaging the gums during oral hygiene
③ Immediately discontinue the drug if a skin rash appears
④ Expect transient joint discomfort on occasion

Test 4

Situation: Jonah Hopkins, age 4, is brought to the pediatric clinic after a week-long history of an upper respiratory infection. A blood workup reveals a hemoglobin of 7g/100 ml, a hematocrit of 20, a WBC of 39,000, and a platelet count of 130,000. He is diagnosed as having acute lymphocytic leukemia (ALL).

282. The physician decides to perform a bone marrow aspiration. When involving Jonah in therapeutic play before the procedure the nurse should help him understand that:
① He did nothing to cause his present illness
② His problem was caused by an environmental factor
③ He needs to have a positive attitude
④ His parents are concerned about him

283. When performing the admission history and physical assessment the common early signs of ALL that the nurse should assess Jonah for are:
① Enlargement of the liver and spleen
② Fever and areas of ecchymosis
③ Abdominal pain and reddened complexion
④ Nosebleeds and papilledema

284. Mr. and Mrs. Hopkins ask the nurse, "Why did the doctor say Jonah has too many white blood cells?" The nurse's best response would be:
① "Your doctor is the best one to answer that question for you."
② "You seem to be focusing on Jonah's white blood cells."
③ "It sounds like you really do not understand what occurs in leukemia."
④ "The bone marrow isn't working properly and makes too many white cells."

285. Platelets are ordered for Jonah, and an IV is started. The nurse should:
① Flush the line with 5% dextrose and normal saline
② Administer the platelets over 2 hours
③ Administer the platelets rapidly
④ Check vital signs 3 hours after the transfusion

Situation: Joan Healy is in the terminal stage of cancer of the colon. She is 43 years old, divorced, and has two sons, ages 18 and 14.

286. A public health nurse visits Mrs. Healy in her home 3 days a week to provide physical care and emotional support. The nurse observes that the children are having difficulty talking with their mother. The nurse suggests family meetings with the hospice nurse, knowing that:
① A deeper level of understanding will help the children comprehend what their mother is going through
② Opening communication systems reduces the intensity of a family's emotional reaction to terminal illness
③ It is important to solve family problems before death occurs
④ They will be unable to deal with their feelings until after their mother dies

287. When assessing Mrs. Healy's potential reaction to grief, the nurse knows that the most important factor in predicting her response is her:
① Social support systems
② Earlier experiences of grief

③ Family interactions
④ Emotional relationships

288. Mrs. Healy is admitted to the hospital in severe pain but refuses medication because it puts her to sleep and she wants to be awake. One day, despite Mrs. Healy's objection, the nurse administers the pain medication saying, "You know that this will make you more comfortable." The nurse in this situation could be charged with:
① Battery
② Assault
③ Invasion of privacy
④ Lack of informed consent

289. Mrs. Healy is furious with the nurse. Over the next several days she becomes very angry and agitated and insists on doing everything herself. A different nurse is assigned to care for her. The nurse's initial step in revising the nursing care plan to meet Mrs. Healy's needs would be to:
① Tell her about the change in staff responsibilities and assess her reaction
② Get a full report from the first nurse and adjust the plan accordingly
③ Assess her present status and capabilities and discuss revisions with her
④ Ask her physician for a report on her condition and plan accordingly

290. The nurse encourages Mrs. Healy to make most of the decisions about her daily activities. The nurse would know that Mrs. Healy had resolved some of her anger when she says:
① "I can do my face, hands, arms, and chest today but I think you'd better do the rest."
② "You've got a busy morning ahead of you! I'm really a mess."
③ "It's so hard to let someone do so much for me. It just doesn't seem right."
④ "What are you going to let me do this morning? You know I can help."

291. Mrs. Healy's oldest son is very concerned about his mother's condition. He asks the nurse, "Will she get better?" The nurse's most appropriate response would be:
① "I don't know. You'll have to ask the doctor when he comes. I'll tell him you are here."
② "Of course she will. You can't give up. You must hope for the best."
③ "Her condition is very serious. Would you like to discuss your concerns with me?"
④ "Her vital signs are stable, so she is holding her own."

Situation: Amy Ross, age 40, attends a program on breast self-examination given by the local women's club. The program includes a demonstration and a return demonstration.

292. The public health nurse presenting the program realizes that certain aspects of the teaching program would have to be reviewed when the nurse observes that Ms. Ross is:
① Observing her breasts for symmetry while holding her arms above her head
② Palpating her breasts while in the sitting position
③ Checking her nipples for alterations in size or shape
④ Palpating her breast with the palmar surface of her extended fingers

293. When reviewing the examination procedure with Ms. Ross, the comment by Ms. Ross that the nurse should consider significant is:
① "My left breast was always slightly larger than my right."
② "My bra feels tight when I am menstruating."
③ "My breasts feel lumpy just before menstruation."
④ "My right breast feels and looks thicker than my left breast."

294. Following the nurse's recommendation, Ms. Ross makes an appointment with her physician. She is subsequently hospitalized for a biopsy and possible mastectomy. As the nurse is preparing her for surgery, Ms. Ross says, "I'm really scared. My mother and sister went through this. It was awful." The nurse's most appropriate response would be:
① "You know most breast lumps are benign."
② "Breast cancer has an excellent cure rate."
③ "You are worried about the results tomorrow?"
④ "What happened with your mother and sister?"

295. A modified radical mastectomy is performed. After the surgery Ms. Ross tells the nurse that what has occurred to her is as "Good as a death sentence and I would rather go now than to suffer." At this time it would be most important for the nurse to:
① Encourage her to admit herself to the psychiatric unit of the hospital
② Explore the possibility of a vacation after hospitalization to reduce her stress level
③ Encourage her to think positively and to try and focus on the good things in her life
④ Determine whether she has experienced self-destructive or suicidal thoughts

296. After an uneventful recovery, Ms. Ross is discharged with a referral to the public health nurse. The nurse knows Ms. Ross understands the schedule for self-examination of her remaining breast when she states she will carry out the procedure:
① Several days before an expected menstrual period
② The same date every month, regardless of when menstruation occurs
③ Two to three days after the completion of each menstrual period

④ Halfway between menstrual periods, preferably after taking a shower

Situation: Sean O'Malley goes to his physician because he has abdominal discomfort and a yellow color to his skin.

297. Because of the jaundice, the nurse would expect Mr. O'Malley to also complain of:
① Pruritus
② Bleeding tendencies
③ Diarrhea
④ Blurred vision

298. The physician performs a thorough diagnostic workup, and cancer of the pancreas is confirmed. The physician explains various treatment modalities but strongly suggests surgery. A Whipple procedure is planned. When arranging for his next appointment Mr. O'Malley says to the nurse, "Wouldn't I be better off with one of those other treatments instead of surgery?" The nurse's best response would be:
① "Why don't you explore the other acceptable treatments for your cancer with the doctor?"
② "Surgery is the recommended approach, but why don't you discuss this further with the doctor?"
③ "Maybe you would be more confident with a second opinion. Would you like a referral to another doctor?"
④ "With your disease your prognosis will improve if surgery is the treatment chosen."

299. Based on Mr. O'Malley's diagnosis the nurse understands that his jaundice is caused by:
① Excessive serum bilirubin caused by red cell destruction
② Impaired liver function resulting in incomplete bilirubin metabolism
③ Necrosis of the parenchyma caused by the neoplasm
④ Obstruction of the common bile duct by the pancreatic neoplasm

300. During the first 36 hours after surgery Mr. O'Malley complains of severe pain. He is medicated every 4 hours with meperidine (Demerol) 75 mg IM. Because he rests or sleeps between injections the nurse can conclude that:
① The Demerol can probably be given orally
② Pain management is effective
③ The dosage of the drug is excessive
④ Another narcotic should be substituted

301. Mr. O'Malley is worried about what to expect in the future. In assisting him to plan, it would be most important for the nurse to know:
① The survival rate for individuals with pancreatic cancer
② Any previous exposure to known carcinogens

③ The state and grade of Mr. O'Malley's cancer
④ Any history of alcohol and/or tobacco use

Situation: Wanda Crane, who has a history of Crohn's disease, is admitted to the hospital with chronic bloody diarrhea, weight loss, and signs of general malnutrition.

302. Mrs. Crane has clinical symptoms including edema, anemia, low serum albumin, and negative nitrogen balance. Her health status is related to a major deficiency of:
① Iron
② Potassium
③ Protein
④ Linoleic acid

303. Mrs. Crane is to have an upper gastrointestinal series. The nurse understands that an upper GI series with barium would be contraindicated if the client had:
① Hyperkalemia
② An inflamed colon
③ Hemorrhoids
④ A perforation

304. Mrs. Crane is started on steroid therapy. The nurse knows that the teaching was effective when Mrs. Crane says that when taking her medication she should:
① "Divide the dose into equal parts and take it with each meal."
② "Take the drug in the early morning with food or an antacid."
③ "Take the drug 1 hour before or 2 hours after eating."
④ "Take the medicine at bedtime with a snack."

305. Realizing that hypokalemia is a side effect of steroid therapy, the nurse should also teach Mrs. Crane to monitor for:
① Hyperactive reflexes
② An increased pulse rate
③ Nausea, vomiting, and diarrhea
④ Leg weakness with muscle cramps

306. Mrs. Crane's physician has also ordered the drug cholestyramine, an anion exchange resin used to treat diarrhea. This drug reduces the absorption of fat, which may produce a deficiency of:
① Vitamin B_6
② Vitamin A
③ Thiamin
④ Riboflavin

307. In light of the fact that Mrs. Crane has Crohn's disease, the teaching plan should focus on:
① Anticipating sexual alteration
② Controlling severe constipation
③ Meeting nutritional needs
④ Preventing increased weakness

Situation: Grace Close, a diabetic since childhood, is pregnant for the third time. Her first child is now 4 years old. Her second pregnancy resulted in a stillbirth at 38 weeks. She is being admitted for an oxyto-cin challenge test (OCT) at 33 weeks' gestation.

308. Mrs. Close's history indicates she is a candidate for an OCT primarily because:
① Her diabetes was probably the major causative factor in the previous stillbirth
② OCT is indicated for high-risk clients with possible placental insufficiency
③ OCT measures plasma levels of maternal estriols, which indicate fetal distress
④ She is past the twenty-eighth week of gestation; OCT has no clinical value before this time

309. During the test the nurse should place Mrs. Close in the:
① Semi-Fowler's position to avoid hypotension
② Trendelenberg position to prevent cervical pressure
③ Sims' position to promote examination
④ Lithotomy position to facilitate visualization

310. Mrs. Close's OCT is positive and indicates potential problems. The nurse knows this means the test:
① Indicated the need for cesarean delivery in order to deliver a viable fetus
② Showed repetitive decelerations of the fetal heart rate
③ Showed a consistent fetal heart rate of 120 to 160 beats per minute
④ Indicated the need for induction of labor

Situation:: Susan Daly is 39 weeks pregnant. She has an active episode of genital herpes.

311. A woman with an active herpes infection can transmit the virus to her infant during a vaginal delivery. The nurse understands that the incidence of infection in the infant following a vaginal delivery is:
① 15% to 20%
② 25% to 35%
③ 40% to 60%
④ 75% to 90%

312. Ms. Daly had a cesarean delivery and is now in the recovery room. When providing direct care to Ms. Daly the nurse should:
① Use pHisoHex hand scrubs
② Wear a gown and gloves
③ Wear a gown, gloves, and a mask
④ Use meticulous hand washing

313. Ms. Daly is to be transferred to the postpartal unit. The nurse should plan to institute:
① Contact isolation
② Enteric isolation
③ Protective, or reverse, isolation
④ Strict isolation

314. The nurse teaches Ms. Daly how to limit transmission of the virus to the baby. The nurse would evaluate that Ms. Daly understands the instructions when she says:
① "I must wear gloves when holding my baby."
② "I should avoid kissing my baby on the lips."
③ "I have to wash my clothes and my baby's clothes separately."
④ "I should wash my hands thoroughly with soap and water."

Situation: Michael Shea, 10 months old, is injured in an automobile accident. He is brought to the emergency room with a fractured right femur and a large hematoma on the left temporal area. He is quiet but does not appear lethargic. He is admitted to the hospital.

315. In assessing Michael, the nurse should be particularly alert for signs and symptoms that may indicate neurologic involvement such as:
① A positive Babinski reflex
② A pulse rate of 110
③ The development of a headache
④ Persistent vomiting

316. Severe head injury is ruled out, and Michael is placed in Bryant's traction. While Michael is in traction, the nurse should frequently monitor him to ensure that his buttocks are:
① Flat on the bed
② Slightly elevated
③ Elevated 3 to 4 inches
④ Resting on a small pillow

317. Mr. and Mrs. Shea ask the nurse about the traction. The nurse explains that with Bryant's traction:
① A system of pulleys keeps the affected leg elevated in a sling
② Moleskin and weights are applied to the affected extremity to keep it extended
③ Traction is placed on both legs, even though the left femur is not fractured
④ A Thomas splint, a sling, and pulleys keep the femur aligned

318. Several days after the accident the nurse notes a slight decrease in Michael's hemoglobin and hematocrit. The most appropriate nursing action would be to:
① Provide additional meat for dinner
② Notify the physician immediately
③ Assess his abdomen for internal bleeding
④ Order a blood type and crossmatch

319. In addition to being nonconstipating, the diet for Michael, while he is in traction, should be:
① High in calories and phosphorus
② Low in calories and purine
③ Adequate in calories and high in calcium
④ Moderate in calories and high in protein

Situation: Brad Liest, a 32-year-old client with schizophrenia, paranoid type, is admitted to the psychiatric unit. His thought processes are marked by ideas of reference and persecutory ideation.

320. The staff of the psychiatric unit conducts a biweekly orientation meeting for newly admitted clients. In planning for this meeting the nurse recognizes that the beginning of the meeting should be directed toward defining the:

① Rules for client behavior
② Purpose of the group meeting
③ Client's role and the leader's expectations
④ Development of trust between staff and clients

321. Mr. Liest frequently displays overt sexual behavior toward female clients and nurses. The nurses can best respond to his behavior by:

① Refusing to speak with him until he stops this behavior
② Ignoring this behavior until he is more in control of his responses
③ Matter-of-factly telling him that his behavior is unacceptable
④ Sending him to his room when the behavior is observed

322. One morning Mr. Liest appears very upset. He tells the nurse that the reporter on television told everyone that he is "a queer." The most therapeutic response by the nurse would be:

① "You seem upset by this. Why do you think he said that about you?"
② "It sounds to me like you're having some frightening feelings."
③ "I will call the station and ask why he said that about you."
④ "Sometimes when we are unsure of ourselves we project our feelings on others."

323. The behavior that would indicate to the nurse that Mr. Liest's mental status was improving would be his:

① Ability to function effectively in activities of daily living
② Development of insight into his problem
③ Decreased need to use defense mechanisms
④ Absence of or freedom from anxiety

Situation: Troy Collins, 46 years old, is presently being treated at the outpatient clinic for mood disorder—major depression. His medical regimen over the past 5 years has included the MAO inhibitors, the tricyclic antidepressants, and for the past 1½ years, trifluoperazine (Stelazine).

324. The nurse should be aware that the statement by Mr. Collins that would indicate an irreversible adverse response to long-term therapy with Stelazine would be:

① "I can't seem to sleep at night."
② "My mouth is always dry."
③ "I'm not eating like I should."
④ "My tongue and lips move themselves."

325. Considering his drug regimen, the nurse should encourage Mr. Collins to:

① Eat a high-carbohydrate diet
② Suck on hard candy
③ Restrict fluid intake
④ Avoid aspirin-containing products

326. Mr. Collins' depression deepens. When Mrs. Collins reports that for the past week he has been unresponsive, stares into space, remains curled up in bed and refuses to get up, it is decided that hospitalization is necessary. To foster a therapeutic relationship with Mr. Collins, the nurse must first break through his withdrawal. Initially, this can best be achieved by:

① Gently touching Mr. Collins on the arm when approaching him
② Informing him that he must dress and go to the dayroom
③ Urging his participation in simple games with other clients
④ Sitting quietly next to Mr. Collins for set periods of time each hour

327. Because Mr. Collins' depression has not responded to any of the antidepressant medications, the psychiatrist decides to initiate a series of electroconvulsive therapy (ECT). Before the treatment the nurse should:

① Have Mr. Collins speak with other clients receiving ECT.
② Give Mr. Collins a detailed explanation of the entire procedure
③ Provide a simple explanation of the procedure and continue to reassure Mr. Collins
④ Limit Mr. Collins' intake to a light breakfast on the days of the treatment

328. The nurse should be aware that the most therapeutic activity for a depressed client such as Mr. Collins would be:

① Putting together a jig-saw puzzle
② Stuffing envelopes for a local charity
③ Participating in an aerobic exercise group
④ Assembling and whip-stitching a wallet

329. Mr. Collins responds to therapy, and with the help of the staff begins to set some immediate goals for himself. The goal that would most indicate his improvement would be his plan to:

① Show the staff that he can do what they want him to do
② Talk with at least one person on the unit daily
③ Stay clear of people who seem to make him anxious
④ Take at least 3 to 4 hours daily to sit alone and think about things

Situation: Brent Meyer, 50 years old, has advanced cancer of the bladder. He is admitted to the hospital for a cystectomy and urinary diversion.

330. A cystectomy and ileal conduit are scheduled. Physical preparation for the surgery should include:

① Administration of neomycin sulfate
② Insertion of a Foley catheter
③ A well-balanced diet with vitamins
④ Administration of urinary antiseptics

331. During the administration of the preopera-

tive enema, Mr. Meyer complains of cramps. The nursing action indicated at this point is to:

① Administer the enema rapidly to permit quicker evacuation

② Discontinue the enema and try at a later time

③ Lower the container to the floor to decrease pressure

④ Narrow the lumen of the tubing until cramps subside

332. After the surgery, Mr. Meyer is admitted to the recovery room. During the first hour of the postoperative period, the nurse should notify the physician if:

① The stoma is swollen

② No urine output is noted

③ Bowel sounds are diminished

④ Vomiting occurs

333. When Mr. Meyer awakes in the recovery room, he asks for a sip of water. The nurse informs him that he cannot have any water by mouth until:

① He returns to his room in a few hours

② The ileal loop begins to drain in 6 hours

③ The nasogastric suction is discontinued in 3 days

④ The intestinal anastamosis heals in 10 days

334. Mr. Meyer complains of postoperative pain. Initially the nurse should:

① Tell Mr. Meyer to take deep breaths

② Measure his current vital signs

③ Administer the prescribed analgesic

④ Interview Mr. Meyer for more data

335. The nurse plans early postoperative ambulation for Mr. Meyer to prevent:

① Wound infection

② Abdominal distension

③ Incisional evisceration

④ Urinary retention

Situation: Elvira King, a primipara in active labor for the past 6 hours, is not making progress. X-ray films are ordered, and a diagnosis of cephalopelvic disproportion is made. An immediate cesarean delivery is scheduled. A spinal anesthetic is administered by the anesthetist.

336. A common adaptation that Mrs. King should be monitored for after receiving the anesthesia is:

① Light-headedness

② Elevated temperature

③ Sensation of chilliness

④ Urticaria

337. A cesarean delivery is performed, and a healthy baby boy is born to Mrs. King. After the surgery Mrs. King is transferred to the recovery room with a Foley catheter in place. Mrs. King's fluid intake should be increased when the nurse notes:

① A blood pressure of 100/60

② A urine specific gravity of 1.030

③ Tinges of blood in the urine

④ Urinary suppression

338. On the day after delivery the nurse ambulates Mrs. King down the hall. Mrs. King asks the nurse, "Why am I being made to walk so soon after surgery?" The nurse's best reply would be:

① "You can get to hold your baby more quickly if you walk around."

② "Walking keeps the blood from pooling in your legs and prevents clots."

③ "Walking about early will prevent your wound from opening."

④ "Early walking lowers the incidence of urinary infection."

339. When doing coughing and deep-breathing exercises, Mrs. King complains of a severe, sharp, localized pain at the site of the wound. The nurse should:

① Tell Mrs. King to splint the wound when she coughs and deep breathes

② Call the physician to secure an order for an abdominal binder

③ Place Mrs. King in a supine position and inspect the incisional site

④ Assess the duration and intensity of pain and give analgesics as ordered

340. The physician's orders for Mrs. King include removal of her Foley catheter and initiation of a regular diet. After the catheter is removed, the nurse can evaluate that Mrs. King's urinary function has returned to normal when:

① A residual urine of 90 ml is obtained after the client voids

② The urinalysis indicates no bacteria present

③ Mrs. King voids at least 300 ml 4 hours after catheter removal

④ Mrs. King's daily urinary output is at least 1500 ml

341. Mrs. King complains of abdominal pain, and her abdomen is distended. The physician orders a Harris drip. The nurse can evaluate the effectiveness of the Harris drip when:

① Mrs. King has a bowel movement

② Mrs. King's returns are finally clear

③ Mrs. King is able to retain 500 ml of fluid

④ Mrs. King's abdomen is less distended

Situation: Jim Laur, 3 months old, is admitted to the unit in severe dyspnea. His temperature is 104° F. A diagnosis of laryngotracheobronchitis (croup) is made. He is placed in a high-humidity tent with cold mist.

342. The main reason cold humidity is preferred to steam is that:

① Cold mist produces a more comfortable environment

② Cold humidity aids in reducing mucosal edema

③ Cold humidity dries up the mucosal secretions
④ Cold water vapor is more readily absorbed by the mucosa

343. Jim is taken out of the high-humidity tent for morning care. During the bath the nurse observes he has increased respiratory distress. The nurse should:
① Suction his nasal passages to clear the airway
② Discontinue the bath and place him in the croupette
③ Do chest clapping and postural drainage
④ Put him in the orthopneic position and call the physician

344. Jim is taken off oral feedings, and intravenous feedings are ordered to:
① Meet his caloric needs
② Decrease vagal stimulation
③ Lessen physical exertion
④ Relieve laryngospasm

345. The nurse notes some erythema at the infusion site. On palpation Jim cries and draws away. There is a blood return in the tubing when the solution container is held briefly below the insertion site. The nurse should:
① Maintain the IV but continue to observe the insertion site
② Decrease the flow rate of the IV solution
③ Realize that additives may have this effect
④ Have the venipuncture site changed to a new area

346. Mr. and Mrs. Laur ask the nurse about caring for Jim at home. The best response by the nurse would be:
① "No specific restrictions are necessary after Jim goes home."
② "No one should be allowed to visit the baby for a while."
③ "Give 2 ounces of water after the feeding of formula."
④ "All allergen producers such as animals should be avoided."

347. Mr. and Mrs. Laur express concern that Jim still has a "soft spot" on the top of his head. The nurse explains that the normal closure time for the anterior fontanel is between the ages of:
① 6 and 8 months
② 9 and 12 months
③ 13 and 18 months
④ 19 and 24 months

Situation: Dan Barton, 47 years old, has aortic stenosis. He is scheduled for a valve replacement in 2 days. He tells the nurse, "I told my wife all she needs to know if I don't make it."

348. The response by the nurse that would be the most therapeutic would be:
① "Men your age do very well."
② "I'll get you a sleeping pill tonight, I know you will need it."

③ "I know you are concerned, but your physician is excellent."
④ "You are worried about dying."

349. During the early postoperative period after open heart surgery, adequate oxygenation is essential because:
① An increased respiratory rate adds to postoperative pain
② Hypoxia can precipitate respiratory alkalosis
③ All clients have a chest tube in place
④ Hypoxia can stimulate dangerous arrhythmias

350. A slow pulse rate during the early postoperative period after open heart surgery can be indicative of:
① Hypoxia
② Heart block
③ Shock
④ Congestive heart failure

351. To decrease or control the sensory and cognitive disturbances that can occur after Mr. Barton's open heart surgery, the nurse should:
① Keep the room light on most of the time
② Withhold analgesic medications
③ Plan for maximal periods of rest
④ Restrict all visitors

Situation: Malcom McMillan, age 58, is admitted to the hospital for a diagnostic workup for possible intestinal carcinoma. He complains of malaise, constipation, and stomach rumbling.

352. When obtaining the health history the nurse should expect Mr. McMillan to report changes in:
① The shape of his stools
② His daily fluid intake
③ His daily intake of fats
④ The use of spices in his diet

353. The nurse should plan to observe Mr. McMillan for signs of:
① Diarrhea
② Abdominal peritonitis
③ Dehydration
④ Intestinal obstruction

354. Mr. McMillan is diagnosed as having cancer of the sigmoid colon. An abdominoperineal resection with a permanent colostomy is planned. In preparation for surgery Mr. McMillan is placed on a low-residue diet to:
① Lower the bacteria in the intestine
② Limit the amount of flatus produced
③ Prevent irritation of the intestinal mucosa
④ Reduce the amount of stool in the bowel

355. Mr. McMillan's surgery results in a permanent colostomy. During the first 24 hours there is no drainage from the colostomy. The nurse should realize that this is a result of the:
① Absence of intestinal peristalsis

② Decrease in fluid intake before surgery
③ Proper functioning of his nasogastric tube
④ Edema following the surgery

356. Mr. McMillan is to be discharged in several days. A primary nursing goal should be to:
① Teach Mr. McMillan about the special precautions concerning his diet
② Demonstrate how to change the dry sterile dressing on his incision
③ Determine Mr. McMillan's ability to care for his colostomy
④ Cajole Mr. McMillan into caring for his colostomy by himself

Situation: Breda Carty, age 5, is admitted to the hospital for a tonsillectomy and adenoidectomy.

357. The nurse can best determine why Breda thinks she is coming to the hospital by asking:
① "You do know why you are in the hospital, don't you?"
② "Why did you come to the hospital?"
③ "Do you know what's going to happen to you?"
④ "Do you know what place this is?"

358. After the operation the nurse observes that Breda is swallowing frequently. The nurse suspects that she is:
① Experiencing pain in the throat
② Reacting from general anesthesia
③ Hemorrhaging from the operative site
④ In need of suctioning to keep the airway patent

359. The nurse, in preparing for Breda's discharge, tells Mr. and Mrs. Carty that Breda may have an objectionable mouth odor, slight ear pain, and a low-grade fever for a few days. The nurse recommends that the parents:
① Let her gargle with warm saline solution
② Give aspirin for pain as necessary
③ Let the child suck on peppermint candies
④ Apply an ice collar for the pain

360. When Breda returns after 6 weeks for a follow-up visit, in addition to assessing Breda's hearing the nurse should include an assessment of her:
① Speech and taste
② Smell and taste
③ Swallowing and speech
④ Swallowing and smell

Situation: Jack Lee, 35 years old and unemployed, is arrested for shoplifting and possession of marijuana and is brought to the psychiatric unit for evaluation. His mother describes her son as intelligent, witty, entertaining, and friendly. She is aware, however, that since childhood he has been unreliable, untruthful, and insincere. Mr. Lee is diagnosed as having a personality disorder.

361. The most accurate nursing diagnosis for Mr. Lee would be:
① Impairment of common sense, feelings of guilt and remorse
② Potential for introverted and mature behavior
③ Antisocial personality disorder
④ Ineffective individual coping

362. In caring for Mr. Lee, the staff should use a consistent approach that is:
① Indifferent and detached but nonjudgmental
② Conditionally acquiescent to his demands
③ Warm and firm without being punitive
④ Clearly communicative of personal resentment

363. During a group therapy session, one of the clients asks Mr. Lee why he is in the hospital. Considering his personality disorder, the nurse might expect him to respond:
① "My life needs straightening out and this might help."
② "I need a lot of help with my troubles."
③ "I decided that it's time I own up to my problems."
④ "Society makes people react in odd ways."

Situation: Inga Gosney, 30 years old, has a 35-day menstrual cycle and is attempting to become pregnant. She and her husband are counseled by the nurse about the optimal timing of intercourse during the cycle.

364. The nurse would know the counseling was effective when Mr. and Mrs. Gosney state they should have intercourse on the:
① Twelfth day of the cycle
② Fourteenth day of the cycle
③ Twenty-first day of the cycle
④ Twenty-fifth day of the cycle

365. Mrs. Gosney becomes pregnant. Later in her pregnancy Mrs. Gosney experiences low back pain and asks the nurse which exercises will provide some relief. The nurse can consider the teaching to have been effective if Mrs. Gosney performs:
① Leg lifts
② Pelvic rocking
③ Kegel exercises
④ Tailor sitting

366. In her eighth month of pregnancy Mrs. Gosney tells the nurse that she is experiencing dyspareunia. The nurse should plan to teach the Gosneys to:
① Avoid intercourse
② Try alternative positions
③ Consult a therapist for sexual counseling
④ Have Mrs. Gosney douche to lubricate the vaginal mucosa

367. The Gosneys attend Lamaze preparation for childbirth classes. The exercise that the

nurse teaches for toning the pelvic floor muscles is:
① Pelvic rocking
② Half sit-ups
③ Pelvic tilt
④ Kegel exercises

368. Mrs. Gosney attends a parent education class in which warning signs that should be reported to the obstetric care practitioner are discussed. Afterward Mrs. Gosney indicates that she understands the information presented by stating that the sign she would report is:
① Low back pain
② White vaginal discharge
③ Braxton-Hicks contractions
④ Leakage of fluid from the vagina

369. In the classes, Mrs. Gosney is taught to control an urge to push until her cervix is fully dilated by:
① Hyperventilating
② Pelvic rocking exercises
③ Panting or blowing breathing patterns
④ Deep breathing between contractions

Situation: Nancy Jones, 36 years old, has a history of rheumatic fever and a heart murmur. In the last few months she has gained weight even though she has nausea and a loss of appetite. Her clothes are tight at the waist, and her shoes feel snug. She wakes up short of breath several times nightly and notices that she gets tired and has trouble breathing while doing normal daily tasks.

370. Mrs. Jones calls to make an appointment with her physician. When hearing Mrs. Jones' symptoms the nurse should immediately seek additional critical data such as:
① Her elimination pattern over the last month
② A retrospective 24-hour calorie count
③ The presence of a recent cough and pulmonary secretions
④ A complete gynecologic and sexual history

371. Mrs. Jones is admitted to the hospital with a diagnosis of congestive heart failure secondary to rheumatic heart disease. The nurse should be aware that the symptoms of heart failure occur because the:
① Heart can no longer pump blood adequately in relation to venous return
② Excessive blood volume increases the workload of the heart muscles

③ Arterial system is less flexible because of hypertension or arteriosclerosis
④ Heart valves have become stenotic or regurgitant and impede blood blow

372. Mrs. Jones is digitalized and placed on a maintenance dose of digoxin 0.25 mg daily. If a therapeutic effect is achieved the nurse would expect to observe:
① Decreased pulse rate, diuresis, decreased edema
② Decreased pulse pressure, increased blood pressure, weight loss
③ Increased pulse rate, stable fluid balance, decreased blood pressure
④ Decreased pulse rate, reduced heart murmur, increased blood pressure

Situation: Patrick Miles, a 56-year-old blond-haired, blue-eyed farmer, goes to the physician because he has a large, crusty patch of skin on his cheek. He states that it bleeds easily and has not gotten better in the last 3 months even after he has used different kinds of lotions.

373. From the history, the office nurse suspects skin cancer, because the major precipitating factor associated with skin cancer is:
① Contact with soil contaminants
② Position of the lesion
③ Self-treatment of lesions
④ Exposure to radiation

374. Mr. Miles' lesion is diagnosed as a basal cell epithelioma, and it is to be removed. He tells the nurse that he is concerned that the cancer has spread. To best reduce his anxiety the nurse should respond:
① "I can understand how you must feel."
② "You are a good surgical risk."
③ "Basal cell tumors usually do not spread."
④ "The physician probably caught it just in time."

375. The cancerous lesion is removed by fulguration. Mr. Miles is given a topical steroid to apply to the surgical site. The nurse would recognize that the teaching regarding steroids and skin lesions was effective when Mr. Miles tells his wife that the purpose of the medication is to:
① Decrease fluid loss from the skin
② Reduce inflammation at the surgical site
③ Prevent infection of the wound
④ Limit itching around the area of the lesion

Answers and Rationales for Review Questions

Medical–Surgical Nursing

1. **1** This is the correct flow rate; multiply the amount to be infused (50 ml) by the drop factor (10) and divide the result by the amount of time in minutes (20). (b) (SU; AN; TC; FE)
   2 This is an inaccurate calculation; this would deliver the solution too rapidly and would irritate the vein.
   3 Same as # 2.
   4 Same as # 2.

2. **2** A new dietary regimen, with a balance of foods from the basic four food groups, must be established and continued for weight reduction to occur and be maintained. (c) (ME; AN; PA; GI)
   1 Although this would be true in a weight reduction diet, this response does not address its relationship to the other three food groups.
   3 Same as # 1.
   4 This is only one part of a weight reduction regimen; usually in obese individuals caloric intake exceeds energy expenditure.

3. **1** Increased exercise builds skeletal muscle mass and reduces excess fatty tissue. (c) (ME; EV; PA; GI)
   2 The metabolic rate will increase.
   3 Appetite is usually increased.
   4 This is unrelated to weight loss; during the aerobic exercise the heart rate will increase, but between periods of exercise the heart rate will decrease because of the development of collateral circulation.

4. **1** These sets of muscles will be used in walking with crutches and therefore need strengthening. (b) (SU; AN; TC; SK)
   2. Although these muscles keep the person erect, the most important muscles for walking with crutches are the triceps, elbow extensors, and finger flexors of the arms, and the muscles in the unaffected leg.
   3 This will do nothing to strengthen the weight-bearing leg.
   4 A pushing motion, not a pulling motion, is used with crutches; the triceps, not the biceps, are used.

5. **3** The palms should bear the client's weight to avoid damage to the nerves in the axilla (brachial plexus). (a) (SU; EV; ED; SK)
   1 This would be unsafe; pressure on the axillary region could injure the nerves in the brachial plexus.
   2 The physician ordered non-weight bearing on the affected leg.
   4 Same as # 1.

6. **3** Using ratio and proportion
   8 mg/10 mg = X minims/15 minims
   $$10\,X = 120$$
   $$X = 12 \text{ minims. (b) (ME; IM; TC; DR)}$$
   1 This is an inaccurate calculation; this is less than the desired dose.

   2 Same as # 1.
   4 This is an inaccurate calculation; this is more than the desired dose.

7. **2** Morphine is a specific central nervous system depressant used to relieve the pain associated with myocardial infarction; it also decreases apprehension and prevents cardiogenic shock. (b) (ME; IM; PA; CV)
   1 The lidocaine given intravenously will accomplish this.
   3 This is not the primary reason for the use of morphine; the Valium prescribed will be used for this purpose as necessary.
   4 This is not the reason for the use of morphine.

8. **3** Oxygen is necessary for the production of fire. (a) (ME; PL; TC; CV)
   1 This is irrelevant to the need for safety precautions.
   2 Same as # 1.
   4 Oxygen does not burn itself; it supports combustion.

9. **3** Creatine phosphokinase (CPK) isoenzyme levels, especially the MB subunit, begin to rise in 3 to 6 hours, peak in 12 to 18 hours, and are elevated for 48 hours after the occurrence of the infarct; they are therefore most reliable in assisting with early diagnosis. (b) (ME; AS; PA; CV)
   1 Serum glutamic oxaloacetic transaminase (SGOT) isoenzyme levels begin to rise later and do not peak until 24 to 36 hours, so they are not as early an indicator.
   2 Lactic dehyrogenase (LDH) isoenzyme levels, especially LDH_1 do not begin to rise until 12 hours after the infarct and peak in 48 hours, so they are a much later indicator.
   4 Serum aspartate amino-transferase (AST) is another name for SGOT.

10. **2** This is a typical early finding after a myocardial infarct because of the altered contractility of the heart. (c) (ME; AS; PA; CV)
    1 Q waves may become distorted with conduction or rhythm problems, but they do not disappear unless there is cardiac standstill.
    3 This occurs in atrial and ventricular fibrillation.
    4 Flattened or depressed T waves indicate hypokalemia.

11. **2** This provides the opportunity for the client to verbalize the feelings underlying behavior. (b) (ME; IM; PE; EC)
    1 Although allowing the client to release feelings is therapeutic, leaving immediately denies the client the opportunity for exploration and discussion.
    3 Explanation will not decrease anxiety so that the client can rest.
    4 This has no effect on decreasing the client's anxiety or allowing ventilation.

12. **4** Fever causes an increase in the body's metabolism, which results in an increase in oxygen consumption; this need for oxygen is met by in-

creasing the heart rate, which is reflected in the increased pulse rate. (a) (ME; AS; PA; CV)

1 Although the respiratory rate may increase slightly, fever will not cause dyspnea.

2 Chest pain is not related to the fever unless its cause is respiratory in nature.

3 Blood pressure elevation will not accompany a fever.

13. **3** The nurse must analyze the feelings that are implied in the client's question and reflect these to help the client verbalize and explore them; the focus is on collecting more data. (a) (ME; IM; PE; EC)

1 This is avoiding the responsibility of helping the client explore feelings; it cuts off communication.

2 Although this may be true, it does not respond to the feelings implicit in the client's comment.

4 No data presented at this time suggests that such a referral is warranted; this also cuts off communication when the client has expressed a need; the nurse is avoiding responsibility to assist the client.

14. **3** Pernicious anemia is caused by the inability to absorb vitamin B_{12} due to a lack of intrinsic factor in gastric juices; for the Schilling test, radioactive vitamin B_{12} is administered and its absorption and excretion can be ascertained. (c) (ME; AS; PA; BI)

1 This is not measured by this test.

2 Same as # 1.

4 Vitamin B_{12} is not produced in the body.

15. **4** First convert milligrams to micrograms and then use ratio and proportion:
$$(0.2 \text{ mg} = 200 \text{ mcg})$$
$$200 \text{ mcg}/100 \text{ mcg} = X \text{ ml}/1\text{ml}$$
$$100 X = 200$$
$$X = 2 \text{ ml. (b) (ME; IM; TC; DR)}$$

1 This is an inaccurate calculation; this is less than the desired dose.

2 Same as # 1.

3 Same as # 1.

16. **3** IM injections bypass B_{12} absorption defect (lack of intrinsic factor, the transport carrier component of gastric juices); a monthly dose is usually sufficient since it is stored in active body tissues such as the liver, kidney, heart, muscles, blood, and bone marrow. (c) (ME; IM; PA; BI)

1 It cannot be taken by mouth because of the lack of intrinsic factor.

2 Since it is stored and only slowly depleted, it is not necessary to give injections this frequently.

4 The Z-track method need not be used as for iron dextran injections; injections once a month are usually sufficient.

17. **4** Since the intrinsic factor does not return to gastric secretions even with therapy, B_{12} injections will be required for the remainder of the client's life. (b) (ME; EV; ED; BI)

1 It must be taken on a regular basis for the rest of the client's life.

2 Same as # 1.

3 Same as # 1.

18. **4** Projection is the attribution of unacceptable feelings and emotions to others. (b) (SU; AN; PE; EC)

1 A reaction formation is the unconscious reversal of feelings or behavior unacceptable to the self-image, and the assumption of opposite feelings or behavior.

2 Sublimation is the substitution of socially acceptable feelings for instincts that, if expressed, would be threatening to the ego.

3 Intellectualization is the use of mental reasoning processes to deny facing emotions and feelings involved in a situation.

19. **1** Irrigation should be performed at the time the client normally defecated before the colostomy to maintain continuity in life-style. (b) (SU; PL; ED; GI)

2 An irrigation cannot be postponed until the client accepts the altered body image because this may take weeks or months.

3 Most people defecate after breakfast because the ingestion of food on an empty stomach initiates the gastrocolic reflex.

4 This may be true for some people; however, irrigations usually can be completed in 1 hour.

20. **3** The irrigation bag should be hung 12 to 18 inches above the level of the stoma; a clothes hook is too high. (a) (SU; EV; ED; GI)

1 Fluid flowing into the intestines can cause distention and discomfort; clamping the tubing is an appropriate intervention.

2 The tip of the catheter should be lubricated to prevent trauma to mucosal tissue and to facilitate insertion.

4 There is not enough information given to choose this response; the amount of fluid ordered is not included.

21. **2** This would indicate stenosis of the stoma and should be reported to the physician. (b) (SU; IM; ED; GI)

1 This is a common response that can be remedied by clamping the tubing until the discomfort subsides.

3 Flatus is always present in the bowel to some degree, and a colostomy irrigation will facilitate its expulsion.

4 This is not indicative of a medical problem; a colostomy irrigation usually can be completed in 1 hour, but some individuals may need a little more time.

22. **2** As long as no one else confirms the presence of the stoma and the client does not need to adhere to a prescribed regimen, the client's denial is supported. (b) (SU; AS; PE; EC)

1 There is no evidence to document that reaction formation is being used.

3 There is no data to support this conclusion; the client should be able to function sexually as before.

4 There is no evidence presented that suicidal thoughts are present or will be acted out.

23. **2** These clients can eat a regular diet; only gas-forming foods that cause distention and discomfort should be avoided. (a) (SU; EV; ED; GI)

1 The amount of stool does not have to be limited; therefore a low-residue diet is not necessary.

3 The affected tissue has been removed, and normal mucosal tissue lines the intestine and forms the stoma; therefore bland foods are not necessary.

4 Nutrients are absorbed by the small, not the large, intestine; a regular diet is usually easily digested and absorbed.

24. **4** These are top priorities in trauma management; basic life functions must be maintained or reestablished. (b) (SU; AS; TC; RE)
    1 This is an assessment for head injury that follows determination of respiratory and circulatory status.
    2 This is an assessment for abdominal injury that follows determination of respiratory and circulatory status.
    3 Pain assessment would follow the appraisal of airway, breathing, and circulation.
25. **3** Nothing is achieved if the equipment is working and the client is not responding. (c) (SU; AS; TC; RE)
    1 Endotracheal intubation does not permit verbal communication.
    2 This is important but not the priority.
    4 This is presumptive; the data base is incomplete for the assessment that surgery is immediate.
26. **2** This assists in moving blood, fluid, or air, which may be obstructing drainage, toward the collection chamber. (b) (SU; IM; TC; RE)
    1 This is a medical decision and would not be done unless the tube could not be made patent.
    3 This is not indicated unless other symptoms, such as dyspnea, are present.
    4 This is contraindicated unless there is a break in the system.
27. **1** The chest tube normalizes intrathoracic pressure, drains fluid and air from the pleural space, and improves pulmonary function. (b) (SU; EV; PA; RE)
    2 This indicates a probable leak in the drainage system.
    3 This indicates that air has entered the subcutaneous tissue (subcutaneous emphysema).
    4 This may be a sign of pain, respiratory obstruction, or bleeding.
28. **1** A rate of 30 ml/hr is considered adequate for perfusion of kidney, heart, and brain. (a) (SU; EV; PA; FE)
    2 A central venous pressure reading of 2 cm H_2O indicates hypovolemia.
    3 This indicates improvement but not necessarily adequate tissue perfusion.
    4 Same as # 3.
29. **4** Drains are usually inserted into the splenic bed to facilitate removal of fluid that could lead to abscess formation. (b) (SU; IM; ED; GI)
    1 Splenectomy has a low mortality (5%) except when multiple injuries are present (15% to 40%).
    2 Bleeding occurs more frequently with splenic repair than with removal.
    3 There is no need to frighten the client unnecessarily, but the operative risk increases with multiple injuries.
30. **2** This prevents atelectasis and collection of secretions and promotes respiratory exchange. (b) (SU; IM; PA; RE)
    1 Activity should be promoted within limits of physical ability.
    3 This is important but not as conducive to improving respiratory status as are coughing and deep breathing.
    4 Observing for dyspnea remains important, but crepitus is unlikely to occur with stabilization of respiratory status.
31. **4** The withdrawal provides time for the client to assimilate what has occurred and integrate the change in the body image. (b) (SU; IM; PE; EC)
    1 The client is not ready to hear these explanations until assimilation of the accident and surgery has occurred.
    2 This does not acknowledge that the client must grieve; it also does not allow the client to express any feelings that may be present that life will never be normal again.
    3 The client would feel that the nurse had no comprehension of the situation or understanding of his feelings.
32. **4** It is not reality, but the client's feeling about the change, that is the most important determinant of the ability to cope. (c) (SU; AN; PE; EC)
    1 The extent of change is not relevant; it is whether the client perceives the change as enormous or minuscule.
    2 This is not relevant to the client's ability to deal with a change in body image.
    3 Same as # 2.
33. **3** Intellectualization is the use of reasoning and thought processes to avoid the emotional aspects of a situation; this is a defense against anxiety. (a) (ME; AN; PE; EC)
    1 Reaction formation is behavior exactly opposite to what the person is feeling.
    2 Sublimation is a defense wherein the person redirects the energy of unacceptable impulses into socially acceptable behaviors or activities.
    4 Projection is denying unacceptable traits and regarding them as belonging to another person.
34. **4** Suppression of red bone marrow increases bleeding susceptibility associated with decreased platelets. (a) (ME; IM; TC; BI)
    1 With bone marrow depression there would be a decrease in red blood cells; rest should be encouraged.
    2 With bone marrow suppression the red blood cells are decreased in number and there is a decreased O_2 carrying capacity of the blood; this position will not increase the number of red blood cells.
    3 This will not affect the bone marrow; citrus juices should be avoided by the client receiving chemotherapy because of the side effects of stomatitis.
35. **3** This results from a recipient's antibodies that are incompatible with transfused red blood cells; also called a type II hypersensitivity; these signs result from RBC hemolysis, agglutination, and capillary plugging. (c) (ME; AS; PA; BI)
    1 There is no transfusion reaction called by this name, although anaphylaxis occurs with an allergic transfusion reaction.
    2 This results from an immune sensitivity to foreign serum protein; also called a type I hypersensitivity; signs include urticaria, wheezing, dyspnea, and shock.
    4 Bacterial pyrogens are present in contaminated blood and can cause a febrile transfusion reaction; signs include fever and chills.
36. **4** This nonjudgmentally points out the client's behavior. (b) (ME; IM; PE; EC)
    1 This is too confrontational and an assumption by the nurse.
    2 This is too judgmental, an assumption, and a stereotypical response.

3 This response is too confrontational; the client may not be able to answer the question.

37. **3** This does not take away the client's only way of coping, and it permits future movement through the grieving process when the client is ready. (b) (ME; PL; PE; EC)
   1 The client's denial should be neither supported nor taken away; encouraging denial is a form of false reassurance.
   2 This is false reassurance.
   4 The client must not be abandoned; the nurse's presence is a form of emotional support.

38. **3** The client's intake was 360 ml (6 oz × 30 ml), and loss was 125 ml of fluid; loss is subtracted from intake. (a) (ME; AN; TC; FE)
   1 This is an inaccurate calculation; the client has a more positive fluid balance.
   2 Same as # 1.
   4 This is an inaccurate calculation; this answer added the output to the intake.

39. **2** Pulmonary congestion and edema occur because of fluid extravasation from the pulmonary capillary bed, resulting in difficult breathing. (a) (ME; AS; PA; CV)
   1 This is a hallmark of a client with myocardial infarction; it is caused by inadequate oxygen supply to the myocardium.
   3 This is a sign of right-sided, not left-sided, heart failure; a weakened right ventricle causes venous congestion in the systemic circulation.
   4 This results from increased pressure in the right atria associated with right-sided heart failure.

40. **4** This is the site of action of Lasix. (c) (ME; AN; PA; DR)
   1 Thiazides act here.
   2 Potassium-sparing diuretics act here.
   3 Plasma expanders and xanthines act here.

41. **3** One liter of fluid weighs approximately 2.2 pounds; therefore, a 4.5 pound weight loss equals approximately 2 liters. (b) (ME; AN; PA; FE)
   1 This is approximately a 1 pound weight loss.
   2 This is approximately a 2.2 pound weight loss.
   4 This is approximately a 7.5 pound weight loss.

42. **4** A cardiac glycoside such as digitalis decreases the conduction speed within the myocardium and slows the heart rate. (b) (ME; EV; PA; DR)
   1 The primary effect is on the kidneys, not the heart.
   2 This could cause tachycardia, not bradycardia, which is an adverse effect.
   3 This does not drastically reduce heart rate.

43. **2** There are 9 calories in each gram of fat and 4 calories in each gram of carbohydrate and protein; this diet contains 1970 calories. (c) (ME; AN; TC; GI)
   1 This is too high for the diet prescribed.
   3 This is too low for the diet prescribed.
   4 Same as # 3.

44. **2** Restriction of sodium reduces the amount of water retention, thus reducing cardiac workload. (a) (ME; PL; TC; CV)
   1 Magnesium is not restricted.
   3 Potassium would not be restricted, especially if a diuretic and cardiac glycoside are ordered.
   4 This is not true for a client with CHF; calcium is restricted for individuals who develop renal calculi with a calcium phosphate base and are placed on an acid-ash diet.

45. **1** Some medications, such as aspirin and prednisone, irritate the stomach lining and may cause bleeding with prolonged use. (b) (ME; AS; PA; GI)
   2 This may be related to intestinal irritation causing diarrhea and intestinal bleeding, not gastric bleeding.
   3 This is not the cause of gastric bleeding; it is important to ascertain dietary habits when teaching about dietary therapy.
   4 Although stress may play a part, the use of some medications has a more direct relationship.

46. **2** The stomach is located within the sternal angle; thus the area is known as the epigastric area. (a) (ME; AS; PA; GI)
   1 This is in the area of iliac bones.
   3 This is the lowest middle abdominal area.
   4 This is the area above the sternum.

47. **2** Presence of food in the stomach at regular intervals interacts with HCl, limiting acid mucosal irritation. (a) (ME; PL; TC; GI)
   1 Small frequent meals or meals with planned snacks would be most appropriate; limiting intake to three large meals would leave the stomach empty for long periods of time.
   3 Food will relieve the pain.
   4 The plan should be specific to try to keep food in the stomach at close intervals to limit mucosal irritation.

48. **2** Antacids may interfere with complete absorption of Tagamet; therefore they should be administered at least 1 hour apart. (b) (ME; PL; TC; DR)
   1 This would interfere with absorption of Tagamet.
   3 Same as #1.
   4 This would interfere with absorption of Tagamet, and orange juice may be irritating and slow the client's recovery; milk may be used because it may enhance the effectiveness of the medication.

49. **2** Hyperventilation results in the increased elimination of carbon dioxide from the blood. (b) (SU; AN; PA; FE)
   1 The carbonic acid will be decreased.
   3 The pH will be increased.
   4 The PO_2 would not be affected.

50. **2** Carbohydrates provide 4 kcal per gram; therefore 3 L × 50 g/L × 4 kcal/g = 600 kcal; only about a third of the basal energy need. (a) (SU; AN; TC; GI)
   1 This is less than the calories provided by the ordered IV fluid.
   3 This is more than the calories provided by the ordered IV fluid.
   4 Same as # 3.

51. **4** Inactivity causes venous stasis, hypercoagulability, and external pressure against the veins, all of which lead to thrombus formation; early ambulation or exercise of the lower extremities reduces the occurrence of this phenomenon. (a) (SU; IM; TC; CV)
   1 Although this may help, the primary intervention is to provide exercise of the extremities until ambulation is permitted.
   2 This will be helpful, but it is not an independent activity; elastic stockings require a physician's order.
   3 Massaging would be contraindicated because any developing clot could be dislodged.

52. **3** Bleeding from the ears occurs only with basal skull fractures. (b) (ME; AS; TC; NM)
    1 This would be a positive response; pupils should react to light.
    2 This would occur only in an infant if there is dehydration present.
    4 This occurs with increased intracranial pressure and pressure on the brain stem; it would be an expected response but not an immediate one; bleeding from the ears is an assessment that assists in diagnosing the location of the injury.

53. **3** Promoting hydration maintains urine production at a higher rate, which flushes the bladder and prevents urinary stasis and possible infection. (b) (ME; PL; TC; RG)
    1 The drainage bag is emptied once every shift unless it fills before then; changing the bag periodically, not emptying it, would help prevent infection.
    2 Although this could help identify a urinary tract infection, it would not prevent it.
    4 Same as # 2.

54. **4** These movements include all possible range of motion for the ankle joint. (a) (ME; IM; PA; SK)
    1 Although the ankle can be moved in a circular motion, flexion and extension are more specifically called dorsiflexion and plantar flexion in relation to the ankle; also, eversion and inversion should be used when manipulating the ankle.
    2 Flexion and extension are more specifically called dorsiflexion and plantar flexion in relation to the ankle; the ankle cannot be abducted or adducted; the ankle can be inverted and everted.
    3 These motions refer to the upper extremity.

55. **1** Shearing force occurs when two surfaces move against each other; when the bed is at an angle greater than 30 degrees, the torso tends to slide and cause this phenomenon. (a) (ME; PL; TC; IT)
    2 This would raise the head of the bed too high to prevent the client from sliding in bed.
    3 Same as # 2.
    4 Same as # 2.

56. **2** An indwelling urethral catheter is used, because surgical trauma can cause urinary retention, leading to further complications such as bleeding. (b) (SU; IM; ED; RG)
    1 Urinary control is not lost in most cases; loss of control is temporary if it does occur.
    3 A cystotomy tube is not used if the client has a transurethral resection; however, it is used if a suprapubic resection is done.
    4 This is usually not affected; sexual ability is maintained if the client was able to perform before the surgery.

57. **3** Patency promotes bladder decompression, which prevents distention and bleeding; continuous flow of fluid through the bladder limits clot formation and promotes hemostasis. (b) (SU; PL; TC; RG)
    1 There is no abdominal dressing with a TURP; surgery is performed via the urethra.
    2 There is no cystotomy tube; a cystotomy tube is used when a suprapubic resection is performed.
    4 There is no wound because there is no abdominal incision.

58. **2** After transurethral surgery, hemorrhage is common because of venous oozing and bleeding from many small arteries in the area. (a) (SU; EV; TC; RG)
    1 Sepsis is unusual and occurs later in the postoperative course.
    3 Leaking around the catheter is not a major complication.
    4 Urinary retention is highly unlikely with an indwelling catheter in place.

59. **2** The pressure of the balloon against the small blood vessels of the prostate causes them to constrict, thereby preventing bleeding. (b) (SU; AN; TC; RG)
    1 It may actually cause discomfort or spasms but is necessary to limit bleeding.
    3 Same as # 1.
    4 It is not the balloon but the Foley catheter that promotes urinary drainage.

60. **2** Milking the tubing will usually dislodge the plug and will not harm the client; no physician's order is necessary to check patency. (b) (SU; IM; TC; RG)
    1 The catheter may be irrigated after milking the catheter and only with a physician's order.
    3 The nurse should not remove a catheter without specific instructions from a physician.
    4 The nurse should call the physician after trying measures to restore patency of the catheter.

61. **2** The urethral mucosa in the prostatic area is destroyed during surgery, and strictures may form with healing. (c) (SU; EV; ED; RG)
    1 The client should be out of bed ambulating; sitting for several hours is contraindicated because it promotes venous stasis and thrombus formation.
    3 The client should void as need arises; straining can cause pressure in the operative area, precipitating hemorrhage.
    4 Although vigorous exercise should be avoided, 6 months is too long a period for this restriction.

62. **3** Classic signs associated with hyperthyroidism are weight loss and restlessness because of increased basal metabolic rate; exophthalmos is due to peribulbar edema. (b) (SU; AS; PA; EN)
    1 Lethargy and weight gain are associated with hypothyroidism as a result of a decreased metabolic rate; forgetfulness is not related.
    2 Although weight loss and exophthalmus occur with hyperthyroidism, the client would be hyperactive, not hypoactive.
    4 These are all associated with hypothyroidism because of the decreased metabolic rate.

63. **2** Remaining thyroid tissue may provide enough hormone for normal function. (a) (SU; AN; PA; EN)
    1 This would be a total, not a subtotal, thyroidectomy.
    3 No parathyroid glands should be removed in a thyroidectomy.
    4 Same as # 3.

64. **2** Acute respiratory obstruction can result from edema, nerve damage, or tetany. (a) (SU; PL; TC; EN)
    1 A cardiac arrest is not an expected response following thyroid surgery.
    3 If the airway was obstructed by postoperative edema, the use of a mechanical airway would be ineffective because it would not reach the point of obstruction; a rebreathing mask would be used for clients with COPD, not a thyroidectomy.

4 Acidosis or cardiac arrest are not expected responses after a thyroidectomy.

65. **3** If the pharyngeal nerve is damaged during surgery, the client will be hoarse and have difficulty speaking. (c) (SU; EV; TC; EN)
   1 This would be an assessment for hypocalcemia resulting from inadvertent removal of the parathyroid glands.
   2 This would not indicate injury to the pharyngeal nerve; this is part of the assessment for a compromised airway.
   4 This assesses for hemorrhage, not pharyngeal nerve injury.

66. **2** Dry skin is most likely caused by decreased glandular function and fatigue caused by decreased metabolic rate. (b) (SU; EV; ED; EN)
   1 This is associated with hyperthyroidism, not hypothyroidism.
   3 Same as # 1.
   4 Same as # 1.

67. **3** The mask may irritate or scratch the eye if the client turns and lies on it during the night. (c) (SU; EV; ED; EN)
   1 Although this will help reduce edema of the eyeball, it will not prevent ulceration of the cornea.
   2 Although this may strengthen the eye muscles, it will do nothing to relieve edema or prevent ulceration of the eye.
   4 Blinking of the eyes will bathe the eyes and prevent corneal ulceration.

68. **4** The entire right lower extremity is 18%; the anterior portion of the right upper extremity is 4.5%. (b) (SU; AS; PA; IT)
   1 This is less than the total percent of body surface burned.
   2 Same as # 1.
   3 Same as # 1.

69. **1** Sulfamylon is effective against a wide variety of gram-positive and gram-negative organisms including anaerobes. (a) (SU; AN; PA; DR)
   2 This is an antimicrobial, not an analgesic; topical application causes pain.
   3 It promotes healing and decreases the need for grafting.
   4 This medication is an antimicrobial; it does not provide chemical debridement.

70. **2** This is the correct flow rate; multiply the amount to be infused (2000 ml) by the drop factor (10) and divide the result by the amount of time in minutes (12 hours × 60 min). (b) (SU; AN; TC; FE)
   1 This is an incorrect calculation; this flow rate is too slow to administer the ordered solution in the 12 hour time frame.
   3 This is an incorrect calculation; this flow is too fast to administer the ordered solution over 12 hours.
   4 Same as # 3.

71. **3** The graft covers nerve endings, which reduces pain and provides a framework for granulation. (c) (SU; AN; PA; IT)
   1 The graft promotes epithelialization; enzymatic preparations or surgery debride wounds.
   2 This is untrue; pig skin grafts are not sutured.
   4 This is contraindicated; topical antimicrobials would soften the graft and impede healing.

72. **3** The orthopneic position lowers the diaphragm and provides for maximal thoracic expansion. (a) (SU; IM; PA; RE)

1 Although this could help, it would not be as beneficial as the orthopneic position.
2 This would not facilitate thoracic expansion because it still permits abdominal organs to press against the diaphragm.
4 Same as # 2.

73. **3** Anabolic agents are synthetic androgenic steroids, which may produce masculinizing effects in women. (c) (SU; EV; PA; DR)
   1 Maxibolin will not cause hyperglycemia; it may cause hypoglycemia in clients with diabetes mellitus.
   2 The client may become hypernatremic, not hyponatremic; the client may become hypercalcemic as well.
   4 With an increase in muscle mass and stimulation of erythropoiesis, the client should have an increase in energy.

74. **3** Tensilon acts systemically to increase muscle strength; with a peak effect in 30 seconds, it lasts several minutes. (c) (ME; IM; ED; NM)
   1 Tensilon produces a brief increase in muscle strength; with a negative response the client would demonstrate no change in symptoms.
   2 Duration of Tensilon's action is about 3 minutes.
   4 Tensilon acts systemically on all muscles, rather than selectively on the eyelids.

75. **3** Until diagnosis is confirmed, the primary goal should be to maintain adequate activity and prevent muscle atrophy. (c) (ME; AN; TC; NM)
   1 This is an intervention, not a goal; it is too early to develop a teaching plan; the diagnosis is not yet established.
   2 This is too early; the client cannot adjust if the diagnosis is not yet confirmed.
   4 This is an intervention, not a goal; presenting symptoms do not indicate the client is near a crisis stage.

76. **4** Respiratory failure will require emergency intervention, and inability to swallow may lead to aspiration. (c) (ME; AS; PA; NM)
   1 These are symptoms of myasthenia that may occur but are not life threatening.
   2 This is a long-term problem that needs attention but is not life threatening.
   3 Same as # 1.

77. **3** Peak response occurs 1 hour after administration and lasts up to 8 hours; the response will influence dosage levels. (c) (ME; EV; PA; DR)
   1 This medication must be administered on time whether the dosage is already established or is being adjusted.
   2 This reduces gastrointestinal upset whether the dosage is established or is being adjusted.
   4 There are no psychologic side effects associated with Mestinon.

78. **4** Dysphagia should be minimized during peak effect of Mestinon, thereby decreasing the probability of aspiration. (b) (ME; IM; TC; NM)
   1 There is insufficient data to know whether this is appropriate because liquids can also be aspirated.
   2 This is a treatment for, rather than prevention of, aspiration.
   3 This action will not prevent aspiration, although it is vital that the respiratory function be monitored.

79. **2** Spacing activities will encourage maximal functioning within the limits of the client's strength

and fatigue. (b) (ME; PL; PA; NM)

1 This is probably unnecessary if the client is closely observed by the nursing staff; it should be permitted if requested by the client or family.

3 Bed rest and limited activity may lead to muscle atrophy and calcium depletion.

4 This is necessary for lifelong psychologic adjustment but more appropriate as the client is moving toward discharge.

80. 4 Exacerbation of myasthenia may occur within 2 weeks of steroid therapy, causing respiratory embarrassment and dysphagia. (c) (ME; EV; PA; DR)

1 This is unnecessary; adequate fluid intake should be maintained.

2 Steroids increase sodium retention, and this would be contraindicated.

3 Although clients should avoid contact with persons having upper respiratory infections, reverse isolation is not required.

81. 3 Results are unpredictable, and symptoms may gradually return over several years. (c) (SU; IM; ED; NM)

1 This may increase the client's anxiety, and details of the actual surgery are not required with informed consent.

2 Thymectomy is a well-established treatment and is not considered experimental.

4 This may actually increase the client's anxiety; although complications will be mentioned, they will not be emphasized.

82. 1 Honest discussion with emphasis on functional and psychologic abilities helps promote adjustment. (b) (SU; IM; PE; EC)

2 This provides false reassurance; there is no guarantee the client will feel better on discharge.

3 This is too soon; this may eventually be necessary if the client continues to have difficulty coping.

4 Postoperative depression is not a characteristic feature of thymectomy.

83. 1 The failing left ventricle cannot accept blood returning from the lungs; this results in increased vascular pressure in the lungs. (c) (ME; AN; PA; CV)

2 Wheezing and coughing are associated with paroxysmal nocturnal dyspnea and right-sided heart failure.

3 Dyspnea on exertion is an early, not an advanced, sign of CHF.

4 A rise in central venous pressure results from right-sided failure.

84. 4 Generalized weakness is a sign of significant hypokalemia, which may be a sequela to diuretic therapy. (a) (ME; EV; ED; DR)

1 Insomnia is not known to be related to hypokalemia or HydroDIURIL therapy.

2 Although this is unrelated to HydroDIURIL therapy, it can occur with other antihypertensive drugs.

3 This may be a sign of hyponatremia, not hypokalemia that accompanies diuretic therapy.

85. 3 Potassium supplements can cause gastrointestinal ulceration and bleeding. (b) (ME; EV; ED; DR)

1 Because they can be irritating to the stomach, potassium supplements should not be taken on an empty stomach.

2 Most salt substitutes contain potassium, and their use with potassium supplements can cause hyperkalemia.

4 Although muscle cramps can indicate hypokalemia, clients should not adjust their own dosage.

86. 4 Carbonated beverages are generally high in sodium and should be avoided. (a) (ME; IM; ED; FE)

1 This contains sodium.

2 Same as # 1.

3 Same as # 1.

87. 2 Stressful situations will increase the body's oxygen demands. (b) (ME; IM; ED; CV)

1 Clients with low cardiac reserve cannot tolerate extremes of temperature; a hot bath will increase the body's oxygen demands.

3 The heart of a client with low cardiac reserve cannot tolerate a pulse rate this high.

4 Hot, humid weather is not good for those with chronic heart disease; these individuals should use an air conditioner.

88. 2 Rest decreases demand on the heart and will also prevent fatigue. (a) (ME; PL; PA; CV)

1 The client should sleep with her head slightly elevated to facilitate respiration.

3 The client needs potassium; low potassium in a client taking digoxin predisposes to toxicity and dangerous arrhythmias.

4 To avoid becoming obsessed with the pulse rate, the client should not be taught to take the pulse so often; once daily is adequate.

89. 4 Shoes that become too tight indicate pedal edema, which is a sign of fluid retention; 2.2 pounds is equal to 1 liter of fluid. (c) (ME; AS; PA; CV)

1 Although left-sided failure can proceed to right-sided failure, the client has given no indication that pulmonary edema may be developing.

2 With fluid retention the rate is not as significant as a bounding characteristic to the pulse.

3 Eventually the physician will be notified, but the nurse should have more data before calling.

90. 3 Morphine sulfate increases spasms of smooth muscle and is contraindicated in all conditions in which there is obstruction of smooth muscle ducts. (c) (SU; AN; PA; DR)

1 Morphine sulfate and meperidine hydrochloride cause respiratory depression.

2 Ingestion of food stimulates pancreatic function; drugs do not have this effect.

4 Morphine sulfate and meperidine hydrochloride are central nervous system depressants.

91. 4 Vagal stimulation slows the heart; because atropine blocks vagal innervation, an increased heart rate would occur. (c) (SU; EV; PA; DR)

1 It may cause urinary retention, not polyuria.

2 It may cause constipation, not diarrhea.

3 It does not cause murmurs; it causes palpitations and tachycardia.

92. 3 This surgery involves the stomach, duodenum, pancreas, and common bile duct; a nasogastric tube removes gastric secretions and prevents distention. (a) (SU; PL; TC; GI)

1 A chest tube is used to remove air or blood from the chest cavity, which is not entered in a Whipple procedure.

2 Intestinal tubes are used for small bowel obstruction; except for the duodenum, the small bowel is not included in the Whipple procedure.

4 Nutrients in the stomach will stimulate pancre-

atic secretions; this is contraindicated until healing takes place.

93. **3** Shallow respirations, bronchial tree obstruction, and atelectasis compromise gas exchange in the lungs; an elevated carbon dioxide level leads to acidosis. (a) (SU; AN; PA; FE)
   1 Metabolic acidosis is seen in diarrhea with loss of base from the lower gastrointestinal tract.
   2 Metabolic alkalosis is caused by excessive loss of hydrogen ions from gastric decompression or excessive vomiting.
   4 Respiratory alkalosis is caused by increased expiration of carbon dioxide, a component of carbonic acid.

94. **3** This is the correct flow rate; to determine the amount of fluid, take the sum of all IV fluid for the period (2750 ml), multiply this by the drop factor (15), and divide the result by the time in minutes (24 hr × 60 min). (b) (SU; AN; TC; FE)
   1 This is too slow a drip rate to infuse the required amount of fluid.
   2 Same as # 1.
   4 This is too rapid a drip rate, and the required fluid will be infused in too short a period.

95. **4** Use ratio and proportion to calculate:
   370 mg/225 mg = X ml/1 ml
   $$225 X = 375$$
   $$X = 1.6 \text{ ml or 25 minims.}$$
   (c) (SU; AN; TC; DR)
   1 This is too little; it would not provide enough drug.
   2 This is too much; it would provide excessive drug.
   3 Same as # 1.

96. **3** The pancreatic enzymes (amylase, trypsin, and lipase) must be present when food is ingested for digestion to take place. (b) (SU; EV; ED; DR)
   1 The client would have no chyme in the duodenum for the enzyme to act on.
   2 Same as # 1.
   4 At this time the food eaten for dinner has already passed beyond the area of action; the enzyme would be given too late to aid in digestion.

97. **1** The Whipple procedure leads to malabsorption because of impaired delivery of bile to the intestine; fat metabolism is interfered with, causing dyspepsia. (c) (SU; IM; ED; GI)
   2 High protein is required for tissue building; there is no problem with the liver in cancer of the pancreas.
   3 High-calorie meals are needed for energy and to promote use of protein for tissue repair.
   4 These clients are anorexic, require small frequent meals, and should eat high-calorie, high-protein, low-fat diets.

98. **4** Polydipsia is characteristic of hypoinsulinism (diabetes mellitus) because of impaired carbohydrate metabolism. (b) (SU; EV; PA; GI)
   1 Polyuria, not oliguria, is characteristic of diabetes mellitus because excess fluid is excreted with the glucose by the kidneys.
   2 Increased appetite is characteristic of diabetes mellitus because of impaired metabolism.
   3 Weight loss characterizes diabetes mellitus because of the use of body mass as a source of energy.

99. **3** This position promotes localization of inflammation and prevents an ascending infection. (a)

(SU; IM; TC; GI)
   1 The risk of an ascending infection may be increased in this position, because it allows fluid in the abdominal cavity to bathe the entire peritoneum.
   2 Same as # 1.
   4 The client would probably prefer a Sims' position, which increases the risk of an ascending infection.

100. **3** The medical history could be obtained during assessment, and a relationship could be established if they were uninterrupted. (c) (ME; IM; PE; EC)
   1 Agency information and data could be obtained after the assessment data had been obtained and rapport established.
   2 Accepting coffee may be an imposition and is not the best way to develop trust.
   4 Assessment of the environment could be less obviously done while obtaining the history and physical data.

101. **4** The client's cardiac condition, increased age, and poor socioeconomic status increase vulnerability; the daughter's condition should be explored in greater detail. (c) (ME; AN; PA; RE)
   1 Children before puberty and adolescence have the least incidence of tuberculosis.
   2 Although the incidence of tuberculosis is increasing, death from tuberculosis has been steadily on the decline because of improved drug therapy.
   3 The incidence of tuberculosis has been on the increase but not at an alarming rate.

102. **2** Placing an aide in the home will allow the grandmother to rest and provide the child with attention. (c) (ME; IM; TC; EC)
   1 Making the client feel guilty will only increase anxiety and will not be constructive.
   3 Elaborate toys need not be employed for sensory stimulation; household objects can serve as well.
   4 The handicapped sibling requires attention, and this may increase jealousy, rivalry, and resentment.

103. **4** This is the schedule for active immunization recommended by the American Academy of Pediatrics. (b) (ME; PL; PA; BI)
   1 This regimen does not follow the schedule for active immunization recommended by the American Academy of Pediatrics.
   2 Same as # 1.
   3 Same as # 1.

104. **2** The Bureau of Child Welfare handles cases of child abuse and neglect, of which the child seems to be a victim.. (b) (ME; IM; TC; EC)
   1 The Bureau of the Handicapped would be concerned with equipment and supplies required for the individual with a handicap.
   3 The hospital would probably not admit the child unless an immediate medical incident required it.
   4 The clinic would observe the client medically but would not deal with social problems.

105. **1** Tubercle bacilli are transmitted through airborne droplets; therefore respiratory isolation with an Ultra-Filter mask is necessary. (a) (ME; IM; TC; RE)
   2 This is not necessary; tuberculosis is spread by airborne droplets.
   3 This would not be necessary unless objects are

contaminated by respiratory secretions.

4 This is unnecessary as long as appropriate isolation precautions are followed.

106. **4** Tubercle bacilli are particularly resistant to treatment and can remain dormant for prolonged periods of time; medication must be taken consistently as ordered for prolonged periods. (a) (ME; AN; TC; RE)
  1 Although this is important, the microorganisms must be eliminated by the use of medication.
  2 Same as # 1.
  3 This is unrelated; the microorganism must be eradicated by the medication.

107. **3** The kidney, an extremely vascular organ, receives a large percentage of the blood flow. (c) (SU; PL; TC; RG)
  1 This may occur later in the postoperative period.
  2 This can occur but is not acute and develops later.
  4 This can occur but is not life threatening.

108. **2** Turning facilitates drainage from the operative site. (c) (SU; PL; TC; RG)
  1 Because clients are prone to develop paralytic ileus, they are kept npo or on clear fluid for at least 24 to 48 hours.
  3 The dressing should be changed frequently because the wound generally drains large amounts.
  4 A nephrostomy tube should never be clamped unless specifically ordered by the physician.

109. **3** The wound will drain urine until healing takes place, sometimes up to several weeks. (c) (SU; AS; PA; RG)
  1 The hourly urine output must be 30 ml or more to be adequate.
  2 A specific gravity this low indicates that the kidneys have lost their ability to concentrate urine.
  4 Urine begins to clear within about 24 hours; urine that remains dark red and contains clots indicates abnormal bleeding.

110. **2** The dressing will need to be changed at home because drainage can persist for several weeks. (a) (SU; IM; ED; RG)
  1 A nephrostomy tube is generally not irrigated unless specifically ordered by the physician.
  3 The client should be up and about at home.
  4 The client should be encouraged to take fluids.

111. **3** Reflection conveys acceptance and encourages further communication. (b) (SU; IM; PE; EC)
  1 This is false reassurance that does not help to reduce anxiety.
  2 This provides false reassurance that also removes the focus from the client's needs.
  4 This is unrealistic, and it is too late to think of this.

112. **1** Oral hypoglycemic agents decrease serum glucose levels. (a) (ME; IM; ED; DR)
  2 Ketoacidosis occurs with insulin-dependent diabetes.
  3 Weight gain is usually present in adult onset diabetes.
  4 Same as # 2.

113. **1** Oral hypoglycemics stimulate endogenous insulin production by the beta cells of the pancreas. (a) (ME; AN; PA; DR)
  2 This occurs when serum glucose drops below normal levels.
  3 This occurs in the presence of insulin and potassium.

  4 Beta cells must have some function to enable Diabinese to be effective.

114. **4** According to the ADA diet, green beans and brocolli are equivalent vegetable substitutes. (b) (ME; IM; ED; GI)
  1 This is a bread exchange.
  2 Same as # 1.
  3 Same as # 1.

115. **4** The nurse needs to know specifically what the client is asking; this response permits clarification. (b) (SU; IM; PE; EC)
  1 This assumes that the client is referring to the diabetes in relation to surgery and sidesteps the question.
  2 Asking what the physician has said collects more information, but it will not clarify what the client wants to know.
  3 The nurse is making an assumption about medical management.

116. **3** Bending increases intraocular pressure and must be avoided. (b) (SU; IM; ED; NM)
  1 Activities do not have to be restricted this long.
  2 This should be avoided because it raises intraocular pressure.
  4 Same as # 1.

117. **1** Safety is a priority; this will keep the client from falling out of bed and will provide a sense of security. (a) (SU; PL; TC; NM)
  2 The affected eye is patched; therefore the level of light is insignificant.
  3 This may increase anxiety and reduce the client's feeling of being in control.
  4 It is not necessary to immobilize the head so rigidly; also, this may increase anxiety.

118. **3** Regular insulin is the only insulin that acts rapidly and is compatible with intravenous solutions. (a) (SU; AN; TC; DR)
  1 This insulin is not compatible with intravenous solutions; it is an intermediate-acting insulin.
  2 Same as # 1.
  4 Ultralente insulin is not compatible with intravenous solutions; it is a long-acting insulin.

119. **3** An antiemetic would prevent vomiting; vomiting increases intraocular pressure and should be avoided. (b) (SU; IM; TC; NM)
  1 This is unsafe; vomiting increases intraocular pressure and aggressive intervention is required.
  2 Same as # 1.
  4 Same as # 1.

120. **4** To protect against physical injury and infection, the dropper tip should not touch the eye. (a) (SU; EV; ED; NM)
  1 This an is incorrect technique; it would squeeze medication out of the eye.
  2 This is an incorrect technique; the lower lid should be retracted for placement of eyedrops.
  3 This is an incorrect technique; drops should be placed within the lower lid.

121. **2** This response focuses on the client's feelings of despair and provides the opportunity to talk about them. (a) (ME; IM; PE; EC)
  1 This abandons the client and leaves the client with no support.
  3 This response avoids a pressing problem and misses an opportunity for discussion of feelings.
  4 This focuses on the nurse's interpretation of the problem, not the client's.

122. **2** This is true; it could be the foundation for devel-

oping a positive mental outlook. (b) (ME; IM; PE; EC)

1 This is probably true, but this response belittles the client's actual concern and physical discomfort.

3 This is a patronizing response that does not recognize the despair.

4 There is no indication that the client needs drugs for depression.

123. **4** Chemotherapy destroys normal erythrocytes, white blood cells, and platelets indiscriminately along with the neoplastic cells. (a) (ME; IM; ED; DR)

1 Although true, this does not explain pancytopenia.

2 This is not a true description of the side effects of steroids.

3 This is not the cause for fewer erythrocytes, white blood cells, and platelets.

124. **2** Reduced platelets increase the likelihood of uncontrolled bleeding; reduced lymphocytes increase susceptibility to infection. (b) (ME; PL; ED; BI)

1 This would be helpful for stomatitis, not pancytopenia; aggressive oral hygiene could precipitate bleeding from the gums.

3 Although fluids may be increased to flush out the toxic byproducts of chemotherapy, this would have no effect on pancytopenia.

4 This is a sign of hypocalcemia that would not apply to pancytopenia.

125. **4** The afferent sensory branch of the trigeminal nerve innervates the cornea. (c) (ME; AS; PA; NM)

1 This would test the function of cranial nerves III, IV, and VI.

2 This would test the function of cranial nerve XI.

3 This would test the function of cranial nerve VII.

126. **4** Visual disturbances such as diplopia and blurred vision are common initial symptoms of optic nerve lesions. (a) (ME; AS; PA; NM)

1 Constipation may occur late in the disease because of immobility.

2 Although a neuromuscular disorder, headaches are not a common symptom.

3 Decubiti may become infected if they occur late in the disease because of immobility.

127. **4** This is a truthful answer that provides hope for the client. (c) (ME; IM; ED; NM)

1. This response avoids the client's question and could increase anxiety.

2 Analgesics are not commonly prescribed unless pain results from some other condition.

3 Avoids the client's question by suggesting a task to complete.

128. **3** This is a truthful answer that provides some realistic hope. (a) (ME; IM; PE; EC)

1 This provides false reassurance; there are frequent remissions and exacerbations that may reduce the life span.

2 This response avoids the client's question; the family did not ask.

4 This avoids the client's question and transfers responsibility to the physician.

129. **4** Assessment is the priority; the nurse should determine if symptoms are caused by a full bladder. (b) (ME; AS; TC; RG)

1 This could be done, but it would not be the initial action.

2 This may be done to reduce urinary bacterial count and stone formation, but it is not the initial action.

3 This may eventually be necessary, but it is not the initial action.

130. **3** It is fact that *E. coli* is commonly found in the bowel and, because of close anatomic proximity and improper hygiene after bowel movements, may spread to the urethra. (a) (ME; AN; PA; RG)

1 *E. coli* is no more virulent than other infective agents.

2 *E. coli* is not commonly found in the kidneys.

4 *E. coli* does not compete with *Candida* organisms for host sites.

131. **3** Complementary mixtures of essential amino acids in plant proteins provide complete dietary protein equivalents. (c) (ME; IM; PA; GI)

1 A total vegetarian does not consume flesh, milk, milk products, or eggs.

2 Same as # 1.

4 Same as # 1.

132. **2** Classic symptoms include gnawing, boring, or dull pain located in the mid-epigastrium or back; pain is caused by irritability and erosion of the mucosal lining. (b) (ME; AS; PA; GI)

1 This type of pain is more characteristic of cholecystitis.

3 This type of pain is more characteristic of the complication of a perforated ulcer.

4 This type of pain is more characteristic of a hiatal hernia.

133. **2** It is necessary to clarify the route of administration because medication can be given po, IV, or IM. (b) (ME; AN; TC; DR)

1 Ranitidine is usually given with meals.

3 Ranitidine is used to decrease gastric acid and is helpful to clients with peptic ulcer.

4 This is the usual dose of ranitidine when given twice a day.

134. **4** A client's knowledge about the treatment program enhances conformity and reduces stress. (a) (ME; IM; PE; EC)

1 This response does not answer the client's question and might produce frustration.

2 This is a general statement that does not focus on the specific client.

3 This does not support the treatment regimen; it may cause more stress if the client interprets it as a conflict between the physician and nurse.

135. **4** These are classic indicators of perforated ulcer, for which immediate surgery is indicated; this should be anticipated. (b) (SU; PL; TC; GI)

1 There are no symptoms indicating that the client is in shock.

2 Black, tarry stools or red stools indicate bleeding, not perforation.

3 Tachycardia and tachypnea are related to pain and possible blood loss; keeping the client npo is the priority.

136. **3** Without an adequate stomach reservoir, the hypertonic concentrated food mass "dumps" into the small intestine, drawing fluid from surrounding blood and tissue and causing hypovolemia and typical shock symptoms. (b) (SU; AN; PA; GI)

1 The opposite is true; the food passes too quickly into the small intestine.

2 The opposite is true; the food mass is more concentrated (hypertonic).

4 Same as # 2.

137. 1 The rapid absorption of sugars from the food mass causes elevation of blood sugar, and the insulin response often causes transient hypoglycemic symptoms. (b) (SU; AN; PA; GI)

2 The insulin-adjusting mechanism is not overwhelmed but responds vigorously, causing rebound hypoglycemia.

3 This is unrelated; usually a bland diet is prescribed following a gastrectomy.

4 The response is a rebound hypoglycemia, not hyperglycemia.

138. 2 In a suprapubic prostatectomy an incision is made into the bladder via the abdomen so that the bladder abnormalities can be corrected concurrently with prostatic resection. (a) (SU; AN; ED; RG)

1 An indwelling catheter is required following surgery to provide for drainage of urine until postoperative edema subsides.

3 This is untrue; resection via the transurethral route would necessitate a shorter convalescence.

4 Radical perineal prostatectomy, when perineal nerves are severed, can result in impotence.

139. 4 This dose could be excessive in the elderly because detoxification and excretion of the drug take longer. (b) (SU; IM; TC; GD)

1 Although this would be appropriate if the medication is administered, the nurse should first question the order because the dosage is excessive for an elderly client.

2 This dosage could excessively depress the elderly client; the nurse has a responsibility to question the order.

3 Same as # 1.

140. 3 Blood glucose needs to be reduced; regular insulin begins to act in 30 to 60 minutes. (a) (SU; PL; PA; EN)

1 Oral hypoglycemics are long acting and begin to act about 1 hour after administration; in addition, the client has Type I, not Type II, diabetes mellitus and an oral hypoglycemic would be ineffective.

2 The rate may be increased because polyuria often accompanies hyperglycemia.

4 Blood glucose levels are far more accurate than urine glucose levels.

141. 4 Emotional and physical stress may cause insulin requirements to remain elevated in the postoperative period. (a) (SU; PL; PA; EN)

1 Insulin requirements would remain elevated, rather than decrease.

2 Fluctuating insulin requirements indicate less than adequate control.

3 An increase in the client's insulin requirements could indicate sepsis, but this is not expected.

142. 2 Because venous stasis is the major predisposing factor of pulmonary emboli, venous flow velocity should be increased. (b) (SU; PL; TC; RG)

1 Increasing the coagulability of the blood would lead to the development of deep vein thrombosis.

3 This would not affect the development of deep vein thrombosis.

4 Same as # 3.

143. 3 More than 90% of pulmonary emboli originate in the deep veins of the pelvis and thighs because of the extensive vascular network. (b) (SU; AN; PA; CV)

1 This is untrue; most pulmonary emboli originate in the pelvis or thighs.

2 Same as # 1.

4 Same as # 1.

144. 4 Green vegetables contain fiber, which promotes defecation. (a) (SU; EV; ED; GI)

1 This has a binding effect and would cause constipation with resultant straining at stool.

2 Same as # 1.

3 Same as # 1.

145. 3 Compression fractures of the vertebrae are the most frequent fractures in clients with osteoporosis; a gradual collapse of vertebrae may be asymptomatic and only observed as kyphosis. (a) (ME; AS; PA; GD)

1 This is untrue; it is not supported by statistics.

2 Same as # 1.

4 Same as # 1.

146. 3 Weight greater than 8 pounds causes excessive tension on the skin, leading to damage. (b) (SU; AN; TC; SK)

1 Covering the malleoli causes skin breakdown.

2 Moleskin is placed on the medial and lateral portions of the leg.

4 The spreader bar should be wide enough to keep materials away from the malleoli.

147. 3 These are correct techniques; deep inhalation promotes alveolar expansion, and exhalation promotes lung recoil. (b) (SU; EV; ED; RE)

1 These are incorrect techniques; inhalation should be through the mouthpiece.

2 Coughing is done after deep breathing.

4 The breaths should not be in succession; they should be spaced by several normal breaths to avoid fatigue.

148. 3 This puts the least strain on the prosthesis, and the hip may be flexed to 90 degrees 10 days after surgery. (b) (SU; PL; TC; SK)

1 Elevation of the leg places increased strain on the prosthesis; a soft chair would permit hip flexion greater than 90 degrees.

2 Elevation of the leg places increased strain on the prosthesis.

4 A soft chair would permit hip flexion greater than 90 degrees.

149. 1 This includes the client in the problem-solving process. (b) (SU; PL; PE; EC)

2 This does not include the client in the problem-solving process; more data should be obtained from the client before deciding on an intervention, which may or may not be appropriate.

3 Same as # 2.

4 Same as # 2.

150. 4 Research demonstrates that women past menopause need 1500 mg of calcium a day, which is almost impossible to obtain through dietary sources because the average daily consumption of calcium is 300 to 500 mg; vitamin D promotes the deposition of calcium into the bone. (b) (ME; AN; PA; GD)

1 This does not contain adequate calcium and vitamin D to meet requirements to prevent os-

teoporosis.

2 These do not contain adequate calcium to meet requirements to prevent osteoporosis; these do not contain vitamin D unless fortified.

3 If large amounts of magnesium are present, calcium absorption is impeded because magnesium and calcium absorption are competitive; vitamin E is unrelated to osteoporosis.

151. **1** Avoidance of strain is essential to provide time for the prosthesis to sit adequately in the socket and not become dislodged; this usually takes 2 months. (b) (SU; PL; TC; SK)

2 This is too long; it is usually up to 2 months for partial weight-bearing, although positional restrictions may go beyond 2 months.

3 Same as # 2.

4 This is inadequate time for healing to take place.

152. **2** To allow for the insertion of the bronchoscope, throat muscles are anesthetized, diminishing the protective gag reflex. (a) (SU; PL; TC; RE)

1 General anesthesia is not usually used; therefore paralytic ileus is not a complication.

3 This is irrelevant; dysphasia is difficulty talking, and dyspepsia is disturbed digestion.

4 This does not occur after a bronchoscopy.

153. **2** There is air in the tissues, and palpation results in a crackling sound referred to as crepitus. (b) (SU; EV; TC; RE)

1 The size of the chest is determined by bony structure; a barrel chest with an increase in the AP diameter is associated with COPD, not cancer of the lung.

3 This is excessive accumulation of fluid in tissue spaces.

4 This is a harsh, vibrating sound usually produced on inspiration because of airway obstruction.

154. **3** Different infusion sets deliver different preset numbers of drops per ml; knowing this is a necessity for calculating the drip rate. (a) (SU; AN; TC; FE)

1 This does not determine the drip rate.

2 Same as # 1.

4 This determines the size of the drop, not the drip rate.

155. **3** A mediastinal shift with airway obstruction may occur because pressure builds up on the operative side, causing the trachea to deviate toward the unoperative side; assessment of the airway takes priority. (c) (SU; AS; TC; RE)

1 This is unsafe; the client needs immediate intervention; the airway is the priority.

2 There is no need for a chest tube when a pneumonectomy is performed.

4 Same as # 1.

156. **1** Lying on the operative side permits ventilation of the remaining lung and prevents fluid from draining into the sutured bronchial stump. (c) (SU; PL; TC; RE)

2 When used all the time, this inhibits respiration because of pressure of the abdominal organs against the diaphragm; there is no chest tube.

3 Lying on the unoperative side restricts left lung excursion and may allow fluid to drain into the right bronchial stump.

4 Although high-Fowler's position promotes ventilation, it is extremely tiring.

157. **3** The skin is the first line of defense; keeping it dry

and safe from injury promotes skin integrity. (a) (ME; PL; PA; IT)

1 This is unsafe; irradiated skin is fragile and subject to blistering and sloughing.

2 This is unsafe; soap film left after rinsing can change the angle and intensity of radiation.

4 This is unsafe; the skin should be free of emollients because they change the angle or degree of radiation.

158. **4** A productive cough indicates mucus is being raised from the lungs. (b) (ME; EV; PA; RE)

1 Rales are unaffected by postural drainage or coughing.

2 Saliva comes from the mouth and does not indicate clearance of lungs.

3 The depth of respirations may not be altered by postural drainage.

159. **3** Serum albumin indicates severe depletion of visceral protein stores; the normal range for serum albumin is 3.5 to 5.5 g/100 ml; white meat turkey (2 slices $4 \times 2 \times \frac{1}{4}$ inch) contains approximately 28 g protein. (c) (ME; EV; ED; GI)

1 A 4 oz serving of beef broth contains approximately 2.4 g of protein.

2 A 6 oz serving of mixed fruit contains approximately 0.5 g of protein.

4 A 3 tablespoon serving of cooked spinach contains approximately 9 g of protein.

160. **4** Tofu products increase protein without increasing vitamin D because unlike milk products, tofu does not contain vitamin D. (b) (ME; EV; ED; GI)

1 This contains milk, which has vitamin D and should be avoided.

2 This contains vitamin D and should be avoided.

3 Eggnog contains milk and should be avoided.

161. **4** All these characteristics are well-established risk factors for gallbladder disease (female, fat, and 40). (a) (ME; AS; PA; GI)

1 Risk factors include being a female and having a family history of gallstones, but clients are usually over 40.

2 The age is correct, but clients are usually female and have elevated serum cholesterol.

3 None of these factors are correctly associated with cholecystitis.

162. **4** A low-fat dinner is given so that large amounts of bile will be stored in the gallbladder when the test is done. (b) (SU; IM; TC; GI)

1 This test is given on 1 day; occasionally it must be repeated if the test results are inconclusive.

2 The contrast medium in the pills often causes diarrhea.

3 Some stones may not be visible because of composition and/or location.

163. **1** Questran depletes vitamins A, D, and K, as well as folic acid. (c) (SU; AS; PA; GI)

2 This is unnecessary; protein would be desirable for wound healing.

3 This is not relevant to the situation.

4 These would be decreased; Diuril depletes K^+, and Questran depletes folic acid.

164. **3** Local fat-stimulated duodenal glands dispatch the hormone, cholecystokinin, that signals the gallbladder to contract and release bile. (a) (ME; AN; PA; GI)

1 Soft-textured foods are unnecessary.

2 This would not be necessary at this time; sur-

gery is to be performed shortly.

4 Although this would be desirable before surgery, it is not the priority.

165. **2** Self-splinting results in shallow breathing, which does not aerate the lungs adequately, particularly the lower right lobe. (a) (SU; AS; TC; GI)

1 The client would be npo for the first 48 hours after surgery.

3 Dressing is not changed by the nurse in the immediate postoperative period; the client's respiratory status takes first priority.

4 The T-tube is never irrigated; it drains by gravity until the edema in the operative area subsides and the tube is then removed by the physician.

166. **4** Sustained diastolic pressure above 90 mm Hg reflects pathology and indicates hypertension. (a) (ME; AS; PA; CV)

1 This is unrelated to the hypertension.

2 This reflects heart rate, not the pressure within the artery.

3 This is not the most significant indicator; an elevated diastolic pressure is more important because it reflects the pressure while the heart is at rest.

167. **3** The client must increase dietary intake of potassium because of potassium loss associated with Diuril; water miscible forms of vitamins A and E should be taken because Questran combines with bile acids to form insoluble complexes; also Questran interferes with absorption of folic acid and iron. (c) (ME; IM; ED; DR)

1 There is no such action by fruits and vegetables.

2 Protein should be obtained from food.

4 This may or may not be true following a cholecystectomy; the client should be taught about medication-induced deficiencies.

168. **4** The Centers for Disease Control have listed several opportunistic infections that must be present along with HIV for the disease to be labeled AIDS. (c) (ME; AN; PA; BI)

1 This places someone at risk but does not constitute a positive diagnosis.

2 This only confirms the presence of HIV antibodies.

3 This indicates AIDS-related complex (ARC).

169. **4** Blood and body fluid precautions require that hands be washed before and after client care to minimize risk of transmission; since this procedure normally does not involve contact with blood or secretions, additional protection is not indicated. (a) (ME; IM; TC; BI)

1 These are necessary only when there is risk of contact with blood or body fluid.

2 Same as # 1.

3 A mask and gown would be indicated only if there were danger of secretions or blood splattering on the nurse (for example, during suctioning).

170. **4** AZT can cause anemia, leukopenia, and granulocytopenia; these blood dyscrasias can be life threatening, so the CBC is monitored. (b) (ME; EV; PA; DR)

1 These are not directly affected by drug.

2 Same as # 1.

3 Once infected, the client will continue to test positive for the antibody.

171. **3** The presence of opportunistic infections is a dis-

tinguishing diagnostic criterion for acquired immunodeficiency syndrome but is not part of the diagnostic criteria for ARC. (c) (ME; AN; PA; BI)

1 Because ARC is not associated with the opportunistic infections, clients are generally less debilitated.

2 Both medical conditions are caused by the same organism.

4 The AIDS virus is present in both AIDS and ARC, thus it can be transmitted in both instances.

172. **3** Equipment used is disposable; the donor does not come into contact with anyone else's blood. (b) (ME; AN; PA; BI)

1 Condoms offer some protection but are subject to failure because of condom rupture or improper use; risks of infection are present with any sexual contact.

2 An individual may be infected for many weeks before testing positive for the antibody; the individual could still transmit the virus.

4 The risk would depend on the spouse's prior behavior.

173. **3** Lesions are characteristic of Kaposi's sarcoma, a cancer associated with AIDS. (c) (ME; AS; PA; BI)

1 This is present in ARC; an associated opportunistic infection or tumor must be present before the diagnosis of AIDS can be made.

2 Same as # 1.

4 Leukopenia, not leukocytosis, is a characteristic of AIDS.

174. **2** Policies relative to DNR orders vary among hospitals, and the nurse must adhere to the policies within the institution. (b) (ME; AN; PE; EC)

1 This may not be true for all hospitals; the information does not indicate this is so in this situation.

3 The decision resides with the client.

4 This is untrue; the wish of the client is the deciding factor.

175. **2** With an inflammatory response the body increases its production of WBCs and fibrinogen, which increases the WBC count and blood sedimentation rate respectively. (a) (ME; AN; PA; GI)

1 This is untrue; this would not affect the white blood cell count or the sedimentation rate.

3 Same as # 1.

4 Same as # 1.

176. **2** Prednisone inhibits phagocytosis and suppresses other clinical phenomena of inflammation; this is a symptomatic treatment that is not curative. (a) (ME; IM; ED; DR)

1 Generally, the response is rapid.

3 The drug suppresses the immune response and increases the potential for infection.

4 The appetite is increased; weight gain may result from this or from fluid retention.

177. **2** Medical treatment is directed toward reducing motility of the inflamed bowel, restoring nutrition, and treating and preventing infection; surgery is used selectively for those who are acutely ill or have excessive exacerbations. (b) (ME; PL; ED; GI)

1 This is untrue; medical treatment is symptomatic, not curative.

3 It is usually performed as a last resort.

4 Although there is an emotional component, the

physiologic adaptations determine whether surgery will be necessary.

178. **3** The solution is hyperosmolar and a very concentrated source of glucose; too rapid infusion can cause hyperglycemia; an infusion pump should be used as an added precaution. (c) (SU; PL; TC; GI)

  1 Although the nurse should be aware of the client's electrolyte values, monitoring is primarily the physician's responsibility.

  2 The nurse should monitor intake and output, but the primary responsibility is to maintain the ordered flow rate.

  4 Although S and A may be performed, finger sticks for blood glucose are done concurrently and are more accurate.

179. **2** Intravenous fluids supply minimal calories; a client on only IV therapy will lose weight and become malnourished. (a) (ME; AN; PA; FE)

  1 This is not related to weight; lack of bulk in the diet results in constipation.

  3 Vitamins are not related to weight loss.

  4 Intracellular electrolytes are not related to weight loss.

180. **4** The less disruptive the procedure, the greater the acceptance by the client. (b) (SU; PL; ED; GI)

  1 Most frequently, total parenteral nutrition is set up to run during sleeping hours.

  2 Someone living with the client can be taught the principles of administration and site care.

  3 The catheter is inserted only by a physician under sterile conditions.

181. **3** An iatrogenic infection is one that is caused by medical personnel, procedures, or environment of the health care facility. (a) (SU; AN; PA; IT)

  1 This is not the cause of an iatrogenic infection.

  2 Same as # 1.

  4 Same as # 1.

182. **2** The pain of renal colic is excruciating; unless relief is obtained the client is unable to cooperate with other therapy. (c) (SU; AN; TC; RG)

  1 Although a culture is generally ordered, it is not a priority when a client has severe pain.

  3 Increasing fluid intake helps mobilize the stone, but a client who has severe pain may be nauseated and unable to drink.

  4 Any urine can be saved and strained after the client's priority needs are met.

183. **4** Pain with ureteral stones is caused by spasm and is excruciating and intermittent; it follows the path of the ureter to the bladder. (b) (SU; AS; PA; RG)

  1 Pain is spasmodic and excruciating, not boring.

  2 This is untrue; pain intensifies as the stone is caught in the ureter and spasms occur in attempt to dislodge it.

  3 This is typical of pain caused by a stone in the renal pelvis.

184. **4** Laxatives remove feces and flatus, providing better visualization. (b) (SU; PL; ED; RG)

  1 A light supper may be indicated; however, there is no restriction as to fat content.

  2 Large amounts of water may dilute the dye, impairing visualization.

  3 A light dinner and beverage are permitted.

185. **3** Purines are precursors of uric acid. (c) (SU; AN; PA; RG)

  1 A struvite stone is sometimes called a magnesium ammonium phosphate stone and is precipitated by recurrent urinary tract infection with coliform bacteria.

  2 Cystine stones are caused by a rare hereditary defect in inadequate renal tubular reabsorption of cystine (inborn error of cystine metabolism).

  4 An oxalate stone would be composed of calcium oxalate.

186. **2** Calculi may obstruct the flow of urine to the bladder, allowing the urine to distend the ureter, causing hydroureter. (c) (SU; AN; PA; RG)

  1 There is insufficient information to come to this conclusion even though output is less than intake; oliguria is present when the output is between 100 and 500 ml in a 24-hour period.

  3 Calculi do not cause renal shutdown directly; they may obstruct the urinary tract and cause damage indirectly as a result of pressure from urine buildup.

  4 If the urethra were obstructed, the bladder would be distended.

187. **1** If the calculus is in the upper two thirds of the ureter, and a ureterolithotomy is performed, the stone is removed via a flank incision. (b) (SU; AN; TC; RG)

  2 Bladder stones may be crushed with a lithotrite that is passed transurethrally (litholapaxy); a ureterolithotomy was performed in this situation.

  3 This would be present if stones are removed from the bladder via a suprapubic incision.

  4 This is not necessary; an incision is made into the ureter at the level of the calculus and it is removed.

188. **2** These occur with a urinary tract infection because of bladder irritability; burning on urination and fever are additional signs of a UTI. (a) (SU; EV; PA; RG)

  1 This is a symptom of urinary calculus, not infection.

  3 This is not related to urinary tract infection.

  4 This is not a sign of a urinary tract infection; this may be caused by altering the diet from acid ash to alkaline ash or vice versa.

189. **1** This uses gravity to allow urine to exert pressure on the area of the trigone, initiating relaxation of the urinary sphincter and facilitating micturition. (a) (ME; IM; ED; RG)

  2 This is important after urination but will not help facilitate micturition.

  3 An acid ash diet may be used to prevent urinary infection and the formation of calcium stones; it will do nothing to facilitate micturition.

  4 Although this may be important so that urine may be strained, it will not facilitate micturition.

190. **1** A client's vital signs, especially the pulse and temperature, will rise before the client demonstrates any of the more severe symptoms of withdrawal from alcohol. (c) (ME; AS; PA; GI)

  2 This is contraindicated initially because it may cause cerebral edema.

  3 This becomes a priority after the problems of the withdrawal period have subsided.

  4 This is not a priority until after the detoxification process.

191. **3** Scar tissue that forms as cirrhosis progresses causes the liver tissue to contract, making the

liver small with a rough surface; little lumps are formed as scar tissue pulls the liver at certain points. (c) (ME; AS; PA; GI)

  1 The client has cirrhosis, not hepatitis.

  2 The liver converts ammonia to urea; therefore the blood ammonia level increases when the liver fails.

  4 This is a manifestation of liver infection.

192. **3** Petechiae are evidence of capillary bleeding; the diseased liver is no longer able to metabolize vitamin K, which is necessary to activate blood clotting factors. (a) (ME; PL; PA; GI)

  1 Vitamin A is not involved in clotting, even though the transformation of carotene to vitamin A takes place in the liver.

  2 Although bile is synthesized and secreted in the liver, bile salts are not involved in the clotting process.

  4 Folic acid is stored in the liver but not involved in the clotting process.

193. **1** This keeps the bladder in the pelvic area and prevents puncture when the abdominal cavity is entered. (a) (SU; IM; ED; GI)

  2 This is unsafe; the bladder will rise into the abdominal cavity and may be punctured.

  3 This is not necessary.

  4 Same as # 3.

194. **3** Bicarbonate solution is soothing and prevents scratching, which can cause abrasions and lead to infection. (a) (ME; PL; PA; IT)

  1 This is irritating and drying to the skin; also, alcohol can be absorbed through the skin and should be avoided.

  2 This would have no effect on the pruritus.

  4 Same as # 2.

195. **2** Administration of SSKI with milk or juice reduces GI distress. (b) (ME; IM; TC; DR)

  1 Adequate fluid intake should be maintained to help liquefy respiratory secretions.

  3 This is not related to administration of SSKI.

  4 It is not necessary before the administration of SSKI.

196. **4** 250 mg is equal to 0.25 g; therefore

$$4 \text{ g}/0.25 \text{ g} = X \text{ ml}/1 \text{ ml}$$
$$0.25 X = 4$$
$$X = 16 \text{ ml. (b) (ME; AN; PA; DR)}$$

  1 This is an inaccurate calculation; the amount is too small to provide the ordered amount.

  2 Same as # 1.

  3 Same as # 1.

197. **3** Corticosteroids act to decrease inflammation, which decreases edema. (b) (ME; AN; PA; DR)

  1 This is an antiinflammatory agent, not a diuretic; it does not cause diuresis by action on the kidney.

  2 Resistance to infection is decreased, but this is not pertinent in this situation.

  4 The problem is not with increased cerebrospinal fluid.

198. **2** Corticosteroids, such as Decadron, have a hyperglycemic effect. (b) (ME; EV; PA; DR)

  1 This is unnecessary; this is required when administering magnesium sulfate.

  3 Corticosteroids would not increase bacterial growth in the lungs.

  4 Corticosteroids are not known to precipitate cessation of gastrointestinal activity.

199. **2** Shortening and eventual atrophy of muscles oc-

curs, resulting in contractures. (c) (ME; AN; PA; NM)

  1 Muscles will atrophy, not hypertrophy, from disuse.

  3 Flexion abnormalities, not extension rigidity, occur, resulting in contractures.

  4 It does not predispose to infection, but to atrophy and contractures.

200. **3** Administration of an anticoagulant to a client who is bleeding would interfere with clotting and increase hemorrhage. (b) (ME; IM; ED; DR)

  1 This is unsafe; it would not be used in this situation because it would increase bleeding; anticoagulant therapy may be used with cerebral thrombosis.

  2 Same as # 1.

  4 Although contraindicated, it would increase signs and symptoms if given.

201. **1** The client has lost vision from the right visual field; scanning compensates for loss. (c) (ME; IM; ED; NM)

  2 This is the approach to be used for apraxia.

  3 This is the approach to be used for denial of the right side (unilateral neglect).

  4 This alleviates neglect of the affected side.

202. **4** If the client exhibits emotional instability, it is usually caused by lesions affecting the thalamic area, the thalamic area is the integral part of the neural system for emotional response to sensory experience over which the client with a CVA has little control. (a) (ME; IM; ED; NM)

  1 The client may have remote memory, but there is no selective process of what events are remembered.

  2 This is associated with consistent behavior and cognitive thinking, of which the client is incapable at this time.

  3 Same as # 2.

203. **1** Emboli, occurring from atrial fibrillation, cause complete occlusion of vessels; usually middle cerebral arteries are involved; the infarct causes hemiplegia, possibly aphasia, or spatial perceptual deficits. (c) (ME; AN; PA; NM)

  2 Hypertension is a disease that may cause spasm of the arteries, but does not cause anatomic occlusion.

  3 Seizures are caused by inappropriate paroxysmal discharge.

  4 Developmental defects of the arterial wall are associated with sacular aneurysms.

204. **3** Recovery from aphasia is a continuous process; the amount of recovery cannot be predicted. (a) (ME; IM; ED; NM)

  1 This response abdicates the nurse's responsibility; the physician cannot predict return of function.

  2 This gives false reassurance; it may take a year or longer or may never return.

  4 Speech return is a continuous process; it may take a year or longer or may never return.

205. **4** In addition to the extent of injury, a factor in relearning speech is the client's motivation and effort; the more the client attempts to talk, the more likely speech will progress to its optimal level; relearning is a slow process. (a) (ME; IM; ED; NM)

  1 Clients with aphasia are not deaf.

  2 The nurse should instruct the wife to approve

and support every effort to communicate.

3 This will cause frustration and anger in the client.

206. **1** Heat inhalation can cause edema of the respiratory lumens, interfering with oxygenation; evaluation of respiratory status is a priority assessment. (c) (SU; AS; TC; IT)

2 This would be done after the client's respiratory status has been evaluated.

3 Burns should be evaluated by the physician, and then the ordered medical therapy should be implemented; airway has priority.

4 Same as # 2.

207. **3** Hoarseness is a sign of potential respiratory insufficiency as a result of inhalation burns, which cause edema in the surrounding tissues, including the vocal cords. (c) (SU; AS; PA; IT)

1 This would indicate metabolic acidosis, not respiratory insufficiency.

2 Same as # 1.

4 Sputum would be sooty, not frothy; pink-tinged, frothy sputum is associated with pulmonary edema.

208. **2** Pain is from the loss of the protective covering of the nerve endings; blisters and redness occur because of the injury to the dermis and epidermis. (a) (SU; AS; PA; IT)

1 Grafting is not done with a second-degree burn unless it becomes infected and converts to third-degree status.

3 Second-degree burns involve only the superficial layers of skin, unless they become infected.

4 Recovery in second-degree burns with no infection occurs in 2 to 3 weeks.

209. **3** This provides for the quickest use of the narcotic so that relief of pain can occur immediately. (c) (SU; PL; TC; DR)

1 Nausea, vomiting, and paralytic ileus may occur post-burn, making oral medication impractical.

2 This route does not provide a uniform absorption; also, relief of pain would be delayed.

4 The medication may be sequestered in the tissues and, with the fluid shifts, it is unknown when the medication will take effect.

210. **3** Albumin given intravenously increases colloid osmotic pressure, resulting in a pull of fluid from the interstitial and intracellular compartments to the intravascular compartment. (c) (SU; AN; PA; FE)

1 The interstitial compartment is part of the extracellular compartment.

2 This is opposite to the actual shift of fluids.

4 Same as # 2.

211. **3** Osmosis is the movement of water from an area of lesser solute concentration to an area of greater solute concentration. (c) (SU; AN; PA; FE)

1 In active transport, molecules move against a concentration gradient; this differs from diffusion and osmosis because metabolic energy is expended.

2 Diffusion is the movement of particles across a semipermeable membrane from an area of greater concentration of particles to an area of lesser concentration of particles.

4 Filtration is the passage of fluid through a material that prevents the passage of certain constituents; hydrostatic pressure the pressure exerted

within a closed system, is known as filtration force; this force moves fluid by pressure and concentration gradients.

212. **2** Urinary output reflects circulating blood volume; it is the most reliable, immediately available information to assess fluid needs. (a) (SU; EV; PA; FE)

1 Daily weights reflect fluid retention or loss; however, other factors beside fluid affect weight; this is not as immediately accurate as hourly urines.

3 This may indicate hypervolemia or hypovolemia; it is not an accurate indicator of fluid balance.

4 Same as # 3.

213. **3** All data is in normal limits; Po_2 is 80 to 100 mm Hg, Pco_2 is 35 to 45 mmHg, and the pH is 7.35 to 7.45. (a) (SU; AN; PA; FE)

1 None of the data provides an indicator of fluid balance.

2 The pH would have to be below 7.35

4 Oxygen is within normal limits of 80 to 100 mm Hg.

214. **2** Care of burns is a painful procedure, and pain medication should be administered before care to limit discomfort. (a) (SU; PL; TC; IT)

1 Surgical asepsis should be used.

3 No dressings are applied when the exposure method is used.

4 This is unnecessary; sulfamylon is not hepatotoxic.

215. **2** Range of motion should be instituted as soon as it will not compromise the individual's cardio-respiratory status. (b) (SU; PL TC; IT)

1 Pain will continue for some time, and if ROM is delayed until it subsides, contractures will have already developed.

3 If ROM is delayed until skin grafts heal, contractures will have already developed.

4 Pain and inability to cope may be prolonged; if ROM is delayed, contractures will have already developed.

216. **4** This diet is low in bulk; after digestion and absorption there is only a small amount of residue and therefore feces to be eliminated. (a) (SU; AN; TC; GI)

1 This diet does not influence the bacterial flora of the intestine; antimicrobials, such as neomycin, are given to do this.

2 This diet increases flatus; peristalsis is decreased and the products of digestion remain in the intestine longer.

3 Although a low-residue diet is less irritating, this is not the primary reason for its use before surgery.

217. **2** This is caused by the trauma of intestinal manipulation and the depressive effects of anesthesia and analgesics. (a) (SU; AN; PA; GI)

1 Edema would not totally interfere with peristalsis, which may be less effective but would still result in some output.

3 Any ingested food or fluid initiates the gastro-colic reflex and would therefore result in some output.

4 A nasogastric tube decompresses the stomach; it does not cause paralytic ileus, in which there is no output.

218. **2** Amount to be infused (850 ml) multiplied by the drop factor (10) divided by total time in minutes

(480) equals 18 gtt/min. (b) (SU; AN; TC; FE)
1 This is less than the desired flow rate; it would take longer to infuse than the time ordered.
3 This is more than the desired flow rate; the fluid would be infused in less than the time ordered.
4 Same as # 3.

219. **3** A nosocomial infection, by definition, is acquired during hospitalization. (a) (SU; IM; ED; IT)
1 This nosocomial infection is a primary infection, not a secondary infection.
2 It may or may not be highly contagious; reverse isolation protects the client from others; in this situation, others need to be protected from the client.
4 Exposure to the pathogen must have occurred after admission to the hospital for classification as a nosocomial infection.

220. **3** This is the correct amount: use ratio and proportion; 250 mg is equal to 0.25 g;
$0.25 g/1g = x ml/3ml$
$x = 0.75 ml$
$0.75 ml = 12$ minims. (b) (SU; AN; TC; DR)
1 This is an incorrect calculation; too little medication will be administered.
2 Same as #1.
4 This is an incorrect calculation; too much medication will be administered.

221. **2** Communication facilitates joint solution of the problem; the nurse must first determine the client's understanding and perceptions before solutions to the problem can be attempted. (b) (SU; AS; PE; EC)
1 This will not collect data about why the client is leaving the room.
3 This abdicates the responsibility of the nurse.
4 This may be done, but not until further assessment is done to determine the reason why the client is leaving the room.

222. **1** The client's feelings, knowledge, and skills concerning the colostomy must be assessed before discharge. (a) (SU; EV; ED; GI)
2 People should not be pressured into performing self-care before they are physically, emotionally, or mentally ready.
3 After a colostomy the client is usually encouraged to eat a regular diet and told only to eliminate gas-producing foods.
4 The client usually does not need a dressing on the incision at the time of discharge.

223. **2** This occurs with stenosis of the stoma; forcing insertion of the tube could cause injury. (b) (SU; EV; ED; GI)
1 This is caused by too rapid infusion of fluid; slowing the flow by clamping the tube relieves discomfort.
3 This is an expected response; feces and flatus accompany fluid expulsion.
4 A colostomy irrigation usually can be completed in 1 hour.

224. **1** Steps are short and dragging; this is seen with basal ganglia defects. (b) (ME; AS; PA; NM)
2 This is a staggering gait often associated with cerebellar disease.
3 This is associated with bilateral spastic paresis of the legs.
4 This is associated with unilateral upper motor neuron disease.

225. **2** Amplitude of the voice is reduced by neuromuscular involvement. (a) (ME; AS; PA; NM)
1 Usually loss of weight occurs because of embarrassment of slowness and untidiness in eating.
3 Constipation is a common problem because of a weakness of muscles used in defecation.
4 The tendency is for the head and neck to be drawn forward by loss of basal ganglia control.

226. **3** There is a lack of neural control of individual muscle fibers, resulting in a characteristic mask-like facies. (a) (ME; AS; PA; NM)
1 Movement usually abolishes the tremor, which is known as a nonintention tremor.
2 This is unrelated to Parkinson's disease; this is often associated with a CVA.
4 This does not occur; both arms fall rigidly to the sides and do not swing with a normal rhythm when walking.

227. **1** This produces bulk, which is a stimulant to defecation; the muscles used in defecation are weak in clients with Parkinson's disease, usually causing constipation. (b) (ME; IM; PA; GI)
2 Cathartics are irritating to the intestinal mucosa, and their regular administration promotes dependence.
3 This will intensify the problem; fluids need to be increased.
4 Bananas are binding and will intensify the problem of constipation.

228. **3** Tachycardia and palpitations, not bradycardia, occur. (c) (ME; EV; PA; DR)
1 Nausea may occur; it reflects a central emetic reaction to Levodopa.
2 Anorexia may occur; decreased appetite results because of nausea and vomiting.
4 Changes in affect, mood, and behavior are related to toxic effects of the drug.

229. **3** Pain is wavelike, colicky, and sharp because of obstruction and localized bowel ischemia. (b) (SU; AS; PA; GI)
1 Flatus would be impeded by strangulation.
2 Vomiting is persistent, not projectile.
4 This is not an early sign of obstruction; decreased bowel sounds occur after gas and fluid accumulate.

230. **4** After general anesthesia, these activities expand alveoli and prevent atelectasis. (a) (SU; IM; TC; RE)
1 This is not necessary; the abdomen has not been entered, and there should be no interference with peristalsis.
2 This is not necessary.
3 This is not necessary; clients can ambulate after recovery from anesthesia.

231. **4** Atropine is an anticholinergic-parasympathetic that interferes with the response of the heart muscle to vagal stimulation. (a) (SU; EV; PA; DR)
1 This is a side effect of sedatives.
2 This is a side effect of tranquilizers.
3 This is a side effect of narcotic analgesics.

232. **3** Because of pain and the proximity of the operative site to the lower urinary tract, voiding problems are common. (c) (SU; EV; PA; GI)
1 This should not be a complication of herniorrhaphy because early ambulation is permitted.
2 This is not a complication of herniorrhaphy.
4 The abdomen was not entered, and there should be no interference with peristalsis.

233. **3** This increases lymphatic drainage, reducing edema and pain. (b) (SU; IM; TC; RG)
   1 This increases circulation to the area, intensifying edema and pain.
   2 Same as # 1.
   4 This is not indicated; scrotal swelling is caused by the trauma of surgery, not infection.

234. **1** The fiber component of complex carbohydrates helps bind and eliminate dietary cholesterol and foster growth of intestinal microorganisms to break down bile salts and release cholesterol component for excretion. (c) (ME; IM; ED; CV)
   2 Fat-binding fiber should be increased.
   3 Of the fats in the diet, saturated fats should be decreased.
   4 It is what the client eats, not when the client eats, that is important.

235. **3** The essential fatty acid, linoleic acid, is necessary for muscle tissue integrity, especially of the myocardium. (b) (ME; IM; ED; CV)
   1 All fats cannot and should not be eliminated from the diet.
   2 Proteins and carbohydrates do not contain the essential fatty acid called linoleic acid.
   4 The body does manufacture cholesterol.

236. **3** The Prudent Diet contains reduced fat with less saturated animal fat, increased carbohydrate with more of it in complex forms, and moderate protein with emphasis on lean forms. (b) (ME; AN; TC; CV)
   1 This caloric distribution does not represent the Prudent Diet proposed by the American Heart Association.
   2 Same as # 1.
   4 Same as # 1.

237. **2** This is caused by the hypervolemia and pulmonary hypertension associated with heart failure. (a) (ME; AS; PA; CV)
   1 This is present in pleurisy, not CHF.
   3 The pulse would most likely be rapid and bounding, not slowed.
   4 Hypertension, not hypotension, would occur because of hypervolemia.

238. **2** Coumadin inhibits vitamin K; therefore vitamin K is the antidote for Coumadin (b) (ME; AN; TC; DR)
   1 This is the antidote for heparin.
   3 This is a blood clotting factor, not the antidote for Coumadin.
   4 Same as # 3.

239. **4** This is a classic sign of denial; by reducing the importance or extent of the problem the individual is able to cope; not acknowledging that it is really a problem is a form of denial. (b) (ME; AS; PE; EC)
   1 This usually indicates displacement of anger, not denial.
   2 There is insufficient evidence to diagnose denial; the husband-wife relationship may be strained, or the husband may be worried about upsetting the wife.
   3 This indicates repression of affect rather than denial.

240. **2** This is necessary for monitoring cardiac function; the drug slows and strengthens the heart rate. (a) (ME; EV; PA; DR)
   1 Hypokalemia increases the potential for digitalis toxicity; potassium intake should be increased.

   3 This is not an appropriate decision for the client; the physician makes this decision.
   4 This is not appropriate; it is not related to digoxin.

241. **1** Rales is the sound of air passing through fluid in the alveolar spaces; in pulmonary edema, fluid moves from the intravascular compartment into the alveoli. (a) (ME; AS; PA; CV)
   2 The blood pressure is usually increased with hypervolemia.
   3 This would occur with angina or a myocardial infarction.
   4 The pulse would be bounding with hypervolemia.

242. **4** Pulmonary capillary wedge pressure is an indirect measure of left ventricular and diastolic pressure, an indication of ventricular contractility. (b) (ME; AN; PA; CV)
   1 Right atrial pressure measures only function of the right heart and indirectly its ability to receive blood.
   2 Cardiac output by thermodilution does not measure intracardiac pressures.
   3 Pulmonary artery diastolic pressure may not be as accurate an indicator of left ventricular pressure if COPD or pulmonary hypertension exist.

243. **4** This drug binds with heparin sodium to form a physiologically inert complex; corrects clotting deficits. (c) (ME; PL; TC; DR)
   1 Vitamin K counteracts the effects of warfarin sodium-type (Coumadin-type) drugs.
   2 This is an alternate name for heparin sodium.
   3 This is an oral anticoagulant that interferes with the synthesis of prothrombin.

244. **4** Dark brown or black stools (melena) could indicate gastrointestinal hemorrhage. (a) (ME; AS; PA; GI)
   1 Frothy stools are indicative of poor fat absorption and are associated with sprue.
   2 Ribbon-shaped stools indicate a bowel mass or obstruction.
   3 Clay-colored stools are usually related to problems causing a decrease in bile.

245. **3** Abdominal distention, nausea, and abdominal pain can be signs of nasogastric tube blockage. (b) (SU; IM; TC; GI)
   1 Although narcotics are usually ordered postoperatively, they tend to decrease peristalsis and may increase abdominal distention and nausea.
   2 No bowel sounds are expected for a time after stomach or intestinal surgery.
   4 There will be no stools for several days; gastric drainage may contain some blood from surgery.

246. **2** Bright bleeding at this point would be a normal finding that should be monitored. (b) (SU; EV; PA; GI)
   1 This is contraindicated; secretions would accumulate and cause pressure on the suture line; this prevents observation of drainage.
   3 If the tube is draining, there is no need to irrigate; also, irrigations should be ordered by the physician.
   4 Reducing suction would allow secretions to accumulate and cause pressure on the suture line.

247. **2** Total volume (1250 ml) times the drop factor (15) divided by total time in minutes (480) equals 39 gtt/min. (b) (SU; AN; TC; FE)
   1 This is too slow; it would not deliver the ordered

amount of fluid in the ordered time period.

3 This is too fast; it would deliver too much fluid too quickly.

4 Same as #3.

248. **1** Symptoms characteristic of the dumping syndrome can be lessened with small, frequent meals that are low in carbohydrates. (b) (SU; EV; TC; GI)

2 Resting after meals might mitigate the symptoms of dumping syndrome, but resting before meals will not prevent them; resting is nonspecific; the client should be lying down to slow the emptying of the stomach.

3 The client may need to avoid these foods to minimize irritating the gastric mucosa, but they are not the cause of the dumping syndrome.

4 Fluids during meals should be limited; increased fluid intake speeds emptying time of the stomach.

249. **3** It is necessary to minimize stress to prevent further ulcer development; this is most effective if the family is involved. (b) (SU; PL; PE; EC)

1 Although pernicious anemia could occur as the result of gastric surgery, there is little that can be done to prevent it.

2 Most clients recover from ulcer surgery without complications.

4 Maximizing changes in life-style can increase stress and is contraindicated for ulcer clients.

250. **4** Teaching for the postoperative period should begin as soon as the client is admitted; knowledge of what to expect decreases anxiety and may improve compliance with the treatment regimen. (a) (SU; PL; ED; IT)

1 This is too late; at this time the client will be in too much discomfort to concentrate on learning.

2 Same as # 1.

3 This is too late; the client must have time to ask questions and demonstrate the ability to care for the wound; teaching begins preoperatively.

251. **3** The infected bone is placed at rest in a cast, splint or traction to reduce pain and limit spread of infection. (b) (SU; PL; TC; SK)

1 This is contraindicated; ambulation may facilitate spread of infection.

2 Osteomyelitis is usually caused by a microorganism traveling through the bloodstream to the bone, not the reverse; the client is already septic.

4 This is contraindicated; this would increase pain and spread of infection.

252. **4** Use ratio and proportion:
1200 mg = 1.2 g;
1.2g/1 = X ml/3 ml
X = 3.6 ml. (b) (SU; AN; TC; DR)

1 This is an incorrect calculation; this amount is too small to deliver the desired dose.

2 Same as # 1.

3 Same as # 1.

253. **3** The nurse epidemiologist acts as a consultant to help devise an infection control strategy. (a) (ME; IM; ED; IT)

1 This is the role of the physician.

2 This is usually done by the primary nurse.

4 This is the role of the laboratory technician.

254. **2** Smoking accelerates oxidation of tissue vitamin C, so smokers need 100 mg/day, whereas adult RDA is 60 mg/day; also, vitamin C helps with wound healing. (c) (ME; IM; TC; GI)

1 It is not oxidized more rapidly in the smoker.

3 Same as # 1.

4 Same as # 1.

255. **4** Oxacillin is a form of penicillin and should be given on an empty stomach; food delays absorption. (b) (ME; EV; ED; DR)

1 This is incorrect; food or milk delays absorption of this drug.

2 Same as # 1.

3 This is not necessary; however, it is appropriate with sulfonamides.

256. **3** The actual reason for the lack of ketonuria in Type II diabetes mellitus (NIDDM) is unknown; one theory is that extremely high hyperglycemia and hyperosmolarity block the formation of ketones, stimulating lipogenesis, rather than lipolysis. (b) (ME; AS; PA; EN)

1 This does not occur with either type of diabetes mellitus.

2 This is impossible; if glycosuria is present, there must first be a level of glucose in the blood above the renal threshold of 160 to 180 mg/dl.

4 This is expected in Type I diabetes mellitus (IDDM).

257. **1** In the overweight individual with Type II diabetes, occasional alcohol can be used with caloric substitution for equivalent fat exchanges in the diet because it is metabolized like fat. (b) (ME; IM; ED; EN)

2 Alcohol can be used as long as it is accounted for in the diet.

3 This is untrue; all regular foods can be used in the ADA diet.

4 Moderation is vital; these may not be used in unlimited quantities; they must be accounted for in the dietary calculations.

258. **3** According to the individual's needs, consistency and regularity in the basic food plan should be maintained; this is a basic principle of dietary management of diabetes mellitus. (b) (ME; IM; ED; EN)

1 This is not necessary; the client can use the ADA food plan to make selections.

2 This is unrealistic; it cannot always be done; it is unnecessary because choices can be made within the ADA diet.

4 The client is not taking insulin and needs to have a monitored intake to keep the blood sugar within limits.

259. **2** Zyloprim may prolong the half-life of Diabinese, producing signs of hypoglycemia. (c) (ME; EV; TC; DR)

1 This is not necessary; the dosage of Diabinese needs to be decreased.

3 Same as # 1.

4 Same as # 1.

260. **1** Intermittent claudication is the pain that occurs during exercise because of a lack of O_2 to muscles in the involved extremities. (b) (ME; AN; PA; CV)

2 This is not the cause of intermittent claudication; legs would feel heavy, not crampy.

3 It is the exercise, not the lack of it, that precipitates the pain.

4 This is related to a venous problem, not an arterial one.

261. **2** Decreasing the demand for oxygen by resting will relieve the pain. (a) (ME; IM; ED; CV)

1 Pain will not resolve as long as exercise and thus muscle hypoxia is continued, regardless of whether ASA is taken or not.

3 This is appropriate only for venous insufficiency, not arterial insufficiency.

4 Nitroglycerine is a coronary artery dilator, not a peripheral vascular dilator.

262. **2** Any client who has been sedated, or who is not fully conscious, may not sign consent for a surgical procedure. (b) (SU; AN; PE; EC)

1 Many clients face contradictory feelings regarding their impending surgery, but their consent is legal unless they withdraw the consent.

3 A second opinion is not required for a consent to be legal.

4 A complete history and physical are needed before surgery, but they do not affect the legality of consent.

263. **2** Use ratio and proportion:
30 U/100 U = X ml/1 ml
100 X = 30 ml
X = 1/3 ml or 5 minims.
(b) (ME; AN; TC; DR)

1 This is an inaccurate calculation; this would deliver too small a dose.

3 This is an inaccurate calculation; this exceeds the ordered dose.

4 Same as # 3.

264. **2** Allowing the client to grieve for the lost limb is an important part of nursing care; remaining with the client conveys empathy and support. (a) (SU; IM; PE; EC)

1 This behavior may be interpreted by the client as rejection.

3 Family visits are important for their value as support, not as distraction; distraction delays confronting the problem.

4 Sedation will prevent the client from facing the problem.

265. **4** Phantom limb pain is a real experience with no known cause or cure. (a) (SU; AN; TC; SK)

1 This may be an appropriate diagnosis for the client with an amputation, but it is not the diagnosis for phantom limb pain.

2 Same as # 1.

3 This is not an appropriate diagnosis for the individual with an amputation.

266. **4** The wrapping of the stump is implemented to reduce swelling and shape the stump for fitting a prosthesis in the future. (c) (SU; AN; TC; SK)

1 Secretion drainage is not promoted by wrapping the limb; portable drainage systems are used for this purpose.

2 The stump sock is used to protect the stump from irritation and injury.

3 Infection is not prevented in this manner; surgical asepsis should be maintained.

267. **1** Because the hospital beds are narrower and higher than the beds clients sleep in at home, side rails frequently create a sense of security. (a) (ME; EV; PE; EC)

2 This relates to the physical status, not the psychologic status, of the client.

3 On the contrary, this will cause the client to feel more dependent.

4 Bed rails are unrelated to proprioception, which is knowing the location of a body part when it is out of the field of vision.

268. **1** This is a true statement; anxiety and/or anger associated with other stages interferes with learning. (c) (ME; AN; ED; EC)

2 Although clients in the acceptance or adaptation phase are less angry, the reason teaching is most effective is not because of their compliance but because new information can be processed more easily.

3 The anxiety associated with mental anguish would interfere with the ability to process new information; mental anguish is associated with an earlier stage.

4 Readiness for discharge is unrelated to the client's readiness for learning.

269. **2** In the obese individual this helps to inject the medication into subcutaneous tissue rather than adipose tissue, where its absorption would be poor. (b) (ME; IM; ED; DR)

1 This will result in the drug being injected into adipose tissue, where it will be poorly absorbed.

3 Same as # 1.

4 Same as # 1.

270. **3** The antibody called rheumatoid factor is present in 90% of clients with advanced arthritic changes; it is not found in the early stages of the disease process. (b) (ME; IM; ED; SK)

1 This denies the client's discomfort and does not deal with the stated confusion.

2 This denies the client's immediate feelings and blocks communication of them.

4 This response reinforces the client's felt discomfort and confusion over negative test results.

271. **2** Aspirin may damage the eighth cranial (acoustic) nerve, causing ringing in the ear and impairing hearing. (c) (ME; EV; PA; DR)

1 Diminished hearing, not ringing, occurs because of mechanical obstruction of the outer ear.

3 Aging may cause decreasing acuity in the extremes of pitch, but would not cause ringing in the ears.

4 Pain, not ringing, is a sign of otitis media; ASA toxicity affects the eighth cranial nerve, not the middle ear.

272. **3** Data supports supplementation in the elderly only in illness or debilitated states to help restore tissue integrity and function. (b) (ME; IM; ED; GD)

1 This is untrue; a well-balanced diet that contains a variety of foods as recommended from the four basic food groups is adequate.

2 The elderly do not need supplemental vitamins and minerals as long as their diet is adequate.

4 This is untrue; the best source of all nutrients is from natural foods rather than supplements; loss of weight results from reduction of calories, not addition of vitamins and minerals.

273. **3** Vitamin E hinders oxidative breakdown of structural lipid membranes in body tissues caused by free radicals in the cells. (b) (ME; AN; PA; GD)

1 This assists in the formation of visual purple needed for night vision.

2 This is used for formation of collagen, which is important for maintaining capillary strength, promoting wound healing, and resisting infection.

4 This is necessary for protein and fat metabolism and normal function of the nervous system.

274. **3** After surgery, abduction is maintained to reduce

the chance of dislocation of the femoral head. (a) (SU; PL; ED; SK)

1 This can lead to dislocation of the femoral head.

2 This causes adduction, which can lead to dislocation of the femoral head and is contraindicated.

4 Same as # 1.

275. **4** The pelvis is elevated by actions involving the unaffected upper extremities and nonoperative leg. (b) (SU; IM; TC; SK)

1 This is not permitted because it causes adduction of the leg and can lead to dislocation of the femoral head.

2 No pressure is permitted on the operative hip because it can cause dislocation of the femoral head.

3 Lifting with the arms requires strength; use of both heels puts pressure on the operative hip.

276. **2** When a client is anxious and has a decreased ability to cope, minor environmental irritants are magnified; eye contact is avoided to decrease additional stimuli. (c) (SU; EV; PE; EC)

1 This would be indicated by complaints of pain, splinting, refusal to move, and alteration in vital signs.

3 If the client were angry, eye contact would be maintained; prolonged eye contact may be used as a form of intimidation or aggression.

4 If this were so, the client would be verbalizing about the need to continue the abduction, not about a variety of other annoyances.

277. **2** The client is not in pain; also, this offers false reassurance. (b) (SU; EV; PE; EC)

1 The nurse inappropriately identifies the problem and never clarifies the need.

3 The nurse's response denies the client's needs; the client needs to discuss concerns and feelings.

4 The nurse's response denies the client's anxiety; it identifies pain as the problem.

278. **1** Increased basal metabolic rate, increased circulation, and vasodilation result in warm moist skin. (c) (ME; AS; PA; EN)

2 This symptom is associated with hypothyroidism.

3 Same as # 1.

4 Same as # 1.

279. **2** The client is hyperventilating and blowing off excessive carbon dioxide, which leads to these symptoms. (c) (ME; AS; PA; FE)

1 Eupnea is normal, quiet breathing; the client has shallow, rapid breathing.

3 Kussmaul respirations are deep, gasping respirations associated with diabetic acidosis and coma, not hyperventilation associated with anxiety.

4 These symptoms are related to a decreased carbon dioxide level in the body.

280. **2** Reassurance decreases anxiety and slows respirations; the mask is used so that exhaled carbon dioxide can be rebreathed to resolve respiratory alkalosis and return the client to acid-base balance. (c) (ME; IM; PA; FE)

1 This is not necessary because there is no evidence of hypoxia.

3 This is not necessary; the client is capable of adequate ventilation if respirations are slowed and/or carbon dioxide is rebreathed.

4 The client is already alkalotic; bicarbonate ions would increase the problem.

281. **3** In respiratory alkalosis the pH is elevated because of loss of hydrogen ions; Pco_2 is low because carbon dioxide is lost by hyperventilating. (c) (ME; AS; PA; FE)

1 This is metabolic acidosis with some compensation.

2 This is respiratory acidosis.

4 This is alkalosis.

282. **2** These are normal respiratory sounds heard on auscultation as inspired air enters and leaves the alveoli. (a) (ME; AS; PA; RE)

1 This is evidence of reduction in the amount of air entering the alveoli, usually caused by obstruction or consolidation.

3 Adventitious sounds is the general term for all abnormal breath sounds.

4 These are fine crackling sounds heard at the end of an inspiration; they are associated with pulmonary edema.

283. **4** This reflects the client's feelings and encourages a further exploration of concerns. (c) (SU; IM; PE; EC)

1 This response does not reflect the feeling tone of the client's statement; also, the client may not be able to answer this question.

2 This is false reassurance; thyroid storm could occur, which is capable of causing death.

3 This could reinforce the client's anxiety, and it avoids discussing the client's concerns and cuts off communication.

284. **1** General anesthesia is delivered via an endotracheal tube that irritates the posterior pharynx and larynx and causes discomfort when swallowing. (b) (SU; EV; PA; RE)

2 This is not an effect of general anesthesia.

3 Same as # 2.

4 Occasionally this may occur; however, it is a systemic, not a local, effect.

285. **1** Bleeding may occur, and blood will pool in back of the neck because the blood will flow via gravity. (a) (SU; EV; TC; EN)

2 This is contraindicated; this would increase pain and would put tension on the suture line.

3 Talking should be avoided in the immediate postoperative period except to assess for a change in pitch or tone, which may indicate laryngeal nerve damage.

4 Activity should be gradually resumed; because of the increased BMR associated with hyperthyroidism, frequent rest periods are encouraged.

286. **3** Hepatitis Type A is transmitted via the fecal-oral route; medical aseptic technique, specifically enteric precautions, must be used when there are articles that have potential fecal and/or urine contamination. (b) (ME; PL; TC; GI)

1 This is necessary only for respiratory (airborne) infections; a private room is not required.

2 Type A hepatitis is not transferred via the airborne route and therefore a mask is not necessary; a gown and gloves are required only when handling articles that may have fecal and/or urine contamination.

4 This is too limited; a gown and gloves should also be worn when handling other fecally contaminated articles, such as a bedpan or rectal thermometer.

287. **4** Hepatitis Type A is primarily spread via a fecal-oral route; sewage-polluted water may harbor

the virus. (c) (ME; AS; PA; GI)

1 Exposure to arsenic or carbon tetrachloride can cause toxic hepatitis, which is not communicable.

2 Hepatitis Type B is more often spread via the blood-borne route; using disposable equipment and proper handling of syringes decrease the risk of spreading the virus.

3 This does not increase the risk of developing the disease but will allow an infected individual to spread the disease to others.

288. **2** Damage to liver cells affects the ability to remove bilirubin from the blood, with resulting deposition in the skin and sclera. (b) (ME; AN; PA; GI)

1 With Hepatitis, the liver does not secrete excess bile.

3 There is no increased destruction of red blood cells in hepatitis.

4 This is unrelated; decreased prothrombin levels cause spontaneous bleeding, not jaundice.

289. **4** High carbohydrates provide calories for energy, high protein provides for tissue repair, and fats are permitted as tolerated. (b) (ME; PL; PA; GI)

1 High carbohydrates are needed for body fuel, otherwise protein will have to be used for metabolism rather than tissue repair; protein will be high and fats permitted as tolerated.

2 This diet does not offer adequate protein, which is required for tissue repair in the client with hepatitis; carbohydrates will be high, and fats are permitted as tolerated.

3 Same as # 2.

290. **4** Hepatitis type A is spread via the fecal-oral route; transmission is interfered with by proper hand washing. (b) (ME; IM; TC; GI)

1 This may increase transmission because no provision is made for the cleaning of equipment or disposal of contaminated wastes.

2 This is untrue; hepatitis can be transmitted via the fecal-oral route and precautions, such as hand washing, must be taken.

3 This is inadequate; transmission is still possible via the roll of toilet tissue unless hand washing is done.

291. **1** The first heart sound is produced by closure of the mitral and tricuspid valves; it is best heard at the apex of the heart. (b) (ME; AS; PA; CV)

2 This border covers a large area; the only auscultatory area near it is the aortic area.

3 This border covers a large area; the auscultatory areas that lie near it are the pulmonic and mitral areas.

4 This is where the second heart sound (S_2) is best heard; S_2 is produced by closure of the aortic and pulmonic valves.

292. **4** Closure of the atrioventricular valves, the mitral and tricuspid, produces the first heart sound (S_1). (c) (ME; AN; PA; CV)

1 These valves do not close simultaneously.

2 These are the semilunar valves; closure of these valves produces the second heart sound (S_2).

3 Same as # 1.

293. **2** Lasix promotes potassium excretion; hypokalemia increases cardiac excitability; digitalis in the presence of low extracellular potassium produces ectopic pacemaker activity. (a) (ME; AN; PA; DR)

1 Lasix causes diuresis and consequent potassium loss regardless of the serum potassium level.

3 Potassium is excreted by the kidneys, not destroyed by the liver.

4 Digitalis does not affect potassium excretion; Lasix promotes potassium excretion.

294. **3** Hypokalemia is suspected when the T wave on an ECG tracing is depressed or flattened; serum potassium below 3.5 mEq/L indicates hypokalemia. (a) (ME; AS; PA; FE)

1 This would have no significance in diagnosing potassium deficit.

2 Same as # 1.

4 Same as # 1.

295. **2** Food and fluids are usually withheld for approximately 6 to 8 hours to prevent vomiting and aspiration. (a) (SU; IM; TC; CV)

1 The procedure takes approximately 2 hours.

3 Bed rest with legs extended and a weight applied to the femoral site is suggested for several hours after the femoral method of entry.

4 A mild sedative is used because the client must be alert enough during the procedure to follow directions.

296. **1** The presence and specific location of pedal pulses are identified as a frame of reference for future readings. (a) (SU; AS; PA; CV)

2 The femoral artery, not a small artery in the foot, is used for cannulation.

3 Pedal pulses reflect the functioning of the arterial system; edema reflects the inadequacy of the venous system or decreased cardiac output.

4 Pedal pulses reflect the functioning of the arterial system, not the venous system.

297. **2** Immobilization of the right leg and pressure over the groin promote coagulation and healing at the puncture site of the femoral artery. (a) (SU; AN; TC; CV)

1 A small amount of radiopaque dye is injected (via the catheter) directly into the heart, where it is diluted by the blood; it does not create a problem at the puncture site.

3 These interventions cannot prevent or limit these symptoms; these symptoms are not usual.

4 The catheterization does not decrease blood pressure in the presence of adequate fluid replacement.

298. **3** An apical pulse is taken to detect dysrhythmias related to cardiac irritability; blood pressure is monitored to detect hypotension, which may indicate bleeding or shock. (a) (SU; EV; TC; CV)

1 This is contraindicated; flexion of the groin may compromise the clot at the femoral insertion site.

2 This is not necessary; the client did not undergo a general anesthetic and will soon be ambulatory.

4 A temperature may indicate a bacterial invasion, but this will not be evident during the first few hours after the catheterization.

299. **3** During inspiration negative pressure in the chest increases, causing fluid to rise in the chamber; during expiration negative pressure in the chest decreases, causing fluid to drop in the chamber. (c) (SU; EV; TC; RE)

1 If the system is closed to the atmosphere, as it should be, no bubbling will occur.

2 If the system is closed to the atmosphere, as it

should be, no bubbles will be present.

4 Changes in intrapleural pressure cause fluid to rise on inspiration and fall on expiration (tidaling).

300. **2** 1000 mcg = 1 mg; 500 ml of the drug added to 500 ml of IV fluid results in a solution where 1 ml contains 1 mg of the drug; the physician's order is for 1 mg/minute, therefore multiply total solution (1 ml) times the drop factor (6) and divide by total time in minutes (1). (b) (SU; AN; TC; DR)

1 This is an incorrect calculation; this would deliver half the desired dose.

3 This is incorrect; this would deliver 50% more than the desired dose.

4 This is an incorrect calculation; this would deliver twice the desired dose.

301. **1** Pain is a cardinal symptom; it is helpful to have as much specific information about it as possible, particularly its description and its relationship to foods ingested. (b) (ME; AS; ED; GI)

2 It is not necessary to save all urine and stools, although changes in color should be reported.

3 The client should be free to question orders that are not understood or agreed with.

4 This would not add any valuable information.

302. **4** Cholecystitis is frequently accompanied by intolerance to fatty foods, including fried foods and butter. (b) (ME; AS; PA; GI)

1 These cause flatulence and pain for clients with lower intestinal problems such as diverticulosis.

2 These foods contain less fat than do fried foods or butter.

3 Neither chocolate nor boiled seafood have as much fat as do fried chicken and butter.

303. **3** If the dye is not retained, the gallbladder cannot be visualized. (b) (ME; IM; TC; GI)

1 This will not affect concentration or visualization of dye in the gallbladder.

2 There is no reason to postpone the examination unless the diarrhea persists.

4 Preparation for oral cholecystogram sometimes includes a fat-free supper before the examination.

304. **3** Air in the secondary line will not enter the vein; fluid from the primary bottle is under pressure and will flow before air from the secondary line could reach the port in the primary line. (a) (SU; IM; TC; FE)

1 This is possibly true, but this answer would increase anxiety.

2 Gentamicin bypasses the large IV bottle because it is piggybacked into the primary line below the drip chamber and check-valve.

4 This is contraindicated; this stops the infusion, which can clog the lumen of the catheter that is inserted into the vein.

305. **1** Because the drug was just administered, the blood level of the drug would be at its highest level. (b) (SU; IM; TC; DR)

2 The result would reveal a drug blood level halfway between the peak and trough levels.

3 This would be done for a trough level when the drug level would be at its lowest.

4 This would result in inaccurate results; peak and trough levels are measured in relation to the time a drug is administered.

306. **3** Gentamicin can cause ototoxicity, resulting in vertigo, tinnitus, and hearing loss. (c) (ME; EV; PA; DR)

1 This is unlikely; the client has not been on prolonged bed rest.

2 Liquid diet and IV therapy may cause weakness because of low calorie intake, but dizziness does not occur.

4 This is unrelated; over 24 hours have passed since anesthesia was administered.

307. **3** Barriers reduce the contact of bile with skin and limit excoriation. (b) (SU; PL; TC; IT)

1 When wet, dressing should be changed, not reinforced; usually T-tube drainage empties into a pouch.

2 Antiseptics are drying and irritating to excoriated skin, and they sting when applied; this would require a physician's order.

4 This action may help, but the excoriation is probably caused by bile, not adhesive tape.

308. **1** Vitamin K, a precursor for prothrombin, cannot be absorbed without bile. (b) (SU; AS; PA; GI)

2 This is frequently related to electrolyte imbalances, not fat-soluble vitamin deficiency.

3 Jaundice results from a backup of bile, not a deficiency of fat-soluble vitamins.

4 This may be related to electrolyte imbalances or deficiency of B vitamins, which are water-soluble.

309. **3** It may take 4 to 6 months, but ultimately most people can eat anything they want. (b) (SU; EV; ED; GI)

1 Although fats may have to be gradually reintroduced, most people can tolerate them after a cholecystectomy.

2 Foods that caused gastric distress before surgery are usually tolerated after surgery.

4 Increased protein is needed only until healing has occurred.

310. **4** Increased intraocular pressure damages the optic nerve, interfering with peripheral vision. (a) (ME; AS; PA; NM)

1 These may be associated with a detached retina.

2 There is difficulty in adjusting to darkness.

3 Same as # 1.

311. **1** This is a miotic that constricts the pupil, permitting fluid drainage, which reduces intraocular pressure. (b) (ME; PL; PA; DR)

2 This is contraindicated; this is a mydriatic that dilates the pupil, obstructing drainage, which increases intraocular pressure.

3 This is contraindicated; this dilates the pupil and paralyzes ciliary muscles.

4 This is a topical anesthetic; it will not reduce the increased intraocular pressure associated with glaucoma.

312. **4** A major goal of early postoperative care is to prevent increased intraocular pressure. (a) (SU; EV; ED; NM)

1 This is contraindicated; this increases intraocular pressure

2 Same as # 1.

3 Same as # 1.

313. **2** Internal self-stimulation increases as external stimuli decrease. (c) (ME; AN; PE; EC)

1 Blindness is an added stress that could increase anxiety, which impairs decision making; lack of visual stimuli limits data for decision making.

3 Blindness would not precipitate neurotic behav-

ior unless other emotional factors are present.

4 Lack of visual stimuli would increase restlessness, lethargy, and apathy.

314. **2** Normal plasma pH is 7.35 to 7.45; the client is in alkalosis; normal plasma bicarbonate is 23 to 25 mEq/L; the client has an excess of base bicarbonate indicating a metabolic cause for the alkalosis. (a) (SU; AS; PA; FE)

1 Normal plasma level of chloride is 95 to 105 mEq/L; the client has hypochloremia because of vomiting of gastric secretions.

3 To be acidotic the plasma pH would have to be below 7.35; in respiratory alkalosis the plasma CO_2 would be decreased below 38 torr; in metabolic alkalosis the plasma CO_2 would be normal or elevated above the normal of 38 to 42 torr.

4 Normal plasma potassium is 3.5 to 5.0 mEq/L; the potassium is within normal limits.

315. **4** The stomach produces about 3 L of secretions per day; fluid lost through vomiting can produce a fluid volume deficit. (b) (SU; AN; TC; FE)

1 This would be true for duodenal ulcer; the gastric acid secretory rate is normal in persons with gastric ulcers; in gastric ulcers there is a decreased resistance of the gastric mucosa to acid-pepsin injury and a reflux of bile-containing duodenal contents back into the stomach; the priority is fluid volume deficit, which can lead to arrhythmias and death.

2 Although this diagnosis is related, it is not the priority.

3 The shallow respirations are not related to a primary respiratory problem or pain; they are a compensatory mechanism to conserve CO_2 to combine with H^+ to form carbonic acid (H_2CO_3) and lower the plasma pH.

316. **4** Both sides of the posterior pharynx should be touched to elicit the gag reflex; absence of the reflex indicates the client is at risk for aspiration of secretions or fluid. (a) (SU; IM; TC; RE)

1 This is unsafe; the client might be able to breathe deeply and cough without an adequate gag reflex.

2 This is unsafe; this could happen even in the absence of a gag reflex.

3 This is unsafe; if the gag reflex is absent, the client would aspirate.

317. **1** There is no respiratory movement in stage 4 of anesthesia; before this stage, respirations are depressed but present. (c) (SU; AN; PA; RE)

2 Consciousness is lost in stage 2.

3 The corneal reflex is lost in the second phase of stage 3 of anesthesia.

4 The gag reflex is lost in the first phase of stage 3 of anesthesia.

318. **3** As a result of the trauma of surgery, some bleeding can be expected for 4 to 5 hours. (c) (SU; EV; PA; GI)

1 Clamping the tube would cause increased pressure on the gastric sutures from a buildup of gas and fluid.

2 Iced saline can cause vasoconstriction and unnecessary local ischemia; if bleeding were excessive, surgical intervention would be necessary.

4 This is not necessary; this is a normal occurrence.

319. **3** Rigidity and pain are hallmarks of bleeding from the suture line and/or of peritonitis; vital signs provide supporting data. (a) (SU; AS; TC; GI)

1 An analgesic may mask the symptoms delaying diagnosis.

2 Ambulation would be indicated if pain were the result of flatulence; however, rigidity is clearly associated with bleeding or peritonitis, and more data is needed.

4 This is unrelated to the symptoms presented.

320. **4** This is absolutely necessary to prevent an acute immunologic reaction if the donated blood is not compatible with the client's blood. (a) (SU; AN; TC; BI)

1 Unless there is a religious consideration, the admitting consent form would cover this procedure.

2 Blood must be kept cold until ready to use; if blood is at room temperature for 30 minutes before administration it should be returned to the blood bank; after it is started, blood must be administered within 4 hours.

3 This is the role of the physician; these laboratory results were part of the data used to determine the need for the blood.

321. **3** Transfusion reactions from mismatched blood will usually occur during the beginning of the transfusion (first 30 ml); initially keeping the infusion at a slow rate decreases the amount of blood infused, so that the nurse has an opportunity to assess the recipient's response. (b) (SU; PL; TC; BI)

1 Blood must be administered within 4 hours to prevent hemolysis from occurring before infusion.

2 Blood should be administered via gravity; volume control and peristaltic infusion devices cause hemolysis.

4 For monitoring the client's reaction, blood would not be drawn until several hours after the infusion.

322. **3** This is a sign of an acute hemolytic transfusion reaction indicating the recipient's antibodies are incompatible with the transfused red cells; pain is caused by hemolysis, agglutination, and capillary plugging in the kidneys. (b) (SU; IM; TC; BI)

1 This is unsafe; blood must be stopped first and then normal saline should be infused to keep the line patent and maintain blood volume.

2 This is unsafe; this is a classic sign of a transfusion reaction, and the blood must be immediately stopped; while the assessment was being made, more incompatible blood would be infused, increasing the severity of the reaction.

4 Same as # 2.

323. **4** Bowel sounds and flatulence indicate the return of intestinal peristalsis; peristalsis is necessary for movement of nutrients through the GI tract. (a) (SU; EV; PA; GI)

1 Dumping syndrome occurs after, not before, the ingestion of food, and would not be an indication that the client was ready to ingest food.

2 Hematocrit levels indicate blood loss; they are not affected by GI functioning.

3 Incisional pain is unrelated to intestinal peristalsis.

324. **4** Over-the-counter antacid preparations are taken to neutralize gastric acid and relieve pain. (b) (SU; EV; TC; GI)

1 Although eating food initially prevents the gastric acids from irritating the gastric walls, it can precipitate acid production and weight gain.

2 This is contraindicated; aspirin irritates gastric mucosa and promotes bleeding by preventing platelet aggregation.

3 Reduction of fluids with meals does not affect pain; it does help control symptoms of dumping syndrome.

325. **3** Excessive hunger, excessive thirst, and frequent urination are caused by the body's inability to correctly metabolize glucose. (a) (ME; AS; PA; EN)

1 Frequent urination occurs throughout a 24-hour period because glucose in the urine pulls fluid with it; the weight loss occurs with insulin-dependent diabetes mellitus, not with non–insulin-dependent diabetes mellitus.

2 Confusion is related to both severe hypoglycemia and hyperglycemia.

4 Lethargy, not irritability, results because of a lack of metabolized glucose for energy.

326. **1** Knowledge of the signs and treatment for hypoglycemia or hyperglycemia is essential for survival and critical to client health and well-being. (c) (ME; AN; ED; EN)

2 A finger stick with serum glucose monitoring is more accurate than urine S & A measurements to identify present serum glucose levels.

3 The client has non–insulin-dependent diabetes mellitus; insulin injections are not necessary.

4 Although this is important, it is not the priority.

327. **4** Improper foot care can lead to skin breakdown, poor healing, and subsequent infection. (a) (ME; IM; ED; EN)

1 This potentially increases anxiety and reduces the client's ability to learn.

2 This is only one aspect of proper foot care; foot care must be more comprehensive.

3 Same as # 2.

328. **3** Sugar provides for a rapid elevation of blood glucose; bread is a complex carbohydrate that produces a more sustained response. (b) (ME; EV; ED; EN)

1 Neither of these are fast-acting sugars; peanut butter crackers can be used to maintain the glucose level after the glucose level has been raised.

2 The fat content of chocolate candy decreases the rate of absorption of glucose.

4 Although these are fast-acting sugars, neither of them will provide a sustained response.

329. **2** Exercise improves glucose metabolism, decreasing the need for insulin production; with exercise there is a risk of developing hypoglycemia, not hyperglycemia. (b) (ME; IM; ED; EN)

1 Exercise is desirable because it improves glucose metabolism.

3 An extra Orinase tablet would probably result in hypoglycemia because exercise alone also improves glucose metabolism.

4 Control of glucose metabolism is achieved through a balance of diet, exercise, and pharmacologic therapy.

330. **1** Physiologic stress increases gluconeogenesis, requiring continued pharmacologic therapy despite an inability to eat; fluids prevent dehydration; monitoring serum glucose permits early intervention if necessary. (a) (ME; IM; ED; EN)

2 These are incomplete instructions; oral hypoglycemics should be taken, and serum glucose should be monitored.

3 Skipping the oral hypoglycemic agent could pre-

cipitate hyperglycemia; serum glucose must be monitored.

4 Food intake should be attempted to prevent acidosis; oral hypoglycemics should be taken, and serum glucose should be monitored.

331. **4** Pressure must be exerted at the arterial insertion site because the intraarterial pressure can promote bleeding. (b) (SU; IM; TC; CV)

1 General anesthesia is not used; therefore voiding is really not a concern.

2 Although this would promote venous return, keeping the client supine for 6 to 8 hours would be adequate; the client has an arterial problem, and perfusion is promoted by keeping the legs dependent, not elevated.

3 This is unsafe; ROM may be done to the unaffected extremities; ROM to the leg with the catheter insertion site could dislodge a clot and result in bleeding.

332. **1** The client is hypertensive, and intraarterial pressure is elevated; increased pressure could cause the arterial suture line to rupture. (b) (SU; AN; TC; CV)

2 The client is hypervolemic, not hypovolemic.

3 This is unlikely because the blood pressure is elevated and the client is at risk for bleeding.

4 With anaphylaxis the client would be in shock and the blood pressure would be decreased, not elevated.

333. **4** Presence of pulses and a normal skin color indicate adequate arterial perfusion and graft viability. (a) (SU; EV; ED; CV)

1 Clients with arterial insufficiency usually have paresthesias and may perceive water as cool when it is actually hot enough to cause tissue damage; the peripheral dilation produced by a hot bath would increase the work load on the heart, which is undesirable in a client with hypertension.

2 This is appropriate for venous, not arterial, problems.

3 This is contraindicated in peripheral vascular disease because it may traumatize vessels; it could cause a thrombus to become an embolus.

334. **1** The length of time a low-grade temperature is present, together with a history of night sweats and other physical findings is valuable in making a diagnosis. (b) (ME; AS; PA; BI)

2 This is not immediately relevant to the presenting signs and symptoms; more should be explored about the temperature itself before investigating causes of the temperature.

3 Same as # 2.

4 Same as # 2.

335. **4** Displacement reduces anxiety by transferring the emotions associated with an object or person to another emotionally safer object or person. (b) (ME; AS; PE; EC)

1 Dissociation is an attempt by the person to detach emotional involvement or the self from an interaction or the environment.

2 Intellectualization is the use of facts or other logical reasoning, rather than feelings, to deal with the emotional impact of a problem; this is a form of denial.

3 In projection, the individual attempts to deal with unacceptable feelings by attributing them to another.

336. **1** The nurse is using facts and knowledge to detach

the self from the emotional impact of the client's problem and decrease the anxiety it is causing. (c) (ME; AS; PE; EC)

2 This is trying to unconsciously imitate the behavior of another who is considered important, in an attempt to incorporate this important other into the self.

3 Substitution is similar to displacement; this reduces anxiety by transferring the emotions associated with an object or person to another, safer object or person.

4 Sublimation is the channeling of unacceptable thoughts or feelings into acceptable activity.

337. **2** This provides an opportunity for the client to explore concerns with the nurse. (b) (SU; IM; PE; EC)

1 The data does not indicate regression; the client is anxious, not regressed.

3 The nurse is basing the response on an incorrect interpretation of the data.

4 The data does not indicate that the client does not understand; the nurse should attempt to provide for consensual validation before coming to this conclusion.

338. **1** Women in the childbearing years should be informed of all options available to preserve ovarian function. (c) (SU; AN; TC; BI)

2 This is an incorrect statement because radiation can influence or destroy ovarian functioning.

3 This is an incorrect statement; always is too absolute.

4 Once ovarian function, including viable ova, has been destroyed, it cannot be restored.

339. **3** Postoperative pain will cause splinting, shallow breathing, and underaeration of the lung's left lower lobe because of close proximity of the spleen to the diaphragm. (c) (SU; PL; PA; BI)

1 This would be true of any surgery and is not specific to a splenectomy.

2 Same as # 1.

4 Same as # 1.

340. **1** The father is siding with his daughter and supports her when the mother accuses her of negative behavior; this is an example of coalitions or alliances; in this instance the mother may also be in denial. (c) (ME; AS; PE; EC)

2 Resignation is evident when someone gives up.

3 Scapegoating is when an individual is labeled or blamed by other family members as the cause of the family's problems.

4 Reaction formation is consciously behaving in a manner that is exactly opposite to what is really felt.

341. **3** Nausea is the most frequent and immediate side effect of Mustargen therapy. (b) (ME; EV; PA; DR)

1 This is not a side effect of Mustargen therapy.

2 Mustargen is more likely to cause urinary retention than urinary incontinence.

4 Same as # 1.

342. **3** A protocol consisting of three or four chemotherapeutic agents that attack the dividing cells at various phases of development is therapy of choice at this stage; alternating courses of different protocols may be used. (c) (ME; AN; TC; BI)

1 This is not a therapy for Hodgkin's disease at any stage; nodes may be removed for biopsy; nodes may be irradiated as part of therapy.

2 This is recommended for use in Stage III A.

4 Radiation, alone or in combination with chemotherapy, is used in stages I A, I B, II A, II B and III A.

343. **3** Congestive heart failure and dysrhythmias are the only life threatening toxic effects unique to Adriamycin. (b) (ME; EV; PA; DR)

1 This is a very uncomfortable side effect but is not life threatening.

2 This is not a side effect of Adriamycin nor of any of the other antineoplastic agents.

4 When bone marrow is depressed to precarious levels, the dose is altered and/or blood components administered before life is threatened.

344. **3** The headaches are the result of fluid retention and hypertension. (c) (ME; AS; PA; RG)

1 The client would have anorexia related to elevated toxic substances in the blood.

2 The client would have a weight gain because of the retention of fluid.

4 The client would have oliguria, not nocturia.

345. **1** Sucking on a hard candy will relieve thirst and increase carbohydrates but does not supply extra fluid. (b) (ME; IM; TC; RG)

2 Broth contains sodium, which can compound the fluid retention problem.

3 A milk shake contains both fluid and protein, which must be restricted.

4 Carbonated beverages are high in sodium and provide additional fluid, which must be restricted.

346. **1** H. streptococci, common in throat infections, initiate an antibody formation that damages the glomeruli. (b) (ME; IM; ED; RG)

2 Any fluid restriction is moderated as the client improves; fluid is allowed to prevent urinary stasis.

3 Moderate activity is helpful in preventing urinary stasis, which could precipitate an infection.

4 The alkalinity of bubble baths has been linked to urethritis, not glomerulonephritis.

347. **2** Hostility and noncompliance are both forms of anger that are associated with grieving. (b) (ME; AN; PE; EC)

1 It is an effort to maintain control over a situation that is really controlling the client; an unconscious method of coping and may be a form of denial.

3 This is a self-destructive method of coping, which could result in death.

4 This is not a conscious attempt to hurt others, but a way to relieve and reduce anxiety within the self.

348. **3** The recipient's own kidneys are not removed unless a chronic infection is present. (c) (SU; IM; ED; RG)

1 It is the left kidney that is preferred as the donor kidney because it has a larger renal vein; in actuality, both of the client's kidneys are nonfunctioning.

2 Both kidneys are left in place unless a chronic infection is present; the new kidney is placed in the right lower quadrant.

4 Same as # 2.

349. **2** An appendectomy is performed to avoid appendicitis in the future, which might be confused with rejection of the renal transplant in the right lower quadrant. (c) (SU; IM; ED; RG)

1 The intestines are not involved in a kidney transplant; therefore an examination of the colon is not necessary.

3 The stomach is not involved with renal function or with kidney transplant.

4 There is usually no problem with the bladder, but only with the kidneys.

350. **3** Hourly output is critical in assessing kidney function; decreasing urinary output is a sign of rejection. (b) (SU; EV; TC; RG)

1 It is not necessary to monitor this frequently.

2 Same as # 1.

4 This is too infrequent to monitor output immediately after transplant; it is essential to monitor output more frequently to evaluate if the new kidney is working or if it is being rejected.

351. **3** Serum creatinine, a test of renal function, measures the kidneys' ability to excrete metabolic wastes; creatinine, a nitrogenous product of protein breakdown is elevated in renal insufficiency. (b) (SU; EV; TC; RG)

1 Although intake and output would be monitored, these would not provide information about the constituents of the urine.

2 A WBC count would not reflect functioning of the new kidney.

4 This would not provide any information about filtering ability of the kidney.

352. **2** The glomerulus is not permeable to large proteins like albumin or to red blood cells. (a) (SU; EV; PA; RG)

1 The proximal tubules are responsible for regulating water, electrolytes including sodium and potassium, urea nitrogen, and pH; the byproducts of this regulation will appear in normal urine.

3 Same as # 1.

4 Same as # 1.

353. **4** Hypertension is caused by a return of the hypervolemia because of the failure of the new kidney. (b) (SU; EV; ED; RG)

1 There will be a weight gain because of fluid retention, which is indicative of failure of the transplanted kidney.

2 The client will have an elevated temperature above 100° F.

3 Urine output will be decreased or absent, depending on the degree of failure.

354. **4** These are the drugs of choice for suppression of normal immunologic response to prevent rejection of the donor kidney. (a) (SU; IM; ED; DR)

1 None of these is used for immunosuppression.

2 Only cyclosporine (Sandimmune) is used for immunosuppression.

3 Methylprednisolone (Solu-Medrol) in large doses is the only drug in this option that is used to prevent kidney rejection.

355. **1** The WBC count can drop precipitously; if leukocytes are below 3000/mm^3, the drug should be stopped to prevent irreversible bone marrow depression. (b) (SU; EV; PA; DR)

2 The WBC count would be elevated, not decreased.

3 The high creatinine level is related to kidney failure, but it does not cause leukopenia.

4 Leukocytosis, not leukopenia, would occur.

356. **1** The Mantoux is the most accurate skin test because of the testing material used and the intradermal method; no other skin test would be ap-

propriate as a follow-up; further tests are now warranted, including a chest x-ray. (a) (ME; EV; PA; RE)

2 Above 10 mm induration is a positive test result, not a doubtful test result.

3 The Tine test is less accurate than the Mantoux and would not be used as a follow-up test.

4 The test result was positive, not negative; further testing is necessary.

357. **1** The tubercle bacilli can be stained with carbol fuchsia, an acid, when the stain is applied with heat; the bacilli resist discolorization when an acid-alcohol wash is applied. (a) (ME; AS; PA; RE)

2 This reflects pulmonary status but does not identify the organism.

3 This indicates presence of antibodies but is not diagnostic for the presence of the disease.

4 Same as # 2.

358. **3** Organism mutation commonly results in drug resistance when treatment is inadequate. (b) (ME; IM; ED; DR)

1 This may raise anxiety and may not be true; combination drug therapy is always used for tuberculosis.

2 High concentrations of at least two antitubercular drugs are necessary for an extended period.

4 Both drugs are specific antitubercular drugs; pyridoxine (B$_6$) is used to prevent neuropathy associated with INH.

359. **1** Rifampin causes the body fluids, such as sweat, tears, and urine, to turn orange. (b) (ME; EV; ED; DR)

2 This is not a side effect of rifampin.

3 It is not necessary to drink large amounts of fluid with this drug; it is not nephrotoxic.

4 Damage to the eighth cranial nerve is not a side effect of rifampin; it is a side effect of another drug sometimes used to treat tuberculosis, streptomycin sulfate.

360. **4** One of the most common side effects of INH is peripheral neuritis, and Vitamin B$_6$ will counteract this problem. (b) (ME; IM; ED; DR)

1 It does help nutrition, but that is not the specific reason it is given.

2 It does not act to kill the tubercle bacilli.

3 It does not speed the destruction of the causative organism.

361. **4** Hepatitis is a toxic effect of isoniazid. (a) (ME; EV; TC; DR)

1 Weight gain would indicate improvement in the client's health status.

2 This temperature is within acceptable limits.

3 Rifampin can produce orange coloration of excretions, which is not harmful.

362. **3** In a comminuted fracture, the bone is splintered or crushed. (b) (SU; AN; PA; SK)

1 This is a compound fracture.

2 This is a green-stick fracture.

4 This is a complete fracture.

363. **2** Absence of pedal pulses indicates a lack of blood supply to the lower extremity. When pedal pulse in inaccessible, the blanching technique should be used. (b) (SU; EV; PA; SK)

1 Decreased circulatory perfusion of the foot would cause the skin temperature to decrease, but the foot could feel cool because of shock or anxiety.

3 Damage to the major blood vessels would more likely cause a decrease in blood pressure from shock.

4 The break is between the knee and the ankle, not the thigh.

364. **2** This subjective symptom is caused by stimulation of retinal cells by ocular movement. (c) (SU; AS; PA; NM)

1 Cerebral concussions do not result in this ocular symptom.

3 Glaucoma causes the perception of halos around lights, not flashes of light.

4 This is a disease of the connective tissue, not of the eye.

365. **4** The thermal inflammatory response, caused by a laser beam, results in a chorioretinal scar that holds the retina in place. (b) (SU; IM; ED; NM)

1 Radiation is not used because it destroys retinal tissue.

2 Burr holes are used in brain surgery.

3 Dermabrasion is used in acne vulgaris.

366. **4** This indicates tissue hypoxia or breakdown and should be reported to the physician. (a) (SU; IM; TC; SK)

1 This is not addressing the cause of the problem; also, other data, such as elevated temperature or increased white cells, is not present to support the presence of an infection.

2 The priority is to notify the physician; this could be done to provide relief to the client before the physician responds.

3 This is not a typical response to a cast and may indicate a complication.

367. **4** Pain is most effectively relieved when analgesia is administered at its onset, before the pain becomes intense; this prevents a pain cycle from occurring. (a) (SU; IM; ED; DR)

1 Analgesia is least effective when it is administered as pain is at its peak.

2 Adequate pain management includes dosing at intervals sufficient enough to promote comfort and prevent peaking of the pain intensity.

3 Same as # 1.

368. **2** Elevation will help control the swelling that normally occurs. (c) (SU; IM; ED; SK)

1 The leg should be put through full range of motion more than once daily.

3 Because the skin has not been exposed, it needs gentle washing to prevent breaking the skin.

4 Because the ankle has been at rest, discomfort and stiffness are expected after the cast is removed.

369. **2** When calculated:
90 ml per hour = 1.5 ml per minute (90 ÷ 60); 1.5 ml × drop factor of 15 gtt/ml = 22.5 or 23 gtt per minute. (b) (SU; AN; TC; FE)

1 This drip rate would infuse too slowly to deliver the amount ordered in the specified time.

3 This drip rate would infuse too rapidly and would deliver the ordered amount too quickly.

4 Same as # 3.

370. **1** Atropine can increase intraocular pressure because of its cycloplegic action, which paralyzes the ciliary muscles and causes pain and blindness. (a) (SU; AN; PA; DR)

2 It does not cause pupillary constriction.

3 Although this is a side effect of the drug, it is not related to glaucoma.

4 It does not affect extrinsic ocular muscles that support the orb.

371. **4** Slight hip flexion reduces tension on the abdominal musculature and the operative site. (a) (SU; PL; TC; GI)

1 This position places pressure on the abdominal wall, causing pain.

2 This position causes tension on the abdominal musculature and operative site.

3 Same as # 1.

372. **1** The inflammatory response occurs because of trauma of surgery; the T-tube maintains patency of the common bile duct until edema subsides. (b) (SU; AN; TC; GI)

2 Surgical asepsis prevents infection at the site of the incision; the T-tube is a portal of entry for microorganisms and places the client at risk for infection.

3 This is the purpose of the portable drainage system, not of a T-tube.

4 It diverts the bile out of the body into a collection bag.

373. **3** This series of diets progress from the one that makes the least metabolic demand on the client (clear liquid) to a regular diet, requiring the capability of unimpaired digestion. (a) (SU; AN; PA; GI)

1 The caloric content is not the focus in a progressive post-surgical diet.

2 Initially, a progressive diet has very little nutritional value; the focus is to rest the gastrointestinal tract immediately after surgery.

4 Initially, a limited variety of fluids is presented to rest the gastrointestinal tract; food is not included until later.

374. **1** This is the first action; the nurse should be aware that the technique is not safe, and it provides an opportunity for the offending nurse to correct the technique being used; the dressing should be immediately and correctly changed; the priority is to protect the client. (c) (ME; IM; TC; EC)

2 This depends on the policy of the institution and might be done later.

3 This may or may not be done by the observing nurse; it could also be done by an inservice educator.

4 Same as # 2.

375. **2** *Respondeat superior* is a doctrine that states employers may be held liable for torts committed by their employees. (c) (ME; AN; PE; EC)

1 *In loco parentis* refers to another person or agency assuming responsibility for a minor in the absence of the minor's parents.

3 The department of health sets standards and evaluates if these are met; the hospital's responsibility for safe care under *respondeat superior* is a legal one.

4 This is unrelated to *respondeat superior* or to a hospital's legal responsibility to its clients.

376. **2** Weight reduction decreases intraabdominal pressure, thereby decreasing the tendency to reflux into the esophagus. (c) (ME; IM; ED; GI)

1 This would increase pressure; fluid should be discouraged with meals.

3 This increases the pressure against the diaphragmatic hernia, increasing symptoms.

4 Fats decrease emptying of the stomach, extend-

ing the time period during which reflux can occur; fats should be decreased.

377. **3** Headache is most common because of the increased pressure within the arterial circulation. (a) (ME; AS; PA; CV)
  1 Flushed face may occur because of increased pressure, but it is not the most common symptom.
  2 Nosebleeds are possible when the blood pressure does reach extremely elevated levels; however, this is not a common indication.
  4 Fatigue can be associated with hypertension in the elderly, but, this is not common.

378. **1** This has a low sodium content. (c) (ME; EV; ED; FE)
  2 These vegetables are high in sodium.
  3 Processed meats are high in sodium.
  4 Shellfish is high in sodium.

379. **4** Lasix may cause hypovolemia, which can result in orthostatic hypotension with sudden position changes. (a) (ME; EV; PA; DR)
  1 Lasix does not cause photophobia.
  2 This has no relationship to Lasix.
  3 Citrus fruits, particularly oranges, are high in potassium and should be encouraged when the client is taking Lasix because this medication can cause hypokalemia.

380. **1** Lasix enhances the excretion of potassium, producing symptoms of hypokalemia, such as hyporeflexia. (c) (ME; EV; PA; DR)
  2 This is not a side effect of Lasix.
  3 Same as # 2.
  4 Same as # 2.

381. **1** Nipride decreases blood pressure by both of these mechanisms. (b) (ME; AN; PA; DR)
  2 It should decrease peripheral resistance by dilating peripheral vessels.
  3 It decreases cardiac workload by decreasing preload and afterload.
  4 Actually, Nipride may increase the heart rate as a response to the vasodilation.

382. **4** This attempts to collect adequate data to plan the most appropriate intervention. (b) (ME; AS; TC; CV)
  1 This alone will not guarantee compliance once the client goes home; the client has the right to accept or reject therapy.
  2 Same as # 1.
  3 Table salt is contraindicated on a 2 g sodium diet.

383. **2** Inderal and Lanoxin both exert a negative chronotropic effect. (b) (ME; AN; PA; DR)
  1 These drugs reduce headache associated with hypertension.
  3 These drugs may cause hypotension.
  4 These drugs may depress nodal conduction.

384. **3** This position will neither raise intracranial pressure nor interfere with respirations and will permit oral secretions to drain from the mouth by gravity. (b) (ME; IM; TC; NM)
  1 This could compromise the airway by permitting the tongue to fall to the posterior pharynx and obstruct the airway.
  2 Elevating the head of the bed could compromise vital functions by compressing the brain stem.
  4 This is contraindicated because it may increase intracranial pressure.

385. **4** Increased intracranial pressure is manifested by

sluggish pupils and elevation of the systolic blood pressure. (a) (ME; AN; PA; NM)
  1 Spinal shock is manifested by a lowered systolic blood pressure with no pupillary changes.
  2 Hypovolemic shock is indicated by a decrease in systolic pressure and tachycardia with no changes in pupillary reaction.
  3 Transtentorial herniation is manifested by dilated pupils and severe posturing.

386. **4** This cancer is usually asymptomatic in the early stages; the stomach accomodates the mass. (a) (SU; AN; PA; GI)
  1 This is untrue; it can be accurately diagnosed by gastric washings or biopsy.
  2 This is untrue; this cancer is painless in its early stages.
  3 This is untrue; this is typical of Hodgkin's disease, not gastric carcinoma.

387. **3** Often the thoracic cavity is entered for a complete resection, necessitating a chest tube. (b) (SU; PL; ED; GI)
  1 There would be no physiologic necessity for this position.
  2 The client would ambulate early to minimize the hazards of immobility.
  4 Fluids are contraindicated until the suture line has healed and nasogastric suction is no longer being used.

388. **1** This response indicates recognition of the client's need to use denial and opens the way for discussion of feelings. (c) (SU; IM; PE; EC)
  2 This forces reality on the client and blocks discussion of feelings.
  3 This reply focuses on the surgery, which is not the concern expressed by the client.
  4 This changes the subject and moves away from the client's feelings.

389. **3** Large amounts of blood or excessive bloody drainage 12 hours postoperatively must be reported immediately. (b) (SU; IM; TC; GI)
  1 This must be ordered by the physician; this is not an independent function of nurse; also, although ice might constrict the vessels, 30 ml would not be effective.
  2 This is contraindicated; accumulation of secretions would cause pressure on suture line; this prevents further observation of drainage.
  4 This is an unsafe intervention at this time; physician should be notified.

390. **3** Well-differentiated cells are associated with a positive prognosis, whereas undifferentiated cells are ominous. (a) (SU; PL; PE; EC)
  1 This is inappropriate because the prognosis is fairly positive.
  2 Although the cancer could recur, a primary lesion in another location would not be expected.
  4 The client's pathology report provides specific data that is more significant than general statistics.

391. **2** Capacity is reduced because of surgery; smaller, frequent feedings with controlled bulk prevent dumping syndrome. (a) (SU; EV; ED; GI)
  1 This is not a realistic plan for a client without a stomach.
  3 This is not usually the case; a more normal diet is the goal.
  4 The diet should be high in protein, low in carbohydrates, and normal in fats.

392. **4** Statistics demonstrate that these are the most likely sites for metastasis of this tumor. (b) (SU; AN; PA; GI)
    1 These are routes of metastasis, not sites.
    2 It is less likely that the tumor will spread to these areas.
    3 Same as # 2.
393. **4** Intrinsic factor is lost with removal of the stomach, and vitamin B_{12} is needed to maintain the hemoglobin level. (b) (SU; PL; PA; GI)
    1 Pancreatic enzymes should be normal because surgery has not altered this function.
    2 This would not be a routine expectation.
    3 Adequate diet, fluid intake, and exercise should prevent constipation.
394. **3** The mechanism is unclear, but this is probably caused by fluid shifts. (b) (SU; AN; TC; RE)
    1 This is untrue; this is done only occasionally to slow development of new effusion in clients with recurrent effusions.
    2 This is untrue; it can provide dramatic relief and improvement.
    4 This is untrue; dyspnea should be immediately relieved; if dyspnea increases, pneumothorax should be suspected.
395. **2** Compression of the lung by fluid that accumulates at the base of the lungs reduces expansion and air exchange. (c) (SU; AS; PA; RE)
    1 Dullness is produced on percussion of the involved area.
    3 If there is tracheal deviation, it is away from the involved side.
    4 There is no fluid in the alveoli, so no rales are produced.
396. **1** Clients with pleuritic disease are prone to develop pneumonia because of impaired expansion, air exchange, and lung drainage. (b) (SU; PL; TC; RE)
    2 Sedation is not therapeutic because the client must be alert for deep breathing and coughing.
    3 Coughing should not be suppressed; it enhances expansion, air exchange, and lung drainage.
    4 Oral fluids are encouraged; pulmonary edema does not develop unless the client has severe cardiovascular disease.
397. **2** Tension is placed on the pleura at the height of inspiration and causes pain. (c) (SU; AS; PA; RE)
    1 This may indicate pulmonary infection.
    3 Same as #1.
    4 This is typical of congestive heart failure.
398. **1** Increased negative pressure on inspiration causes fluid to rise; decrease in the negative intrapleural pressure on expiration causes fluid to fall. (b) (SU; EV; PA; RE)
    2 Suction is too high; bubbling should be gentle.
    3 This would indicate an air leak.
    4 This would indicate that there is an obstruction in the drainage tubing or the suction is too low; there should be a slight increase in fluid in this chamber postoperatively.
399. **2** Restlessness is an early sign of cerebral hypoxia. (b) (SU; AS; PA; RE)
    1 Lightheadedness is a sign of respiratory alkalosis.
    3 Tachycardia, not bradycardia, would occur.
    4 Tachypnea, not bradypnea, would occur.
400. **3** The urinary system compensates by retaining

H^+ ions, which become part of bicarbonate ion; the bicarbonate becomes elevated and raises the pH to near normal; the normal HCO_3 is 22 to 26 mEq/L, and the normal pH is 7.35 to 7.45. (c) (SU; AS; PA; FE)
    1 The normal Po_2 is 80 to 95 mmHg; this is within normal range.
    2 The normal Pco_2 is 35 to 45 mmHg; although in compensated respiratory acidosis the Pco_2 may be elevated, it is the elevated HCO_3 level that indicates compensation.
    4 This K^+ level is 3.5 to 5.0 mEq/L, which is within normal range; serum potassium is not significant in identifying compensated respiratory acidosis.
401. **3** This pause allows added time for gaseous exchange at the alveolar capillary beds. (c) (SU; EV; ED; RE)
    1 Inhalation should be through the nose to moisten, filter, and warm the air.
    2 This decreases the effectiveness of respirations.
    4 The expiratory phase should be lengthened, and exhalation should be through pursed lips.
402. **4** The enlarged liver is caused by long-term respiratory acidosis with increased pulmonary pressures that eventually cause right-sided heart enlargement and failure (cor pulmonale); the elevated pressures cause backup pressure in the hepatic circulation. (c) (SU; AN; PA; RE)
    1 Liver hypoxia would cause atrophy and necrosis of cells, not enlargement.
    2 Right-sided heart failure with increased pressure in the ascending vena cava causes increased pressure in the hepatoportal system, causing an enlarged liver, not acidosis.
    3 These are the result of hepatic portal hypertension, not the cause of an enlarged liver.
403. **2** Moist heat increases circulation and decreases muscle tension, which helps relieve chronic stiffness. (a) (ME; IM; PA; SK)
    1 Inactivity promotes stiffness.
    3 This is related to muscle fatigue, not to stiffness of joints.
    4 Although this is advisable for someone with arthritis, it will not relieve morning stiffness.
404. **1** This is caused by inflammation of the synovium, resulting in edema, vascular congestion, fibrin exudate, and cellular infiltrate. (a) (ME; AN; PA; SK)
    2 This is unrelated to rheumatoid arthritis.
    3 Although autoimmunity is believed to be a factor in rheumatoid arthritis, it causes inflammation of the synovial lining, not interstitial fluid.
    4 Rheumatoid arthritis does not cause fluid to collect in interstitial spaces, but it causes edema of the synovial joints.
405. **3** This is necessary because ibuprofen is nephrotoxic and hepatotoxic and prolongs bleeding time. (b) (ME; EV; ED; DR)
    1 This is important for all clients with arthritis; it is not related to ibuprofen.
    2 Ibuprofen causes epigastic distress and occult bleeding; it should be taken with meals or milk to reduce these adverse reactions.
    4 Motrin does not cause postural hypotension.
406. **1** Palpation will elicit tenderness because pressure stimulates nerve endings and causes pain. (a) (ME; AN; PA; SK)

2 It is already swollen, and the pressure causes pain.

3 Nodules associated with rheumatoid arthritis are not caused by pressure; they occur spontaneously in about 25% of individuals with rheumatoid arthritis and are formed of collagen fibers, exudate, and cellular debris.

4 These are present in gout, not arthritis; they are composed of sodium urate.

407. **2** The *Salmonella* organism thrives in warm, moist environments; washing, cooking, and refrigeration of food limits the growth of or eliminates the organism. (a) (ME; AS; PA; GI)

1 Salmonellosis is unrelated to cancer.

3 Salmonellosis is caused by the *Salmonella* organism, not stress.

4 The *Salmonella* organism is ingested; it is not an airborne or blood-borne infection.

408. **2** This medical aseptic technique contains contaminated articles and reduces the possibility of transmitting the organisms to others. (b) (ME; PL; TC; GI)

1 Enteric precautions for adults can be handled in a semi-private room as long as fecally contaminated articles are disinfected or double bagged and sent for appropriate disposal.

3 Type of exposure, not length of exposure, increases risk of transmission; visitors are allowed, as long as those having close contact wear gowns and gloves.

4 The organism is not transmitted via the airborne route.

409. **3** The *Salmonella* bacilli can be visualized via microscopic examination. (a) (ME; AS; PA; GI)

1 Although this test might be done, it is not definitive for the diagnosis of salmonellosis.

2 Same as # 1.

4 Same as # 1.

410. **3** Fluids of dextrose and normal saline are administered to prevent profound dehydration caused by an excessive loss of water and salts through diarrheal output. (c) (ME; PL; PA; GI)

1 These are not used when there is a possibility of bacterial infection because slowed peristalsis decreases excretion of the *Salmonella* organism.

2 Same as # 1.

4 This is not necessary; salmonellosis is an infection, not a condition caused by hyperacidity.

411. **3** The body fights acidosis by H^+ exchange, which results in excretion of excess H^+ in the urine, a compensatory mechanism to raise serum pH. (c) (ME; AN; PA; FE)

1 In acidosis the pH of the blood is decreased.

2 Plasma bicarbonates are decreased; this is a classic indication of metabolic acidosis.

4 In acidosis the respiratory center in the medulla is stimulated to increase respiration and blow off CO_2, which is carried to the lung as carbonic acid (H_2CO_3); lowering carbonic acid raises serum pH.

412. **4** A cold environment limits growth of microorganisms. (a) (ME; EV; TC; GI)

1 This promotes the growth of microorganisms because they thrive in warm, moist environments.

2 This promotes the growth of microorganisms because the stuffing would still be warm for a period of time before the refrigerator's cold environment cooled the center of the bird; poultry should be stuffed immediately before being cooked.

3 All food should be refrigerated before and after it is cooked to limit the growth of microorganisms.

413. **4** Incomplete oxidation of fat results in fatty acids that further break down to ketones. (c) (ME; AN; PA; EN)

1 Carbohydrates do not contain fatty acids, which are broken down into ketones.

2 Potassium is not oxidized; in hypokalemia or hyperkalemia no ketones are formed.

3 Protein metabolism results in nitrogenous waste production, causing an elevated blood urea nitrogen (BUN).

414. **2** Potassium is the principal intracellular cation, and during ketoacidosis it moves out of cells into the extracellular compartment to replace K^+ lost due to glucose-induced osmotic diuresis; overstimulation of the cardiac muscle results. (c) (ME; AS; PA; EN)

1 P waves are abnormal because the PR interval may be prolonged and the P wave may be lost; however, the T wave is peaked, not depressed; the T wave is depressed in hypokalemia.

3 Initially, the QT segment is short and as the K^+ level rises, the QRS complex widens; the ST segment becomes depressed.

4 The PR interval is prolonged and the P wave may be lost; QRS complexes and thus T waves become irregular, and the rate does not necessarily change.

415. **4** These are classic signs of hypokalemia that occur when potassium levels are reduced as potassium reenters cells with glucose. (c) (ME; EV; PA; EN)

1 Symptoms of hyponatremia are nausea, malaise, and changes in mental status.

2 Symptoms of hypoglycemia are weakness, nervousness, tachycardia, diaphoresis, irritability, and pallor.

3 Symptoms of hypercalcemia are lethargy, nausea, vomiting, parasthesias, and personality changes.

416. **4** These vegetables are under the vegetable exchange, as are asparagus, broccoli, and mushrooms. (a) (ME; EV; PA; EN)

1 These are starchy vegetables and are listed as bread exchanges.

2 Same as # 1.

3 These food items are from the bread exchange.

417. **3** NPH insulin's onset of action is 1 to 2 hours, peak action is 8 to 12 hours, and duration of action is 18 to 24 hours; if hypoglycemia were to occur it would happen between 4 PM and 8 PM. (a) (ME; EV; PA; DR)

1 Regular insulin peaks in 2 to 4 hours.

2 Semilente insulin peaks in 4 to 7 hours.

4 No insulin peaks in 12 to 14 hours; however, protamine zinc insulin and ultralente insulin peak in 16 to 18 hours.

418. **1** These signs of hypoglycemia are related to increased sympathetic nervous system activity. (b) (ME; EV; PA; DR)

2 These are signs of hyperglycemia.

3 Same as # 2.

4 Same as # 2.

419. **1** Increased activity and stress precipitate exacerbation of symptoms because nerve impulses fail

to pass to muscles at the myoneural junction; theories include inadequate acetylcholine, excessive cholinesterase, or a nonresponse of the muscle fibers to acetylcholine. (b) (ME; AS; PA; NM)

2 Strength decreases with progressive activity.

3 Rest promotes a decrease in symptoms because the demand for muscle contraction is reduced.

4 Muscle weakness and fatigue come on quickly and disappear rapidly with rest in the initial stages of the disease.

420. **3** Facial muscles innervated by the cranial nerves are often affected; dysphagia, ptosis, and diplopia are common. (b) (ME; AS; PA; NM)

1 This is associated with Parkinson's disease.

2 This is associated with multiple sclerosis.

4 It is a neuromuscular disease with lower motor neuron characteristics, not CNS symptoms.

421. **4** This drug is a cholinergic and an anticholinesterase; it blocks the action of cholinesterase at the myoneural junction and inhibits the destruction of acetylcholine. (b) (ME; AS; PA; DR)

1 Results will be added to the data base, but they are non-specific.

2 Same as # 1.

3 This is a slower-acting anticholinesterase drug that is frequently ordered to treat myasthenia gravis; Tensilon is used, instead of this drug, to diagnose myasthenia gravis because when injected IV it immediately increases muscle strength.

422. **2** The drug should be taken as ordered, usually before meals, to limit dysphagia and possible aspiration. (a) (ME; EV; TC; DR)

1 This is unsafe; the drug should be taken with milk to prevent GI irritation; it is usually taken about 30 to 60 minutes before meals.

3 Action will begin within 30 minutes and start to peak in an hour.

4 This is not necessary; it may be kept at room temperature.

423. **4** A positive response to the administration of Tensilon indicates myasthenic crisis, whereas an increase in the severity of symptoms indicates cholinergic crisis. (c) (ME; PL; TC; DR)

1 This is the treatment for cholinergic crisis.

2 This is the antidote for heparin.

3 This is a narcotic antagonist.

424. **3** Excessive weakness and impaired diaphragmatic innervation result in a depressed ability to breathe; maintaining effective breathing and a patent airway take priority. (c) (ME; AN; TC; NM)

1 This is not the priority nursing diagnosis at this time.

2 Same as # 1.

4 Same as # 1.

425. **3** Remissions and exacerbations are common; a decrease in symptoms is related to rest and adequate blood levels of anticholinesterases; an increase in symptoms is related to physical activity, stress, and inadequate blood levels of anticholinesterases. (c) (ME; AS; PA; NM)

1 Anticholinesterase drugs will increase muscle strength.

2 The proximal muscles are more involved than the distal muscles.

4 Exercise decreases muscle strength.

426. **2** Respiratory infections place people with myas-

thenia gravis at high risk because they do not cough effectively and may develop pneumonia or airway obstruction. (a) (ME; EV; ED; NM)

1 Activity should be done earlier in the day before the energy reserve is depleted; periods of activity should be alternated with periods of rest.

3 This is unsafe; the client should eat sitting up to prevent aspiration.

4 This is contraindicated; these potentiate weakness because of their effect on the myoneural junction.

427. **4** The least amount of breast engorgement occurs at this time, limiting lumps that may occur because of fluid accumulation. (a) (ME; AS; PA; IT)

1 Breast engorgement begins before ovulation and does not subside until after menses; engorgement interferes with accurate palpation.

2 Inaccurate assessment could result because examination would occur at different times of the menstrual cycle; accurate comparisons could not be made from month to month; this is appropriate for postmenopausal women.

3 Same as # 1.

428. **1** Serous or bloody discharge from the nipple is abnormal. (b) (ME; AS; TC; IT)

2 The right hand should examine the left breast because this allows the flattened fingers to palpate the entire breast including the tail (upper, outer quadrant toward the axilla) and axillary area.

3 A small pillow or rolled towel should be placed under the scapula of the side being examined.

4 The flat part of the fingers, not the palm or fingertips, should be used for palpation.

429. **2** Compression of the breast flattens mammary tissue and maximizes the penetration of the breast by x-rays; this is especially important for the dense breast tissue of adolescents, young nulliparous women, and women with large breasts. (a) (ME; IM; ED; IT)

1 This is usually done with sonography.

3 This is not necessary.

4 The American Cancer Society recommends that women at high risk for breast cancer (the client's sister had breast cancer) should have routine mammography regardless of age or relationship to menopause.

430. **2** A needle attached to a syringe is advanced into the lump, which has been manually immobilized by the examiner's fingers, and fluid is withdrawn for cytologic examination. (a) (SU; EV; ED; IT)

1 This approach is still used for clients who do not want to wait between examination of tissue and a necessary mastectomy.

3 This is sometimes done with early, small, or nonpalpable lesions to facilitate localization of the area targeted for surgical biopsy.

4 This is a tissue biopsy.

431. **2** This identifies the client's feelings and provides an opportunity for further discussion. (b) (SU; IM; PE; EC)

1 Although this echoes the client's statement, it does not identify a feeling.

3 This denies the client's feelings and focuses on information; the client may be too emotionally distraught to be able to construct or verbalize questions.

4 This provides false reassurance and cuts off com-

munication; introduction of the word *cancer* could increase anxiety.

432. **4** The negative pressure of a portable wound drainage system exerts a sucking force that pulls fluid toward the collection chamber. (a) (SU; AN; PA; IT)

   1 Gravity is the environmental force that pulls weight toward the center of the earth; an indwelling urinary catheter allows urine to flow by gravity from the bladder to a collection bag placed below the level of the bladder.

   2 Osmosis occurs when solvent moves from a solution of lesser concentration to one of greater solute concentration when the two solutions are separated by a semipermeable membrane; fluid moving from the interstitial compartment into the intracellular compartment uses osmosis.

   3 Active transport occurs when ions move across a cell membrane against a concentration gradient with the assistance of the expenditure of metabolic energy; the sodium-potassium pump uses active transport.

433. **2** Once the drugs that interfere with cell division are stopped, the hair will grow back; sometimes the hair will be a different color or texture. (a) (SU; IM; PE; EC)

   1 Alopecia is a common side effect of chemotherapy.

   3 Hair loss persists while the drugs are being received; once the drugs are withdrawn, the hair grows back.

   4 Although ice caps on the head and rubber bands around the scalp have been used to try to limit alopecia, they have not been particularly effective.

434. **2** Putting the upper arm and leg toward the side to be turned uses body weight to facilitate turning; the spine is kept straight. (c) (SU; AN; ED; NM)

   1 This could be done if another person were turning the client; however, when turning alone in this position the client would have no leverage and turning would probably result in twisting the spinal column.

   3 This would interfere with turning because the bent leg almost becomes an obstacle and provides a force opposite to the leverage needed to turn.

   4 This is unsafe; this would result in twisting the spinal column.

435. **2** This identifies the underlying client concern in a non-judgmental way by not actually addressing the behavior; it provides the opportunity for an exploration of concerns and feelings. (b) (SU; IM; PE; EC)

   1 Although it points out behavior, this is aggresive and may produce a defensive response instead of an exploration of concern and feelings.

   3 This response minimizes the client's feelings and provides false reassurance.

   4 Same as # 3.

436. **2** These drugs tend to irritate the gastric mucosa and should be taken with food or milk. (b) (SU; EV; TC; DR)

   1 This could result in toxicity; the dosage should be prescribed by the physician.

   3 This is an expected side effect; safety precautions are indicated, but the drug should not be discontinued.

4 To limit GI irritation these drugs should be taken with food or milk.

437. **2** This is contraindicated; the prolonged sitting position places excessive body weight and stress on the surgical area. (b) (SU; EV; ED; NM)

   1 This maintains lordosis of the small of the back and provides proper support.

   3 This prevents excessive pressure on the musculature and vertebral column.

   4 This relieves pressure on the back and promotes comfort in bed.

438. **2** This is done while in the supine position before the body is subjected to the force of gravity in a vertical position; anatomic landmarks are easier to locate for correct appplication of the brace, intraabdominal organs have not shifted toward the pelvic floor by gravity, and the brace is applied before transferring from supine to standing position. (b) (SU; PL; PA; NM)

   1 This is unsafe; it should be applied while in the supine position before getting out of bed and should be worn the entire day for support.

   3 The brace should be applied while in the supine position, not the sitting position.

   4 Twisting exercises are contraindicated because they exert excessive pressure on the operative site.

439. **1** As the heart contracts, an expanding midline mass can be palpated to the left of the umbilicus. (b) (SU; AS; PA; CV)

   2 There is no disease in the intestinal tract; this finding is associated with intestinal obstruction.

   3 These are not definitive for abdominal aortic aneurysm; shock and pallor and probably death would occur if the aneurysm ruptured.

   4 This is not definitive for abdominal aortic aneurysm.

440. **2** Immediate surgical intervention to clamp the aorta is necessary for survival; the aneurysm has ruptured. (a) (SU; IM; TC; CV)

   1 Sedatives mask important signs and symptoms.

   3 This may be initiated in anticipation of surgery, but notifying the physician is the priority.

   4 This may be intiated, but notifying the physician is the priority.

441. **4** When the aneurysm ruptures, shock ensues because fluid volume depletion occurs as the heart continues to pump blood out of the ruptured vessel. (b) (SU; AN; PA; FE)

   1 This type of shock results from humoral or toxic substances acting directly on the blood vessels and causing vasodilation.

   2 This type of shock results from decreased neuromuscular tone, which causes decreased vasoconstriction.

   3 This type of shock results from a decrease in cardiac output.

442. **4** The respiratory process is essential to life and therefore is the first priority. (a) (SU; AS; TC; RE)

   1 The Trendelenburg position decreases respiratory functioning and should be avoided.

   2 This may eventually be done, but respiratory assessment is the priority.

   3 Same as # 2.

443. **2** In shock the heart rate accelerates to increase blood flow and oxygen to body tissues. (a) (SU; AS; PA; CV)

1 With shock there would be hypotension.

3 In shock respirations would be increased and shallow.

4 For a client in shock there would be a decreased urinary output because of the lowered glomerular filtration rate.

444. **2** Decreased O_2 increases conversion of pyruvic acid to lactic acid, resulting in metabolic acidosis. (c) (SU; AN; PA; FE)

1 Respiratory alkalosis could occur in early shock because of rapid, shallow breathing, but in late shock metabolic acidosis occurs.

3 Pco_2 will be increased in profound shock.

4 Hyperkalemia would occur because of renal shutdown; hypokalemia could occur in early shock.

445. **2** Blood replacement is needed to increase the O_2 carrying capacity of the blood; normal hematocrit for women is 37% to 47%. (a) (SU; PL; TC; BI)

1 Dextran does expand blood volume, but it causes cell aggregation, which aggravates existing decreased tissue perfusion.

3 Serum albumin helps maintain volume but does not affect hemoglobin.

4 Ringer's lactate does not increase the O_2 carrying capacity of the blood.

446. **3** With increased intraabdominal pressure the abdominal wall will become rigid and tender. (b) (SU; AS; PA; GI)

1 The WBC count would increase because of the inflammatory process.

2 The pulse rate will increase in an effort to compensate for impending septic shock.

4 Peristalsis and associated bowel sounds will decrease or be absent in the presence of increased intraabdominal pressure.

447. **1** The nurse at the scene of an accident should function in a responsible and prudent manner; the use of a soiled cloth on an open wound is not prudent, nor is the independent transfer of an accident victim from the scene. (b) (ME; EV; PE; EC)

2 Although the Nurse Practice Act defines nursing, it does not provide detailed standards for practice; the nurse's action was not prudent.

3 The nurse's action was not what a reasonably prudent nurse would do and is therefore not protected.

4 The nurse's intervention was not prudent and placed the client in jeopardy; the nurse was not practicing medicine, but attempting to provide first aid.

448. **4** The amount of irrigant instilled into the bladder must be deducted from the total output to determine the amount of urine voided. (a) (SU; IM; TC; RG)

1 This is unnecessary; the bladder is constantly being irrigated with GU irrigant.

2 Unless irrigant is subtracted from the output, the total would be inaccurate.

3 Specific gravity measurement would be inaccurate; urine is diluted with GU irrigant.

449. **1** The client who is confined to bed should be encouraged to move in the bed to prevent prolonged pressure on any one skin surface. (b) (SU; PL; PA; IT)

2 Range-of-motion exercises move joints to prevent contractures; they do not relieve prolonged pressure.

3 This does not prevent prolonged pressure although it can help decrease skin breakdown by allowing air to circulate beneath the client.

4 This will help promote peripheral circulation, but prolonged pressure must be avoided.

450. **2** Reliving the experience brings back the feelings, such as anxiety and fear, associated with it; the symptoms described reflect sympathetic nervous system activity. (b) (ME; AN; PA; EC)

1 These symptoms are indicative of a sympathetic, not a parasympathetic, response.

3 The increased pulse and restlessness could indicate bleeding; however, the other data presented supports anxiety; additional assessment would be necessary to identify bleeding.

4 Not enough data is present to recognize the client's usual method of seeking sympathy.

451. **1** Stress ulcers are asymptomatic until they produce massive hematemesis and rectal bleeding. (b) (ME; AS; PA; GI)

2 A gradual drop in hematocrit indicates slow blood loss.

3 Sudden massive bleeding occurs; not the slow oozing that causes melena.

4 Shock is the outcome of massive hemorrhage; it would not be unexplained because the sudden gastrointestinal bleeding would be seen.

452. **3** Increased acidity caused by the stress occurring during burns and crushing injuries contributes to the formation of Curling's ulcer; Tagamet, a histamine$_2$ antagonist, decreases the formation of gastric acid, and Maalox, an antacid, neutralizes it once it is formed. (a) (ME; IM; ED; DR)

1 This does not explain how the drug works and why it is prescribed for this client.

2 Same as # 1.

4 These drugs do not decrease irritability of the bowel; their purpose is to decrease gastrointestinal irritation.

453. **3** Maalox can cause diarrhea and sometimes needs to be given alternately with another more constipating antacid. (b) (ME; AN; PA; DR)

1 Although diet can affect elimination, no data supports this conclusion.

2 Diarrhea is not a side effect of cimetidine; constipation is.

4 Immobility causes constipation, not diarrhea.

454. **2** A patent nasogastic tube prevents distention and compression in the surgical area. (b) (SU; IM; TC; GI)

1 The client is prone to skin breakdown; movement should be encouraged.

3 Replacement of vitamins is a dependent function; the physician must order or adjust the dosage.

4 Tube feedings are contraindicated because peristalsis is absent, and the feeding would place pressure on the suture line.

455. **4** Formation of lipase necessary for digestion of fats is an exocrine function; the endocrine function is to secrete insulin, which is a hormone essential in carbohydrate metabolism. (c) (SU; IM; TC; GI)

1 Although it is necessary to avoid alcohol, this is

not related to exocrine functioning of the pancreas.

2 Deficiencies of both may occur because of poor intake, but these deficiencies are not specifically related to exocrine or endocrine pancreatic functioning.

3 Fluid and electrolyte problems are not related specifically to exocrine or endocrine pancreatic functioning.

456. **3** Rapid administration can cause glucose overload, leading to osmotic diuresis and dehydration; slowing the infusion decreases glucose overload. (b) (SU; IM; TC; GI)

1 The client's headache should disappear with oral fluid replacement; analgesics are not indicated.

2 Signs of bowel obstruction are not present.

4 Stopping the flow would jeopardize the central line; slowing the infusion will give the client's body a chance to handle the excess glucose.

457. **3** These are realistic, productive, and constructive ways of using this time. (a) (ME; AN; PE; EC)

1 These are signs of depression.

2 Going from physician to physician shows disbelief, denial, or desperation.

4 This indicates anger, not acceptance.

458. **4** This is a legal requirement of participating institutions to protect the individuals involved. (a) (SU; AN; PE; EC)

1 Active euthanasia is a direct act to shorten a person's life and is illegal.

2 This is untrue; no age restrictions exist.

3 Legal statutes make certain the opposite is true.

459. **1** These tests provide a measure of thyroxine production, a disturbance of which is associated with the client's symptoms. (a) (SU; AS; PA; EN)

2 Prothrombin time (PT) and partial thromboplastin time (PTT) assess blood coagulation.

3 VDRL test is for syphilis; the CBC assesses the hematopoietic system.

4 This measures the kind and amount of circulating barbiturates; the client's symptoms would not be associated with barbiturate intake.

460. **1** This drug does not interfere with thyroxine already stored in the gland; symptoms remain until the hormone is depleted. (c) (SU; PL; ED; DR)

2 Absorption is not affected by the presence of food in the stomach.

3 This drug is not irritating to mucosal tissue, and no special precautions are necessary.

4 Duration of therapy varies from several months to several years, with 1 year being the average.

461. **3** This relieves tension on the incision and limits the risk of dehiscence. (b) (SU; IM; ED; EN)

1 Coughing should be avoided during the early postoperative period to prevent trauma to the operative site.

2 This should be avoided until advised by the physician, usually after the sutures or skin clips are removed.

4 Pressure against the operative area is not necessary to promote the integrity of the incision, and it may inhibit swallowing.

462. **3** Injury to the parathyroid gland results in a deficiency of parathormone, which decreases calcium levels in the blood. (c) (SU; EV; PA; EN)

1 This is characterized by a weak, thready pulse and hypotension.

2 This is characterized by tachycardia, hyperpyrexia, and exacerbation of thyroid symptoms.

4 Symptoms are generalized weakness, decrease in reflexes, shallow respirations, and cardiac arrythmias.

463. **1** Thyroid crisis is severe hyperthyroidism; excessive amounts of thyroxine increase the metabolic rate, thereby raising the pulse and temperature. (b) (SU; AS; PA; EN)

2 Because of the increased metabolic rate the pulse and respiratory rates increase to meet the body's oxygen needs.

3 The blood pressure will rise to meet the oxygen demand caused by the increased metabolic rate during thyroid crisis.

4 During thyroid crisis there is usually no increase in the difference between the apical and peripheral pulse rates (pulse deficit).

464. **2** Dry, thickened skin and cold intolerance are characteristic adaptations to low serum thyroxine. (a) (SU; EV; ED; EN)

1 Low thyroxine levels reduce the metabolic rate, resulting in weight gain and bradycardia, not tachycardia.

3 Muscle cramping is associated with hypocalcemia.

4 Low thyroxine levels reduce the metabolic rate, resulting in fatigue, and should not increase the pulse rate.

465. **3** After thyroidectomy the thyroxine output is usually inadequate to maintain an appropriate metabolic rate. (a) (SU; AN; PA; EN)

1 Hypothyroidism is a decrease in thyroid functioning.

2 In hypothyroidism the level of thyroid stimulating hormone (TSH) from the pituitary is usually increased.

4 Atrophy of the thyroid tissue remaining after surgery does not occur.

466. **1** Alkylating drugs frequently cause severe bone marrow depression because they affect rapidly dividing cells. (c) (ME; EV; PA; DR)

2 These are common side effects with the administration of steroids.

3 These are complications of hormonal therapy.

4 These are complications more common with antimetabolites.

467. **4** Stomatitis and hyperuricemia are possible complications of therapy; therefore oral care and hydration are very important. (a) (ME; PL; PA; DR)

1 This is false reasssurance; CML is not curable.

2 Abnormal bleeding is a common problem and thus injections are contraindicated; rest is important for increased fatigability.

3 Hot substances are avoided because of frequent occurrence of stomatitis.

468. **2** Aspirin is contraindicated in the presence of bleeding tendencies because of its inhibitory effect on platelet aggregation. (b) (ME; IM; TC; DR)

1 The antacid will reduce the gastric irritation common with aspirin but will not alter its effect on platelets.

3 The dosage is within acceptable limits.

4 Action needs to be taken when the temperature is above 101° F.

469. **4** Because of the client's history and the site of the

surgery, thrombi are likely to develop; activity is a preventive measure. (b) (SU; PL;TC; CV)
1 Getting out of bed will provide little exercise if the client only sits in a chair; also, an order is needed.
2 This alone will not prevent thrombi; activity is necessary.
3 Although body alignment is important for all clients, it will not discourage thrombus formation.

470. **3** Muscle contraction associated with walking prevents edema and pooling of blood in the extremities. (a) (ME; IM; ED; CV)
1 This is inactivity, and movement is required.
2 This is an inactive position, and no exercise is involved; this will not prevent thrombus formation.
4 This does not include movement, which is essential to prevent thrombus formation.

471. **4** This helps the client express concern and examine feelings. (a) (ME; IM; PE; EC)
1 The client's apprehension is legitimate and should be explored; the misconception that the clot will hurt the heart can be explored later.
2 This was not the client's concern and would not meet the need to explore feelings; this could be done later.
3 This is inappropriate; it disregards the client's expressed fears and would increase anxiety.

472. **1** Seeing the exercise demonstrated will reinforce the verbal explanation. (b) (ME; IM; ED; CV)
2 This statement is too vague; it does not explain how to move them.
3 This statement is too vague and thus may be ineffective; the time period should be stipulated.
4 This is open to interpretation and therefore may be ineffective.

473. **4** This provides support and promotes venous return; applying stockings while legs are horizontal before arising ensures that stockings are applied before dependent edema occurs. (b) (ME; IM; ED; CV)
1 Although helpful, it will not provide continuous support for the veins, which is mandatory.
2 These need to be ordered by the physician.
3 Warm soaks resolve inflammation; they do not prevent development of thrombophlebitis.

474. **1** Sorbitrate dilates the coronary vasculature, improving the supply of oxygen to the hypoxic myocardium. (b) (ME; IM; ED; DR)
2 This is not the action of Sorbitrate.
3 Same as # 2.
4 Same as # 2.

475. **3** Sorbitrate may produce vasodilation, resulting in postural hypotension from sudden changes in position. (b) (ME; PL; ED; DR)
1 This drug may cause tachycardia, not bradycardia.
2 This drug results in a more efficient cardiac output; therefore the lungs will not have to compensate for inadequate cardiac output by increasing the respiratory rate.
4 The only gastrointestinal complications may be nausea and vomiting.

476. **1** The carotid artery is located along the anterior edge of the sternocleidomastoid muscle at the level of the lower margin of the thyroid cartilage. (a) (ME; AS; PA; CV)

2 This is not the anatomic landmark for locating the carotid artery.
3 Same as # 2.
4 Same as # 2.

477. **4** A direct relationship exists between the strength of cardiac contractions and the electrical conductions through the myocardium. (c) (ME; AN; PA; CV)
1 Heart rate is related to factors such as the SA node function, partial pressures of oxygen and carbon dioxide, and emotions.
2 This is the period when the heart is at rest, not when it is contracting.
3 Pulmonary pressure does not influence action potential; it becomes elevated in the presence of left ventricular failure.

478. **1** A direct relationship exists between the systolic blood pressure and the force of left ventricular contraction. (b) (ME; AN; PA; CV)
2 This would indicate decreased cardiac sufficiency.
3 This would be indicated by dysrhythmias and tachycardia.
4 This would be indicated by hypertension, not a decreased pulse pressure.

479. **2** This is the cardinal reason for PVCs. (b) (ME; AS; PA; CV)
1 This is a type of arrhythmia, not the cause of PVCs; the source is the atrium, not the ventricles.
3 This type of arrhythmia is associated with interference with the conduction system, not cardiac irritability.
4 This is a type of arrhythmia, not the cause of PVCs.

480. **2** This type pacemaker synchronizes impulses to the atria and ventricles to more closely simulate the normal action of the heart. (b) (SU; IM; ED; CV)
1 The physiologic pacemaker stimulates both the atria and ventricles to contract.
3 It affects the electrical conduction system of the heart, not the anatomic structures.
4 It will increase the heart beat to a more normal rate.

481. **3** This is the primary indication for a pacemaker because there is an interference with the electrical conduction system of the heart. (a) (SU; AN; TC; CV)
1 The primary treatment is medication; this is not an indication for a pacemaker.
2 Same as # 1.
4 Same as # 1.

482. **1** Milliamps are used, not volts of electricity; higher voltages are needed to electrocute. (a) (SU; IM; ED; CV)
2 The voltage used can never cause electrocution; all pacemakers are pretested for accuracy.
3 Technology is not directly related to the problem; the voltage used in pacemakers can never cause electrocution.
4 This is a patronizing response.

483. **1** Meat can react with reagents used in the test to cause false-positive results. (b) (SU; AS; ED; GI)
2 This may apply for testing for ova and parasites but not for occult blood.
3 If the correct procedure is followed, discarding

the first specimen is unnecessary.

4 Random stool testing can be done, but must be on three different bowel movements during the screening period.

484. 1 When intestinal continuity cannot be restored after removal of the anus, rectum, and adjacent colon, a permanent colostomy is formed. (b) (SU; PL; ED; EC)

    2 This segment of colon lies on the right side of the abdomen and has no anatomic proximity to the rectum.

    3 This procedure is performed to allow a segment of colon to heal; intestinal continuity can be restored.

    4 This procedure is commonly performed for inflammation of the colon when intestinal continuity can be restored.

485. 2 Refusal to recognize anticipated loss in an attempt to protect oneself against the overpowering stress of illness is called repudiation. (b) (SU; AN; PE; EC)

    1 There is no data to support that the client is demonstrating behavior characteristic of an earlier stage of development.

    3 The data does not suggest the client has made a realistic adjustment to illness.

    4 The data does not suggest the client has contemplated consequences related to the illness.

486. 2 According to Erikson, poor self-concept and feelings of despair are conflicts manifested in the 65-and-older age-group. (c) (SU; EV; PE; GD)

    1 These are conflicts manifested in early childhood between ages 3 and 6 years.

    3 These are the conflicts manifested during the ages from 6 to 11 years.

    4 These conflicts are manifested during middle adulthood, 45 to 65 years.

487. 3 This is the correct amount:

$$0.8 \text{ mg}/0.4 \text{ mg} = X \text{ ml}/1 \text{ ml}$$
$$0.4 X = 0.8$$
$$X = 2 \text{ ml. (b) (SU; AN; TC; DR)}$$

    1 This is unsafe; too little of the preoperative medication would be administered.

    2 Same as # 1.

    4 This amount is unsafe; too much of the preoperative medication would be administered.

488. 1 The client receives 1000 ml + 500 ml + 1500 ml from the main IV and 150 ml in piggybacks (3 × 50 ml). (a) (SU; AN; TC; FE)

    2 This is an incorrect computation; this is more than the amount of fluid ordered.

    3 Same as # 2.

    4 Same as # 2.

489. 3 Irrigations regulate the bowel to function at a specific time for the convenience of the client. (b) (SU; AN; PA; GI)

    1 This is not the function of the irrigation; most of the fluid already has been absorbed in the large intestine by the time it reaches the sigmoid.

    2 Irrigations will facilitate expulsion of flatus but will not decrease the amount; avoidance of gas-forming foods will accomplish this.

    4 Although irrigations will limit pushing, this is not the purpose of the irrigation.

490. 3 Before a teaching plan can be developed, the factors that interfere with learning must be identified. (b) (SU; AS; ED; GI)

    1 This is premature; assessment comes before intervention; written instructions may not be the most appropriate teaching modality.

    2 This may be an unrealistic expectation; the client may never accept the change but must learn to manage care.

    4 Although family members can be helpful, client involvement in care is important for promoting independence and self-esteem.

491. 4 Left or right side-lying position puts the least strain or pressure on the perineal suture line. (b) (SU; IM; TC; GI)

    1 This position is difficult to maintain for any time and would place stress on the suture line.

    2 Flexion of one hip and knee would increase tension on the perineal suture line; the Sims' position would result in the client lying on the new colostomy, which would be traumatic.

    3 This position places undue stress on the suture line and is the most uncomfortable position.

492. 4 There is no need to irrigate before stool is formed. (b) (SU; IM; ED; GI)

    1 The perineal wound may take weeks to heal, and irrigations must be started when the stool is formed.

    2 This is premature; stool is not yet formed.

    3 If proper technique is used, fecal elimination should flow through the sleeve of the colostomy bag to the commode.

493. 2 This is the point at which a client is generally hypoglycemic; however, if the client's typical level is well above the norm of 90 to 120 mg/100 ml, a level higher than 70mg/100 ml could produce signs of hypoglycemia. (b) (ME; AS; PA; EN)

    1 This is within the norm of 90 to 120 mg/100 ml.

    3 Same as # 1.

    4 This is not a sufficient drop to be hypoglycemia; hypoglycemia is usually 50 to 70 mg/100 ml.

494. 3 The dose of exogenous insulin causes a rapid drop in blood glucose, especially if food is not eaten; the oral hypoglycemic acts slowly, and there is time to take evasive measures if hypoglycemia begins to develop. (c) (ME; AN; PA; EN)

    1 Although stress could contribute to hypoglycemia, the primary reason for this client's precipitous fall in blood glucose was because insulin had been taken and the client had not eaten at all.

    2 When glycogenolysis is inhibited, it would lead to hypoglycemia.

    4 Although adjustment in insulin dosage must be made according to activity and life-style, the use of insulin over long periods does not build up tolerance or cause blood glucose levels to fluctuate dramatically.

495. 3 This occurs with low serum glucose levels because of sympathetic nervous system activity. (b) (ME; AS; PA; EN)

    1 This is a sign of hyperglycemia and is related to metabolic acidosis; it is a compensatory response in an attempt to blow off CO_2 and raise the pH.

    2 This is a sign of hyperglycemia; it is caused by dehydration associated with osmotic diuresis related to glycosuria.

4 This is a sign of hyperglycemia and is related to metabolic acidosis and inadequate energy production.

496. **2** The client with liver disease has a decreased ability to metabolize CHO because of a decreased ability to form glycogen (glycogenesis) and to form glucose from glycogen (glycogenolysis). (c) (ME; AN; PA; EN)
  1 This is not related to decreased blood glucose.
  3 Clients with type II diabetes do not depend on exogenous insulin, nor are they prone to ketosis; the blood glucose levels fall much more slowly, and there is ample time to monitor signs and symptoms before insulin shock can develop.
  4 Same as # 1.

497. **1** This is the correct flow rate; 500 mg of the drug added to 100 ml of IV produces a solution in which 1 ml contains 5 mg of the drug; the required amount of the drug is contained in 0.3 ml of fluid; to calculate the dosage to be delivered, multiply the amount to be delivered (0.3 ml) by the drop factor (60) and divide the result by the amount of time in minutes (1). (b) (ME; AN; TC; DR)
  2 This is too slow; this would not deliver the ordered amount of lidocaine.
  3 Same as # 2.
  4 Same as # 2.

498. **3** Morphine is a narcotic analgesic that acts on the central nervous system by a sympathetic mechanism; it decreases systemic vascular resistance, which decreases left ventricular afterload, thus decreasing myocardial oxygen consumption. (b) (ME; IM; TC; CV)
  1 Oxygen administration elevates arterial oxygen tension with the potential for improving tissue oxygenation; however, oxygen administration usually does not deliver enough oxygen to the myocardium to reverse the infarction and thus relieve the pain.
  2 Nitroglycerine sublingually is effective in relieving anginal pain but not myocardial infarction pain.
  4 Lidocaine is an antiarrhythmic, not an analgesic.

499. **4** Tremors are a precursor to the major adverse effect of seizures or convulsions. (c) (ME; EV; PA; DR)
  1 Hypotension, not hypertension, occurs.
  2 Bradycardia, which can lead to heart block, occurs, not tachycardia.
  3 Although this can occur, it is not a serious side effect.

500. **1** Nitroglycerine does this by its vasodilating effect; it dilates coronary arteries, reduces myocardial ischemia, strengthens contractility, and increases efficiency of cardiac output. (c) (ME; AN; PA; DR)
  2 Decreasing the pulse rate does not strengthen cardiac contractility.
  3 Cardiac output is increased, not decreased.
  4 Peripheral resistance is not affected by dilating coronary arteries but by dilating peripheral arteries.

501. **2** The speed of conduction is decreased when digoxin is given, and this can result in premature beats, atrial fibrillation, and first degree heart block. (a) (ME; EV; PA; DR)
  1 There is no need to give digoxin with food; if

gastrointestinal upset occurs, this can be a sign of toxicity.
  3 The purpose of the drug is to reduce this fast rate; the drug should be withheld if the rate is below 60.
  4 Insulin and digoxin can be given at the same time.

502. **2** Orthopnea at night is a symptom of left-sided cardiac failure; the orthopneic position, a compensatory mechanism, limits venous return, which decreases pulmonary congestion and promotes ventilation, easing the dyspnea. (b) (ME; AS; PA; CV)
  1 This occurs with right-sided failure because of portal hypertension and liver congestion.
  3 Anorexia and nausea occur with right-sided failure because of the venous stasis and venous engorgement of abdominal viscera; weight gain would occur because of fluid retention.
  4 This occurs with right-sided failure because of hypervolemia.

503. **1** The bladder must be empty to decrease the chance of puncturing it during the paracentesis. (a) (SU; IM; TC; GI)
  2 This is not necessary.
  3 Same as # 2.
  4 This is usually performed in the Fowler's position to assist the flow of fluid by gravity.

504. **4** Sharing concerns and talking about problems often releases anxieties; giving the client the ordered hypnotic would produce relaxation. (a) (SU; IM; PE; EC)
  1 This might relax the client but would do little to reduce the level of anxiety.
  2 The client is not in pain at this time but needs to share concerns.
  3 The procedure is over; this might be appropriate before the paracentesis; also, there is no data to support that this is the client's concern.

505. **3** Nerves for arm innervation are above the injury level at C4. (c) (SU; AS; PA; NM)
  1 Diaphragm innervation is not affected by this injury; it is innervated above C4.
  2 Innervation for pain sensation of the hands is not affected by this injury; they are innervated above C7.
  4 Innervation of muscles used to move the lower arm is not affected by this injury; they are innervated above C7.

506. **3** The T6 level is the sympathetic visceral outflow level, and any injury above this level results in autonomic dysreflexia. (c) (SU; AN; PA; NM)
  1 The reflex arc remains after spinal injury.
  2 The important point is not that the cord is totally transected but the level at which the injury occurs.
  4 This is not related to autonomic dysreflexia; all cord injuries result in flaccid paralysis during the period of spinal shock; as the inflammation subsides, spasticity gradually increases.

507. **4** These symptoms occur as a result of exaggerated autonomic responses, and if autonomic dysreflexia is identified, immediate intervention is necessary to prevent serious complications. (c) (SU; AS; PA; NM)
  1 Paralysis is related to transection, not dysreflexia; the client will have no sensation below the injury.

2 Profuse diaphoresis occurs.

3 Bradycardia occurs.

508. **1** The client has the capability; this maintains a positive identity and is necessary for progression to long-term goals. (b) (SU; PL; PE; EC)

2 This is a long-term goal.

3 Same as # 2.

4 Same as # 2.

509. **2** Arm strength is necessary for transfers and activities of daily living and for the use of crutches or a wheelchair. (b) (SU; IM; ED; NM)

1 The client has no neurologic control of this activity.

3 Equilibrium is not a problem.

4 Same as # 1.

510. **2** This is the young adult task associated with intimacy vs isolation. (b) (SU; AN; PE; GD)

1 This is a toddler's task associated with autonomy vs shame and doubt.

3 This is a school-ager's task associated with initiative vs guilt.

4 This is a toddler's task associated with autonomy vs shame and doubt.

511. **1** Drug hypersensitivity and anaphylaxis are most common with antimicrobial agents. (a) (ME; IM; TC; BI)

2 This is an important assessment, but it is not crucial to starting antibiotic therapy.

3 This is a dependent function; it is not crucial to starting antibiotic therapy.

4 Withholding treatment until culture results are available may extend the infection.

512. **1** Pyrexia increases fluid loss through the skin; to maintain balance, the body compensates by reducing urinary output. (a) (ME; AN; PA; FE)

2 This represents a possible, but not probable, side effect of antimicrobial agents; also, nephrotoxicity would not be evident so soon.

3 This is unlikely; the client would have to become septic before this could occur.

4 The data does not indicate anything that would result in a declining blood pressure.

513. **4** This would promote extension of a local infection into the circulation, causing septicemia. (c) (ME; AN; TC; IT)

1 This is not accomplished by bed rest.

2 Although bed rest does this, it is not the purpose for it in this situation.

3 Same as # 2.

514. **4** Controlling the diabetes decreases the risk of infection; this is the best prevention. (a) (ME; EV; TC; IT)

1 If not completely absorbed, these may provide a warm, moist environment for bacterial growth.

2 Coexisting neuropathy may result in injury from heat application.

3 Protein, carbohydrates, and fats must be in an appropriate balance; high carbohydrate intake could provide too many calories.

515. **4** Incompetent valves result in retrograde venous flow and subsequent dilation of veins. (a) (SU; IM; ED; CV)

1 These are considered a result of, rather than a cause of, varicose veins.

2 Plaque formation is considered an arterial, rather than a venous, problem.

3 Pressure is increased, not decreased.

516. **4** Impaired venous return causes increased pressure, with subjective symptoms of fatigue and heaviness. (b) (SU; AS; PA; CV)

1 Homan's sign is indicative of thrombophlebitis.

2 Symptoms of hypoxia are related to impaired arterial, rather than venous, circulation.

3 Ecchymosis may occur in some individuals, but there is insufficient bleeding into tissue to cause hematomas.

517. **2** This results from venous pooling with increased hydrostatic pressure; fluid moves from intravascular to interstitial space. (b) (SU; AS; PA; CV)

1 Pigmentation, not pallor, occurs.

3 This occurs with arterial, not venous, insufficiency.

4 Same as # 3.

518. **1** After ligation, the saphenous vein is removed. (a) (SU; IM; ED; CV)

2 Plaque is considered an arterial, rather than a venous, problem.

3 They are normally attached by communicating veins; surgery involves ligation to isolate the saphenous vein.

4 Although a common therapy, this is not a surgical procedure.

519. **4** Ambulation is essential to promote venous return and prevent thrombus formation. (a) (SU; PL; TC; CV)

1 This causes increased popliteal pressure and impairs venous return.

2 Same as # 1.

3 Pressure dressings with elastic bandages remain in place postoperatively until the surgeon removes them.

520. **4** Nutrition by intravenous route eliminates pancreatic stimulation, therefore reducing the pain experienced in pancreatitis. (a) (SU; IM; ED; GI)

1 Administration requires the competence and skill of an experienced nurse.

2 Route and type of solution creates many safety risks for the client.

3 Hunger can be experienced with parenteral nutrition therapy.

521. **4** The Valsalva manuever produces a positive phase in central venous pressure that will lessen the risk of air entering the circulation. (b) (SU; IM; TC; CV)

1 This is irrelevant to the procedure.

2 This is not necessary; a local, rather than a general, anesthetic is given.

3 These are inappropriate instructions; this would create a negative central venous pressure.

522. **3** Morphine sulfate should be avoided because it causes spasms at the sphincter of Oddi, thereby increasing pain. (c) (SU; EV; TC; DR)

1 Cimetidine (Tagamet) is useful in reducing gastric acid stimulation of pancreatic enzymes.

2 Promethazine HCl (Phenergan) is useful as an antiemetic for pancreatitis.

4 Meperedine HCl (Demerol) would be useful for pain relief in pancreatitis.

523. **1** Rapid infusion of concentrated glucose into the vascular system does not allow time for adequate insulin release to transport glucose to the cells. (c) (SU; AN; TC; GI)

2 A hyperconcentrated solution usually results in hypervolemia rather than hyperglycemia.

3 If this were true, the blood glucose would not be 240 mg/100 ml.

4 This finding is not an expected response.

524. **3** A mask and sterile gloves protect the infusion site against contamination with airborne and other pathogenic organisms. (b) (SU; PL; TC; GI)

1 Sterile gloves will not protect against airborne pathogens.

2 A gown and gloves will not protect against airborne pathogens.

4 A gown would serve no useful purpose during site care.

525. **3** These characteristics describe steatorrhea often occurring in pancreatitis and resulting from impaired fat digestion. (c) (SU; AS; PA; GI)

1 This is descriptive of acholic stools occurring with biliary obstruction and resulting from absence of urobilin.

2 This would be descriptive of upper and lower gastrointestinal bleeding.

4 This is descriptive of stools resulting from constipation and fecal impactions.

526. **2** Tuberculosis must be suspected if an individual has spent a length of time in an undeveloped country; also, one of the symptoms is diaphoresis at night. (b) (ME; AS; PA; RE)

1 Recurrent fever is present; however, frothy sputum is present with pulmonary edema, not tuberculosis.

3 The cough would be productive, not dry.

4 A productive cough may occur, but engorged neck veins are symptomatic of congestive heart failure.

527. **1** It takes this length of time for antibodies to respond to the antigen and form an indurated area. (a) (ME; AS; PA; BI)

2 This is longer than necessary; the site will reveal induration in 2 to 3 days.

3 Same as # 2.

4 Same as # 2.

528. **4** The specimen must represent phlegm containing the mycobacterium, which is in the lung, not the oronasopharynx. (a) (ME; IM; ED; RE)

1 This is not necessary.

2 Same as # 1.

3 Same as # 1.

529. **1** This medication causes hyperuricemia, leading to joint swelling and pain; fluids dilute the urine and help remove the uric acid. (b) (ME; EV; ED; DR)

2 This medication causes GI irritation and should be taken with food.

3 This is not a side effect of this medication.

4 This is a side effect of rifampin (Rifadin), not pyrazinamide.

530. **3** Clients with tuberculosis tend to lose weight and have anorexia; this will encourage food intake and provide calories for weight gain. (a) (ME; PL; TC; GI)

1 This is not necessary; protein can be obtained through natural foods.

2 This is not possible; carbohydrates contain calories.

4 Proteins are needed for tissue building.

531. **4** Fresh airflow into the house changes the air and lowers the concentration of microorganisms. (c) (ME; IM; ED; RE)

1 This is not necesssary.

2 This is not necessary; only articles contaminated with infected sputum, such as used tissues, should be contained.

3 It is permissible to do this because the extremely hot water used to process the dishes kills the myobacterium.

532. **3** This is secondary to cerebral hypoxia, which accompanies ARDS; cognition and level of consciousness are reduced. (c) (ME; AS; PA; RE)

1 Hypotension occurs because of the hypoxia of the heart.

2 Sputum is not tenacious, but it may be frothy if pulmonary edema is present.

4 Breathing will be fast and shallow.

533. **1** Increased rate and depth of breathing results in excessive elimination of CO_2; acid is blown off, and respiratory alkalosis results. (a) (ME; EV; TC; RE)

2 This results from excess hydrogen ions caused by a metabolic problem, not a respiratory problem.

3 With hyperventilation, CO_2 levels will be decreased (hypocapnea).

4 Hypoxia is associated with respiratory acidosis, not respiratory alkalosis, which is related to hyperventilation.

534. **1** This position promotes respirations by removing the pressure of abdominal organs on the diaphragm, it requires the least amount of energy to maintain, and it helps reduce edema at the tracheostomy site. (b) (SU; IM; TC; RE)

2 It requires too much energy to maintain this position.

3 Same as # 1.

4 This position promotes collection of fluid around the operative site, which impedes healing.

535. **4** The drug paralyzes voluntary skeletal muscles, including those involved with respiration; the client will die without mechanical ventilation. (b) (ME; IM; TC; DR)

1 This is not the priority.

2 Same as # 1.

3 Same as # 1.

536. **3** These cuffs do not compress the capillary beds and thus do not cause tracheal damage. (b) (SU; AN; TC; RE)

1 Surgical asepsis, not the use of these cuffs, prevents infection.

2 A minimal air leak is desirable to assure the lowest possible pressure in the cuff.

4 Secretions will be increased because the cuff is a foreign body in the trachea.

537. **3** This method obtains a specimen uncontaminated by environmental organisms. (c) (ME; IM; TC; RG)

1 This is not as accurate as obtaining the purulent discharge from the site of origin.

2 This would contaminate the specimen with organisms external to the body.

4 This would dilute and possibly contaminate the specimen.

538. **2** Anal itching and irritation result from erythema and edema of the anal crypts from the gonococcus. (c) (ME; AS; PA; RG)

1 Frank rectal bleeding, not upper GI bleeding, occurs.

3 Diarrhea, not constipation, occurs.

4 The shape of formed stool does not change; however, diarrhea does occur.

539. **2** This is a description of a chancre, which is the initial sign of syphilis. (c) (ME; AS; PA; RG)
   1 These are condylomata lata (venerial warts), which are typical of the secondary stage.
   3 This is typical of the secondary stage of systemic involvement from disappearance of chancre to 2 to 4 years later.
   4 This is typical of the secondary stage.
540. **4** Dryness inactivates the *Treponema pallidum*, making it incapable of causing disease. (a) (ME; AN; PA; RG)
   1 The organism is transferred by sexual contact; warm, moist body contact supports growth of organism.
   2 This is not true; nothing chelates the organism.
   3 This supports growth of the organism.
541. **3** Correct calculation:
   2,450,000 U/300,000 U = X ml/1 ml
   $$300,000 X = 2,450,000$$
   $$X = 8.2 \text{ ml.}$$
   (b) (ME; AN; TC; DR)
   1 This would deliver less than the ordered amount.
   2 Same as # 1.
   4 This would deliver more than ordered amount.
542. **1** Neurotoxicity, as manifested by ataxia, is evidence of tertiary syphilis, which may involve the CNS; other CNS signs include confusion, paralysis, delusions, impaired judgment, and slurred speech. (b) (ME; AS; PA; RG)
   2 This is not a sign of late-stage syphilis.
   3 This occurs in the secondary stage.
   4 Same as # 3.
543. **1** The catheter must be passed through the highly vascular liver to reach the gallbladder. (b) (SU; PL; TC; GI)
   2 Pressure on the operative site is desirable.
   3 This is unsafe; pressure must be maintained against the catheter insertion site.
   4 Same as # 2.
544. **1** Colic may occur in the postoperative period as a result of passage of pulverized fragments of the calculi; this may occur 3 or more days after lithotripsy. (c) (SU; IM; ED; GI)
   2 Fever would indicate pancreatitis, which is a rare occurrence.
   3 The delivery of shock waves during the procedure is synchronized with the heartbeat to avoid initiation of arrhythmias.
   4 Sedation with Valium or epidural or general anesthesia may be used to keep the client comfortable and as still as possible.
545. **4** During the procedure, Valium is administered as required intravenously to help the client stay calm. (c) (SU; IM; ED; GI)
   1 This is not used during this procedure.
   2 The client is awake during this procedure.
   3 Same as # 1.
546. **4** Narrowing of arteries supplying the brain causes temporary neurologic defects that last for a short time; between attacks the neurologic examination is normal. (b) (ME; AN; PA; NM)
   1 This occurs with multiple small cerebrovascular accidents; TIAs do not cause permanent damage.
   2 This is not the description of a TIA; remissions and exacerbations occur with progressive degenerative neurologic disorders, such as multiple sclerosis.

   3 Emboli result in a cerebrovascular accident; damage is permanent.
547. **3** The cause of the hypotension must be evaluated by the physician. (c) (SU; IM; TC; FE)
   1 This is a dependent function, and the physician must be notified first.
   2 This is contraindicated; it would further decrease blood flow to the brain.
   4 This is contraindicated; the physician must be notified first.
548. **3** Muscles used for swallowing are innervated by the ninth (glossopharyngeal) and tenth (vagus) cranial nerves. (c) (SU; EV; PA; NM)
   1 This is unrelated to cranial nerves; this is associated with neck edema and potential compromise of the airway.
   2 This is unrelated to cranial nerves; some edema is expected because of the inflammatory process at the site of surgery.
   4 Alterations in blood pressure will occur but are not caused by cranial nerve dysfunction.
549. **2** Aspirin interferes with platelet aggregation and will impede the formation of thrombi. (b) (ME; EV; PA; DR)
   1 Although aspirin has antiinflammatory properties, 1 month after the surgery the edema has already subsided.
   3 This is not an expected response following surgery, and it would indicate infection; a prescription for antibiotics would be more appropriate.
   4 At this point, there should no longer be discomfort at the surgical site.
550. **4** This detergent action promotes addition of fluid into stool to soften feces. (b) (ME; AN; PA; DR)
   1 This is the action of lubricant laxatives such as mineral oil.
   2 This is the action of peristalsic stimulants such as cascara and castor oil.
   3 This is the action of saline laxatives such as milk of magnesia.

Psychiatric–Mental Health Nursing

1. **1** This is a theoretic explanation for the development of anorexia nervosa. (b) (PS; AN; PA; BA)
   2 This does not play a role in the development of anorexia nervosa.
   3 The basis is the struggle between dependence and independence, not a desire for independence alone.
   4 Same as # 2.
2. **2** In behavior modification, positive behavior is reinforced and negative behavior is punished or not reinforced. (b) (PS; PL; TC; TR)
   1 This may be a part of the program, but it is not a major component.
   3 Same as # 1.
   4 Same as # 1.
3. **4** Clients with anorexia nervosa have a disturbed self-image and always see themselves as fat and needing further reducing. (b) (PS; AS; PE; BA)
   1 The relationship is usually not supportive but is disturbed.

2 There is usually high achievement and great concern about grades.

3 There is usually dissatisfaction with weight and a desire to lose weight.

4. **3** It is most therapeutic for the staff to control food needs, thus removing parents from the struggle. (c) (PS; IM; TC; BA)

1 This is nontherapeutic; it only continues the struggle between parents and client.

2 This is nontherapeutic; it cuts off parents from future involvement.

4 This increases parents' guilt.

5. **4** The client's security is increased by limit setting; guidelines remove responsibility for behavior from the client and increase compliance with the regimen. (b) (PS; PL; PE; BA)

1 The client needs control, not empathy.

2 Simply maintaining control is not therapeutic and increases the power struggle.

3 Emphasis on dietary intake increases the power struggle between the client and the staff.

6. **4** All food issues should be discussed with the dietician, thus removing a potential source of conflict between nurse and client. (b) (PS; PL; PE; BA)

1 This may be self-defeating because discussion of food would be the major focus of all nurse-client interactions.

2 This would increase the conflict between nurse and client.

3 This would accomplish little because the client's failure to eat is not based on likes or dislikes.

7. **3** Clients with anorexia nervosa use manipulation to divide the nursing staff; sharing this knowledge alerts health team members. (c) (PS; AN; PE; BA)

1 This would be counterproductive because it supports the client's manipulative behavior.

2 Same as # 1.

4 The client is attempting to manipulate the staff; this is not how trust is established.

8. **4** The client is fearful and suspicious, and feeling he is in a powerful position helps him deal with anxiety. (b) (PS; AN; PE; SD)

1 The client is not out of touch with his real identity; he has given his real identity an important role.

2 This is incorrect; the client is compensating for feelings of inadequacy.

3 Same as # 2.

9. **2** The recommended approach for working with suspicious clients is to allow them to set the pace for the relationship. (c) (PS; PL; TC; SD)

1 This would be threatening and add to feelings of paranoia.

3 Same as # 1.

4 Same as # 1.

10. **3** Clients with paranoia often feel safer selecting foods from a cafeteria-type display that is prepared for the general population rather than eating from a tray specifically prepared for them. (c) (PS; IM; PE; SD)

1 This would not provide security because part of the food could still be poisoned.

2 Same as # 1.

4 Same as # 1.

11. **2** Anticonvulsants and Haldol exert a synergistic CNS depressant effect. (b) (PS; EV; TC; DR)

1 This is untrue; the effect is potentiated.

3 Anticonvulsants do not affect absorption or metabolism of Haldol.

4 Same as # 3.

12. **4** This acute dystonic reaction is a severe side effect of Haldol and requires intramuscular or intravenous administration of antiparkinsonian medication. (b) (PS; EV; TC; DR)

1 The dosage would not be increased but discontinued, and antiparkinsonian medication would be administered.

2 At this point symptoms are so severe that medication must be discontinued.

3 These symptoms are more severe than pseudoparkinsonism and require more than adjustment in this medication.

13. **2** Motivation is necessary to assist the client in withstanding the pain of giving up his defense; motivation is more influential in facilitating change than any external factor. (b) (PS; AN; PE; SA)

1 Most families of individuals with alcoholism are enablers; enabling behavior does not help the individual to deal with the drinking problem but denies that problems exist.

3 This can be of assistance, but internal factors will have a greater impact on rehabilitation than will external factors.

4 Self-esteem will be useful if it precipitates abstinence behavior; however, people with alcoholism frequently have low self-esteem.

14. **4** Alcohol causes both physical and psychologic dependence; the individual needs and depends on the alcohol to function. (b) (PS; AN; PE; SA)

1 This is a myth often associated with alcoholism; the individual needs to learn how to use other coping mechanisms more consistently and effectively.

2 This is untrue; alcoholism is a disease that entails physical and psychologic dependence.

3 People with alcoholism frequently drink alone or feel alone in a crowd.

15. **4** The client must learn to develop and use more healthful coping mechanisms if drinking is to be stopped; the responsibility is with the client because the client must do the changing. (b) (PS; PL; PE; SA)

1 This will increase guilt and place the client on the defensive; it usually does not foster the development of a trusting relationship.

2 Medications do not provide the motivation for change; this must come from within the client.

3 This would tell the client what to expect but would not instill responsibility for change.

16. **4** This statement recognizes the feeling of ambivalence associated with admitting that a problem with alcohol exists; this occurs early in treatment. (b) (PS; IM; PE; SA)

1 This places the client on the defensive and interferes with communication.

2 Same as # 1.

3 Same as # 1.

17. **1** This behavior indicates that the client lacks insight and is denying that alcohol is the problem. (a) (PS; AN; PE; SA)

2 There are no data to support this conclusion.

3 Same as # 2.

4 Same as # 2.

18. **1** The client is still denying the illness and has not resolved the basic problem that led to the alcoholism. (b) (PS; EV; PE; SA)
    2 This is incorrect because the client is still denying the illness; willpower alone will not keep the client away from alcohol.
    3 This may be true, but it does not ensure compliance or successful rehabilitation.
    4 This is not helpful unless the client understands the basis of the conflicts and his role in resolving them.

19. **4** These products often contain an alcohol base and can cause a severe reaction in the presence of Antabuse. (b) (PS; IM; ED; DR)
    1 These do not contain alcohol and need not be avoided.
    2 Only wine vinegar should be avoided.
    3 Same as # 1.

20. **1** This assists the client in decision making; new situations may be stressful and lead to ambivalent feelings. (b) (PS; IM; PE; OR)
    2 This would make the client feel guilty and add to anxiety.
    3 This is not sharing decision making; hurrying the client will lead to feelings of frustration and resentment.
    4 The client may perceive this action as punishment.

21. **3** This allows the client to exercise the right to decide which articles to keep and provides for safety and cleanliness. (b) (PS; PL; TC; OR)
    1 This deceives the client, limits judgment, and creates mistrust toward the staff.
    2 This does not help because harmless objects do not have to be removed.
    4 Explanation alone will not provide safety for this client because of decreased attention span and memory.

22. **1** Routines and familiarity with activities or environment provide for a sense of security. (b) (PS; PL; TC; OR)
    2 Change is poorly tolerated; frustration and the inability to accomplish tasks lead to lowered self-esteem.
    3 Decreased physical capacity and attention span limit active participation; frustration can result.
    4 Challenging activities can be frustrating and can lead to hostility or withdrawal.

23. **4** Confabulation is used as a defense mechanism against embarrassment caused by lapse of memory. (b) (PS; AN; PE; OR)
    1 Regression is a defense mechanism in which the individual moves back to earlier developmental defenses.
    2 Although the elderly fear being forgotten or losing others' affection, this is not the main reason for confabulation.
    3 This may be accomplished but is usually not the purpose of reminiscence or confabulation.

24. **2** This encourages verbalization, gives the client a feeling of security, and decreases the sense of isolation. (a) (PS; IM; PE; OR)
    1 This discourages verbalization of feelings and will lead to feelings of being unwanted.
    3 This action discourages verbalization between client and nurse; the client may be unable to function in a small group because of increased anxiety.

4 Same as # 3.

25. **2** This response accepts the client's behavior (desires) but lets the client know the nurse is not going to give up attempts to establish a relationship. (b) (PS; IM; PE; SD)
    1 This statement on initial encounter does not show respect for client's space and is inappropriately interpretive.
    3 This response requests insight that the client does not have at this point.
    4 This does not respect the client's wish for space at the present time.

26. **1** The fetal position represents regressed behavior; regression is a way of responding to overwhelming anxiety. (a) (PS; EV; PE; SD)
    2 There are no data to substantiate this; further assessment is necessary to make this interpretation.
    3 Same as # 2.
    4 Making this interpretation assumes that the nurse controls the client's behavior; the client is not responding to the nurse any differently than to anyone else who tries to establish reality contact.

27. **3** This response accepts the client at the client's present level and, in addition, allows the client to set the pace of the relationship. (c) (PS; PL; TC; SD)
    1 This approach to any client can be misinterpreted and may precipitate an aggressive response.
    2 This response asks the client to reach out to the nurse; in the therapeutic relationship the nurse must reach out to the client.
    4 Even if the client is too withdrawn to respond, the nurse's physical presence can be reassuring.

28. **3** The state in which the client feels unreal or believes that parts of the body are distorted is known as depersonalization, or loss of personal identity. (a) (PS; AN; PE; SD)
    1 The client's statement does not indicate any feelings that others are out to do harm, are responsible for what is happening, or are in control of the client.
    2 The statement is not an example of autistic verbalization.
    4 This is not an example of a hallucination; a hallucination is a sensory experience for which there is no external stimulus.

29. **4** Depersonalization is the result of high anxiety levels; projecting empathy to the client will facilitate exploration of concerns. (b) (PS; IM; TC; TR)
    1 This response belittles the client's feelings and will make establishment of a therapeutic relationship difficult.
    2 This response points out reality to the client from the nurse's perception, but does not acknowledge the frightening experience for the client.
    3 This is irrelevant; the nurse must deal with what the client is experiencing now.

30. **3** These client behaviors indicate increased trust and comfort in the nurse-client relationship. (a) (PS; EV; TC; TR)
    1 This tells nothing about the client's behavior in the therapeutic nurse-client relationship.
    2 Same as # 1.

4 In a therapeutic relationship, the client is prepared in advance for the nurse's days off; the client may act out on these days but it cannot be attributed solely to the nurse's absence.

31. **4** In most instances, the abusing parent attempts to avoid talking about the situation as a means of reducing guilt and repressing the action. (b) (PS; AS; PE; CS)
  1 Denying the beating requires the parent to fabricate a story about how the obvious physical injury occurred.
  2 Little concern is expressed for the child because this would require verbal expression and acceptance of the action.
  3 A mother's concern for the unabused children without the expression of concern about the abused child would document a different feeling about the abused child, which the parent would try to avoid.

32. **4** These underlying feelings frequently precipitate trying to improve the child's behavior by the beating. (b) (PS; AS; PE; CS)
  1 This would be an unusual request because abusing parents do not usually ask to see their children.
  2 These parents offer many vague explanations of how the child was injured; rarely is the explanation detailed.
  3 These parents usually do not admit their behavior, so they do not have a need to rationalize it.

33. **1** The nurse feels that her own inability to deal with her daughter could have resulted in a loss of control, leading to possible abuse. (c) (PS; AN; PE; CS)
  2 Nothing in the data presented leads to this conclusion; the argument could have been justified.
  3 Same as # 2.
  4 The nurse is uncomfortable because the client's situation reflected her own feelings.

34. **3** This is the best response that reflects back the feelings being expressed at this time. (a) (PS; IM; PE; TR)
  1 False reassurance avoids the real issue.
  2 This does not address the real concern; the mother's argument may have been justified and the daughter's behavior should not be rewarded.
  4 This avoids the issue; the fear may be that next time control may be lost and abuse may occur.

35. **3** By learning how the child's behavior provokes frustration, parents may develop more acceptable ways of responding. (c) (PS; IM; ED; CS)
  1 The abusing parent responds to both negative and acceptable behavior with abuse.
  2 Although these parents need to learn what behavior is appropriate for a given age level, they must also learn how to respond correctly to less appropriate behavior.
  4 Punishment of a child for behavior is always wrong; it is an act of retribution, not an act of discipline.

36. **4** This child would distrust any approach because approaches frequently result in pain; abused children remain alert in an attempt to ward off an attack. (b) (PS; AS; PA; CS)
  1 This child would not be open to an approach by a stranger; basic trust of others has not developed in abused children.
  2 This child would be acutely aware of anyone coming near; abused children attempt to defend themselves by keeping alert to the possibility of attack.
  3 This child would usually not cry out; abused children learn not to expect comforting or soothing of pain by others.

37. **3** Such stimuli encourage the client to remain reality oriented; research has shown that competing stimuli are useful in controlling hallucinations. (b) (PS; PL; ED; CS)
  1 This is not very realistic and fosters greater dependency; it focuses on the client's inability to deal with the problem and increases his fear of being alone.
  2 Same as # 1.
  4 This does not assure that the client's needs will be met.

38. **1** Denial may be handled by seeking other opinions in an attempt to prove an unacceptable one incorrect. (a) (PS; AS; PA; CS)
  2 This is not associated with the initial stage; this behavior usually occurs after the client recognizes the outcome and is fearful of being alone.
  3 This occurs during the stage of anger, which is a later stage.
  4 This occurs during the stage of depression, which is a later stage.

39. **2** Rationalization is offering a socially acceptable or logical explanation to justify an unacceptable feeling or behavior. (a) (PS; AS; PA; CS)
  1 Sublimation is the substitution of a socially acceptable behavior for an unacceptable feeling or drive.
  3 Projection is the denial of emotionally unacceptable feelings and the attribution of the traits to another person.
  4 Compensation is making up for a perceived deficiency by emphasizing another feature perceived as an asset.

40. **4** This approach is positive because it attempts to deal with the staff's feelings and the problem without singling out people for guilt; the nurse therefore is taking ethically sound action without being moralistic or authoritarian. (a) (PS; PL; TC; CS)
  1 This abdicates the nurse's responsibility and may create anger and guilt in the staff.
  2 Same as # 1.
  3 Same as # 1.

41. **1** It is important for the couple to discuss their feelings to maintain open communication and support each other. (b) (PS; PL; ED; CS)
  2 This may be useful in the future but is most likely premature; they need to deal with their own feelings first.
  3 This may elicit feelings but will not improve communication; this is a rather long-term goal.
  4 This action would not meet the needs of this couple; it focuses only on the client's needs and ignores the partner's; psychotherapy is long-term.

42. **3** Without an awareness of personal beliefs the nurse may unconsciously stop listening if the client expresses deviant beliefs. (a) (PS; AN; PE; TR)
  1 Although this may create some anxiety, it usually does not interfere with accurate listening.
  2 Same as # 1.
  4 Same as # 1.

43. **2** Private confrontation with reported facts provides for verification; a calm, direct manner is most assertive. (b) (PS; IM; PE; PR)
    1 This action places control in the hands of the client rather than the nurse, which could lead to aggressive confrontation.
    3 This is not assertive intervention; it is manipulation and is not truthful.
    4 This is aggressive confrontation, not assertive intervention.

44. **3** The client is unable to control impulses at this time, so controls must be provided for the client; the nurse's behavior provides a role model. (b) (PS; PL; PE; PR)
    1 The client is not able to set his own controls; freedom could prove frightening to a client who is not in control.
    2 This is nontherapeutic; this would probably provoke even more acting-out behavior.
    4 Same as # 2.

45. **4** Emotionally immature individuals are often unable to deal with the role changes associated with parenthood. (b) (PS; AN; PE; CS)
    1 This may have contributed to the crisis but did not precipitate it.
    2 Same as # 1.
    3 Same as # 1.

46. **4** These clients are threatened by reality; withdrawal from reality and the use of magical thinking reduces anxiety. (b) (PS; AS; PE; SD)
    1 Clients with schizophrenia have poor self-esteem and a low self-image and usually have feelings of guilt and self-blame.
    2 Clients with schizophrenia are not preoccupied with suicidal thoughts.
    3 The loosening of associative links that occurs in schizophrenia makes these impossible.

47. **1** Depersonalization is a feeling of change or unreality about the self or the environment caused by a loss of ego boundaries and a loss of reality testing. (c) (PS; AN; PE; SD)
    2 Ideas of reference are false beliefs that the words and actions of others are concerned with or are directed toward the individual.
    3 Loose associations are verbalizations that are difficult to understand because the links between thoughts are not apparent.
    4 Paranoid ideations are beliefs that the individual is being singled out for unfair treatment.

48. **4** These are the classic premorbid symptoms of schizophrenia. (b) (PS; AS; PE; SD)
    1 These symptoms are usually not associated with schizophrenia.
    2 Same as # 1.
    3 These symptoms are not associated with any particular type disorder.

49. **4** The presence of ego strengths is demonstrated by the level of adjustment before the occurrence of the precipitating event; these ego strengths can be used to help the client reorganize the personality. (a) (PS; AS; PE; SD)
    1 This would tend to contribute to a poor prognosis.
    2 Same as # 1.
    3 Same as # 1.

50. **3** Because making decisions is frequently difficult, the nurse can best help the client by limiting the number and scope of choices. (b) (PS; IM; PE; SD)
    1 This is an unstructured question leaving too many choices; it would create great anxiety in the client.
    2 Same as # 1.
    4 Same as # 1.

51. **2** Ambivalence describes the existence of two conflicting emotions, impulses, or desires. (b) (PS; AN; PE; SD)
    1 Inappropriate affect is not two conflicting emotions but the inappropriate expression of emotions.
    3 Loose association is not two conflicting emotions but the loosening of connections between thoughts.
    4 Double bind is two conflicting messages, not emotions, in a single communication.

52. **3** This response focuses on the client's feelings rather than the statement, and it serves to open channels of communication. (b) (PS; IM; PE; MO)
    1 Such a response simply echoes the client's statement and does not reflect feelings or stimulate further communication.
    2 This response asks the client to decide why she feels the way she does; most people are unable to answer why they feel as they do.
    4 This response does nothing to stimulate further communication; in fact, it tells the client to talk about feelings with someone else.

53. **3** The nurse must accept the client's statement and beliefs as real to the client to develop trust and move into a therapeutic relationship. (b) (PS; PL; PE; TR)
    1 Redirecting the client's conversation whenever negative topics are brought up adds to the client's feelings that thoughts are correct.
    2 These feelings and thoughts are constant; this would result in an overdose.
    4 Clients cannot be argued out of any delusions.

54. **3** Because clients cannot be argued out of their feelings, it is best to initially accept them; it also encourages communication. (b) (PS; PL; PE; MO)
    1 This delays discussing the client's feelings and has little value.
    2 This has little effect on the depressed client; it can increase depression.
    4 The depressed client does very little talking and needs to be encouraged to communicate.

55. **4** This removes the necessity of making the decision from the client and demonstrates that the client is worth spending time with. (b) (PS; IM; TC; MO)
    1 This requires the client to make a decision the client may be unable to make; if the client says "no," communication is blocked.
    2 Same as # 1.
    3 This requires an action the client may be unable to take.

56. **2** Depression is contagious; it affects the nurse as well as the client. (b) (PS; AN; PE; MO)
    1 These clients usually do not offer negative responses; they offer no responses.
    3 The client's lack of energy really does not make nursing care difficult.
    4 Same as # 3.

57. **2** Allowing the client to make those decisions that can be handled helps improve confidence. (b)

(PS; PL; TC; MO)

1 This action would demoralize the client; also, it is impossible for one individual to make all the decisions for another.

3 The client is depressed, and this would probably result in total inactivity.

4 Same as # 3.

58. **4** This action demonstrates to the client that the nurse feels the client is worth spending time with, and it helps restore and build trust. (b) (PS; PL; TC; MO)

1 This action would be impossible to carry out on a regular basis unless the client was potentially suicidal.

2 The depressed client may never get around to speaking to the nurse and, left alone, will withdraw even further.

3 This action does little to establish communication between nurse and client and might be threatening.

59. **3** This drug creates a general sense of well-being, increases appetite, and helps lift depression. (b) (PS; EV; ED; DR)

1 Symptomatic relief usually begins after 2 to 4 weeks of therapy.

2 The client might not know the reason for depression, and the drug does not cause amnesia.

4 Concomitant use of monoamine oxidase inhibitors and tricyclic antidepressants is usually contraindicated.

60. **4** The parents are focusing their feelings about their child's prognosis on someone or something else—in this case each other. (a) (PS; IM; PE; CS)

1 Projection is the attribution of one's own feelings to another person.

2 Compensation is a defense in which one makes up for a perceived deficiency by emphasizing another feature perceived as an asset.

3 Denial is ignoring, avoiding, or refusing to recognize painful realities.

61. **3** Family therapy tries to view the whole (Gestalt) within the context in which the emotional problems are occurring. (c) (PS; PL; TC; TR)

1 Time efficiency is not an adequate rationale for choosing a therapeutic approach.

2 Promotion of truthfulness is a secondary gain achieved through this mode.

4 This may or may not be true; an astute nurse can control manipulation and alliance in any situation.

62. **4** Early notification provides an opportunity to prepare for change. (c) (PS; PL; TC; TR)

1 This may be a secondary gain but not the primary purpose.

2 Same as # 1.

3 Same as # 1.

63. **2** Reasonable limits are necessary because they provide security and help to keep the child's behavior in acceptable bounds. (c) (PS; PL; ED; CS)

1 This is an unrealistic approach that allows the child to manipulate the total situation.

3 Care should be directed to help the child, not the staff.

4 Relationships, not special privileges, should provide the necessary security.

64. **1** Children frequently use denial of parents as a

stage of coping with separation; they avoid the fact that separation is real. (a) (PS; IM; ED; CS)

2 Undoing is a behavior or communication technique calculated to neutralize earlier behavior or communication.

3 Repression is the involuntary exclusion of painful thoughts, impulses, or memories; the child's behavior is voluntary.

4 Sublimation is the act of substituting socially acceptable behavior for an unacceptable feeling or drive.

65. **3** The client has the right to expect that all records of care will remain confidential; permission must be sought for use. (a) (PS; AN; TC; TR)

1 This right was not violated; this applies to the concept of holding clients against their will.

2 This right was not violated; this applies to the humane aspect of care, that is, care given with respect for the client's rights.

4 This right was not violated; this applies to procedures and treatments to be performed on the client.

66. **2** This ethically sound response clearly defines who is involved in decision making, but allows for parental expression of ideas and thoughts. (b) (PS; AN; PE; TR)

1 The abruptness of this answer conveys negativeness and abdicates nursing responsibility.

3 Although the answer promotes the physician-client relationship, it stops the nurse-client interaction.

4 Discussion of the implication of a no-code should not be done until after the family has spoken with the physician.

67. **4** This verifies family and physician agreement and uses institutional policy developed by the ethics committee. (b) (PS; IM; PA; TR)

1 The nurse should not accept this inappropriate burden.

2 Same as # 1.

3 The order must be part of the written record.

68. **4** This is the psychoanalytic explanation for the development of obsessive-compulsive symptomatology. (b) (PS; AN; PE; PR)

1 This is not related to rituals but rather to phobias.

2 The client is unable to consciously stop the behavior because anxiety would become overwhelming if the defense was not used.

3 Compulsive rituals frequently result in interference with activities of daily living, and the individual becomes dysfunctional; rituals cannot be controlled.

69. **2** This limits the time and still allows the rituals; rituals should be allowed as much as possible until the underlying cause of anxiety can be dealt with. (b) (PS; PL; TC; PR)

1 One ritual cannot be substituted for another; this would interfere with the performance of the original ritual and could result in overwhelming anxiety.

3 This provides for only one time period and probably would result in increased anxiety.

4 This is the client's decision; the nurse should not recommend this action.

70. **4** Paraphrasing encourages further ventilation by the client. (b) (PS; IM; PE; PR)

1 This response denies the client's feelings.

2 This is a negative response that may increase the client's fears about being crazy.

3 This provides false reassurance and implies that the client is out of control, which may increase her fears.

71. **4** By observing the client the nurse is able to adjust care and communications to reflect assessment of individual needs. (a) (PS; AS; TC; SD)

1 This is not vital to initially help the client; the nurse should meet the client where the client is now.

2 Same as # 1.

3 Specific clients differ; the nurse should meet the client where the client is now.

72. **1** The nurse must deal with these feelings and establish basic trust to promote a therapeutic milieu. (b) (PS; PL; PE; SD)

2 Continuous pacing is not really a problem because the nurse can walk back and forth with the client.

3 This may be of long-range importance but has little influence on the nurse's response to the client.

4 Same as # 3.

73. **1** Failure to accept the client and the client's fears establishes a barrier to effective communication. (a) (PS; AN; TC; SD)

2 Family cooperation is helpful but not an absolute necessity; the client can get well in spite of the family.

3 ECT is not effective in clients with schizophrenia; in fact, it makes them more confused.

4 Today, mental health therapy is directed toward returning the client to the community as rapidly as possible.

74. **4** This helps the client explore underlying feelings and allows the client to see the message the verbalizations are communicating. (c) (PS; IM; PE; SD)

1 Attempting to divert the client denies feelings rather than accepting and working with them.

2 This denies the client's feelings rather than accepting and working with them.

3 This focuses on the delusion itself rather than the feeling causing the delusion.

75. **3** This response reflects the client's feelings and avoids focusing on the delusion. (b) (PS; IM; PE; SD)

1 This will not change the client's feelings because the belief is real to the client.

2 This will not change the client's feelings because the other pitcher could also be poisoned.

4 This will not change the client's feelings; the client would believe that the nurse was not really drinking the juice.

76. **1** The manic phase is the mirror image of the depressed phase; the behavior is an attempt to ward off depression by racing into reality. (b) (PS; AS; PE; MO)

2 It is not an incorrect interpretation but an incorrect response to the stimuli.

3 It does not have to be an elating situation; the situation itself matters little, and the client responds to any stimuli.

4 It is an attempt to block feelings of depression, not an acting out of innate drives.

77. **4** The excited, overactive client needs a calm environment; external stimulation only serves to cause further excitation. (b) (PS; IM; PE; MO)

1 The client needs reduced, not increased, external stimulation.

2 Same as # 1.

3 Same as # 1.

78. **2** A firm voice is most effective; the statement tells the client that it is the behavior, not the client, that is upsetting to others. (b) (PS; IM; TC; MO)

1 Demanding that the client stop the current behavior is a useless action; the client is out of control and needs external control.

3 The client does not know what is bothering her, and the question would be frustrating.

4 This should only be done when there is real danger from exhaustion; external controls must be set.

79. **1** The elated client expends a great deal of energy; dehydration, oxygen deficits, cardiac problems, and death can occur. (b) (PS; AS; PA; MO)

2 The elated client usually does not take time to eat while expending a great deal of energy, so weight loss is the problem.

3 The elated person does not withdraw from reality but continues to run headfirst into it.

4 The elated client has little difficulty verbalizing needs.

80. **4** This response simply states a fact and delivers praise without making demands. (c) (PS; IM; PE; MO)

1 The client may not recall what happened yesterday and would not know why today's behavior was better.

2 This does not help the client separate the self from the behavior; it tells the client that acting out behavior will result in rejection.

3 This puts the total responsibility for control on a client who needs external controls set.

81. **2** Medication should be discontinued immediately if these symptoms of lithium toxicity occur. (a) (PS; EV; TC; DR)

1 These are symptoms of toxicity, and a stimulant will not alter them.

3 There is no special diet required; the client is encouraged to maintain a normal diet with normal salt and fluid intake.

4 The client receiving lithium is encouraged to maintain a normal salt and fluid intake.

82. **4** Blood levels must be checked monthly when the client is on maintenance therapy because there is only a small range between therapeutic and toxic levels. (a) (PS; IM; ED; DR)

1 The client receiving lithium is encouraged to maintain a normal diet.

2 There is no need to take lithium with milk because it does not normally cause gastrointestinal problems.

3 Lithium does not cause changes in the blood cells.

83. **2** One of the symptoms an autistic child displays is a lack of responsiveness to others; there is little or no extension to the external environment. (b) (PS; AS; PE; BA)

1 Music is nonthreatening, comforting, and soothing.

3 Repetitive visual stimuli, such as a spinning top, are nonthreatening and soothing.

4 Repetitive behavior provides comfort.

84. **2** If religion is a family concern, then the nurse

should allow discussion of the family's thoughts and feelings on the subject. (b) (PS; PL; PE; TR)

1 The role of the nurse is to facilitate and listen, not to have a mutual discussion.

3 The minister is not part of the family unit; the minister would be invited only if requested by the family.

4 If religion is a family concern, its discussion should be encouraged, not limited.

85. 2 Seeing their daughter as soon as possible will validate her death for them and initiate the grieving process. (b) (PS; IM; PE; CS)

1 This will delay and prolong the grieving process; the response offers no explanation for waiting.

3 This is unnecessary; the parents have asked to see their child now.

4 This is untrue; it would be more traumatic to wait and delay the reality of her death.

86. 3 Deaths that are perceived as preventable cause more guilt for the mourners and therefore increase the intensity and length of the grieving process. (b) (PS; AN; PE; CS)

1 It may prolong and intensify the mourning process but will not necessarily result in a pathologic reaction.

2 Same as # 1.

4 This is untrue; it is usually more difficult.

87. 3 This provides support until the individuals' coping mechanisms and personal support systems can be mobilized. (c) (PS; IM; PE; CS)

1 The individuals need time before the full reality of the death can be accepted.

2 The individuals, not the nurse, must mobilize their support systems.

4 This is not the role of the nurse.

88. 3 Because the client refuses to talk, pertinent data must be obtained from the spouse. (b) (PS; AS; TC; MO)

1 The client is not responding to questions; the client may not know the reason.

2 Presence of scars is an inaccurate way to determine past behavior.

4 This may or may not have influenced current behavior.

89. 1 In 3 days the client should understand that the staff cares enough to prevent suicidal acting out. (c) (PS; AN; PE; MO)

2 This is unrealistic within the stated time period.

3 Same as # 2.

4 Same as # 2.

90. 4 The expression of these feelings may indicate that this client is unable to continue the struggle of life. (b) (PS; AS; TC; MO)

1 The client attempting suicide usually sees death as a release.

2 These are not indications of potential suicide; the client is still responding to the world, not attempting to leave it.

3 These are usually not sufficient to precipitate a suicidal attempt.

91. 2 The client will be most likely to eat if accompanied and encouraged by an individual with whom a trusting relationship has been established. (a) (PS; IM; PE; MO)

1 This will not encourage the client to eat and will promote isolation.

3 This is inappropriate at this time; the client is

not interested in maintaining health, nor is she ready for any teaching.

4 This would be ineffective at this time; the client is too introspective to care.

92. 1 The fact that the nurse spends time with the client conveys a feeling of importance and helps build the client's self-esteem. (c) (PS; IM; TC; MO)

2 This infers agreement with the client's statement that the client is not worthy; the nurse should stay to convey a sense of self-worth to client.

3 This places the client on the defensive and does not respond to the feelings of worthlessness communicated by the client.

4 This response cuts off communication; the client responds better to actions than to words.

93. 1 Silence is a tool employed during therapeutic communication that indicates the nurse is listening and receptive; it allows the client time to collect thoughts, gain control of emotions, or speak without hurrying. (b) (PS; IM; TC; TR)

2 The nurse's facial expression should be projected outward, not inward.

3 Silence should be comfortable and should not create a feeling of pressure to talk to break it.

4 This is incorrect; this would close communication.

94. 3 This provides structure and helps the client learn acceptable behavior. (b) (PS; PL; TC; MO)

1 The client may not be ready for this at the present time.

2 Same as # 1.

4 No environment will be stress free.

95. 4 As with other tricyclics, optimal therapeutic effects take 1 to 3 weeks to occur. (b) (PS; EV; PA; DR)

1 This is untrue; maximum therapeutic effect of tricyclics takes up to 3 weeks to occur.

2 Same as # 1.

3 Same as # 1.

96. 1 Because of the individuality of people, the response to retirement may vary, but it is a task representing a developmental milestone for all people. (b) (PS; AN; ED; CS)

2 This may or may not be true; it depends on the individual and the circumstances.

3 Same as # 2.

4 Same as # 2.

97. 1 The client's physical appearance and presentation, as well as the feelings of paranoia, are indicative of this diagnosis. (a) (PS; AN; PE; SD)

2 The individual with a paranoid disorder usually remains organized in the other areas of functioning; the paranoia is usually isolated to only one area.

3 There is no evidence in the history to demonstrate that the client's feelings are shared by anyone else.

4 The individual usually has generalized feelings of suspiciousness and awareness of imagined wrongs, but delusions and disintegration are rarely present.

98. 2 Clients use a structured delusional system to justify and compensate for their feelings of worthlessness and low self-esteem. (b) (PS; AN; PE; SD)

1 This is not the purpose of the delusional system.

3 Clients experiencing delusions of a paranoid nature are isolated and need contact with people to increase their contact with reality.

4 There is nothing in the situation to indicate this client is not accepted by others.

99. **2** The client has low self-esteem, which forms the basis for the delusion that others do not see him as worthy and wish to be rid of him; a delusion is a fixed, false belief. (a) (PS; AN; PE; SD)

1 The client is not experiencing hallucinations, which are false sensory perceptions without external stimuli.

3 The client is not exhibiting ideas of reference; no data indicate that the client feels everything that is happening or is being said refers to him.

4 The client is not coining words with unusual meanings.

100. **1** This will help the client develop self-esteem and reduce the feeling that people are out to get him. (b) (PS; AN; TC; SD)

2 It is impossible to remove all stress in any situation.

3 This will only succeed in supporting the client's ideas of persecution and will lower the client's self-esteem.

4 Because people must function in a social environment, it is almost impossible to avoid placing some demands on others.

101. **3** Attempting to approach the client in a nonthreatening manner and using a calm, consistent, nonviolent approach often helps the agitated client to gain more self-control. (b) (PS; IM; PE; SD)

1 This is premature; medication should not be used before trying to verbally calm the client down.

2 This action would increase, not decrease, agitation.

4 Action should not be postponed; escalation must be prevented.

102. **4** This is all the staff can do until trust is established and the client is able to give up some of these defenses; forcing the client to attend will disrupt the group. (b) (PS; IM; PE; SD)

1 This will serve little purpose and will result in a confrontation; behavior cannot be altered by arguing.

2 This will serve only to create a confrontation between clients.

3 Same as # 1.

103. **1** This demonstrates that the staff believes that what the client has to say is important; this also encourages verbalization. (b) (PS; IM; TC; TR)

2 This would accomplish little if anything; individuals cannot be talked out of feelings.

3 Feelings cannot always be explained; this also forces the client to further develop the delusional system.

4 This would only increase feelings of worthlessness and persecution and would cut off communication.

104. **3** Helping the client to develop feelings of self-worth would reduce the client's need to use pathologic defenses. (b) (PS; PL; PE; SD)

1 This is not the basic underlying problem but merely a symptom of it.

2 Same as # 1.

4 Insight can only develop when the need to use the defense is reduced.

105. **4** This approach gives the client and spouse an opportunity to discuss their feelings together and clarifies their expectations. (b) (PS; IM; PE; SD)

1 This is the nurse's responsibility and should not be passed to someone else.

2 This is not the nurse's role; the spouse may never be reassured.

3 This would do little to reassure the spouse.

106. **1** Because rape is a threat to the sense of control over one's life, some control should be given back to the client as soon as possible. (c) (PS; PL; TC; CS)

2 This takes control away from the client; the client could view this as an additional assault on the body that increases feelings of vulnerability and anxiety and does not restore control.

3 Same as # 2.

4 This is a normal form of ventilating emotions; the client should be told medication is available if desired.

107. **2** Partners may themselves feel angry and abused; these feelings should be rapidly and openly discussed. (c) (PS; AN; TC; CS)

1 This may be reassuring, but it leaves the partner alone to deal with feelings.

3 This should not be done yet; rape counselors deal with the victim and partner together.

4 The partner's feelings must be resolved before the partner can really help the client.

108. **2** Focusing is indicated when communication is vague; the nurse attempts to concentrate or focus the client's communication on one specific aspect. (b) (PS; IM; TC; TR)

1 Touch would invade the client's space and would do nothing to help focus the client's communication.

3 Silence would only prolong the rambling communication; client needs to be focused.

4 Until the concern is identified and explored, summarizing would be impossible.

109. **2** In projection a person faults another person for having the unacceptable impulses, thoughts, or behaviors that are too uncomfortable to accept as one's own. (a) (PS; AN; PE; SA)

1 Denial is a method of resolving conflict or escaping unpleasant realities by ignoring their existence.

3 Displacement refers to the transfer of an emotion from one object or situation to another, usually safer, object.

4 In compensation the person makes up for personal inadequacies by emphasizing attributes to gain social approval.

110. **1** Alcohol is a central nervous system depressant; these symptoms are the body's neurologic adaptation to the withdrawal of alcohol. (b) (PS; AS; PA; SA)

2 These are late signs of severe withdrawal that occur with delirium tremens; tachycardia results from autonomic overactivity.

3 Fever and diaphoresis may be seen during prolonged periods of delirium and are a result of autonomic overactivity.

4 Grand mal seizures are not early signs of alcohol withdrawal; they would not occur before 48 to

72 hours of abstinence.

111. **3** This strengthens the client's link with reality and reassures the client of safety because the hallucinations are usually frightening. (b) (PS; IM; TC; SA)
1 Validation reinforces the client's distorted perceptions of reality, is not helpful, and may even be unsafe.
2 It is not helpful to argue or try to explain the hallucinations away because they are real to the client.
4 The nurse must respond to the client's behavior by attempting to point out reality and reduce anxiety.

112. **1** Chlorpromazine suppresses central sympathetic activity, which reduces the discomfort of withdrawal and the risk of seizures. (c) (PS; AN; PA; DR)
2 The ability of the client to accept treatment depends on readiness to accept the reality of the problem.
3 Although these may occur, they are not the primary objectives for using the drug.
4 This drug helps to reduce the risk of convulsions but does not prevent physical injury during a convulsion.

113. **2** A hypotensive reaction is a common adverse effect of chlorpromazine. (b) (PS; AS; PA; DR)
1 Restraints of any type may increase the client's anxiety and result in struggling and increased agitation.
3 Tardive dyskinesia and akathisia usually result from prolonged large doses of phenothiazines in susceptible clients.
4 Photosensitivity occurs most frequently when clients are taking large doses and are spending time outdoors in the sun.

114. **4** Recognizing the family's feelings and giving simple factual information helps to allay anxiety. (b) (PS; IM; ED; TR)
1 This is an inappropriate statement, especially during this time of stress; it also gives little assurance to the family.
2 This is false reassurance and does not allow the family to verbalize their anxieties or fears.
3 This discourages further verbalization of concerns and promotes feelings of isolation and helplessness.

115. **1** These are good sources of thiamine; other sources include legumes, whole and enriched grains, and lean beef. (b) (PS; EV; ED; SA)
2 Most vegetables contain only traces of thiamine; this list contains good sources of vitamin C.
3 In this list, only eggs are considered a fair source of thiamine; this list contains good sources of protein.
4 In this list, only fish is considered a fair source of thiamine.

116. **3** Peripheral neuropathy is present, and this measure will limit tactile stimulation. (b) (PS; IM; PA; SA)
1 This would do little to relieve discomfort or reduce the occurrence of neurologic symptoms.
2 Same as # 1.
4 This may be done periodically; however, these symptoms are not caused by impaired circulation but rather by peripheral neuropathy.

117. **2** This supports the partner of the addicted indi-

vidual and allows the partner to continue on with life by reducing guilt. (b) (PS; IM; TC; TR)
1 This is enabling behavior, which does not help the abuser or the partner.
3 This places the burden for preventing drinking on the partner and will create feelings of resentment and guilt.
4 The partner has already stated this is impossible.

118. **2** This will enable the client to begin speaking about the spouse and resolve the loss. (b) (PS; PL; PE; CS)
1 Psychiatric consultation is not indicated by the data at this time.
3 Although this may be beneficial, the primary focus should be on expression of feelings.
4 Data do not indicate ambivalence toward the spouse.

119. **3** This is the most important assessment to make because suicide is a possibility with every depressed client. (b) (PS; AS; TC; MO)
1 The client has already said this and it responds to only part of the client's statement.
2 This is a philosophic approach that would not encourage discussion of feelings.
4 The nurse does not have enough information to have this understanding; this response does not encourage communication.

120. **4** At this point the client may have enough energy to plan and execute an attempt. (a) (PS; AN; TC; MO)
1 The motor retardation accompanying depression usually limits the client's acting out on impulse.
2 Same as # 1.
3 Loss of interest in the environment is an early sign of depression, and the client would not have the energy to act out.

121. **4** These are the defining characteristics of dysfunctional grieving. (c) (PS; AS; PE; CS)
1 Eight months does not constitute a prolonged period of mourning.
2 The client's communication does not lead to this conclusion.
3 Same as # 2.

122. **1** If nurses are unaware of their biases about rape, they will be unprepared to evaluate objectively and meet the client's needs. (a) (PS; AN; PE; TR)
2 It is not necessary to know these to effectively respond to the client in a therapeutic manner.
3 The nurse should be able to deal with this client without assistance.
4 This would interrupt communication; information can be solicited later.

123. **1** Identification of support networks and relationships is a priority if the victim is to be helped after the immediate crisis is over. (c) (PS; AS; PE; TR)
2 This is not necessary for evaluation of the client's condition or support network.
3 This may eventually be of value, but at this time it is irrelevant to assessing the client's condition or needs.
4 Same as # 3.

124. **2** Anxiety is a threat to the identity of the individual; the client is seeking assurance that the fear and panic being experienced will not mean loss of control. (b) (PS; AN; PE; AX)
1 This is not evidence of insightfulness but a plea

for help in reducing the anxiety.

3 The client is not exhibiting depression but severe anxiety and panic.

4 The client is not testing the nurse; she is asking for help.

125. **4** The nurse's presence may provide the client with support and feelings of control. (b) (PS; IM; TC; AX)

1 The client is too distraught to sit; to be therapeutic the nurse would have to be where the client is.

2 It is evident that the client is upset; this question is not therapeutic and may lead to anger, which would interfere with the development of a therapeutic nurse-client relationship.

3 The client is in a panic; anger is not primary; there is no need to work off aggression.

126. **3** Freedom to ventilate feelings acts as a safety valve to reduce the anxiety. (a) (PS; PL; PE; AX)

1 The suppression of anger or hostility would add to the client's anxiety.

2 This may or may not be true; the client's family may provide support to the client.

4 This would not be therapeutic; it might add to the anxiety the client is feeling.

127. **4** This is a technique that avoids misunderstanding so that both the client and the nurse can work toward a common goal in the therapeutic relationship. (b) (PS; AN; PE; TR)

1 This would not provide for clarification or understanding.

2 Same as # 1.

3 Same as # 1.

128. **3** Regression is the defense mechanism commonly used by clients with schizophrenia to reduce anxiety by returning to earlier behavior. (b) (PS; AN; PE; SD)

1 Rationalization, in which the individual blames others for problems and attempts to justify actions, is seldom used by clients with schizophrenia.

2 This unconscious forgetting is not a major defense used by clients with schizophrenia; if it were they would not need to break with reality.

4 This organized defense is used by clients with schizophrenia, paranoid type, in which the delusional system is well systemized.

129. **3** This provides a stimulus that competes with and reduces hallucinations. (b) (PS; IM; PE; SD)

1 This is a direct question that the client probably could not answer; it would also increase anxiety.

2 In addition to setting unrealistic standards, this response fails to recognize that the client believes the hallucinations are real.

4 If the nurse waits for the client to stop hallucinating, there may be no chance for contact with this client.

130. **4** This lets the client know the nurse is trying to understand; it increases the client's feeling of self-esteem and points out reality. (c) (PS; IM; PE; SD)

1 Clients with schizophrenia have problems with associative links, and these same problems will occur regardless of the topic.

2 This statement cuts off communication and tells the client that the nurse will only speak if the client's communication makes sense.

3 Same as # 2.

131. **1** This statement points out reality, prevents the nurse from getting caught up in the client's illness, and recognizes feelings. (b) (PS; IM; PE; SD)

2 This is an attempt to argue the client out of feelings by denying they exist.

3 This is nontherapeutic; it supports and focuses on the hallucination.

4 Same as # 3.

132. **3** All behavior has meaning; the nurse must try to understand what the behavior means to the client. (c) (PS; AS; TC; TR)

1 The nurse cannot explain the meaning of the client's behavior; only the client can.

2 The isolation of a client may increase anxiety and precipitate more acting-out behavior.

4 Ignoring behavior does little to alter it and it may even cause further acting out.

133. **3** Phenothiazine potentiates the action of alcohol and can cause death if the drug and alcohol are taken together. (a) (PS; IM; ED; DR)

1 This medication should be taken consistently to prevent recurrence of symptoms and maintain blood drug levels.

2 Medication should be taken as ordered; taking it all at one time can interrupt the consistency of therapeutic blood levels.

4 Same as # 1.

134. **4** Thorazine reduces emotional tensions, excessive psychomotor activity, panic, and fear. (b) (PS; AN; PA; DR)

1 Clients exhibiting excited-depressed behavior do not respond well to Thorazine because it tends to increase the depression.

2 Thorazine appears to have few stimulating effects and in fact increases feelings of lassitude and fatigue.

3 Clients exhibiting manic behaviors do not respond well to Thorazine, and it can exacerbate their underlying feelings of depression.

135. **2** The medication should be stopped immediately because liver damage is a possible severe side effect of Thorazine. (a) (PS; EV; TC; DR)

1 Liver damage can result from even small doses of Thorazine.

3 Milk does not change the hepatotoxic effect of Thorazine.

4 The symptom will not disappear but will be exacerbated if the drug is continued.

136. **3** This ritual is a process of undoing arising from unconscious conflicts from the anal stage in which dirt, or soiling oneself, is associated with an aggressive act against authority; the rage is controlled by rituals such as handwashing. (b) (PS; AN; PE; PR)

1 There is usually no problem with gender identity.

2 There is initiative; the rebellion is against authority, not autonomy.

4 There is a desire for freedom and independence; the ritual is an act against authority.

137. **3** In the early part of treatment before new defenses are developed, enough time must be allowed for the client to complete the ritual to keep anxiety under control. (b) (PS; IM; PE; TR)

1 The ritual is a defense that cannot be interrupted or delayed; it is used until new defenses are developed.

2 Same as # 1.

4 Same as # 1.

138. **3** Before deciding how to decrease the client's fears of addiction, the nurse must explore the full extent of the client's knowledge and feelings about taking the drug. (a) (PS; AS; PE; PR)

1 Information may or may not be helpful; the client's feelings are what must be addressed.

2 It is too early; exploration to find the basis of the fear is necessary first.

4 Same as # 2.

139. **3** This is a serious charge, and confrontation should occur in the presence of the supervisor. (c) (PS; IM; PE; SA)

1 This is an assumption that may result in an altercation; a witness should be present.

2 This is unnecessary; as a professional the nurse has enough information to confront the other nurse.

4 This is not a professional approach; the nurse has a legal responsibility to intervene.

140. **4** This is a nonpunitive approach that attempts to salvage the nurse as an individual and as a professional. (b) (PS; IM; TC; SA)

1 This is a punitive, nontherapeutic response that offers no chance for rehabilitation.

2 This may be necessary for long-term therapy but would not be the initial approach.

3 The client is addicted; promises will not keep the client from abusing drugs.

141. **1** The user has an emotional and physiologic dependence on the drug, and the phenomenon of tolerance (more drug needed to achieve the same effect) occurs. (b) (PS; AN; PA; DR)

2 There is an emotional dependence.

3 Tolerance, even to levels that would be lethal in the nonaddicted individual, occurs.

4 There is a physiologic dependence.

142. **3** This allows the client to use the staff as a support system and removes an opportunity to deny the problem. (c) (PS; PL; ED; SA)

1 This supports and permits denial; both the client and the staff know a problem exists, and the client must admit it.

2 This is a nonprofessional approach that would be nontherapeutic for the client.

4 Same as # 2.

143. **3** Unless staff can share both positive and negative feelings, resentment, anger, and frustration will develop. (c) (PS; IM; ED; TR)

1 This response attacks the speaker and cuts off communication in the group.

2 This response does little to foster communication and relationships among staff members.

4 Same as # 1.

144. **3** This is a psychiatric disease in which there is no prior history of depression; it is related to age, changes in life-style, and feelings of not contributing and being worthless. (a) (PS; AS; PE; MO)

1 Involutional melancholia, which was usually characterized by depression with agitation, is no longer considered a specific disorder.

2 In bipolar disorders, depression alternates with periods of extreme restlessness, hyperactivity, and flamboyance in dress and behavior; this is not evident here.

4 There is no inconsistency between the behavior

and the mood.

145. **2** Before therapy can begin, a trusting relationship must develop. (b) (PS; PL; TC; TR)

1 A client with major depression would not have the impetus or energy to investigate new leisure activities.

3 This would not be successful unless the client had developed a trusting, comfortable relationship with the nurse.

4 This is not appropriate initially; a trusting one-to-one relationship must be developed first.

146. **1** Some success is important to increase the client's self-esteem. (c) (PS; IM; PE; MO)

2 This would support the client's feelings of uselessness.

3 The client who is in a major depression would not have the interest or energy to act independently.

4 Same as # 3.

147. **4** Before onset of depression, these clients usually have very narrow, limited interests. (b) (PS; AS; PE; MO)

1 Many individuals have been conforming, conscientious, and hardworking in an attempt to feel needed; feelings of guilt, anger, worthlessness, and hopelessness occur with the depression.

2 Same as # 1.

3 Same as # 1.

148. **1** An illusion is a misinterpretation of an actual sensory stimulus. (b) (PS; AN; PE; SD)

2 A hallucination is a false sensory perception without a stimulus being present.

3 A delusion is a false fixed belief.

4 Confabulation is filling in blanks in memory.

149. **4** The usual age of onset of schizophrenia is adolescence or early adulthood. (b) (PS; AS; PE; SD)

1 Symptoms usually do not appear this early.

2 Same as # 1.

3 Same as # 1.

150. **3** A somatic delusion is a fixed false belief pertaining to part of the body. (b) (PS; AN; PE; SD)

1 An illusion is a misinterpretation of an actual sensory stimulus.

2 Depersonalization is a feeling of unreality concerning the self.

4 Hallucinations are false sensory perceptions without stimuli being present.

151. **4** This is very helpful in decreasing hallucinations because it provides another stimulus to compete for the client's attention. (b) (PS; PL; TC; SD)

1 This would foster and support the hallucinations.

2 Same as # 1.

3 Connections should be made to decrease the use of hallucinations.

152. **2** Participating with one trusted individual gradually diminishes the need for withdrawal. (b) (PS; PL; TC; SD)

1 This would not increase socialization but rather would promote withdrawal.

3 This activity fosters competition, which would not be helpful at this time.

4 Same as # 1.

153. **1** This client needs toileting every 2 hours to prevent soiling; physically seating the client on the toilet often prevents accidents and negates the use of diapers. (c) (PS; IM; TC; OR)

2 The client needs to be physically placed on the toilet; confusion limits effectiveness of other actions.

3 Same as # 2.

4 Same as # 2.

154. **2** Clients with organic mental disorders have the greatest loss in the area of recent memory. (b) (PS; PL; PA; OR)

1 Memory of remote events usually remains fairly intact.

3 Same as # 1.

4 Same as # 1.

155. **1** When the client is unable to perform a task, frustration occurs and results in more disorganized behavior. (c) (PS; PL; TC; OR)

2 The client's disorientation is documented and will not change although some day-to-day variations may occur; most important is the assessment of the client's ability to function.

3 There is no documentation of disruptive behavior; frustration must to be avoided.

4 The client will probably never adjust any further.

156. **4** The data presented indicate developmentally related struggles and specific situations that are extremely stressful; multiple stresses can produce a crisis situation for the individual when past coping mechanisms are ineffective. (a) (PS; AS; TC; CS)

1 A crisis is not an age-related problem; a crisis results when the individual's past coping mechanisms are no longer effective for dealing with a present stressful situation.

2 It is not the experience, but the individual's response to the experience, that determines a crisis.

3 The extent of stress, although a factor, is not the most significant factor in identifying the presence of a crisis; the individual's inability to cope indicates a crisis.

157. **1** The major goal of crisis intervention is to resolve the present crisis and return the client to the pre-crisis level of functioning. (a) (PS; AN; PE; CS)

2 This would be a short-term goal.

3 Same as # 2.

4 This is a goal of psychotherapy, not crisis intervention.

158. **2** According to Erikson, adolescents are struggling with identity versus role diffusion. (b) (PS; AN; PE; BA)

1 This is untrue; most adolescents do not use drugs and alcohol to escape.

3 This reflects part of the struggle for independence; it does not indicate failure to achieve the developmental task of adolescence; "all" is too inclusive.

4 Adolescents tend to be group oriented, not isolated; they struggle to belong, not to escape.

159. **3** Adolescents learn about who they are by assuming and experiencing a variety of roles; experimentation results in the retention or rejection of behavior and roles. (b) (PS; EV; PE; BA)

1 Continuous sublimation would not be constructive; this would delay and interfere with the successful completion of the struggle to formulate one's identity.

2 This is not constructive; this would not allow for experimentation with a variety of roles.

4 This is not constructive; it does not allow for the development of independence.

160. **1** Personal internal strengths and supportive individuals are critical factors that can be employed to assist the individual to cope with a crisis (b) (PS; AS; TC; CS)

2 This is unrealistic; identifying unconscious conflicts takes a long time and is inappropriate for crisis intervention.

3 This is a goal of psychotherapy, not crisis intervention; it is usually not necessary to restructure the personality to resolve a crisis.

4 Although this information may be helpful, it is not essential; factors concerning the present situation are paramount.

161. **2** The assessment of the client's present status and ability to perform ADL is the priority because it will influence the choice of an appropriate therapeutic regimen. (c) (PS; AS; TC; CS)

1 Although significant, it is not the priority.

3 Concern now is for the client, not how the client's behavior affects others.

4 The present crisis must be dealt with first.

162. **4** A situational crisis is a sudden unexpected event with which the individual is unable to cope using past coping behaviors; this time frame provides an opportunity for the individual to learn new coping behaviors. (b) (PS; AN; PE; CS)

1 This would be too short a period for the individual to develop new successful coping mechanisms.

2 Same as # 1.

3 Same as # 1.

163. **2** It is important to know if the client is considering suicide so that the nurse can provide a safe environment and therapeutic care. (c) (PS; AS; PE; CS)

1 Concern for the client's safety takes priority at this time over present feelings or past relationships.

3 Same as # 1.

4 Same as # 1.

164. **4** Discussing the partner and the partner's death will help the client work through the grief process. (c) (PS; PL; PE; CS)

1 This would refocus the client's attention away from dealing with feelings; the client would probably not have the physical or emotional energy to get involved with group activities.

2 Same as # 1.

3 The client must deal with the past and present before dealing with the future.

165. **3** Helping a client deal with unresolved grief involves assisting the client to express thoughts and feelings about the lost object or person as a necessary part of grief work. (a) (PS; IM; PE; CS)

1 This would be too threatening; at this point the client needs a therapeutic one-to-one interaction.

2 The current nonverbal behavior indicates that the client is dealing with feelings; an opportunity should be provided for a verbal exploration.

4 This is the responsibility of the nurse; another client would not have the expertise to help the client.

166. **3** As the depression lifts, the client's energy will in-

crease, which permits the person to act out suicidal thoughts. (a) (PS; PL; TC; MO)

1 This is unsafe; the priority is to protect the client from self-harm.
2 The opposite is true.
4 Same as # 1.

167. **2** Sleep and appetite disturbances are clues that the client is anxious; a history of suicidal ideation indicates that the client is thinking about self-harm; the client may attempt suicide to obtain relief from the anxiety. (b) (PS; AS; TC; MO)

1 Severe anxiety would interfere with client's ability to focus energy and act out a suicidal plan.
3 The severely depressed client would not have the energy to act on a suicidal plan.
4 The client who is out of contact with reality would not have the ability to develop or follow through with a suicide plan.

168. **3** The answer to this question will provide the nurse with an idea of the client's hopes and frustrations without being threatening or probing. (c) (PS; AS; PE; TR)

1 This question is probing, disregards the client's statement, and provides little information for the nurse to use in planning care.
2 Same as # 1.
4 Same as # 1.

169. **3** The client's statement is an example of the use of denial, a defense that blocks problems by unconsciously refusing to admit they exist. (b) (PS; AS; PE; AX)

1 The client is not using displacement, a defense mechanism that is used to allow the shifting of feeling from an emotionally charged person or object to a safe substitute person or object.
2 The client is not using projection, a defense that is used to deny unacceptable feelings and emotions and attribute them to others.
4 The client is not using sublimation, a defense that is used to substitute socially acceptable behavior for unacceptable instincts.

170. **4** The client has been able to function well up to this time, and the client's usual behavior and routines should be supported. (b) (PS; PL; TC; TR)

1 At this time the data presented do not identify this as a need.
2 Same as # 1.
3 Same as # 1.

171. **4** The development of confusion would indicate that the client's ability to regain equilibrium has not been achieved and that further disequilibrium was occurring. (b) (PS; EV; TC; AX)

1 This would not indicate the plan needed to be changed; the client's history demonstrates the use of this defense.
2 Same as # 1.
3 This would be a positive response to any plan of care.

172. **2** Establishment of a therapeutic relationship begins with introductions. (b) (PS; IM; PE; TR)

1 This does not provide the client with any information about who the speaker is; use of the client's first name demonstrates lack of respect.
3 In addition to not providing any information and using the client's first name, this greeting is probing and would place the client on the defensive.

4 This provides no information except the speaker's name.

173. **3** This response addresses the reality that the client is on the mental health unit and offers assistance. (b) (PS; IM; PE; TR)

1 On the basis of the information available, it would be too early to make this decision.
2 This is a rather hostile response that assumes the client is unable to follow conversation.
4 This response assumes the client is disoriented as to place; it sounds like the beginning of a lecture.

174. **4** This response addresses the client's misconceptions about mental health services and specific fear of being crazy. (b) (PS; IM; PE; TR)

1 This response ignores the feeling tones behind the client's statement and focuses on facts.
2 Same as # 1.
3 Same as # 1.

175. **2** Value clarification is a technique that uncovers individuals' values so that the individuals can be more aware of them and their effect on others. (b) (PS; AN; TC; TR)

1 This is untrue; it merely helps the individual become aware of values and their effect on others.
3 Same as # 1.
4 Same as # 1.

176. **2** This response is optimistic and supportive and clarifies the purpose of the relationship. (b) (PS; IM; PE; TR)

1 This statement diminishes the client's response and sets up a challenge; it does not foster a therapeutic relationship.
3 Same as # 1.
4 Same as # 1.

177. **3** The ability to discuss feelings about others and life situations is necessary for positive mental health. (b) (PS; AN; TC; TR)

1 This is a long-term, not a short-term, goal.
2 Same as # 1.
4 Same as # 1.

178. **2** These are positive coping behaviors that can consciously be used to promote mental health. (a) (PS; PL; TC; AX)

1 These are not healthy coping behaviors, and their frequent use can lead to distortions of reality.
3 Same as # 1.
4 Same as # 1.

179. **4** Clients frequently respond in this manner when they feel threatened; this behavior supports the client's ego integrity. (b) (PS; AN; TC; AX)

1 The nurse's actions play only a minor role in these situations.
2 This is not true; the client's feelings, not the situation, precipitate this response.
3 Same as # 1.

180. **1** Unless the nurse answers the question, the client will continue to focus on the nurse rather than on the self; the nurse can best redirect after a brief answer. (b) (PS; IM; TC; TR)

2 This moves the focus to the nurse's opinions rather than the client's feelings.
3 Same as # 2.
4 This is not therapeutic; the client is being asked to share, and the nurse should also be willing.

181. **2** This is the task of the older adult; this client has not adapted to triumphs and disappointments,

so there is no acceptance of what life is and was, and this results in feelings of despair and disgust. (b) (PS; AN; ED; CS)

1 This is the task of the preschool period.

3 This is the task of the young adult.

4 This is the task of the adolescent.

182. **1** This allows the client to accept what life is or was and helps avoid feelings of despair. (c) (PS; AN; ED; CS)

2 This would be impossible to accomplish and denies the reality of what was or is in life.

3 Same as # 2.

4 This would require a total reversal in the client's past life-style; this is unlikely, if not impossible, for the client at this age.

183. **1** The client cannot be expected to accept or even respond to a plan that would be incompatible with the family's life-style. (a) (PS; PL; TC; TR)

2 The family should not have to adjust to the nurse's biases; the nurse must deal with biases before they interfere with care.

3 There is no documentation that misconceptions are present.

4 All individuals respond differently to situations.

184. **3** Past experiences are important and must be recognized because they set the parameters for the individual's values throughout life. (a) (PS; AN; TC; TR)

1 This is untrue; past experiences play an important role in an individual's life.

2 This is untrue; past experiences would not affect inherited traits.

4 Nothing establishes how an individual responds forever; new experiences continue to influence future responses.

185. **4** Psychoactive drugs have been shown to be capable of interrupting the acute psychiatric process, making the client more amenable to other therapies. (a) (PS; AN; PA; DR)

1 Clients with schizophrenia usually have little insight into their problems; confronting the client with insight will increase anxiety.

2 This is untrue; ECT is more effective in treating depressed clients.

3 Family therapy is effective but is a long-term, costly therapy; symptoms must be reduced before the client can participate.

186. **1** This would facilitate a one-to-one interaction and the development of a trusting relationship. (c) (PS; PL; TC; SD)

2 This activity would allow the client to withdraw.

3 Same as # 2.

4 This activity would foster competition and could increase the client's anxiety.

187. **3** The client truly believes the voices are real, and because the voices reflect the client's thoughts, they are usually accusatory and derogatory and therefore very frightening. (b) (PS; IM; PE; SD)

1 This would be too late; competing stimuli must be present to block the occurrence.

2 This is incorrect; the client cannot be talked out of a hallucination.

4 Soft music played either before hallucinations begin or after they have started will not be strong enough to compete for the client's attention.

188. **3** The delusional system contains grandiose ideation that allows the client to feel important

rather than inferior. (b) (PS; PL; PE; SD)

1 These individuals are usually able to express aggressive feelings without difficulty.

2 Data show no evidence of feelings of persecution.

4 Although these individuals often feel guilty, feelings of inferiority, not guilt, precipitate delusions.

189. **2** Extreme photosensitivity is a common side effect of Thorazine. (c) (PS; PL; ED; DR)

1 Once the client's medication is adjusted and CNS response is noted, driving may be permitted; drowsiness usually subsides after the first few weeks.

3 Although this drug can cause hypotension, it does not consistently lower blood pressure; a sudden drop can be dangerous to a client with hypertension.

4 This is untrue; energy is usually decreased.

190. **3** Infection can indicate agranulocytosis, a serious side effect that can occur with therapy and can cause death. (c) (PS; EV; PA; DR)

1 This would be unsafe because the client may be developing agranulocytosis, a potentially life-threatening side effect that needs immediate treatment.

2 Same as # 1.

4 Same as # 1.

191. **2** The client needs constant reassurance because forgetfulness blocks previous explanations; frequent presence of staff serves as a continual reminder. (b) (PS; PL; TC; OR)

1 This client will not remember the explanation from one moment to the next.

3 The client needs continual reassurance and would not remember times for planned interactions or activities.

4 This client would be unable to explain the reasons.

192. **2** This response recognizes problems of the care-giver without a hint of blame for admission; it opens the channel of communication. (b) (PS; IM; TC; TR)

1 This is a somewhat hostile response that would place the care-giver on the defensive.

3 Same as # 1.

4 Same as # 1.

193. **2** These clients require external controls to minimize danger of injury and to preserve human dignity. (b) (PS; PL; TC; OR)

1 The client will not have excessive energy.

3 Further deterioration usually cannot be prevented in this disorder.

4 The staff cannot prevent all gross motor activity; the client needs to use muscles, or atrophy will occur.

194. **2** The preinteraction phase is the period before the nurse begins the interaction; it is the preparatory phase of a planned therapeutic relationship. (b) (PS; AN; TC; TR)

1 The orientation phase is the initial period of the actual interaction; it is the introductory or exploratory phase.

3 The working phase is the period in a relationship when the individuals are occupied with achieving goals and sharing facts and feelings.

4 The termination phase is the period in a relationship when the individuals are beginning to separate and move toward independent paths.

195. **2** This is a correct description of the working phase of a relationship; trust has been established, and a relationship has been developed based on mutual respect. (b) (PS; AN; TC; TR)
1 This behavior would occur during the orientation phase before trust is established.
3 Same as # 1.
4 Same as # 1.

196. **2** The withdrawn pattern of behavior prevents the individual from reaching out to others for sharing; the isolation produces feelings of loneliness. (b) (PS; AN; PE; TR)
1 Feelings of anger may result in withdrawal, but withdrawal does not produce feelings of anger.
3 Repression is an unconscious defense whereby the individual excludes ideas, feelings, or situations from the conscious level of thought; this is not the result of withdrawal.
4 Feelings of paranoia may result in withdrawal, but withdrawal does not produce these feelings.

197. **1** Withdrawal provides a temporary defense against anxiety because it limits contact with reality and decreases the client's world. (b) (PS; AN; PE; TR)
2 Withdrawal does not accomplish this, because feelings and anxieties are still present and little attempt is made to work through problems.
3 Same as # 2.
4 Same as # 2.

198. **2** The client expends a great amount of energy running headlong into reality in an attempt to ward off or avoid facing feelings of depression. (c) (PS; AN; PE; MO)
1 This client is not attempting to compensate for an imagined loss but is trying to avoid feelings of depression.
3 The behavior is not an expression of innate desires but an attempt to avoid feelings of depression.
4 The client has no difficulty relating to others; this behavior is an attempt to avoid feelings of depression.

199. **4** These clients are acutely aware of and sensitive to the environment; they need a structured environment in which stimuli are reduced and a feeling of acceptance and support is present. (a) (PS; PL; TC; MO)
1 This client is acutely aware of reality and does not need to have it clarified.
2 The client needs reduced, not increased, stimuli.
3 Although important, this can best be achieved by establishing a supportive, structured environment.

200. **2** These are common side effects of lithium. (b) (PS; EV; ED; DR)
1 This is a side effect of the phenothiazine group of medications.
3 Neither problem is associated with lithium intake.
4 Lithium can cause polyuria and incontinence, not retention.

201. **1** For clients with bipolar disorders, it has been shown that long-term lithium therapy flattens the highs of the euphoric phase and the lows of the depressed phase. (a) (PS; EV; ED; DR)
2 This is untrue; clients should never adjust their own dosage of medication.
3 This is untrue; the physician should be notified before medication is stopped.

4 This is not true; the therapeutic level and the toxic level are very close, and serious side effects do occur.

202. **2** Children usually blame themselves for their parents' marital problems, often believing that they are the reason one parent leaves. (b) (PS; AN; ED; BA)
1 No data are presented to lead to this conclusion.
3 The child's response is not typical of grief work.
4 Same as # 1.

203. **4** Comparison over time is the only way for the nurse to accurately assess the mental status of a child. (b) (PS; AS; ED; PA)
1 This may be unrealistic and biased; the nurse should take the parents' description of behavior into consideration but should mainly rely on personal assessment and observation over time.
2 This would not be an accurate method because the child's ability to discuss feelings is limited.
3 This would be threatening and may increase the child's anxiety.

204. **3** Children with emotional problems usually have difficulty dealing with reality and tend to withdraw; they are afraid to use reality testing. (b) (PS; AS; ED; BA)
1 Behavior is more often disorganized rather than deliberate, and aggressive rather than passive.
2 There is usually a withdrawal from the peer group.
4 The anxiety level is usually severe, often approaching the panic level.

205. **2** This is the family constellation as it is now constructed; without prior discussion and permission, an invitation to anyone else would be an intrusion of privacy. (c) (PS; AN; ED; BA)
1 The father cannot be invited without prior discussion with and permission of the mother.
3 In addition to needing the mother's permission to invite the father, the nurse must also include the child in family therapy.
4 The teacher is not part of the family constellation.

206. **3** This is a nonjudgmental response that does not pressure the client but does clearly indicate that treatment is necessary. (b) (PS; IM; TC; TR)
1 This is an unrealistic response that gives approval to the client's behavior.
2 This is an unrealistic response that is unsupported by any data.
4 This nonsupportive response tells the client that the physician knows best.

207. **4** This statement provides clues that the client feels no one cares, so there is no reason the client should care. (b) (PS; AN; PE; MO)
1 The clues presented do not lead to this conclusion.
2 Same as # 1.
3 Same as # 1.

208. **4** An individual's ability to handle stress develops through experience with life; aging does not reduce this ability but often strengthens it. (a) (PS; PL; ED; TR)
1 The senses of taste and/or smell are often diminished in the aged individual.
2 Gastrointestinal motility is slowed in the aged individual.
3 Muscle or motor strength is diminished in the aged individual.

209. **2** The individual who can reflect back on life and

accept it for what it was and is and who can adjust and enjoy the changes retirement brings is less likely to develop health problems, especially stress-related health problems. (b) (PS; AN; ED; TR)

1 These changes are usually not reversible.

3 This is untrue; most emotionally healthy older individuals do not focus on these thoughts.

4 This is not true; dependency is often more threatening to this age-group.

210. 2 Clients usually respond with better motivation for self-care if they feel someone is depending on them and they are needed. (b) (PS; PL; PE; TR)

1 This is untrue; emotionally healthy individuals do not feel better simply because others have more problems.

3 Clients need to feel needed, not just to establish new social contacts.

4 Same as # 3.

211. 3 Without the development of trust the child has little confidence that the significant other will return; separation is considered abandonment by the child. (a) (PS; AN; ED; BA)

1 Without autonomy, the individual has little self-confidence, develops a deep sense of shame and doubt, and learns to expect defeat.

2 Without identity, the individual will have a problem in forming a social role and a sense of self; this results in identity diffusion and confusion.

4 Without initiative, the individual will experience the development of guilt when curiosity and fantasies about sexual roles occur.

212. 2 This is the developmental task of the school-aged child; the child will feel inferior if recognition is not given. (b) (PS; AN; ED; BA)

1 This is the task of the preschool child.

3 This is not a developmental task identified by Erikson.

4 Same as # 3.

213. 3 This action would provide the child with a constant caregiver with whom the child could relate. (a) (PS; IM; TC; BA)

1 Although this may provide some comfort, the child needs to receive love and attention from an adult.

2 Same as # 1.

4 This would increase the parents' guilt and anxiety; data given assume parents have been unable, not unwilling, to visit the child.

214. 3 The preschooler is terrified by intrusive procedures and views them as a punishment for curiosity and fantasies. (b) (PS; AN; ED; BA)

1 This age child does not fear loss of control.

2 This age child can localize pain even if unable to express it.

4 This age child would be unlikely to recall the procedure merely by the appearance of the technicians.

215. 1 This action would not call attention to the accident and would minimize the child's embarrassment. (b) (PS; IM; PE; BA)

2 The child would probably be unable to accomplish this task without assistance; failure to complete the task would add to embarrassment.

3 This would add to the child's embarrassment.

4 Same as # 3.

216. 1 This would permit the 8-year-old to investigate and become familiar with the equipment to be

used. (b) (PS; IM; PE; BA)

2 This would be beyond the ability of the average 8-year-old and would do little to reduce anxiety.

3 Same as # 2.

4 This would be supportive but is not always possible; even with the parent present the child should be given an opportunity to handle the equipment.

217. 1 The 9-year-old needs an opportunity to express emotions in private; talking about feelings after the child has regained control would be therapeutic. (b) (PS; AN; PE; TR)

2 This is not of great concern to the child at this moment.

3 This action would give the child a feeling that crying was wrong.

4 Same as # 2.

218. 2 Although the client's facial expression suggests happiness, the client's tone of voice gives the message of anger; the behaviors do not go together. (a) (PS; AS; PE; CS)

1 The data given do not support this assessment.

3 Same as # 1.

4 Same as # 1.

219. 3 The client is using intellectual reasoning to block confronting the unconscious conflict and the stress of having to deal with his girlfriend's pregnancy. (b) (PS; AS; PE; CS)

1 No data demonstrate the shifting of emotions from an emotionally charged object or person to a neutral one.

2 No data demonstrate that the client is concentrating thoughts and emotions on his inner self.

4 No data demonstrate that the client is projecting blame on anyone else.

220. 1 The use of self is often the only tool available to the nurse to help a client cope; the nurse must be present, actively listening, and attentive to be therapeutic. (a) (PS; IM; TC; TR)

2 The environment is important, but it is not the most basic tool.

3 The nurse must first use self before the helping process can begin.

4 The client's intellect is not necessarily a therapeutic tool used by the nurse.

221. 2 Empathy is the projection of self into another's emotions to share the emotions and the other's state of mind; this technique helps the nurse understand the meaning and significance of the experience to the client. (a) (PS; IM; TC; TR)

1 This approach does not require the nurse to project the self into the client's emotions, but rather just to accept the client and the emotions.

3 Projection is an unconscious defense, not a therapeutic technique.

4 Sympathy is a shared expression of sorrow over a real or imagined loss.

222. 3 An individual must feel a sense of control over self and the environment to feel secure, reduce anxiety, and function at an optimal level. (c) (PS; AN; PE; TR)

1 This is untrue; most emotionally ill people are too introspective to empathize with others.

2 No one functions optimally in all settings; the healthy individual can accept and handle temporary periods of confusion and loss of control.

4 This is not true; many individuals with mental illness do not demonstrate observable signs or socially inappropriate behavior.

223. **3** When all the members of a family blame one member for all their problems, scapegoating is occurring. (b) (PS; AN; PE; BA)
   1 There are no data to support identifying this pattern of relating.
   2 Same as # 1.
   4 Same as # 1.
224. **4** This action would set a foundation for trust because it allows the child to see that the nurse cares. (b) (PS; IM; PE; TR)
   1 Although this is necessary, limit setting really does not support the development of a trusting relationship.
   2 This would be too infrequent to develop thrust.
   3 This would be threatening at this stage of a relationship.
225. **4** This response would be most successful because it provides a time period for the hyperactive child to regain control; it is neither a positive nor a negative reinforcement of acting-out behavior. (c) (PS; IM; TC; BA)
   1 This action would reward acting-out behavior by providing special attention.
   2 Ignoring behavior can force the child to act out even more to gain attention.
   3 The child would interpret removal of tokens as a punishment.
226. **3** This would help the child develop insight into reasons for acting-out behavior. (c) (PS; IM; PE; BA)
   1 This denies that the child's problem behavior is continuing and does not help the child develop insight.
   2 Same as # 1.
   4 Same as # 1.
227. **1** A child usually assumes a role in the family and, as in this instance, the child's symptoms reflect the pathology that develops to fill that role. (c) (PS; AN; PE; BA)
   2 This may create problems, but these problems usually develop later in life.
   3 Same as # 2.
   4 Same as # 2.
228. **3** This would provide a trial opportunity for the client and the family to reunite outside the confines of the hospital. (b) (PS; PL; PE; BA)
   1 It is too late; this should have been done much earlier.
   2 Same as # 1.
   4 This is not the responsibility of the nurse.
229. **1** The client's verbalization reflects feelings that others are blaming the client for negative actions. (a) (PS; AN; PE; SD)
   2 No data demonstrate that the client is hearing voices at this time.
   3 No data demonstrate feelings of greatness or power.
   4 No data demonstrate the client is experiencing confusing misinterpretations of stimuli.
230. **3** This response demonstrates that the nurse understands the client's feelings; reflection opens channels of communication. (b) (PS; IM; PE; TR)
   1 The client cannot be talked out of delusions by pointing out reality.
   2 Focusing on delusional content only reinforces false beliefs.
   4 This does not reflect the content of the client's statement.

231. **3** Any other approach would be threatening, increase anxiety, and probably result in a physical confrontation. (c) (PS; PL; TC; SD)
   1 This would increase the client's anxiety and probably result in a physical confrontation.
   2 This would increase anxiety, not increase self-esteem.
   4 This would increase anxiety, not foster decision making.
232. **2** This statement demonstrates recognition and acceptance of the client's feelings and also points out reality. (b) (PS; IM; PE; SD)
   1 This provides false reassurance; the client has no reason to trust that the nurse can provide protection.
   3 This is nontherapeutic; it denies the client's feelings and would increase anxiety.
   4 Encouraging the client to focus on hallucinations tends to strengthen and confirm them.
233. **1** The client cannot reach out to others because of lack of trust; withdrawal is used to defend against interpersonal threats and results in isolation. (b) (PS; AN; PE; SD)
   2 Sleep disturbances are not common because clients tend to use sleep to withdraw from reality.
   3 Most clients with schizophrenic disorders are not violent.
   4 This is usually not associated with this disorder.
234. **4** The client and the family should be included in discussion so that concerns can be addressed openly; this increases trust and fosters relationships. (b) (PS; PL; TC; TR)
   1 This may be useful for the family later, but it would not help the immediate problem.
   2 This provides false reassurance; the client has had periods where the behavior was acceptable, only to once again become disturbed.
   3 This may be helpful, but the client should be made aware of the family's present feelings and concerns.
235. **2** This response identifies the child's feelings and lets the child know the nurse can understand them. (c) (PS; IM; TC; TR)
   1 This is an unrealistic response; the nurse cannot be sure that weight loss will improve the child's ability in gym.
   3 This is an unrealistic response; the child would probably be unable to express his feelings to peers.
   4 This denies the child's feelings and really does not offer support.
236. **1** This action would foster the development of an improved self-image. (b) (PS; IM; TC; TR)
   2 The child already is doing this, and the measure has diminished self-esteem.
   3 A problem does exist; their child is unhappy.
   4 Parents cannot avoid talking about the sibling but should avoid any comparisons.
237. **4** This is an achievable goal that will bolster the child's self-esteem. (b) (PS; AN; PE; TR)
   1 This would not improve the child's self-esteem.
   2 Same as # 1.
   3 Same as # 1.
238. **3** This would demonstrate a movement toward peer group activity and interests; exercise would also demonstrate an interest in an improved physical condition. (b) (PS; EV; PE; TR)
   1 This would not demonstrate an increase in self-

esteem.
2 The child was doing average schoolwork before any intervention.
4 Same as # 1.

239. **3** This response interprets the client's behavior to the aide without belittling the aide's feelings; it encourages the aide to get involved with plans for future care. (c) (PS; IM; ED; TR)
1 This statement does not help the aide with the situation or demonstrate any understanding of the client's feelings.
2 Although this response recognizes the client's feelings, it does nothing to assist the aide in dealing with the client.
4 This assumes the aide has nothing to contribute and only the nurse can deal with the problem.

240. **4** This action provides continuity and demonstrates to the client that the nursing staff is concerned; frequent contact reduces client's need to call staff in. (b) (PS; PL; TC; AX)
1 Telling the client is not the same as doing it; the client would not believe staff would come in frequently.
2 This would increase the client's anxiety and need for contact with staff.
3 This would not provide continuity of care.

241. **3** This would document that the client feels comfortable enough to discuss the problems that have motivated the behavior. (b) (PS; EV; TC; AX)
1 This does not demonstrate a resolution of problems underlying the behavior.
2 Same as # 1.
4 Without discussion of the problems underlying the behavior, little would be accomplished.

242. **4** This is an open-ended response that encourages further discussion without focusing on an area that the nurse, not the client, feels is the problem. (c) (PS; IM; PE; AX)
1 This is too specific; the nurse does not have enough information to come to this conclusion.
2 This response denies the client's feeling and can cause feelings of guilt for questioning the partner's love.
3 Same as # 1.

243. **2** In planning a group the nurse must ensure that clients have similar needs in order to foster relationships and interactions; diverse needs do not foster group process. (b) (PS; PL; TC; TR)
1 Although important, this is not a primary consideration.
3 Behavior and needs, rather than diagnosis, are of primary importance.
4 This has little effect on group process.

244. **1** Members have not established trust and are hesitant to discuss problems; the behaviors observed reflect anxiety and insecurity. (b) (PS; AS; PE; AX)
2 This would add to the anxiety and insecurity of group members.
3 These behaviors are expected in the early stage of the group.
4 Same as # 2.

245. **4** Members must feel comfortable to discuss things in the group; there must be an awareness that what is discussed in the group will remain in the group. (b) (PS; PL; PE; TR)
1 This will not establish trust and will increase anxiety because the members will feel their turn for exposure will come whether they want it or not.
2 Talking about trust does little to foster it.
3 Same as # 1.

246. **3** This behavior is typical of the working stage of the group; trust has been established and a willingness to discuss any problems or needs is present. (b) (PS; EV; PE; TR)
1 This can occur at any stage; it occurs in social, as well as therapeutic, relationships.
2 This would occur in the early phase of the group before trust is established and when everyone is trying to fit in.
4 Same as # 2.

247. **3** The client's response demonstrates an inability to deal with the other member's confrontive approach at this time. (b) (PS; EV; PE; AX)
1 The group has reached the working stage, and if the client was able to deal with this area, the nurse would expect the client to state the feeling generated by the statement.
2 Same as # 1.
4 There is not enough information to make this evaluation.

248. **4** This response does not attack the client for behavior but places responsibility for allowing behavior to continue on the group; the client will recognize the message without feeling increased anxiety. (c) (PS; IM; TC; TR)
1 This is not therapeutic; it allows behavior to continue without limits being set.
2 This would increase anxiety by placing demands on other members; it does not deal with the identified problem.
3 This is not a confronting approach but an attack.

249. **3** This response focuses the client on the behavior and what the client is trying to achieve by such behavior; it also helps the client to see how such behavior affects others. (c) (PS; IM; TC; TR)
1 The group would not know what the client was trying to tell the nurse; only the client would know and should be asked directly.
2 This response uses a nondirect approach to attack the client.
4 This is an attacking, defensive response made without really knowing what the client was attempting to accomplish.

250. **2** The leader should not intervene at this point; the client addressed the statement to the group, and the group response should be fostered. (b) (PS; IM; TC; TR)
1 This response would be viewed as an attack and would make other members fearful of contributing because they may be attacked.
3 Same as # 1.
4 Same as # 1.

251. **3** This is an open-ended, nonjudgmental response that points out incongruity between the client's verbal and nonverbal communication. (b) (PS; IM; PE; TR)
1 This would not help the client recognize the incongruity.
2 Same as # 1.
4 Same as # 1.

252. **3** These symptoms are all associated with opiate withdrawal, which occurs after cessation or reduction of prolonged moderate or heavy use of

opiates. (b) (PS; AS; PA; SA)

1 Lacrimation and vomiting are present; but insomnia, not drowsiness, occurs with opiate withdrawal.

2 Nausea is present, but diarrhea, not constipation, and constricted pupils rather than dilated pupils, occur with opiate withdrawal.

4 Rhinorrhea is present, but fever rather than a subnormal temperature, and muscle aches rather than convulsions, occur with opiate withdrawal.

253. **3** Individuals usually take drugs because they cannot deal with the pain of reality; the drug blurs the pain. (a) (PS; AN; PE; SA)

1 Drugs increase dependency rather than fostering independence.

2 Although this factor may encourage initial use by some adolescents, it is not the most frequent reason for use.

4 The use of drugs fosters social isolation rather than social relationships.

254. **4** Tolerance is a phenomenon that occurs in addicted individuals and increases the amount of drug needed to satisfy their need; because this phenomenon is not permanent and may disappear without warning, overdose frequently occurs. (a) (PS; AN; PA; SA)

1 The problem is not related to dependence and addiction; the failure to respond to an adult dose of an opiate is related to tolerance.

2 Same as # 1.

3 Same as # 1.

255. **1** Opiates cause central nervous system depression, resulting in severe respiratory depression, hypotension, and unconsciousness. (b) (PS; AS; PA; DR)

2 These findings, particularly the respirations, are not indicative of an overdose of an opiate.

3 Same as # 2.

4 Same as # 2.

256. **3** This drug is a narcotic antagonist that displaces narcotics from receptors in the brain, reversing respiratory depression. (b) (PS; PL; PA; DR)

1 This is a synthetic opiate that causes CNS depression; it would add to the problem of overdose.

2 This drug would have no effect on respiratory depression related to the presence of an overdose of a narcotic.

4 Same as # 2.

257. **1** Addicted individuals usually use a substance to increase their feelings of worth; the substance helps them appear bigger in their own eyes; they usually have strong unmet dependency needs. (b) (PS; AN; PE; SA)

2 Although anger is present and internalized, there is no struggle for independence.

3 Although guilt about breaking society's code may be present, there is no rejection of reality, just an inability to deal with it.

4 Although there is a need for acceptance, there is no underlying feeling of hostility.

258. **4** These clients are usually severely malnourished and have severe fluid and electrolyte imbalances; unless these imbalances are corrected, cardiac irregularities and death can occur. (b) (PS; PL; PA; BA)

1 This is important, but it is not the highest priority at this time.

2 Same as # 1.

3 Same as # 1.

259. **2** These clients have severely depleted levels of potassium and sodium because of their starvation diet and energy expenditure; these electrolytes are necessary for proper cardiac functioning. (b) (PS; AN; PA; BA)

1 Although this may occur, it is not a major health problem.

3 Same as # 1.

4 Same as # 1.

260. **1** This is a non-threatening, open-ended response that focuses discussion and leaves channels of communication open. (b) (PS; IM; PE; BA)

2 Although this does not quite accuse the client of lying, it is a threatening response that questions the client's truthfulness.

3 Same as # 2.

4 Same as # 2.

261. **2** This action would be neither a positive nor negative reinforcement of specific behavior; it would provide rewards for achievement of specific goals. (b) (PS; PL; TC; BA)

1 This would not be included in a behavior modification program.

3 Same as # 1.

4 Clients talk freely about food; the problem is with ingestion not discussion.

262. **3** By talking to the client on the telephone at mealtimes, the family is enabling the client to continue destructive behavior; the client and family must be included in discussion of and possible solutions to the problem. (b) (PS; PL; PE; BA)

1 This would be a punitive approach that would not deal with the underlying problem.

2 Same as # 1.

4 Same as # 1.

263. **3** This would demonstrate a change in behavior, as well as a positive approach to meals. (b) (PS; EV; PE; BA)

1 This would not demonstrate a change of behavior.

2 The problem is not a lack of interest about food but a deliberate failure to ingest food.

4 This would be a continuation of the same behavior used before hospitalization.

264. **4** Foods such as chocolate, aged cheese, pickled herring, and those containing excessive caffeine contain high levels of tyramine and cause dangerous hypertension in clients taking MAO inhibitors. (b) (PS; EV; ED; DR)

1 There is no need to limit intake of this food while taking MAO inhibitors.

2 Same as # 1.

3 Same as # 1.

265. **3** Monoamine oxidase uptake is inhibited by the medication, increasing concentrations of endogenous epinephrine, norepinephrine, serotonin, and dopamine in CNS storage sites; high levels of these transmitters in the presence of tyramine can cause hypertensive crisis. (b) (PS; PL; ED; DR)

1 This is not related to drug-food interaction.

2 Same as # 1.

4 This may be an adverse reaction to the drug but is not related to drug-food interaction.

266. **1** Crying is an expression of an emotion, that, if not expressed, increases anxiety and tension; the increased anxiety and tension use additional

psychic energy and hinder coping. (b) (PS; AN; PE; CS)

2 This is not universally true; in most instances the client's defenses should not be taken away until they can be replaced by more healthful defenses; the nurse must always interfere with behavior and defenses that may place the client in danger; the client's current behavior creates no threat to the client.

3 Crying does not relieve depression, nor does it help a client face reality.

4 This is not always true; many clients are embarrassed by what they consider to be a "show of weakness" and have difficulty relating to the individual who witnessed it; the nurse must do more than just accept the crying to strengthen the nurse-client relationship.

267. **1** The client has difficulty accepting the inevitability of death and attempts to deny the reality of it. (a) (PS; AN; PE; CS)

2 In this stage the client attempts to bargain for more time; the reality of death is no longer denied, but the client attempts to manipulate and extend the remaining time.

3 In the anger stage the client strikes out with the "why me" and the "how could God do this" type of statements; the client is angry at life and still angrier to be removed from it by death.

4 In the acceptance stage the client accepts the inevitability of death and peaceably awaits it.

268. **4** This is the client's desire, and the nurse should do everything possible to assist the client to achieve it. (b) (PS; PL; PE; TR)

1 This would not be therapeutic; the client has an unmet need, and the nurse should not try to refocus the client away from the objective.

2 The client should be encouraged, not discouraged; mental activity should not be too taxing and it is not unrealistic if the client wishes to do it.

3 No data support the conclusion that the client needs to work through anger.

269. **2** This is true; the client's goal is meaningful, and the nurse should do everything possible to help the client achieve it. (b) (PS; AN; PE; TR)

1 There is no reason to attempt to move the client away from this meaningful goal.

3 No evidence demonstrates the client is using denial.

4 If the client wants to work toward a goal, the energy expenditure is justified.

270. **3** The spouse is expressing the normal feelings of guilt associated with the death of a loved one; there is always initial guilt over what might have been. (a) (PS; AN; PE; CS)

1 No evidence supports this conclusion.

2 Same as # 1.

4 The spouse is expressing guilt, not shame.

271. **1** With the medication the individual does not face the reality of the loss and merely delays the onset of the pain associated with it; because most support is available at the time of the death and the funeral, tranquilizers at this time deny the individual the opportunity to use this assistance. (b) (PS; AN; PE; CS)

2 This is untrue; tranquilizers do not magnify the risk of suicide.

3 Although tranquilizers may initially cause some lethargy, this is not the reason they are not or-

dered.

4 Brain activity does not cause depression.

272. **4** This client needs firm, realistic limits set on behavior; this statement permits the client to make the choice and clearly states the consequences of behavior. (b) (PS; IM; TC; PR)

1 This is an unrealistic response; the client and visitors do not want to socialize with other clients and visitors.

2 This is an unrealistic response; this client would care very little about rules; clients with this diagnosis do not learn from past errors.

3 Same as # 2.

273. **3** Both clients must be included in a discussion about this behavior to make certain that limits on future behavior are understood by both of them. (b) (PS; PL; PE; PR)

1 This action would not set any limits on behavior but merely put staff in the policing role.

2 Although this may be necessary, the nurse must respond directly to the clients involved in this situation.

4 This action would merely cause the clients to find another place to meet; the response sets no limits on behavior but only addresses location.

274. **3** The expression of feelings by this individual would demonstrate the development of some insight and a willingness to at least begin to look at underlying causes of behavior. (b) (PS; EV; PE; PR)

1 These words would probably have little meaning to the client.

2 Same as # 1.

4 Same as # 1.

275. **2** This would be the most therapeutic thing the parents could do; the client must be made accountable for behavior and must know that manipulation and acting out will not be tolerated. (b) (PS; PL; ED; PR)

1 This would probably be a continuation of the parent's previous response to the client and would be of little value.

3 This would probably cause the client to continue to act out to test the limit of her parents' endurance.

4 Same as # 1.

Pediatric Nursing

1. **2** In view of the smoky urine and the other symptoms, the nurse may suspect glomerulonephritis, which usually occurs after a recent streptococcal infection. (b) (PE; AS; PA; RG)

1 Weight loss generally occurs with children who have developed diabetes, not nephrotic syndrome.

3 This rash would be related to scarlet fever, with which there is no smoky-colored urine.

4 This pain would be related to rheumatic fever, which never results in smoky-colored urine.

2. **2** Acute hypertension, which may occur in these children, must be anticipated and identified early to prevent any unpredictable complications. (b) (PE; PL; TC; RG)

1 This should be noted, but identifying hypertension is the priority.

3 This does not occur with glomerulonephritis.

4 Same as # 3.

3. **2** Because of glomerular dysfunction, there is decreased filtration of plasma, leading to excessive water accumulation and sodium retention; this leads to congestion and edema. (c) (PE; AS; PA; RG)
   1 There is usually a decrease in urine volume.
   3 This does not occur with glomerulonephritis.
   4 Same as # 3.

4. **3** KCl is always restricted in the presence of oliguria to prevent cardiac arrhythmias associated with hyperkalemia. (c) (PE; PL; TC; FE)
   1 Glucose and fat are not restricted; they are usually prime sources of calories.
   2 Same as # 1.
   4 Protein restriction is used only when severe azotemia with prolonged oliguria is present.

5. **1** This is an appropriate medication for hypertension because it acts to relax the smooth muscles of the arterioles. (b) (PE; PL; PA; DR)
   2 Diazepam is inappropriate; this relaxes the skeletal muscles, not the smooth muscles of the arterioles.
   3 This is an anticonvulsant that might be prescribed later in the course of the disease if the antihypertensives were not effective and hypertensive encephalopathy caused convulsions.
   4 This increases the contractility and output of the heart.

6. **4** A decreased urinary output is expected with dehydration in a young infant because of decreased circulating fluid volume. (b) (PE; AS; PA; FE)
   1 This is associated with an adequate fluid balance.
   2 This is associated with increased intracranial pressure, not dehydration; the fontanel would be depressed with dehydration.
   3 Because of loss of fluid and electrolytes the infant would be lethargic, not restless.

7. **3** This is a classic sign of fluid volume deficit in infants. (a) (PE; AS; PA; FE)
   1 This is within normal limits of 1.010 to 1.030.
   2 This indicates adequate hydration; the urinary output would be decreased in dehydration.
   4 This is unrelated to allergies.

8. **1** Loss of weight is the best way to evaluate the magnitude of fluid loss in the infant; 1 liter of fluid weighs 2.2 pounds. (b) (PE; AS; PA; FE)
   2 Although this would indicate dehydration, it is not an effective monitoring method for assessing fluid loss.
   3 This is a subjective assessment; measurement of weight is an objective assessment.
   4 This is a subjective and inaccurate assessment.

9. **3** 2.2 lb = 1 kg; 13 lb = 5.9 kg; 150 × 5.9 = 885 ml. (b) (PE; AN; TC; DR)
   1 This is inaccurate; this is less than the ordered amount of fluid.
   2 Same as # 1.
   4 This is inaccurate; this exceeds the ordered amount of fluid.

10. **4** Extremities should be restrained; the child will use all extremities in an attempt to dislodge the needle. (b) (PE; IM; TC; FE)
    1 Pupillary responses are unrelated to dehydration and fluid replacement.
    2 Scalp veins used for IVs are not located in these areas.
    3 The parents can be taught how to hold a child with an IV infusing via a scalp vein.

11. **3** The organisms causing gastroenteritis are eliminated along with the feces; gloves provide a protective barrier and are used for medical asepsis. (b) (PE; EV; ED; GI)
    1 This is required in respiratory isolation, not enteric precautions.
    2 This is required in respiratory and strict isolation, not enteric precautions.
    4 This is not necessary for enteric precautions; this is necessary for an accurate measure of intake and output.

12. **2** One liter of fluid weighs 2.2 pounds; this is the most objective and accurate way to assess fluid loss or gain; weights measured at the same time each day provide for daily comparisons. (b) (PE; EV; TC; FE)
    1 This would be appropriate for assessing the progression of ascites, not for assessing rehydration.
    3 Color of stools is unrelated to fluid balance; noting consistency would be more important, although subjective.
    4 Although this would be done, it is subjective and inaccurate.

13. **1** The purpose of administering lactobacilli, normally found in the GI tract, is to help recolonize this normal flora excreted with the diarrheal stools. (a) (PE; AN; PA; DR)
    2 This is not the action of this medication.
    3 Same as # 2.
    4 Same as # 2.

14. **4** The 3-month-old infant is interested in recognizing himself and playing with the baby in the mirror. (c) (PE; IM; ED; GD)
    1 This is appropriate for a toddler.
    2 Same as # 1.
    3 Same as # 1.

15. **1** Before the sex of the unborn child is known, the odds are 25%; 50% of pregnancies will result in boys and each has a 50% chance of having hemophilia. (c) (PE; AN; ED; BI)
    2 This is too high; there is only a 25% chance that the baby will be affected.
    3 Because the disease is genetically transmitted, this is not likely.
    4 Same as # 2.

16. **4** Joints are the most commonly involved areas, probably because of weight bearing and constant movement of joints. (c) (PE; AS; PA; BI)
    1 This is not the most common site; however, bleeding can occur here.
    2 Same as # 1.
    3 Same as # 1.

17. **1** Toddlers play individually, although side by side (parallel play). (a) (PE; AN; ED; GD)
    2 This kind of play is characteristic of older children.
    3 Same as # 2.
    4 Dramatic play or acting is characteristic of older children; they assume and act out roles.

18. **4** The meningococcal organism is rendered inactive after 24 to 72 hours of antibiotic therapy; therefore isolation is required at least for this time. (b) (PE; PL; TC; NM)
    1 Meningococcal meningitis is a serious contagious disease; isolation is required for at least 24 to 72 hours after beginning antibiotics.
    2 Treatment with antibiotic therapy for 24 to 72 hours will render the microorganism inactive; after that, isolation is usually not required.

3 Disease is not evident in the incubation period; because disease is undiagnosed, isolation would not have been instituted.

19. **1** This precaution reduces the transmission of infection from client to client (cross-infection). (a) (PE; AN; TC; NM)
    2 The act of isolation has no effect on the infectious process.
    3 Thorough hand washing and careful aseptic technique limits nosocomial infections.
    4 This is reverse isolation; it is not used for infectious clients but rather to protect clients with lowered resistance, for example, clients on chemotherapy.

20. **1** The child is old enough to be asked a direct question. (b) (PE; IM; PE; EC)
    2 The parents are too emotionally involved with the child and may not be trained in principles of mental health and therapeutic communications.
    3 A younger child, about 8 to 10 years old, would benefit from this.
    4 This may be productive with a younger child.

21. **1** Unless the child has an episode of acute illness, the home is the best place for the child; this prevents nosocomial infection and promotes family interaction. (b) (PE; PL; ED; GD)
    2 This should be used only if a home environment is not available.
    3 This is required only for episodes of acute illness that cannot be handled at home.
    4 This is not required unless illness exacerbates.

22. **4** HIV has been isolated from blood and other body secretions; the Centers for Disease Control recommend body secretion isolation or universal precautions. (a) (PE; IM; TC; BI)
    1 Enteric precautions will not protect others from blood or other body fluids, only feces.
    2 This is unnecessary; HIV is not known to spread by droplets, and masks, which are part of strict isolation, are not required.
    3 This type of isolation protects the child from others; its purpose is not the protection of others; it might be used if the child were severely immunosuppressed.

23. **4** This is inappropriate for an 8-month-old; this is appropriate for a toddler to promote imitative play. (c) (PE; EV; ED; GD)
    1 A stuffed animal is appropriate; it promotes manipulative play.
    2 A hanging mobile is appropriate; it promotes visual stimulation.
    3 A textured book is appropriate; it promotes tactile stimulation and touch discrimination.

24. **3** Constipation is a common side effect of vincristine because gastric motility is slowed. (c) (PE; EV; TC; DR)
    1 This is not likely; a drug other than vincristine would be used if this were present.
    2 An enlarged spleen would put pressure on the stomach and diaphragm, not on the large bowel.
    4 This is not a toxic effect of prednisone.

25. **4** The 15-year-old is normally preoccupied with appearance; the side effects of the antineoplastics and prednisone will result in the client's feeling different and may cause a poor body image. (a) (PE; AN; PE; EC)
    1 This may be a possible concern but is not likely to be the outstanding concern or feeling.
    2 Same as # 1.

3 A normal 15-year-old enjoys and strives for independence; the sick role would force the client to be dependent.

26. **1** Children with leukemia are immunosuppressed; the chickenpox virus can cause death in the individual without an intact immune system. (b) (PE; PL; TC; BI)
    2 Prednisone does not confer immunity to the chickenpox virus.
    3 There is no immunization against chickenpox.
    4 Chickenpox can be spread by airborne droplets in the prodromal stage and by fomites that have come in contact with pox that are oozing.

27. **1** Eschar is rigid and may restrict circulation and lead to loss of limb perfusion. (c) (PE; AS; TC; IT)
    2 This is unnecessary.
    3 Although this would be done, adequate arterial perfusion is the priority.
    4 This is not the role of the nurse; blisters are a protective adaptation.

28. **2** Because parents are trying to hide the fact of abuse, the explanations are fabricated and vague. (b) (PE; AS; PE; EC)
    1 This is no surprise; parents do not discuss them because this would be an admission of child abuse.
    3 This is expected; the parents are unable to provide emotional support.
    4 The child behaves in this manner because in past experiences adults have inflicted pain rather than provided comfort.

29. **4** Abusers lack personal strengths and adequate support systems, which could help them handle stress and frustration. (a) (PE; AN; PE; EC)
    1 Most abusers were abused as children; physical discipline was probably excessive.
    2 Abusers tend to be young, immature, and dependent.
    3 Abusers have an incorrect concept of what the small child can do; their expectations are unrealistic.

30. **3** This is a truthful statement; the nurse recognizes the fact that this might hurt and requests expected behavior. (b) (PE; IM; PE; GD)
    1 This would be too threatening for the child.
    2 The child may not have the experience to answer the question.
    4 This denies the child's feelings.

31. **3** Streptomycin is potentially ototoxic and nephrotoxic. (c) (PE; PL; TC; DR)
    1 Penicillin reactions are usually allergic reactions.
    2 Tetracycline causes discoloration of forming teeth.
    4 Chloramphenicol may cause blood dyscrasias.

32. **3** With specific manipulation, an audible click may be heard or felt as the femoral head slips into the acetabulum. (a) (PE; AS; PA; SK)
    1 This is not Ortolani's sign; this is associated with bilateral dislocation.
    2 This is Allis' sign.
    4 This is Trendelenburg's sign; it is associated with weight bearing.

33. **2** This position promotes hip abduction and flexion. (a) (PE; PL; ED; SK)
    1 This practice limits hip abduction and puts stress on the hip joint; if mild dysplasia is present, it will be aggravated.

3 Same as # 1.

4 This allows free movement in the flexed position but does not promote abduction.

34. **3** This is the preferred method of protecting the cast from soiling by excreta. (b) (PE; PL; ED; SK)

1 Special precautions are definitely required to keep the cast clean.

2 Plaster needs to "breathe" and should not be completely covered with occlusive material.

4 They should not be used together because clumping of powder, with resultant irritation, may occur.

35. **1** This supplies iron and some protein; it can be eaten with a spoon, encouraging mastery of fine motor muscles. (a) (PE; PL; TC; BI)

2 This is poor in protein and iron.

3 This provides some protein and iron but has a spicy taste that is not generally a favorite of this age-group.

4 Same as # 2.

36. **2** This sign is indicative of increased intracranial pressure, which is caused by the fluid accumulation associated with hydrocephalus. (a) (PE; AS; PA; NM)

1 This is a normal finding; a baby does not do this before 1 to 1½ months of age.

3 This is a normal finding; the head is the largest part of the body at this age.

4 This is a normal finding; conjugate gaze does not occur until 3 to 4 months of age when eye muscles are mature.

37. **1** This will avoid sudden increases in intracranial pressure. (b) (PE; PL; TC; NM)

2 Young infants, especially with this health problem, tolerate a demand schedule better, and it may diminish the possibility of vomiting.

3 This is inappropriate; it may be frightening for the parents.

4 This is inappropriate for a 1-month-old infant.

38. **3** This prevents pressure on the valve, which is on the right side; flat position prevents too rapid drainage of cerebrospinal fluid. (c) (PE; EV; ED; NM)

1 This is inappropriate in the immediate postoperative period; the infant should be kept flat.

2 Neck supports should not be used with infants; they may cause airway occlusion.

4 The support could push the head to the right and exert pressure on the valve, which is on the right side, possibly causing it to close; this would heighten the risk of increased intracranial pressure.

39. **3** This may help to reduce the infant's temperature; chilling should be avoided. (b) (PE; IM; TC; NM)

1 This fever requires more frequent readings than every 2 hours.

2 This is not a priority; temperature reduction should be done first; recording can be done later.

4 Alcohol should never be used with infants or children; it causes severe chilling, which can lead to increased metabolic activity and higher temperature.

40. **1** Pinworms emerge nocturnally to lay eggs in the perianal area; eggs are caught on Scotch tape in the morning before toileting. (a) (PE; IM; TC; GI)

2 A culture will not reveal the presence of parasites.

3 There is no such test to diagnose pinworms.

4 Ova cannot be seen with the naked eye; the parasite is rarely observed in the stool.

41. **3** This is expected; clients should be advised so that they do not become alarmed and can protect clothing and bedding. (a) (PE; PL; TC; DR)

1 The drug will not affect rectal itching; it will eliminate the pinworms, and this takes some time to accomplish.

2 All family members need to be treated.

4 Reinfestation is common; the drug may be needed again.

42. **4** Going to a stranger without protest usually indicates the lack of a meaningful relationship with the mother. (a) (PE; AS; PE; EC)

1 This is a healthy, normal reaction to strangers that is uncommon in children with failure to thrive syndrome.

2 Same as # 1.

3 Children who fail to thrive avoid eye contact with their mothers and do not prefer them over others.

43. **1** These are classic signs of dehydration and hyponatremia; a physician's order to increase fluids is needed. (b) (PE; EV; TC; FE)

2 It is not common for the condition of these infants to continue to deteriorate once therapy is implemented.

3 The nurse must have a physician's order for this; also, dehydration can be corrected with fluids via IV or feeding tube.

4 The symptoms indicate dehydration, not undernutrition.

44. **4** This position limits the potential for aspiration; the infant will be partially upright, and fluid is held in the stomach by gravity. (b) (PE; IM; TC; GI)

1 This position allows gastric reflux and may lead to aspiration.

2 Same as # 1.

3 Same as # 1.

45. **2** Surgery before school age reduces concerns about body image in relation to peers. (b) (PE; AN; PE; RG)

1 Maturation of testes starts about age 5; surgery should be done before maturation to prevent sterility.

3 The puboscrotal ring has nothing to do with the outcome of this surgical procedure.

4 Malignancy may develop with or without surgical correction.

46. **4** In cryptorchidism, sperm-producing abilities of testes are destroyed, resulting in sterility. (a) (PE; AN; ED; RG)

1 This is enlargement of the scrotum with fluid; it is not related to cryptorchidism.

2 This is an abnormal dilation and tortuosity of the scrotal veins; it is not caused by undescended testicles.

3 Inflammation of the epididymis may occur whether or not cryptorchidism is corrected.

47. **4** A visual display, which simulates a suture holding the testes to the thigh, aids in explanation and understanding; it may help the child express feelings about surgery. (c) (PE; PL; ED; EC)

1 A binder will not be used in this surgery.

2 This is used to explain IVs, but it is not specific to this surgery.

3 This is used to explain abdominal surgery such

as appendectomy; it would not apply to this situation.

48. **3** This is a side effect of scopolamine that is seen especially in the young and the elderly. (a) (PE; EV; PA; DR)
    1 This is a side effect of narcotic analgesics.
    2 This can cause respiratory depression, not hyperventilation or rapid respirations.
    4 This a side effect of tranquilizers.

49. **3** Although none of the choices is always indicative of pain, a change in behavior is the indicator that occurs most often in children. (b) (PE; AS; PE; GD)
    1 Vital signs are often normal in children, even in the presence of pain.
    2 Children often hide their pain; they may perceive it as punishment, or they may fear the injection that would be given to relieve the pain.
    4 Many things can cause crying, including pain, fear, separation, and unhappiness; crying does not always indicate pain.

50. **3** This is the best source of the complete protein that is needed to maintain nitrogen balance. (b) (PE; PL; TC; GI)
    1 This is a source of protein, but not the best source.
    2 Same as # 1.
    4 This is high in vitamin C, which is needed for healing but not for nitrogen balance.

51. **1** This reduces activities, allows the intestines to rest, and provides for early follow up. (a) (PE; IM; ED; GI)
    2 Wrapping elevates temperature; sugar water does not include electrolytes and may cause further gastric irritation; there is no emergency.
    3 This does not provide for rest nor for continuing contact with a health professional.
    4 Food may increase the diarrhea; the immediate intervention does not support the mother's attempt to manage the situation at home; there is no emergency.

52. **2** A low blood pH and bicarbonate level indicate metabolic acidosis. (c) (PE; AS; PA; FE)
    1 These findings indicate metabolic alkalosis.
    3 These findings indicate respiratory acidosis.
    4 Same as # 1.

53. **4** This is a normal adaptation to a state of dehydration; the urine will be concentrated. (b) (PE; AS; PA; FE)
    1 There is no indication of celiac disease.
    2 The initial response to decreased circulating fluids would be an increased pulse rate.
    3 One of the signs of dehydration in an infant is a sunken, not a bulging, fontanel.

54. **3** In metabolic acidosis the lungs try to compensate by blowing off excess carbon dioxide in the form of carbonic acid. (c) (PE; AN; PA; FE)
    1 This indicates renal compensation for respiratory alkalosis.
    2 This is not an adaptation to metabolic acidosis; fever with dehydration results from inadequate fluid for perspiration and cooling.
    4 This is a compensatory mechanism to reduce fever by evaporation.

55. **4** This contains milk, which irritates the gastrointestinal tract; milk products are usually withheld for at least 1 week. (b) (PE; PL; TC; GI)
    1 This is an appropriate soft food; it also replaces the potassium lost in diarrhea.

2 These are an appropriate bland food; they are not irritating to the GI tract.
3 These are an appropriate soft food; they also replace the sodium lost in diarrhea.

56. **2** This is characteristic of a child in nephrotic syndrome; large amounts of protein in the urine cause it to have a dark, frothy appearance. (b) (PE; AS; PA; RG)
    1 These children are usually pale.
    3 The child may be somewhat lethargic but usually not severely so.
    4 Blood pressure is normal or decreased; hypertension is associated with glomerulonephritis.

57. **4** In children with nephrotic syndrome, infection is always a threat because of anemia and lowered resistance; the child with a fractured femur is noninfectious so is appropriate as a roommate; in addition, the closeness of age will provide for preschool socialization. (c) (PE; IM; TC; RG)
    1 This disorder is caused by a pathogen; it exposes the client to infection.
    2 Same as # 1.
    3 Same as # 1.

58. **3** The massive edema predisposes the skin to breakdown. (c) (PE; PL; TC; RG)
    1 Carbohydrates are not restricted; proteins may be limited.
    2 This is far too much fluid; damaged kidneys would not be able to handle this amount.
    4 These children usually do not receive blood transfusions.

59. **3** This is incorrect; weight gain must be monitored carefully because it could be indicative of an accumulation of fluid. (a) (PE; EV; ED; RG)
    1 This is a correct statement; this is to determine if kidney functioning is impaired.
    2 This is a correct statement; the child should be monitored for edema.
    4 This is a correct statement; steroids are given with milk or food to prevent gastric irritation.

60. **3** This is correct; this is an indication that kidney function is impaired. (a) (PE; EV; ED; RG)
    1 This is unnecessary; this was an old method of testing the urine of a child with diabetes, not nephrotic syndrome.
    2 A 4-year-old is not old enough to reliably test the urine.
    4 A cloudy urine is indicative of the presence of protein; this is actually a positive, not a false-positive result.

61. **4** Metabolic acidosis results from an excess concentration of hydrogen cations; potassium increases; the kidneys cannot convert ammonium (NH_3) to ammonia (NH_4); there is inadequate base bicarbonate to maintain an appropriate acid-base balance. (c) (PE; AN; PA; FE)
    1 This child will have an excess of hydrogen ions, resulting in metabolic acidosis; carbonic acid blown off as CO_2 results in respiratory alkalosis, not respiratory acidosis.
    2 This child will have an excess of hydrogen ions, the opposite of an excess of base bicarbonate.
    3 This child has an excess of hydrogen ions from a metabolic problem rather than an excess of carbonic acid due to retained CO_2.

62. **4** Down's syndrome (Trisomy 21) results from an extra chromosome 21. (a) (PE; AN; PA; NM)
    1 This is not a cause of Down's syndrome, although translocation of chromosomes 15 and 21

or 22 is a genetic aberration found in 4% to 6% of the children with Down's syndrome.

2 Down's syndrome is not infectious in origin.

3 Down's syndrome is not related to an X-linked or Y-linked chromosome.

63. **1** Forty percent of the children with Down's syndrome have cardiac anomolies. (b) (PE; AN; PA; NM)

2 This is not a characteristic finding in children with Down's syndrome.

3 Same as # 2.

4 Same as # 2.

64. **1** The child should be rolled as one unit, with shoulders and hips turned at the same time to prevent injury. (a) (PE; IM; ED; SK)

2 The crossbar is not used to turn because it may dislodge and weaken the cast.

3 This would not be helpful for turning.

4 The child will not be able to sit up because the cast immobilizes the hips.

65. **1** Lymphadenopathy and the development of a rash after a day of fever, sneezing, and coughing characterize rubella. (b) (PE; AS; PA; IT)

2 The spots in the mucous membrane of the soft palate in rubella are called Forscheimer spots; Koplik spots are present with measles.

3 These are symptoms of rubeola, not rubella.

4 These are symptoms associated with meningitis and encephalitis, not rubella.

66. **2** An unimmunized woman who is exposed to the rubella virus may contract the disease and transmit it to the fetus; there is a potential for pregnancy in this cousin. (a) (PE; PL; TC; IT)

1 If the neighbor should contract the rubella from the child, the disease would probably be mild and confer immunity.

3 Rubeola has no relationship to rubella; the aunt would be at risk only if she were pregnant.

4 There is less risk if a young male adult contracts rubella than if a young adult female, who may be pregnant, does.

67. **1** This is one of the most prevalent diseases in young children; approximately 70% have otitis media at least once, and one third of the children under the age of 3 have had at least three episodes. (a) (PE; AN; PA; NM)

2 This is not the causative agent.

3 Same as # 2.

4 Same as # 2.

68. **3** The eustachian tube in young children is shorter, lacks tone, and opens inappropriately, allowing a reflux of nasopharyngeal secretions. (c) (PE; IM; ED; GD)

1 There is no difference in the functioning of the eustachian tube among age-groups.

2 The size of the middle ear does not play a role in the frequent occurrence of otitis media in very young children.

4 Immunologic differences are not a factor in the development of otitis media.

69. **4** The canal curves upward in children, and this straightens the canal so that medication will reach the inflamed ear drum. (c) (PE; IM; ED; GD)

1 This is an incorrect technique for children under 3 years of age because it will not straighten the ear canal.

2 This is not advised; it can only add more pressure within the ear and prevent drops from reaching the middle ear.

3 This is an incorrect technique; the auditory canal must be pulled down and back to straighten it and facilitate cleansing.

70. **4** The incision allows for drainage, which produces relief of pressure and results in immediate relief of pain. (b) (PE; IM; ED; NM)

1 A myringotomy is performed to prevent the trauma of perforation.

2 This incision is very small and heals spontaneously within 24 hours.

3 This incision does not leave any scar because healing by primary intention occurs within 24 hours.

71. **2** Movement by the child will impede the procedure and may cause additional injuries to the surrounding structures. (b) (PE; IM; TC; NM)

1 This will not guarantee that the child will keep still during the procedure.

3 This is not essential to the accomplishment of the procedure.

4 The child should have had the local anesthetic applied before the procedure.

72. **1** This position facilitates drainage by gravity. (a) (PE; IM; ED; NM)

2 This position will not allow proper drainage.

3 This position will promote pooling of drainage in the operative site and may lead to reinfection.

4 This is rare and should not occur from this tiny incision.

73. **2** These may indicate the need for a repeat myringotomy because of ineffective drainage. (b) (PE; EV; TC; NM)

1 This is characteristic of otitis media and does not indicate an infection.

3 Bleeding is not seen in otitis media or after a myringotomy.

4 These are not expected complications of a myringotomy.

74. **3** A vocabulary consisting of a minimum of six words with telegraphic-type speech is normal for this age child. (b) (PE; AS; PA; GD)

1 Babbling is normal communication for an 8-month-old infant, even one with a moderate hearing loss.

2 The child with hearing impairment communicates in this way because the child has not acquired the rudiments of language.

4 This language skill is seen in the 5-year-old child.

75. **2** The infectious and mechanical changes narrow the bronchial passages and make it difficult for air to leave the lungs. (b) (PE; AS; PA; RE)

1 As a result of increased respiratory effort and decreased oxygen exchange, tachycardia may develop.

3 Breath sounds may be diminished because of the swelling of the bronchiolar mucosa and filling of the lumina with mucus and exudate.

4 Intercostal retractions are unlikely because of the overinflation of the chest with air and the shallow, rapid breathing.

76. **2** Adequate hydration and high humidity are essential to loosen tenacious secretions and minimize fluid loss. (a) (PE; PL; TC; RE)

1 Bronchodilators are not used because the bronchial tree is not in spasm.

3 Antibiotics are ineffectual because the etiologic agent is viral.

4 Corticosteriods are not used because they have not proved effective.

77. **1** The infant is having difficulty with breathing; disturbing the infant frequently causes an excessive expenditure of energy and increases oxygen demands. (b) (PE; AN; TC; RE)

2 Cool mist helps to liquify secretions and keeps temperature down; cool mist does not maintain hydration.

3 Too frequent auscultation will disturb the infant's rest, causing an excessive expenditure of energy and increased oxygen demands.

4 Constant observation, not constant physical disturbance, is important; the infant needs to rest to minimize oxygen demands.

78. **2** These observations are vital to assess the child's hydration status. (b) (PE; AS; TC; RE)

1 The child is too ill to be involved in stimulating activities; energy should be conserved and oxygen demands kept at a minimum.

3 The child needs the parents to limit separation anxiety.

4 Strict isolation is not required although a gown may be worn; cap, mask, and gloves are not required.

79. **4** These easily digested foods have usually been introduced by 6 months of age; breast milk or formula is recommended for the first year of life. (b) (PE; PL; PA; GD)

1 Ham makes this incorrect; it is too high in fat content for a 6-month-old.

2 Whole milk makes this incorrect; breast milk or formula, rather than cow's milk, is recommended for the first year of life.

3 Corn is too difficult for a child this age to digest; formula is recommended for the first year of life.

80. **1** A stuffed animal is the most appropriate toy for the 6-month-old because it is safe and cuddly and requires only gross motor movement. (a) (PE; PL; PA; GD)

2 These are inappropriate; a child at this age puts toys in the mouth; playing with blocks requires motor development beyond this age.

3 A push-pull toy is appropriate for the older infant (9 to 12 months) and the toddler because it encourages walking.

4 Shape-matching toys require intellectual and motor development beyond that of this age-group.

81. **4** The Babinski reflex, present at birth, should remain positive throughout the first 12 months of life. (b) (PE; AS; PA; GD)

1 This reflex, present at birth, disappears by 4 months of age.

2 Same as # 1.

3 Same as # 1.

82. **2** These abilities are age appropriate for the 6-month-old. (b) (PE; PL; PA; GD)

1 These abilities should be developed by 10 months of age.

3 Same as # 1.

4 Same as # 1.

83. **2** Stress of surgery causes release of epinephrine and also glucocorticoids, which raise blood sugar. (b) (PE; AN; PA; EN)

1 Hypoglycemia can result because the client has

taken nothing by mouth and body fluids are being lost.

3 Urine test results are affected by many variables such as renal threshold, so they are not accurate enough when control is precarious.

4 Most clients with diabetes who are diet controlled require insulin for a short period, especially when receiving IV glucose.

84. **2** This position utilizes gravity to drain fluid from the head and prevent fluid accumulation. (a) (PE; IM; TC; NM)

1 Cardiac workload is not reduced in the semi-Fowler's position, but it is in the supine position; semi-Fowler's position does facilitate oxygenation.

3 The semi-Fowler's position has no effect on chemicals, but it does reduce subdural pressure.

4 This is true, but it is primarily done to prevent cerebral edema.

85. **3** Mannitol is an osmotic diuretic that is used to relieve cerebral edema. (b) (PE; AN; TC; DR)

1 Mannitol is an osmotic diuretic that has no effect on the body's glucose.

2 The bladder is a storage basin and is not involved with filtration; mannitol acts in the kidneys.

4 Mannitol is an osmotic diuretic that does not reduce peripheral edema.

86. **4** Pressure on the hypothalamus, the temperature-regulating mechanism of the brain, causes temperature imbalances. (b) (PE; AN; PA; NM)

1 After an operation, a temperature from the inflammatory response rarely exceeds 101° F; this temperature is not slight.

2 These would not cause such a high temperature unless infection were present.

3 This is not true when aseptic technique is observed.

87. **2** Children with diabetes need to be treated normally; they need discipline and should have limits set for their behavior. (a) (PE; EV; PE; EC)

1 This is correct; the parent should foster independence in the child with diabetes.

3 This statement is correct; it is realistic to think that the family will have ups and downs.

4 This is correct; the child with diabetes should be encouraged to maintain normal interests and activities.

88. **4** Proper hand washing is the best infection-prevention technique and should always precede preparation of an injection. (a) (PE; PL; ED; EN)

1 The abdomen, not the upper extremities, is the preferred site for self-administration of insulin; sites should be rotated.

2 Shaking causes air bubbles, which can interfere with preparing the dosage accurately; the bottle should be gently rotated.

3 The injection site should not be rubbed because this affects absorption of the insulin and also causes reactions at the site.

89. **3** Because paresthesias may be present and circulation may be compromised, adequate inspection of the feet is necessary and is the quickest and easiest measure to identify pressure sites and prevent infection. (a) (PE; IM; ED; EN)

1 Strong antiseptics are too harsh and should not be used because they can cause injury to the skin.

2 Feet should be patted dry, not rubbed vigorously; rubbing can cause abrasion and injure the skin.

4 Hot water should never be used because it can cause injury by burning the skin.

90. **3** The legs must be kept perpendicular to the trunk in order for the child's body weight to serve as countertraction. (b) (PE; AS; TC; SK)

1 In this position, the child's body weight and the angle of pull would be insufficient to supply traction.

2 Same as # 1.

4 Same as # 1.

91. **3** Because elastic bandages affix the apparatus to the limbs, the danger of circulatory impairment is always present. (b) (PE; AS; TC; SK)

1 The child in Byrant's traction does not have pins in place; skin traction is utilized.

2 The skin is not punctured, so topical or antibiotic ointment would not be ordered.

4 Removing the bandages would discontinue the traction and would never be done without a physician's order.

92. **2** In the toddler, two- and three-word phrases are used with an increased vocabulary; attributing lifelike qualities to inanimate objects is also associated with preconceptual thought. (c) (PE; EV; PE; GD)

1 This is related to infants.

3 This is related to school-age children.

4 This is a phase of concrete operations seen in school-age children.

93. **2** Ulceration of the oral mucosa occurs as a result of the antineoplastic effect on the rapidly dividing GI epithelium. (b) (PE; PL; TC; DR)

1 Although pain may be present, aspirin would be avoided because doxorubicin is also being used, and a side effect of this medication is thrombocytopenia.

3 These would aggravate the stomatitis that is a side effect of Cosmogen.

4 This is not related to the administration of Cosmogen.

94. **3** This is the correct flow rate; multiply the sum of all IV fluid to be infused for the period (750 ml) by the drop factor (60); divide the results by the amount of time in minutes (24 hr × 60 min); thus, 45,000 ÷ 1440 = 31 gtt/min. (b) (PE; AN; TC; FE)

1 This rate of flow is too slow to deliver the required amount of fluid in 24 hours.

2 Same as # 1.

4 This rate of flow is too fast; the fluid will be infused before 24 hours.

95. **1** Antineoplastic drugs exert their effect on rapidly dividing tissues such as hair follicles, resulting in alopecia. (b) (PE; IM; PE; EC)

2 This is not related to any of the side effects of the antineoplastics that are being used.

3 Same as # 2.

4 Same as # 2.

96. **1** People living in poverty have long-term feelings of powerlessness because they do not have buying power or social status to influence change. (a) (PE; AN; PE; EC)

2 The opposite is true; they are focused on the present, not the future.

3 Their anger is covert and not direct; in addition, the anger rarely resolves their situation, resulting in feelings of powerlessness and hopelessness.

4 People in poverty tend to focus on today; health recommendations may not be delivered under optimal circumstances or may be misunderstood, confusing, or of little value.

97. **4** Cystic fibrosis is a genetic disorder affecting all mucus-secreting (exocrine) glands. (b) (PE; AN; PA; RE)

1 Cilia are not involved in cystic fibrosis.

2 Exocrine glands, not sweat glands (epocrine glands), are involved with cystic fibrosis; children with cystic fibrosis lose excessive amounts of sodium via perspiration.

3 Exocrine, not endocrine, glands are involved in cystic fibrosis.

98. **3** Abdominal cramping and distention are associated with inadequate pancreatic enzyme replacement because foods are not being digested. (b) (PE; EV; PA; DR)

1 The opposite is true; they would have a voracious appetite.

2 Diarrhea, not constipation, would result.

4 There would be a weight loss because of decreased digestion and absorption, not a weight gain.

99. **3** This explanation illustrates that the child can understand cause-effect relationships and offers information to increase the child's understanding of the illness. (b) (PE; IM; ED; GI)

1 This is too authoritarian; the child needs information that will increase understanding and compliance with the regimen.

2 This is too general and does not explain why the child will feel better.

4 Same as # 1.

100. **4** Whole grains, legumes, and meat are excellent sources of thiamine, an essential coenzyme factor in energy metabolism, with an RDA standard of 0.5 mg/1000 kcal intake. (c) (PE; IM; ED; GI)

1 Fruits do not contain thiamine.

2 Vegetables are only a fair source of thiamine.

3 Eggs are only a fair source of thiamine.

101. **1** A toddler's increasing mobility and growing independence in behavior, including food behavior, are normal aspects of psychologic development; slowed physical growth at this age requires relatively less caloric intake. (c) (PE; IM; ED; GD)

2 A toddler's growth rate and energy requirements decrease in comparison to the first year of life.

3 Same as # 2.

4 Nutritious snacks between meals should be encouraged if the child is not eating adequate meals.

102. **1** Stuttering occurs because the child's advancing mental ability and level of comprehension exceed the vocabulary acquisitions in the preschool years. (b) (PE; AN; PA; GD)

2 This is not true; stuttering is common in the preschool years.

3 Same as # 2.

4 Same as # 2.

103. **4** This prevents placing undue emphasis on the speech pattern, thus preventing inadvertent reinforcement of the pattern. (c) (PE; IM; ED; GD)

1 This is demeaning; it may decrease self-esteem

and increase stuttering.

2 Same as # 1.

3 Same as # 1.

104. **3** Family strengths must be identified and utilized by the nurse. (c) (PE; AN; PE; EC)

1 The family members and their problems must be viewed as a whole.

2 The opposite is true.

4 This is untrue; values, beliefs, and attitudes greatly influence perceptions.

105. **1** Lead blocks formation of normal RBCs because it is very toxic to the biosynthesis of heme; this leads to anemia, an initial sign of the disease. (b) (PE; AN; PA; NM)

2 This does not occur; the child usually has anemia and some CNS disturbances.

3 Same as # 2.

4 Same as # 2.

106. **2** Young children have an increased propensity for putting things in their mouths; this age-group uses this as a means of exploring the environment. (a) (PE; AN; ED; GD)

1 This is untrue; normal toddlers do not have a fragile vascular system; children with a fragile vascular system are severely compromised.

3 Although this may be true in older homes or in the inner city, it is the activity of putting things into the mouth that is the primary cause.

4 This is not true; although gas fumes in areas of heavy traffic have increased pollution, most gasoline used today does not contain lead.

107. **1** This is related to lead toxicity or buildup that causes fluid shifts into brain tissue, producing cell ischemia and destruction; this ultimately results in convulsions, mental retardation, and death. (b) (PE; AN; PA; NM)

2 The child is not necessarily malnourished; the child usually eats the paint or plaster chips containing lead (pica) in addition to the diet.

3 Although abdominal cramps and headache may be symptoms of chronic lead poisoning, these are not the primary problems as lead poisoning progresses and central nervous system symptoms appear.

4 This is not related to this disorder; it is related to hemianopia or hemiparesis.

108. **1** Kidney function must be adequate to handle the lead being excreted; if kidney function is not adequate, nephrotoxicity or kidney damage may result. (b) (PE; PL; TC; DR)

2 A normal protein intake is adequate; excessive protein is not lost unless kidney damage is present.

3 There is no skin breakdown with chelation therapy.

4 This would not be a nursing function; liver damage does not occur with chelation therapy.

109. **2** EDTA removes calcium along with lead; serum calcium levels need to be monitored periodically. (c) (PE; EV; TC; DR)

1 This does not happen with chelation therapy.

3 Same as # 1.

4 Same as # 1.

110. **1** Reye's syndrome affects the liver, causing problems with blood coagulation because the liver-dependent clotting factors such as prothrombin are diminished. (c) (PE; AS; PA; NM)

2 There is no rash with Reye's syndrome.

3 Liver, not bladder, function is impaired.

4 The liver, not the kidneys, is involved in Reye's syndrome.

111. **3** This is the correct flow rate; multiply the amount to be infused (700 ml) by the drop factor (60) and divide the result by the amount of time in minutes (24 hr × 60 min). (b) (PE; AN; TC; FE)

1 This rate is too slow; less than the ordered amount would be infused.

2 Same as # 1.

4 This is too fast; the fluid would be administered in a shorter period of time than ordered.

112. **2** These behaviors are associated with separation anxiety; parental contact should be encouraged. (a) (PE; PL; PE; GD)

1 This would increase feelings of anxiety; the same nurse should care for the child to promote consistency, continuity, and the development of trust.

3 Separation anxiety can be minimized by increasing contact with parents, not peers.

4 Separation anxiety can be minimized by increasing contact with parents, not by distraction with toys.

113. **4** The affected leg appears to be shorter because the femoral head is displaced upward. (b) (PE; AS; PA; SK)

1 There is an inability to abduct, not adduct, the affected leg.

2 When the femoral head slips out of the acetabulum, it is easily palpable.

3 This does not occur with congenital hip dysplasia.

114. **3** These age-appropriate games help the infant's social development by fostering a sense of object constancy and object permanency. (b) (PE; PL; ED; GD)

1 This is age-appropriate play for an older child; it promotes psychomotor, not social, development.

2 This is age-appropriate play for the toddler; it promotes gross and fine motor development, not social development.

4 This is age-appropriate play for preschoolers; it helps develop motor, not social, skills.

115. **3** This usually occurs by age 8 months. (a) (PE; AS; ED; GD)

1 Whereas the posterior fontanel is closed by age 2 months, the anterior fontanel closes between ages 18 to 24 months.

2 A two- to three-word vocabulary is an expectation of a 12-month-old child.

4 This is accomplished by the 2-year-old, not the 9-month-old.

116. **2** The American Academy of Pediatrics recommends that infants be given the MMR combination vaccine at 15 months of age. (a) (PE; PL; TC; BI)

1 The infant should have received this immunization at 2 months, 4 months, and 6 months of age; the next booster will be at 18 months.

3 Same as # 1.

4 Same as # 1.

117. **3** In most states, the age of majority is 18 years; however, mothers under 18 years of age are considered emancipated minors and can sign consents for themselves and their children. (b) (PE; AN; ED; EC)

1 This is not an emergency in which the legally responsible person cannot be reached; the 16-year-old mother can give consent.

2 Same as # 1.

4 This is unnecessary; the client is an emancipated minor, and this confers adult status.

118. **3** This response is accepting of the individual and communicates concern. (c) (PE; IM; PE; EC)

1 There is no indication that the injuries were deliberate abuse.

2 This response interprets the client's statement as guilt, which may or may not be the true interpretation.

4 This is the nurse's responsibility and should not be transferred to the client's family.

119. **2** The chest was opened during surgery for the sternal repair, and air was allowed into the thorax; the air must be removed for the lungs to expand properly. (b) (PE; IM; ED; RE)

1 The baby did not have a punctured lung.

3 Chest tubes are uncomfortable; also, this response discounts the importance of the chest tube to the baby's respiratory status.

4 The chest tube is unrelated to the baby's ability to retain feedings.

120. **4** Because steroids are irritating to the gastric mucosa, a peptic ulcer with bleeding may occur; stools should be checked for occult blood. (c) (PE; EV; TC; DR)

1 Steroids do not cause this to occur.

2 Same as # 1.

3 Same as # 1.

121. **2** Protein (albumin) is present in the urine in nephrotic syndrome and is evidence of kidney injury or disease; if the urine is gently shaken, it will foam if protein is present. (b) (PE; AS; PA; RG)

1 Only rarely do RBCs or RBC casts get through the glomerular basement membrane in nephrotic syndrome.

3 A large amount of protein in the urine would result in a high specific gravity.

4 Crystals are not found in the urine of clients with nephrotic syndrome.

122. **1** In nephrotic syndrome a large proportion of the child's body weight is composed of retained fluid; the loss of fluid would be readily reflected by a loss of weight. (c) (PE; AS; TC; FE)

2 It is very difficult to get an accurate recording of output in a young child, especially if vomiting and diarrhea also occur.

3 With nephrotic syndrome it would be difficult to evaluate return to fluid balance in this way because the edema is generalized, not concentrated in the abdomen.

4 Osmolality reflects kidney activity, not the reduction in edema.

123. **2** This allows the child to get a full cup (1 oz medicine cup) without long waits; a full cup, even if it is a small cup, creates the illusion of receiving more. (c) (PE; PL; TC; FE)

1 When fluid is limited, a smaller amount should be apportioned to sleeping hours.

3 If the child were allowed to drink as much as desired until the limit is reached, 15 to 20 hours might elapse before any fluid would be permitted again.

4 Although fluids can be limited more easily during sleeping hours, 12 hours is too long for a young child to tolerate.

124. **2** This would give the child the opportunity for free expression; its free-form nature can give the child a sense of mobility. (c) (PE; PL; PE; GD)

1 This is less than optimal because coloring within lines of pictures in a coloring book requires more skill than most 4-year-olds possess; also this does not allow freedom of expression or movement.

3 Checkers is a game with too many rules for a 4-year-old to comprehend.

4 Playing dominoes requires the ability to count and conserve numbers, which most 4-year-olds do not possess.

125. **2** A 4-year-old can manage large buttons on a pajama top. (a) (PE; AS; ED; GD)

1 A child of 4 years will be able to comb but not part the hair.

3 A child of 4 years can put on shoes but is usually unable to tie them until age 5.

4 A child of 4 can handle a fork and spoon but cannot hold the meat with the fork to cut it with the knife; the child is usually 7 years old before this can be managed.

126. **4** The gonococcus organism is present in the genitourinary tract of males and is easy to identify. (a) (PE; IM; PA; RG)

1 Although urine may contain gonococcus organisms, the urine would dilute the concentration; the organisms are more concentrated in the urethral discharge.

2 Gonococcus organism is in the genitourinary tract, not the blood; VDRL is a test for syphilis, not for gonorrhea.

3 This may identify sexual activity and partners; it does not confirm the diagnosis.

127. **2** Absorption of tetracycline is enhanced when the stomach is empty. (c) (PE; EV; ED; DR)

1 Food interferes with absorption.

3 Same as # 1.

4 Same as # 1.

128. **2** Diarrhea is initially related to GI irritation; later, overgrowth of drug-resistant microbes can result in superinfection, which also causes diarrhea. (b) (PE; EV; ED; DR)

1 The opposite occurs because GI irritation increases motility.

3 Vertigo is unrelated to tetracycline.

4 Tinnitus is unrelated to tetracycline; this is associated with ASA toxicity.

129. **4** A chancre is the earliest symptom of syphilis; a dark-field examination of the scraping will reveal the *Treponema* organism. (c) (PE; AS; PA; RG)

1 This is associated with gonorrhea.

2 A rash is found in the secondary stage of syphilis; if a rash is found, it is too late for early diagnosis.

3 These are late manifestations of syphilis.

130. **4** Probenicid results in better utilization of the penicillin by delaying the excretion of the penicillin through the kidneys. (c) (PE; IM; ED; DR)

1 This is untrue; the penicillin destroys the *Treponema* during all stages of its development; the probenicid delays the excretion of penicillin.

2 Probenicid does not prevent allergic reactions.

3 The probenicid does not treat the urethritis, it delays excretion of the penicillin.

131. **1** A bulging fontanel is the most significant sign of

increased intracranial pressure in an infant. (c) (PE; EV; TC; NM)

  2 This is not a significant indicator of increased intracranial pressure.

  3 Same as # 2.

  4 Same as # 2.

132. **3** Sodium lactate is converted to sodium bicarbonate; it helps correct the sodium deficit and the metabolic acidosis. (c) (PE; PL; TC; FE)

  1 Saline results in the chloride combining with the hydrogen ion, intensifying the acidosis.

  2 Potassium is not administered until urinary function is restored.

  4 Plasmanate is a colloid used as a substitute when plasma is needed; it is not used in the treatment of metabolic acidosis.

133. **1** The passive antibodies received from the mother would be diminished by age 8 weeks and would not interfere with the development of active immunity after this time. (b) (PE; IM; ED; BI)

  2 The spleen does not produce antibodies.

  3 This is untrue; infants are often exposed to infectious diseases; passive immunity from the mother offers some protection.

  4 This is untrue; these immunizations are attenuated; they may cause irritability and fever, but they will not cause the related disease.

134. **4** Fever is a common reaction to the immunizations; Tylenol helps to reduce fever; both loss of consciousness and convulsions are rare, but serious, complications of the pertussis vaccine. (b) (PE; IM; TC; BI)

  1 Infants do not respond well to the application of ice; fever is expected and requires no intervention other than administration of Tylenol.

  2 This would cause an extension of the inflammatory response and should be avoided.

  3 Aspirin should not be given to children because it is associated with Reye's syndrome.

135. **3** Shortened attention span and fussy behavior may indicate a change in intracranial pressure and/or shunt malfunction. (b) (PE; EV; ED; NM)

  1 This is normal behavior for a 2½ year old.

  2 Same as # 1.

  4 Same as # 1.

136. **3** This is the correct amount; use ratio; desired : have = desired : have; no conversion necessary because desired and available dosage are both in milligrams; it is more accurate to convert less than 1 ml to minims. (b) (PE; AN; TC; DR)

  1 This is too much; 0.6 ml = 9 minims.

  2 This is too much; 0.9 ml = 13.5 minims.

  4 This is too much; the child should receive 6 minims.

137. **2** It is most often found in infants at about 2 to 4 months of age. (a) (PE; AN; PA; IT)

  1 It is not associated with any respiratory infections.

  3 The age of the child, the elusive causative factor, and the multifaceted modalities used for therapy make it very difficult to treat.

  4 It is not contagious.

138. **1** The skin integrity of these children is highly compromised because of their constant scratching; they are prone to streptococcal and staphylococcal infections. (a) (PE; AN; TC; IT)

  2 This is the physician's, not the nurse's, responsibility.

  3 This is always important for infants, but the priority is prevention of secondary infection.

  4 Same as # 3.

139. **3** All of these contain protein to which the eczematous child is allergic. (b) (PE; AN; PA; IT)

  1 Environmental inhalants cause eczema in the older child; in infants, protein is the offender.

  2 Fruit does not contain protein, the food element to which the child is allergic.

  4 Woolens provoke itching but do not cause the child to break out.

140. **1** 6-month-olds are capable of holding their bottles. (b) (PE; AS; ED; GD)

  2 This is a skill of older infants.

  3 Same as # 2.

  4 Same as # 2.

141. **1** The baby's nails should be cut very short to minimize injury from scratching. (a) (PE; EV; TC; IT)

  2 This is a correct statement; this kind of clothing seems to be less irritating.

  3 This is a correct statement; milk is one of the foods eczematous infants must avoid.

  4 This statement is correct; woolens tend to further irritate the eczematous rash.

142. **1** Injuries in various stages of healing are the classic sign of child abuse. (a) (PE; AS; TC; SK)

  2 This can be evaluated after child abuse has been ruled out.

  3 Same as # 2.

  4 Same as # 2.

143. **2** Nurses must believe this; otherwise there is little to encourage giving analgesics to children. (c) (PE; AN; TC; GD)

  1 This is a myth; it may be difficult for children to communicate pain.

  3 Some sources suggest this may be a child's way of coping with unrelieved pain; it is no reason to withhold medication, however.

  4 This is a common, but unsound, belief; addiction and respiratory depression are rare.

144. **3** This type of play is characteristic of 5-year-olds. (b) (PE; AN; ED; GD)

  1 This type of play is characteristic of 2-year-olds.

  2 This is a type of behavior, not a type of play.

  4 Same as # 2.

145. **3** Hypertrophy of the circular muscle of the pylorus forms this palpable mass. (a) (PE; AS; PA; GI)

  1 There are visible peristaltic waves that move from left to right across the epigastric area, not the lower abdomen.

  2 Discomfort is felt because of hunger, but there is no pain or tenderness.

  4 Abdominal distention is not seen; food never reaches the intestines because of the gastric obstruction.

146. **2** This corrects the metabolic alkalosis; fluid and electrolytes should be in balance when the child is undergoing the stress of anesthesia and surgery. (b) (PE; IM; ED; GI)

  1 Conservative treatment rather than surgery would be used if vomiting were not severe and projectile.

  3 This may help restore protein, but it will not balance fluids and electrolytes.

  4 This does not include the necessary fluid replacement.

147. **1** Vomiting is a classic sign of digoxin toxicity, and the physician must be notified. (c) (PE; EV; ED; DR)

 2 This need not be given because Aldactone spares potassium; also, orange juice is not given to a newborn.

 3 This is rarely necessary except when the defect is severe; infants are usually not overactive.

 4 There is no restriction on taking aspirin with Aldactone; however, children are generally not given aspirin because of its association with Reye's syndrome.

148. **2** Because the mechanism of CHF is the same in all children, the same basic treatment of a cardiac glycoside (Digoxin) and a loop diuretic (Lasix) is used, although the dosage may vary. (a) (PE; AN; TC; CV)

 1 This is untrue; the treatment of CHF is basically the same whether the client is an infant or a senior citizen.

 3 Children can develop CHF just as adults can; if there is cardiac decompensation, the treatment is the well-established combination of Digoxin and Lasix.

 4 CHF in infants is not in itself a congenital defect but results from a congenital defect of the heart.

149. **3** The parents will probably be anxious and will benefit most from short teaching sessions and written material to review at their leisure. (a) (PE; PL; ED; EC)

 1 The nurse could recommend, but not insist, that both parents attend the teaching sessions.

 2 This would be overwhelming, and the parents would not be able to retain everything presented.

 4 The most effective teaching and learning sessions occur in an area with minimal distractions; being in the room with their child at this time would present a major distraction to the parents.

150. **1** This defect causes blood to bypass the lungs; surgery increases blood flow to the lungs. (c) (PE; AN; PA; CV)

 2 This would not improve the oxygen content of the blood.

 3 Same as # 2.

 4 Same as # 2.

151. **4** Although all of these signs may eventually appear, widespread petechiae appear first as a result of the low platelet count. (b) (PE; AS; PA; BI)

 1 This occurs later, with anemia resulting from erythropoietic failure and blood loss.

 2 These often occur from chemotherapy.

 3 Same as #2.

152. **2** Cystitis is a potentially serious adverse reaction to Cytoxan, which can sometimes be prevented by increased hydration because the fluid flushes the bladder. (c) (PE; PL; TC; DR)

 1 This is an expected but not serious side effect of Cytoxan.

 3 Irritability may be present but will not directly affect Cytoxan administration.

 4 This is unrelated to Cytoxan administration; it occurs with Dilantin therapy.

153. **2** Good nutrition is extremely important to the child's overall health; best results are attained when the child is allowed to eat as desired. (b) (PE; EV; ED; BI)

 1 Although activities are important to the child's health, these should be provided according to the child's interest and should not always be structured.

 3 The child should be isolated only from other children with known or possible infections.

 4 Mouthwashes can irritate the fragile mucosa, so saline should be used; nutrition is the priority.

154. **3** Many vitamins contain folic acid, which is contraindicated with methotrexate, a folic acid antagonist. (a) (PE; IM; ED; DR)

 1 Vitamins would be contraindicated because folic acid interferes with the action of methotrexate.

 2 This is true but does not answer the question; it permits vitamin use in the near future, which long-term chemotherapy contraindicates.

 4 This is inaccurate; vitamin use is contraindicated.

155. **3** Foam is soft, so it will not damage the oral mucosa. (a) (PE; EV; ED; IT)

 1 A toothbrush will injure the oral mucosa.

 2 Hydrogen peroxide will irritate the mucosa and has an offensive taste.

 4 Mouthwash may irritate the oral mucosa and should always be diluted.

156. **2** This is the most accurate and age-appropriate response to the question. (c) (PE; IM; ED; GD)

 1 This response is insensitive to the question and does not provide any explanation.

 3 This is inaccurate; not being truthful interferes with the development of trust.

 4 This is inaccurate and may instill more fear.

157. **4** Chemotherapy causes severe alteration in mucous membranes; a rectal thermometer may damage delicate rectal tissue. (b) (PE; IM; TC; IT)

 1 Although this may be true, it is not the primary reason to avoid taking rectal temperatures in children with leukemia.

 2 This is incorrect; axillary temperatures are frequently used.

 3 Oral temperatures are accurate, provided the child can hold the thermometer in the mouth correctly.

158. **4** Cranial radiation destroys leukemic cells in the brain because chemotherapeutic agents are poorly absorbed through the blood-brain barrier. (c) (PE; AN; TC; NM)

 1 This is inaccurate; this is not the reason for cranial radiation.

 2 This is not the primary reason for the treatment; it is a curative measure.

 3 This is inaccurate; ALL is an abnormality of the bone marrow and lymphatic system.

159. **1** The child learned to think and solve problems in a very different culture and used a different language and may feel helpless in the new classroom. (a) (PE; AN; PE; EC)

 2 Most 5-year-olds adapt well to kindergarten.

 3 This is untrue; 5-year-olds are inquisitive and adapt well to school.

 4 There is not enough data to substantiate this.

160. **2** With each age-group, there are different means of communication; the approach used with a school-age child should differ from that used with a toddler or a teenager. (a) (PE; AS; ED; GD)

1 This might modify the approach, but knowing the child's developmental level is the most important factor.

3 This would be related to the child's developmental level.

4 Although a 5-year-old may fear authoritarian figures, this is only one aspect included in the assessment of developmental level, a more inclusive assessment.

161. **2** Measles is another name for rubeola. (a) (PE; AN; PA; IT)

1 This is known as varicella.

3 This is rubella.

4 This is pertussis.

162. **1** Measles starts with a discrete maculopapular rash on the face and spreads downward, eventually becoming confluent. (b) (PE; AN; PA; IT)

2 This occurs with whooping cough.

3 This occurs with mumps.

4 This occurs with chickenpox.

163. **2** Because of the anomalous structure of the upper lip, the neonate may have difficulty sucking on a nipple; duckbill nipples and other modifying devices may have to be used. (a) (PE; PL; TC; GI)

1 The cleft lip does not predispose the neonate to infection, difficulty in feeding is the main problem.

3 This is not an immediate concern before surgery; it is necessary after surgery to prevent tension on the suture line.

4 The infant should be cuddled like any newborn.

164. **2** Because of the cleft (opening) in the lip the infant tends to suck in more air than usual; burping will prevent frequent regurgitation of formula. (a) (PE; PL; ED; GI)

1 The neonate should be held while being fed.

3 Thickened formula is given to an infant with reflux problems such as vomiting after each feeding.

4 The infant's bottle should never be propped; the infant can aspirate.

165. **1** Surgeons prefer to do surgery as soon as possible; if the infant is in good health it can be done right after delivery or at 6 to 12 weeks of age. (b) (PE; IM; ED; GI)

2 This is incorrect; cleft palates, not cleft lips, are repaired at this time.

3 This is incorrect; surgery is done much earlier; babies begin to have teeth at about 7 to 8 months of age.

4 This would indicate a health problem because the infant should not lose weight; the infant's weight should be stabilized before surgery.

166. **3** Feeding the infant this way does not put any stress or pressure on the suture line. (a) (PE; IM; TC; GI)

1 A plastic spoon may be too hard against the lip; also, it is inflexible and it may be difficult to get formula into the side of the infant's mouth; this is necessary so that the infant does not try to suck on the spoon.

2 This is unnecessary and nonnutritious; the infant can be fed formula with a rubber-tipped syringe as soon as it can be tolerated.

4 A nasogastric tube may be uncomfortable and cause the infant to cry; the infant can be fed with a rubber-tipped syringe.

167. **4** Meticulous care of the suture line is necessary because inflammation and sloughing of tissue disrupt healing. (a) (PE; IM; TC; GI)

1 The infant can be cuddled at all times; priority care after feeding is cleansing the suture line.

2 This is contraindicated; the infant may rub her face on the sheet and irritate the suture line.

3 This would be done throughout feeding; priority care after feeding is cleansing the suture line.

168. **1** This is important; crying would put tension on the suture line. (b) (PE; PL; TC; GI)

2 The infant should be out of restraints periodically.

3 This is unnecessary; the infant should have no respiratory difficulty.

4 The infant needs to be cuddled frequently; parents are encouraged to pick the baby up as much as possible.

169. **2** Parents need to recognize that their child must be taught responsibility for self-care. (b) (PE; IM; ED; EN)

1 This supports the parents' need to keep the child totally dependent.

3 This denigrates the parents and does not allow for further expression of feelings.

4 This demeans the child and inhibits the parents from expressing additional feelings.

170. **2** A quick check of blood sugar level will confirm if the client is hypoglycemic. (b) (PE; AS; TC; EN)

1 Although this might be appropriate to counter hypoglycemia, it does not determine if the client is hypoglycemic or is manipulating.

3 This would not reflect present status but past status.

4 Same as # 3.

171. **1** The client's trouble stems from perceptual difficulties; the preset syringe removes the need to differentiate between 24 and 42 units. (b) (PE; PL; TC; EN)

2 This would not solve the transposition of the numbers; the problem is not caused by the inability to see the numbers but by the child's perception of them.

3 Same as # 2.

4 Same as # 2.

172. **4** Respiratory compensation to acidosis involves increased CO_2 elimination through hyperventilation, with a resulting increase in pH to normal limits. (b) (PE; AN; PA; EN)

1 Hypoventilation would not increase expiration of CO_2 with the ultimate increase in pH.

2 If the client is hyperventilating, blood $H+$ ions would increase because of CO_2 retention; pH would decrease.

3 With hyperventilation there would be an increase in CO_2 elimination, not a decrease; pH would increase, not decrease.

173. **3** NPH insulin is an intermediate-acting insulin that peaks approximately 6 to 8 hours after administration. (a) (PE; AN; TC; EN)

1 This is the time when a reaction from a short-acting insulin could be expected.

2 Same as # 1.

4 This is the time when a reaction from a long-acting insulin could be expected.

174. **2** These are the most common signs of hypoglycemia in children. (b) (PE; AS; PA; EN)

1 These are signs of hyperglycemia.

3 Same as # 1.

4 Same as # 1.

175. **4** The child's confidence, readiness, and skill for giving his own injection is essential for long-term management of diabetes. (c) (PE; PL; ED; EN)

   1 The recommended procedure is to draw up the regular insulin first and then the NPH to prevent contamination of the multidose vial of regular insulin by the long-acting NPH insulin.

   2 Sites must be rotated at all times.

   3 Learning responsibility for injections should be a gradual process with continuous support and guidance.

176. **2** Impetigo may develop as a secondary bacterial infection because of breaks in the skin from scratching. (c) (PE; AN; PA; IT)

   1 This is an extended inflammation that is not commonly found in children with pediculosis.

   3 Eczema is an allergic response, not an infection.

   4 This is a fungal infection of the scalp; it usually occurs by itself, not as a secondary infection to pediculosis.

177. **2** The impression is made on the sticky side of the tape; the specimen is collected before toileting so the ova deposited in the perianal area during the night have not been removed. (b) (PE; IM; ED; GI)

   1 The eggs are deposited in the perianal area, not in the stool.

   3 This will wash away the eggs; they must be directly recovered from the perianal area.

   4 This will prevent the female worm from migrating to the perianal area and laying her eggs.

178. **2** The external auditory canal curves downward and forward in a child older than 3 years of age and is approximately 1 inch long; to adequately view the tympanic membrane in a child this age, the pinna must be pulled up and back; in a child younger than 3 years of age the pinna should be pulled down and back. (c) (PE; AS; PA; GD)

   1 This positioning would impede visualization of the tympanic membrane; it is exactly the opposite of what should be done in a child older than the age of 3 years.

   3 This positioning would impede visualization of the tympanic membrane; the pinna should be pulled backward, not forward.

   4 This is how the pinna of a child younger than 3 years of age should be positioned for otoscopic examination.

179. **2** The gag reflex is elicited by pressing on the posterior pharynx resulting in glossopharyngeal stimulation; inserting the tongue blade on the side of the mouth avoids this stimulation. (a) (PE; IM; TC; RE)

   1 Although this is important, it is not the reason for inserting the tongue blade on the side of the tongue.

   3 Same as # 1.

   4 Same as # 1.

180. **2** 5 ml = 1 teaspoon; therefore 2.5 ml = ½ (0.5) teaspoon. (b) (PE; AN; TC; DR)

   1 This is too little; 0.5 ml = 0.10 teaspoon.

   3 This is too much; 3.75 ml = 0.75 teaspoon.

   4 This is too much; 7.5 ml = 1.5 teaspoons.

181. **1** Because of expanded experiences and developing cognitive ability the 4-year-old should have a vocabulary of approximately 1500 words. (b) (PE; AS; ED; GD)

   2 At 3 years of age, children use 3- or 4-word sentences.

   3 At 5 years of age, children ask the definitions of new words.

   4 At 2½ to 3 years of age, children can name colors.

182. **2** A positive antistreptolysin titer is present with rheumatic fever because of previous infection with streptococci. (c) (PE; AN; PA; CV)

   1 A positive, not a negative, C-reactive protein would be present; this is indicative of an inflammatory process.

   3 The ESR would be elevated, not decreased, indicating the presence of an inflammatory process.

   4 This is usually related to a decrease in mature RBCs caused by hemorrhage or other blood diseases; it is unrelated to an infectious or inflammatory process.

183. **3** Positioning on the side permits flow of oral secretions that could block the child's airway; a patent airway takes precedence; if the client is not able to take air in, all other measures are futile. (a) (PE; AN; TC; RE)

   1 This becomes important after a patent airway is established; the client can receive warm or cool liquids.

   2 Airway patency is of primary importance.

   4 After airway patency is established, deep breathing can be encouraged; coughing is contraindicated because it could dislodge a clot.

184. **3** These tests would confirm glomerulonephritis mainly because they identify the causative organism and its pathologic effects; also, the ASO titer confirms past presence of streptococci. (b) (PE; AN; PA; RG)

   1 A urinalysis would be done, but a chest x-ray film, a blood sugar level test, and an IVP would not confirm a diagnosis of glomerulonephritis.

   2 A blood chemistry and nasopharyngeal culture may be done; an upper GI series and 24-hour urinalysis are not specific.

   4 A urinalysis would be done, but a chest x-ray film, an electrocardiogram, and a heterophile antibody test are not specific for the symptoms described.

185. **4** The beta-hemolytic streptococcus immune complex becomes trapped in the glomerular capillary loop, causing glomerulonephritis. (b) (PE; AN; ED; RG)

   1 The cause is known; prevention depends on treating infected individuals with antibiotics to eliminate the organism.

   2 This is not an inherited but an acquired disease; incidence in males outnumbers that in females by 2:1.

   3 The precipitating streptococcal infection is usually a localized pharyngitis, and clots do not form in the small renal tubules.

186. **3** All these foods are permitted on low-sodium, low-potassium diets. (a) (PE; PL; TC; RG)

   1 Carrots are high in sodium, a banana is high in potassium, and buttermilk is high in both sodium and potassium.

   2 All but the peach are high in sodium; all but butter are fairly high in potassium.

4 All are fairly high in sodium and/or potassium.

187. **2** The glomerular filtration rate is reduced; this results in sodium retention, protein loss, and fluid accumulation, producing these symptoms. (b) (PE; AS; TC; RG)
1 Blood pressure and specific gravity are elevated; proteinuria would be greater than 1+.
3 Blood pressure would be elevated; proteinuria would be greater than 1+; glycosuria is unrelated; anorexia would be present.
4 Blood pressure would be elevated; proteinuria would be greater than 1+; anorexia and hematuria would be present.

188. **1** Reserpine and hydralazine are used to control hypertension. (b) (PE; PL; TC; DR)
2 Digitalis is not used because there is no cardiac involvement.
3 Phenobarbital may be used only if hypertensive encephalopathy causes convulsions.
4 Furosemide is used as a diuretic; phenobarbital would be used only if hypertensive encephalopathy caused convulsions.

189. **2** Bed rest conserves energy; a diet with no added salt is permitted; the other care monitors the response to therapy. (b) (PE; PL; TC; RG)
1 Isolation is unnecessary because the disease is not communicable; fluids would not be forced but limited or permitted as desired.
3 Vital signs do not need to be monitored every 2 hours, a no-sodium diet is not possible, and bed rest is maintained to conserve energy.
4 Blood pressure is not monitored every hour, and IV therapy is not used unless there is no oral intake or convulsions occur.

190. **1** Sodium is usually limited to control or prevent edema and/or hypertension until the child is asymptomatic. (b) (PE; PL; ED; RG)
2 The nurse would not give a home phone number; the mother should contact the physician for follow-up care.
3 The child should not be kept active for long periods because rest is needed; the child will not usually need a long convalescence.
4 Glomerulonephritis does not cause such severe kidney damage that a kidney transplant would be necessary.

191. **3** These are classic signs of celiac disease caused by pathologic mucous cells and atrophy of intestinal villi, which result in poor absorption of nutrients and increased stools. (b) (PE; AS; PA; GI)
1 Constipation leading to fecal impaction is not expected, although this may occur because of decreased peristalsis; rickets is not seen.
2 There is an inability of the villi to absorb vitamin K, with a tendency toward inadequate or prolonged blood coagulation.
4 Rickets is not seen because bone growth is arrested in celiac disease; the remainder of the symptoms do occur.

192. **2** These grains, mainly wheat, are major dietary sources of gluten, the gliadin fraction of which causes celiac syndrome. (a) (PE; IM; ED; GI)
1 There is no gluten in milk and dairy products.
3 Corn and rice are good substitute grain foods because they contain no gluten.
4 There is no gluten in saturated or unsaturated fats.

193. **1** After the removal of gluten, most children demonstrate a favorable personality change within 48 hours. (b) (PE; EV; TC; GI)
2 Weight is not affected for several days or weeks.
3 Diarrhea usually persists for several days or weeks.
4 Steatorrhea usually persists for several days or weeks.

194. **3** Because mucosal lesions cause diarrhea and limit nutrient absorption, loss of nutrients required for hemoglobin synthesis (iron and folic acid) causes anemia. (a) (PE; AN; PA; GI)
1 This causes pernicious anemia.
2 This problem is caused by poor absorption rather than the quantity consumed.
4 Same as # 2.

195. **3** Foods high in folic acid, iron, and vitamin B_{12} promote hemopoiesis. (c) (PE; PL; ED; GI)
1 Of these supplements, only vitamin K is related to blood coagulation.
2 Potassium and magnesium, necessary elements, are lost during celiac crisis but are not related to hemopoiesis.
4 Fat is not absorbed in celiac disease; therefore a low-fat diet is indicated.

196. **1** This child needs help adjusting; often the goals of care neglect individual needs and focus on physical condition. (b) (PE; PL; PE; EC)
2 Teaching the relationship of diet to the disease process does not ensure compliance to the diet.
3 Occasional noncompliance is not permitted; it eventually causes a relapse.
4 In general, the diet is limited to simple carbohydrates; bowel inflammation necessitates avoidance of high-roughage foods.

197. **4** Lifelong adherence to dietary restrictions prevents complications and celiac crisis. (b) (PE; PL; PE; EC)
1 This statement is incomplete; celiac crisis usually develops as a result of nonadherence to the diet, so adherence would be a primary goal.
2 Respiratory involvement is not a primary problem in celiac disease.
3 Regardless of adherence to diet, there is an interference with normal growth.

198. **3** Weight gain, improved appetite, improved behavior, and the disappearance of diarrhea and steatorrhea should have occurred. (a) (PE; EV; PA; GI)
1 It is important to assess this, but it does not guarantee the child will select the foods on the diet.
2 Even with understanding of the disease process, adherence to the diet may be relaxed; in time, symptoms may recur.
4 This is not a stress-related disease; it is caused by a basic defect in metabolism or an immunologic response.

199. **4** Atropine is an anticholinergic drug that can precipitate a celiac crisis; questioning the order is essential. (b) (PE; EV; TC; GI)
1 Giving the medication would precipitate a celiac crisis; calling after administration is unsafe.
2 Prevention of a celiac crisis is primary; the child would be placed in jeopardy if the medication were given.
3 The child would be sent to the OR unprepared;

questioning the order first would permit other orders to be written.

200. **2** There is high occurrence of Reye's syndrome in children who have just recently recovered from chickenpox. (a) (PE; AS; PA; NM)
1 Reye's syndrome does not occur after rubella (German measles).
3 Reye's syndrome is associated with viral, not bacterial, illnesses.
4 Same as # 3.

201. **1** These are some of the symptoms that bring the child to the hospital; they reflect central nervous system involvement. (b) (PE; AS; PA; NM)
2 Fever is usually high.
3 There is no rash or diarrhea with Reye's syndrome.
4 These are not early symptoms; these may occur later in the disease.

202. **2** These children are critically ill and need the constant supervision available in an intensive care unit. (a) (PE; IM; TC; NM)
1 Reye's syndrome is not contagious.
3 These children are critically ill and need intensive care nursing.
4 Surgery is not a treatment used in Reye's syndrome.

203. **3** Reye's syndrome is associated with viral infections, such as influenza or varicella, and frequently follows the ingestion of aspirin during the prodromal stage of these diseases. (a) (PE; IM; ED; NM)
1 Alcohol sponge baths are never used with children; the temperature may be decreased too quickly and this may shock the child; in addition, a fever of 101° F is not high enough for sponge bathing.
2 The child's metabolism is increased during illness; the child should have a high caloric intake.
4 There is no inoculation against Reye's syndrome.

204. **2** The palms will not damage the cast; using fingertips on a wet cast may leave impressions and alter the configuration of the cast. (a) (PE; IM; TC; SK)
1 The child may get burned with a hairdryer; also, the outside of the cast dries, leaving the inside wet and weakened; the cast should be permitted to air dry.
3 The crossbar of a spica cast is used as an abduction bar; it may break if used for turning.
4 The child must be turned every 2 hours.

205. **2** Priority care for any cast application includes checking the color and the temperature of the area surrounding the cast; this ensures that the cast is not too tight, impairing circulation. (a) (PE; PL; TC; SK)
1 If a trapeze is to be used, this teaching would have been done preoperatively or delayed until the child is stabilized and the cast is dry; it is unlikely that a child this small will use a trapeze bar.
3 The child has had general anesthesia; fluid will be given later to avoid any vomiting and aspiration.
4 This is important, but priority intervention in the immediate postoperative period is checking circulation.

206. **3** This is appropriate for the child's age and suited to the child's limited motion. (a) (PE; AN; ED; GD)
1 Because of the spica cast, the child will not have enough mobility to play with this type of toy.
2 The child will not have enough mobility to engage in this type of play and is too young for this activity.
4 The child is too young for this activity; children of 7 or older are able to play checkers.

207. **2** This may be indicative of an infection under the cast and would probably cause a fever. (a) (PE; EV; TC; SK)
1 This would not cause a fever; it may indicate neurovascular impairment.
3 This would not cause a fever.
4 Respirations may increase but do not become irregular with a fever.

208. **1** Alcohol is a drying agent; it may temporarily diminish the stimulation of the itchy areas and inhibit the release of histamine. (b) (PE; EV; ED; SK)
2 Scratching stimulates release of histamine, which makes the area more itchy; scratching may also break the skin and open up an avenue for infection.
3 Powder may become caked, slip under the cast, and cause additional discomfort.
4 Antihistamines are generally not given unless all other measures fail.

209. **1** Difficulty with abduction may indicate a congenital hip problem. (a) (PE; AS; PA; SK)
2 Flexion of extremities is the normal position for a young infant.
3 This is a normal finding in a young infant.
4 Same as # 3.

210. **1** This is the basis for abduction devices and spica casts when the infant is very young. (a) (PE; AN; PA; SK)
2 This may be true, but the easy moldability of the bones at this age favors corrective devices.
3 This is incidental; other forms of traction can be used if necessary.
4 Congenital hip dysplasia usually is not painful and does not limit ambulation for the young child.

211. **1** Regardless of age, parenthood confers the rights of an adult on the teenager. (b) (PE; PL; ED; GD)
2 It is unnecessary and not legal for the grandmother to sign the consent; the mother is present.
3 This would apply only if the hospital or some other party decided to declare the mother incompetent.
4 The mother alone is an adequate source.

212. **3** Safety is the priority during the seizure. (b) (PE; IM; TC; NM)
1 It would be unsafe to leave the child having the seizure.
2 Attempting to open clenched jaws could result in injury to the child's teeth and jaw.
4 This may cause airway occlusion by forcing the neck onto the chin; a small flat blanket is more effective.

213. **2** The child will not breathe until the seizure is over; cyanosis should subside at that time. (a) (PE; IM; TC; NM)
1 Attempting to open clenched jaws could result in

injury to the child.

3 Oxygen will be useless until the child breathes when the seizure is over.

4 The physician can be notified later; provision of safety and observation are the priorities.

214. **4** This may reduce the risk of gingival hyperplasia, a common side effect of Dilantin. (b) (PE; EV; ED; DR)

1 This may occur normally during drug excretion; it causes no physiologic problems.

2 The drug is strongly alkaline and should be administered with meals to avoid gastric irritation.

3 Avoidance of overeating and of overhydration may result in better seizure control.

215. **3** This behavior is a form of denial that may occur once the seizures are controlled; status epilepticus may occur when medication is not taken regularly. (b) (PE; EV; PA; DR)

1 Toxic reactions to Dilantin are not manifested by constant seizures.

2 This is desired and indicates that the drug is effective; would prevent status epilepticus.

4 Dosage is not based on activity but on type of seizure.

216. **4** A high-calorie, low-residue, high-protein diet is important to build the child up for surgery. (a) (PE; EV; ED; GI)

1 Isotonic, not soap suds, enemas are given.

2 A high-protein diet is important to promote nutritional status.

3 Because the obstruction is in the large intestine, there is no indication for nasogastric feedings.

217. **4** Most raw fruits are high-residue foods; the colon cannot handle this type of food. (a) (PE; EV; ED; GI)

1 A ripe banana is a raw fruit not classified as high residue.

2 This is a low-residue food.

3 Same as # 2.

218. **3** Intrusive procedures threaten the developing body image of the preschooler. (b) (PE; PL; PE; GD)

1 The preschooler can tolerate short periods of separation from parents.

2 Routines are still important to the preschooler, but some deviations in structure of activities can be tolerated.

4 The preschooler is more tolerant of strangers than is a younger child.

219. **1** Colostomy care may seem overwhelming to the parents, and it may reassure them to know that a therapist is available. (a) (PE; PL; ED; EC)

2 Increased fluids are often needed to compensate for fecal fluid loss.

3 Mealtime should be a pleasant time; also, this assumes that eating habits are poor.

4 This is untrue; physical activity will probably not be limited.

220. **3** The degree of dehydration is correlated with weight loss; continued fever aggravates fluid losses through evaporation. (b) (PE; AS; PA; FE)

1 This is not relevant because the child has been vomiting and will most likely be NPO to rest the gastrointestinal tract.

2 This is not relevant; the neurologic status is not altered; the urinary output may show signs of decreasing.

4 Poor skin turgor may not occur after only 48 hours of vomiting.

221. **1** The schedule for active immunization is 3 doses of DPT at 2-month intervals beginning at 2 months of age. (b) (PE; AN; PA; BI)

2 Measles vaccine is not given until age 15 months because maternal antibodies block the formation of the infant's antibodies.

3 TOPV booster is due at 18 months; it is given at the same time as the DPT booster dose.

4 This is given at 18 months, or approximately 1 year after the third dose that is given at 6 months of age.

222. **1** During the oral stage, infants tend to complete the exploration of all objects by putting the objects in the mouth as a final step. (b) (PE; AS; ED; GD)

2 9- to 10-month-olds play this way as they learn that objects continue to exist even though they are not visible.

3 These are the random reflexive movements of 1- to 2-month-olds whose voluntary control of distal extremities has not developed.

4 This is the momentary grasp reflex of neonates before the development of eye-hand-mouth coordination.

223. **3** The infant has not yet recognized boundaries between himself and his mother and is not particular about who meets and resolves needs. (a) (PE; EV; ED; GD)

1 Because the concept of self-boundaries has not yet developed, the infant does not really know or fear separation from the mother.

2 The infant does not yet differentiate familiar faces from those of strangers.

4 This behavior is that of a younger infant and does not indicate recognition of a specific person but only a human face.

224. **3** When all vesicles are dried, chickenpox is no longer transmissible; dried vesicles do not harbor the varicella virus. (b) (PE; IM; ED; IT)

1 Vesicles present are mature vesicles that occur in successive crops; these vesicles contain the varicella virus.

2 Chickenpox is not associated with a high fever unless a bacterial complication such as pneumonia is present.

4 This is not true; dry scabs do not transmit the virus.

225. **4** Individuals taking steroids have lowered resistance and may become fatally ill if exposed to the varicella virus. (a) (PE; IM; ED; IT)

1 This does not lower body resistance; therefore it does not increase susceptibility.

2 This may increase resistance rather than decrease it.

3 This does not affect body resistance because immune defense is a systemic response.

226. **2** Patting the lesions will not disturb them, and baking soda is an effective drying agent. (a) (PE; IM; ED; IT)

1 This may tear off the vesicles and lead to scar formation.

3 This may prevent secondary infection but has no drying effect.

4 This may minimize scratching but will not relieve pruritis.

227. **1** Radiation, or the transferring of heat from a warm object to the atmosphere, is prevented by reducing the surface and covering the child with a blanket. (b) (PE; AN; TC; IT)
2 Active transport is not related to loss of heat; this is a process that moves ions or molecules across a cell membrane against a concentration gradient.
3 Conduction is the transfer of heat from one molecule to another with contact between the two; very little body heat is lost by conduction.
4 Vaporization is the conversion of liquid or solid into a vapor; it would occur if a person were perspiring.

228. **1** This is the critical period of organogenesis, during which fetal development is most likely to be adversely affected. (a) (PE; IM; ED; RG)
2 The fetus is less vulnerable to major anomalies during this period because all major organ systems are already formed.
3 The fetus is less vulnerable during this period because development is almost complete.
4 At the time of implantation, cellular differentiation has not occurred; the genital bud appears in the seventh week.

229. **2** At this age the phallus is large enough for surgical repair and the child has not reached the age at which fear of mutilation develops. (c) (PE; IM; ED; RG)
1 The phallus would still be underdeveloped; surgery is done between 3 and 4 years of age.
3 The child is in the oedipal stage of development, which is accompanied by fear of mutilation; surgery is inadvisable.
4 The phallus is not developed enough for surgery to be completed.

230. **4** Circumcisions are never done because the foreskin may be needed for repair and reconstruction of the penis. (b) (PE; PL; ED; RG)
1 Hypospadias is not a genetic disorder although there appears to be some evidence that it may be familial.
2 A cystotomy tube is not inserted because there is no interference with voiding.
3 The penis does not need to be wrapped in petrolatum gauze because no surgery has been done.

231. **4** Mild reactions are redness and induration at the injection site, slight fever, and irritability. (b) (PE; EV; PA; BI)
1 Serious reactions are not common.
2 Induration at the site of injection may occur, but deep ulceration does not.
3 Occasionally a DPT injection may precipitate a febrile seizure, but it does not cause permanent brain damage.

232. **4** Neurotoxicity is a specific common side effect to this drug; the client can become numb and ataxic. (c) (PE; AS; PA; DR)
1 Vincristine causes adynamic ileus, resulting in constipation; diarrhea occurs with other antineoplastics and radiation therapy.
2 Alopecia is an expected side effect rather than a toxic response; it is not considered serious, and hair will regrow.
3 This is not a side effect of this drug but a toxic response to cytoxan.

233. **1** Elevated uric acid levels from destroyed cells may lead to renal problems; increased fluid intake helps dilute urine. (c) (PE; AS; TC; DR)
2 This will have to be monitored, but it is not of primary importance at this time.
3 Same as # 2.
4 Same as # 2.

234. **4** The platelet count is reduced as a result of the bone marrow depression associated with leukemia. (c) (PE; IM; TC; BI)
1 The uric acid level affects urinary output, not blood clotting.
2 Prothrombin time is influenced by vitamin K factors, not lack of platelets.
3 The red blood cell count will indicate the hematocrit and hemoglobin levels, which would neither provide the reason for nor cause the bleeding.

235. **3** Blood tests indicate response to therapy; if the WBC count drops severely, therapy may be temporarily halted. (b) (PE; PL; TC; BI)
1 These children receive therapy for extended periods, and prolonged isolation from their peers may lead to destructive social isolation.
2 This is a very radical and painful procedure and is not done weekly.
4 Nausea commonly occurs with this therapy; although antiemetic measures are instituted, the drug is not withdrawn.

236. **3** The child with abdominal pain may assume the side-lying position with the knees flexed to the abdomen and/or may self-splint when moving. (a) (PE; AS; PA; GD)
1 A 4-year-old may be unable to define the exact location of the pain; in addition, the pain may be generalized rather than localized.
2 This might be included in the health history, but it is not specific to the assessment of pain.
4 This might be included in the physical assessment, but it is not specific to the assessment of pain.

237. **2** Drainage is promoted by the principle of gravity preventing fluid accumulation and possible abscess formation. (b) (PE; PL; TC; GI)
1 Lungs aerate well in any position if a subdiaphragmatic abscess does not form; with an abscess the child will splint breathing.
3 Splinting of an abdominal wound is best accomplished by direct external pressure to the site, not by positional changes.
4 Deep breathing and coughing, leg exercises, and ambulation must be employed to prevent problems with immobility; maintaining a constant position does not provide mobility.

238. **3** The parents need assistance in exploring their feelings and their family relationships with a professional. (a) (PE; EV; PE; EC)
1 The gifts are attempts to relieve guilt feelings; the parent still feels responsible.
2 The parent is assuming the martyr role and accepting the responsibility for the child's illness.
4 This is a gift to the child that helps the parents relieve their guilt feelings.

239. **4** Prevention of infection and assessment of fluid balance and peristalsis are important aspects of care after surgery. (a) (PE; PL; TC; GI)
1 Dumping syndrome is a phenomenon associated with a gastrectomy.
2 Mouth care is not specific, and following appendectomy there is little drainage.

3 A low-residue diet is considered to be one of the factors leading to appendicitis because it tends to decrease peristalsis.

240. **4** Once a sterile object comes into contact with any object that is not sterile, it is no longer considered sterile. (a) (PE; AN; TC; GI)
1 This is untrue; the object is considered contaminated.
2 This is untrue; dry wounds are considered clean.
3 This is untrue; a 1-inch border around the sterile field is considered contaminated.

241. **1** During sickle cell crisis, the RBCs are sickled and clumped and the hemoglobin is ineffective in providing oxygen; therefore fluids to liquify the clumping cells and additional oxygen are necessary. (a) (PE; PL; TC; BI)
2 Hydration is important at this time; even if counseling were needed, it would not be done until the client was out of crisis.
3 Neither one of these is required during sickle cell crisis.
4 Oxygenation is needed; factor VIII is used in hemophilia.

242. **3** Hemolysis of RBCs, which carry the heme component, leads to sickle cell anemia. (b) (PE; AN; PA; BI)
1 It is not the iron intake but ineffective hemoglobin which causes the anemia.
2 The WBCs are not increased unless infection is present.
4 There is no electrolyte imbalance; more fluid is given to decrease the hypertonicity of the blood plasma, thus reversing the sickling process; when the client is adequately hydrated and oxygenated, RBCs tend to appear normal.

243. **2** To prevent crises, the child and family must be taught to prevent sickling by maintaining hydration, promoting adequate oxygenation, and avoiding strenuous exercise. (a) (PE; IM; ED; BI)
1 There are no prophylactic medications used.
3 Blood transfusions are frequently, not rarely, given.
4 It is the lack of oxygen that contributes to sickling.

244. **2** The teenage child is concerned with body image and fears change or mutilation of body parts; in sickle cell anemia, bone weakened because of hyperplasia and congestion of the marrow can cause lordosis and kyphosis. (a) (PE; AN; PE; EC)
1 Although this could be a concern at this time for a teenager, altered body image is a more fearful threat.
3 Teenagers can easily tolerate extended periods of separation from the family.
4 Restriction of movement is not a major problem because when the pain is relieved and the crisis is over, activity can be resumed; for the teenager, the change in body image produces greater anxiety.

245. **3** Cool fingers are a sign of circulatory impairment caused by the pressure of the cast; however, if both hands feel cool it indicates some factor other than circulatory impairment is responsible. (a) (PE; EV; TC; SK)
1 Further assessment should be done before informing the physician.
2 This should not be done without a physician's order.

4 Further assessment to determine the cause of temperature change is indicated before taking immediate remedial action.

246. **4** These are typical behaviors of an 8-month-old. (b) (PE; AS; ED; GD)
1 These are typical behaviors of a 12-month-old.
2 These are typical behaviors of a 3-month-old.
3 These are typical behaviors of an 18-month-old.

247. **1** A damp cloth will remove surface soil but will not damage the plaster cast. (a) (PE; IM; ED; SK)
2 Plastic will cause condensation and wetness, which would soften the cast.
3 Excessive water would soften and damage the cast; cleansing agents could injure the skin.
4 Same as # 3.

248. **4** Potatoes, pancakes, and whole milk are not adequate sources of iron; at age 8 months, fetal iron stores are depleted. (b) (PE; AN; PA; GD)
1 Potatoes are a rich source of potassium.
2 The infant is receiving Poly Vi-Sol, which contains vitamins but no iron; Poly Vi-Sol with iron exists, but the data indicate plain Poly Vi-Sol is being used.
3 There are some amino acids in the foods that are being eaten.

249. **3** Lips and teeth closed around the finger create suction and can move permanent teeth forward, causing malocclusions. (a) (PE; IM; PA; GD)
1 If thumbsucking is practiced only in relation to sleep, no treatment is necessary because it involves only a short period of time.
2 The continued use of a pacifier may decrease the child's ability to imitate sounds, as well as cause malocclusions when permanent teeth appear.
4 There is no indication that first teeth are loosened by thumb sucking.

250. **2** Brief messages, with only essential words included (telegraphic speech), are a normal pattern for a child 18 months to 2½ years of age. (b) (PE; AN; ED; GD)
1 A child advanced for this age would have a larger vocabulary and would use 3- to 4-word sentences rather than telegraphic speech.
3 A child slow for this age would have a smaller vocabulary and would use only single words to identify familiar objects.
4 A child with a severe developmental lag would have no obvious recognizable speech pattern and would only make a few sounds.

251. **1** Maintenance of a patent airway is always the priority. (b) (PE; IM; TC; RE)
2 An IV can be started later; suctioning to ensure airway patency is the priority.
3 The primary focus now is to establish breathing; the child has a pulse of 50, which will be addressed later.
4 The ICU can be called once the ER has stabilized the child's vital signs and a patent airway is ensured.

252. **2** The degree of the hypoxia and asphyxia the child had will determine the extent of the neurologic, liver, and renal damage. (c) (PE; AN; PA; RE)
1 The child is hypothermic, not hyperthermic.
3 Although initially severe, aspiration pneumonia does not result in long-term sequelae as does hypoxia.
4 Although emotional trauma can be all encom-

passing, it usually does not influence the ultimate physical prognosis as does hypoxia.

253. **4** The nurse must emphasize that everything possible is being done because the outcome cannot be predicted. (c) (PE; IM; PE; EC)

    1 The outcome is still in doubt; encouraging the parent's positive interpretation of the child's reflexive behavior raises false hope.

    2 Same as # 1.

    3 The outcome is still in doubt; this response by the nurse confirms the parent's feeling that a miracle is in progress and raises false hope; the parent's statement did not ask for the nurse's religious viewpoint.

254. **3** Because of the drying nature of oxygen, most oxygen is humidified before it is administered. (b) (PE; PL; PA; RE)

    1 Oxygen is combustible and supports fire; it does not ignite; it is not flammable.

    2 Oxygen is considered a drug and therefore must be prescribed.

    4 Oxygen is not warmed before administration; it is cool on administration.

255. **3** This would not affect the potency of the solution. (c) (PE; AN; TC; DR)

    1 The drug should not be used 24 hours or more after it is reconstituted from its powdered form.

    2 The drug should be void of sediment; contamination is indicated if it is present.

    4 The drug should not be used if the solution is discolored.

256. **4** Epinephrine is a sympathetic nervous system stimulant that causes tachycardia. (c) (PE; EV; PA; DR)

    1 Epinephrine is more likely to cause hypertension.

    2 The pupils will be dilated, not constricted.

    3 Hyperglycemia, not hypoglycemia, may result.

257. **4** A child this age loves to collect and manipulate; this meets the need to develop fine motor skills. (b) (PE; IM; ED; GD)

    1 This is below the child's developmental level.

    2 The child is too young for scissors and fragile toys.

    3 The fuzzy fabric is contraindicated because it harbors microorganisms.

258. **3** The nurse needs to gather information regarding the symptoms because they can be related to many factors. (b) (PE; AS; PA; IT)

    1 A developmental screening is not necessary in an acute situation; no rash should exist after chickenpox.

    2 A child in good health would not be in a high-risk group and receive an influenza vaccination; a rash is unusual after a sunburn.

    4 This is unnecessary; this information is not related to the situation.

259. **3** This is a straightforward, truthful answer at a level that a 12-year-old would comprehend. (b) (PE; IM; ED; IT)

    1 This identifies a feeling but avoids answering the question.

    2 This identifies a feeling but disregards the fact that the child has already asked a question.

    4 The answer is full of medical jargon that the child might not understand.

260. **3** The tick must be carefully removed with tweezers or forceps so that the tick does not further inoculate the individual. (a) (PE; IM; ED; IT)

    1 This is an unsafe method of removing a tick; the tick may further inoculate the individual, and the method may hurt the child.

    2 Same as # 1.

    4 Same as # 1.

261. **1** This response identifies concern and presents an appropriate protective intervention; regular and prompt removal of ticks decreases the chances of the spread of Lyme disease to humans. (b) (PE; IM; ED; EC)

    2 The response centers on camping, not on the fear of ticks.

    3 This is an inappropriate response because it focuses on the wrong fear.

    4 This response belittles the child's feelings and attempts to increase guilt because of fear.

262. **4** Bacteria are spread by contaminated stool; thus to protect others, isolation procedures must be initiated immediately on admission. (b) (PE; AN; TC; GI)

    1 This is part of the initial assessment and would have been accomplished before admission.

    2 Although this will be done, the priority is to establish appropriate isolation precautions.

    3 Same as # 1.

263. **3** With a microdrip setup (60 gtt/ml) the number of ml/hr equals the number of micro gtt/min; thus 27 ml/hr = 27 gtt/min; this can be calculated by multiplying the amount to be infused by the drop factor (60) and dividing the result by the amount of time in minutes. (b) (PE; AN; TC; FE)

    1 It is impossible to deliver a half of a drop.

    2 This rate is too slow; less than the ordered amount would infuse.

    4 This is too fast; the fluid would be delivered in a shorter period of time than ordered.

264. **3** Orthopnea is shortness of breath in any position but the erect sitting or standing position. (b) (PE; AS; PA; RE)

    1 This is labored or difficult breathing regardless of the position.

    2 This is an increased respiratory rate, not shortness of breath.

    4 This is a temporary cessation of breathing.

265. **1** The medulla oblongata contains the respiratory center, and the neurons that supply the respiratory muscles originate here; they produce the rhythmic pattern of inspiration and expiration. (b) (PE; AN; PA; RE)

    2 This is unrelated to respirations; this is the thin surface layer of the cerebrum.

    3 This links the nervous system to the endocrine system and functions as a relay station between the cerebral cortex and the lower autonomic centers.

    4 This is concerned with the control of skeletal muscles.

266. **2** Normal arterial blood gas values are pH 7.35 to 7.45; Po_2 83 to 108 mmHg; Pco_2 35 to 45 mmHg; base excess -3 to $+3$. (b) (PE; AS; PA; FE)

    1 The pH is acidotic, the arterial oxygen is low, the Po_2 is high, and the base excess is in the normal range.

    3 The pH is alkalotic.

    4 The Po_2 is low (hypoxic); the Pco_2 is low (hypocapnic); the base excess is high.

267. **4** Capillary beds are closest to the surface in a finger or earlobe; this proximity allows for more

accurate measurement of the arterial oxygen saturation. (a) (PE; IM; TC; CV)

1 Capillary beds are closest to the surface in a finger, toe, or earlobe and not on the abdomen or upper thigh.

2 The pulse oximeter requires no routine calibration.

3 An almost instantaneous accurate readout can be obtained with the pulse oximeter.

268. **3** Children who are mentally retarded can learn concrete concepts faster than they can learn abstract concepts. (a) (PE; AN; ED; GD)

1 This is an abstract concept that a child begins to learn between the ages of 7 to 11 years.

2 Same as # 1.

4 Same as # 1.

269. **3** This follows the normal course of growth and development skills and is no different with a child who is mentally retarded. (b) (PE; PL; ED; GD)

1 This would not be taught before self-feeding.

2 Same as # 1.

4 Same as # 1.

270. **4** Compromised heart function and inadequate oxygen reserve in the infant often result in feeding problems such as cyanosis and fatigue while sucking and swallowing. (b) (PE; AN; PA; CV)

1 Poor sucking is always significant.

2 This may be true in the first days of life but is not true as the infant grows unless there is a major health problem.

3 Same as # 2.

271. **1** Hypoxia leads to poor peripheral circulation; clubbing occurs as a result of additional capillary development and tissue hypertrophy of the fingertips. (b) (PE; AS; PA; CV)

2 Respirations will be increased.

3 The child's problems are related to decreased oxygenation, not to a clotting deficit.

4 The body attempts to compensate for the hypoxemia by increased erythropoiesis.

272. **2** Postprocedure hemorrhage is a major life-threatening complication following cardiac catheterization because arterial blood is under pressure and an artery has been entered by the catheter. (b) (PE; PL; TC; CV)

1 The child has an oxygen deficit; rest would be encouraged; flexion of the insertion site should be avoided to prevent disturbance of the clot.

3 Blood pressure should not be unstable unless a problem developed; fluids should be administered as ordered.

4 This is unnecessary; the distal pulses would be monitored.

273. **4** This position has the same effect as squatting, which decreases venous return from legs; the blood returning to the heart and lungs has a higher O_2 content. (a) (PE; IM; TC; CV)

1 Although this would reduce pressure of abdominal organs on the diaphragm, it does not put enough pressure on the femoral veins and vena cava to sufficiently reduce venous return to the heart.

2 This position does not reduce venous return to the heart.

3 Same as # 1.

274. **3** Preschoolers generally have learned to cope with parents' absence; however, emotions associated with separation—perhaps anger at being left—are difficult to hide when parents arrive or leave.

(b) (PE; IM; ED; EC)

1 Preschoolers usually are quite docile and cooperative because they are afraid of being totally abandoned.

2 The child would demonstrate despair long before the week was over.

4 The presence of others' parents would be unrelated to their relationship with peers.

275. **2** Death is a separation; preschoolers believe they will return to life and former activity; this is part of the fantasy world of the child. (b) (PE; AN; PE; GD)

1 At about 9 or 10 years of age, the child develops an adult concept of death and views it as inevitable, irreversible, and universal.

3 This is true for all age-groups.

4 This is true of the 6- to 7-year-old child.

Maternity Nursing

1. **2** The score at 5 minutes evaluates the adequacy of the cardiac and respiratory systems' response to the environment. (a) (OB; AS; ED; NN)

1 The score represents the neonate's response to the environment and has no relationship to the actual process of labor and delivery.

3 Respiratory distress syndrome is a condition that does not appear until 24 to 48 hours after birth.

4 The Dubowitz score relates to gestational age.

2. **2** Research strongly supports the theory that there is a sensitive period during the first few hours of life that is extremely important in the promotion of parent-infant attachment. (b) (OB; PL; PE; NN)

1 Encouraging rooming-in is also helpful because it increases the amount of contact between the parents and the newborn; however, this contact is after the first few critical hours.

3 Contact with the entire family unit is important during the taking-in phase of postpartum adjustment.

4 Contact with the baby can be achieved with breastfeeding or bottle feeding; it is the contact, not the method, that promotes bonding.

3. **1** Stimulating the rooting reflex is effective in making the infant grasp the nipple. (a) (OB; IM; PA; NN)

2 Allowing the infant to suck indefinitely will contribute to sore nipples.

3 For milk to be expressed the infant must grasp the entire areola, which contains the secretory ducts.

4 Bottle feeding will interfere with the infant's learning to accept the breast.

4. **1** Increased pressure during the birth process causes increased intravascular pressure, which may result in capillary rupture. (b) (OB; AN; PA; NN)

2 Bloody stools or oozing from the umbilicus is the most frequent sign of vitamin K deficiency.

3 This is caused by the collection of eosinophils.

4 These are intact capillaries; they may be distinguished from petechiae if they disappear when the area is blanched.

5. **2** The concentration of propylthiouracil excreted in breast milk is 3 to 12 times higher than its

level in maternal serum; this may cause agranulocytosis or goiter in the infant. (c) (OB; IM; EV; DR)

1 Heparin is not excreted in breast milk.

3 The amount of breast milk excretion of gentamicin is unknown, but it can be given to infants directly without adverse effects.

4 Diphenhydramine is excreted in breast milk, but it does not adversely affect the infant when therapeutic doses are given to the mother.

6. **2** The most vigorous sucking will occur during the first few minutes of nursing when the infant would be on the unaffected breast; later sucking is less traumatic. (c) (OB; IM; PA; PP)

1 A breast shield confuses an infant because it is necessary to use a different sucking pattern to obtain milk.

3 Stopping nursing for 2 days is unnecessary and would interfere with lactation by causing breast engorgement.

4 Manual expression may not completely empty the breast, interfering with lactation.

7. **1** This is a normal Moro response, which indicates an intact nervous system. (b) (OB; IM; ED; NN)

2 This is the Moro response, which is an involuntary reflex to environmental stimuli.

3 This is the Moro response and has no relationship to hunger.

4 This is the Moro response, which is normally not present after the third month of life; if it persists, there may be a neurologic disturbance.

8. **3** Proper cleansing and frequent changing will limit the presence of irritating substances. (a) (OB; IM; ED; NN)

1 Having the nurses change the diaper may lower the mother's self-esteem.

2 Powder and lotion will cake and maintain moisture in the area.

4 This is a nursing, not a medical, problem.

9. **4** During the taking-in phase, a woman is primarily concerned with being cared for and being cared about. (b) (OB; PL; PE; EC)

1 This is not a primary concern during the immediate postpartum period.

2 Infant feeding is best taught during the taking-hold phase of postpartum adjustment.

3 Same as # 2.

10. **3** The detection of the fetal heartbeat may be impeded by a full bladder. (a) (OB; IM; TC; PN)

1 The client should be in semi-Fowler's position to avoid supine hypotension.

2 The client should eat so that the fetus does not become hyperactive.

4 Only external monitoring is done.

11. **2** This is a normal occurrence caused by the action of the sympathetic and parasympathetic nervous systems. (c) (OB; IM; TC; IP)

1 This is not an abnormal finding.

3 There is no need for this intervention because this is a normal response.

4 Unless the fetal heart decelerates, indicating hypoxia, there is no need to change the client's position.

12. **1** Effective pushing will hasten the passage of the baby through the birth canal. (a) (OB; EV; PA; IP)

2 The mother will breastfeed in the fourth stage of labor.

3 Fetal position should have been established before the second stage.

4 Delivery is imminent, and medication given at this time will depress the infant's respirations at birth.

13. **2** Mild toxic reactions occur because of vasodilation from direct action of these medications on maternal blood vessels; vertigo, dizziness, and hypotension may occur. (c) (OB; EV; TC; IP)

1 Local anesthesia will not lower the level of consciousness, thus the loss of the swallowing reflex is avoided.

3 Labor is not affected because there is no systemic effect.

4 Local anesthesia does not affect the respiratory center in the central nervous system.

14. **3** A perfect score is 10; one point is deducted for lessened muscle tone and one point for acrocyanosis, which is manifested by bluish hands and feet. (b) (OB; AS; PA; NN)

1 The infant must have a higher score based on the data.

2 Same as # 1.

4 This infant would not have a perfect score of 10; the muscle tone is somewhat lessened, and there is acrocyanosis.

15. **2** A distended bladder impedes uterine contractions, predisposing the client to hemorrhage. (a) (OB; AS; PA; PP)

1 Love grows with care and responsibility.

3 Relaxation is a priority before delivery; in the fourth stage the client is often euphoric.

4 The mother is egocentric at this point and is not yet totally involved with the infant.

16. **1** Estrogen in the contraceptive may cause hypertension and place the client at risk for the development of a CVA. (b) (OB; AS; TC; FS)

2 Oral contraceptives are contraindicated in women older than age 40 because of an increased risk of myocardial infarction.

3 This is questionable; many physicians believe that oral contraceptives can be given to a client who smokes up to two packs per day.

4 There is no relationship between oral contraceptives and multiple births.

17. **3** Maintenance of serum progesterone levels keeps cervical mucus thick and hostile to sperm at all times. (a) (OB; IM; ED; DR)

1 Fertility drugs are often taken during the first part of the cycle to encourage ovulation, not contraception.

2 Progesterone-only pills do not interfere with ovulation.

4 Combined estrogen and progesterone oral contraceptives are taken during the second, third, and fourth weeks of the cycle.

18. **1** Nausea and vomiting are related to excessive amounts of estrogen; these symptoms can usually be controlled by reducing the dose. (a) (OB; EV; TC; DR)

2 Amenorrhea is associated with pregnancy and excess progesterone.

3 Depression is related to excess progesterone; estrogen causes irritability, not lethargy.

4 Hypomenorrhea is caused by estrogen deficiency.

19. **2** Oral contraceptives should be discontinued with any symptom that could be related to emboli. (a)

(OB; EV; TC; DR)

1 This may be a sign of infection, not a side effect of oral contraceptives.

3 Mittelschmerz is pain midway in the menstrual cycle, usually at ovulation.

4 Menorrhagia is a side effect related to excessive amounts of estrogen; immediate discontinuance of contraceptives is unnecessary.

20. **4** This is the characteristic symptom of eclampsia due to CNS irritation. (b) (OB; AS; PA; HP)

1 This is a symptom of preeclampsia.

2 Same as # 1.

3 Same as # 1.

21. **1** Near-toxic levels of magnesium sulfate are indicated by the disappearance of the knee-jerk reflex and by depressed respirations. (c) (OB; EV; TC; DR)

2 This is unsafe; this would cause an overdose.

3 Waiting could put the client in jeopardy of respiratory arrest; toxic symptoms require medical intervention.

4 This is given as an antidote only when ordered by the physician.

22. **2** Unplanned cesarean delivery can result in guilt, disappointment, anger, and a sense of failure as a woman. (a) (OB; AN; PE; EC)

1 This is not usually a common concern.

3 Mothers who deliver by cesarean delivery can assume the mothering role.

4 The hospital stay is not prolonged; the client usually is discharged within 4 to 5 days.

23. **4** This is a classic sign of respiratory distress in the newborn. (a) (OB; AS; PA; NN)

1 This is associated with neurologic impairment, not respiratory distress.

2 The respiratory rate increases, not decreases.

3 This is within normal limits.

24. **3** This is done because any attempt by the infant to maintain temperature further compromises physical status by increasing metabolic activity and O_2 demands. (b) (OB; PL; PA; HN)

1 This is not accurate; the O_2 percentage will vary with Po_2 values of the infant.

2 Increased activity will increase oxygen demands.

4 Same as # 2.

25. **2** In respiratory acidosis, pH falls and CO_2 levels rise. (b) (OB; AN; PA; HN)

1 This is normal.

3 The arterial oxygen level may or may not change with acidosis.

4 This is very high but is unrelated to acidosis.

26. **1** O_2 has a cooling effect, and the baby should be kept warm. (a) (OB; IM; PA; HN)

2 O_2 concentration is determined by blood gas levels and is changed accordingly.

3 This would tire the baby, as well as defeat the use of O_2.

4 This may cause an overload of fluid in an infant already having respiratory distress.

27. **3** Amniotic fluid is alkaline and turns nitrazine paper blue; acidic fluid turns nitrazine paper yellow. (b) (OB; AN; TC; IP)

1 Amniotic fluid does not turn nitrazine paper this color.

2 Same as # 1.

4 Same as # 1.

28. **3** By discussing the experience, the client is bringing it into reality; this is characteristic of the taking-in phase. (c) (OB; AN; PE; EC)

1 The taking-hold phase is marked by an increased desire to resume independence; this statement reveals the client is still in the taking-in phase.

2 The working-through phase is not a separate phase of adjustment to parenthood; this is not relevant.

4 The client is not ready to assume the tasks of the letting-go phase until completing the tasks of the taking-in and taking-hold phases.

29. **2** The infant would be classified as small for gestational age because the weight is below the 10th percentile on the growth curve for a term infant. (a) (OB; AN; PA; HN)

1 This is untrue; the infant's weight is below the 10th percentile for a term infant; the infant is SGA.

3 Same as # 1.

4 An infant is considered to be preterm if born before the end of the thirty-seventh week of gestation; the term *small for gestational age* rather than *immature* is used.

30. **1** SGA infants may exhibit hypoglycemia, especially during the first 2 days of life, because of depleted glycogen stores and inhibited gluconeogenesis. (b) (OB; AN; PA; HN)

2 Hypercalcemia is uncommon in newborns.

3 Decreased BP, pallor with cyanosis, tachycardia, retractions, lethargy, and weak cry are present in hypovolemia.

4 These are unrelated to hypothyroidism; symptoms of hypothyroidism are difficult to identify in the newborn.

31. **3** This is like binding the breasts; it reduces pain and prevents further engorgement. (a) (OB; IM; ED; PP)

1 Prescribing drugs is the physician's responsibility; medication would reduce pain but would not prevent further engorgement.

2 Cold compresses would prevent further engorgement in the nonnursing mother; this is not an independent function of the nurse; it would require a physician's order.

4 Milk and fluids should not be restricted after delivery.

32. **2** This is the content of childbirth classes to adequately prepare parents for childbirth. (b) (OB; IM; ED; PN)

1 This is only part of the class content.

3 Same as # 1.

4 This is not an absolute; most childbirth methods inform parents that drugs are available if necessary.

33. **3** There is much to be learned and practiced so that the client can vary the techniques through the stages of labor. (c) (OB; IM; ED; PN)

1 The Read method focuses on naturalness and denial of pain.

2 This is untrue, because small amounts of medication can be used if required.

4 The Read method can be quickly taught to an "unprepared" woman in labor.

34. **4** Effleurage is gentle massage of the abdomen. (a) (OB; EV; ED; PN)

1 This is a technique of breathing.

2 This is the pelvic rock; it is used during pregnancy to relieve backache.

3 Same as # 1.

35. **3** Kegel exercises develop and strengthen the pubococcygeal muscle; they are done through repeated contractions of the vagina. (c) (OB; EV; ED; PN)

    1 This is effective in relieving backaches.
    2 Same as # 1.
    4 Tailor sitting aids in relaxing the muscles of the pelvic floor.

36. **1** Bed rest keeps the pressure of the fetal head off the cervix; the side-lying position keeps the gravid uterus from impeding major vessels, thus enhancing uterine perfusion. (b) (OB; PL; TC; HP)

    2 These are used only when the cord is prolapsed or the client is in shock.
    3 This may aid in relieving pressure of the fetus on the cervix, but it will not enhance uterine perfusion.
    4 Sitting up in bed increases pressure on the cervix; this may lead to further dilation.

37. **2** The therapeutic regimen includes bed rest; peace of mind can best be achieved if the children are adequately cared for. (c) (OB; IM; PE; EC)

    1 This explores feelings without including a therapeutic regimen.
    3 Complete bed rest has been prescribed.
    4 This is giving solutions rather than exploring the situation with the client.

38. **2** Prostaglandins in semen may stimulate labor, and penile contact with the cervix may increase myometrial contractability. (a) (OB; IM; ED; HP)

    1 Sexual intercourse may cause labor to progress; delivery is not desired in the thirty-third week of pregnancy.
    3 Same as # 1.
    4 Same as # 1.

39. **1** Hypotension is an expected side effect of ritodrine, a sympathomimetic drug; the client is kept in the side-lying position to minimize hypotension. (c) (OB; EV; TC; DR)

    2 Ritodrine is not given for diuretic action; this is necessary when using magnesium sulfate.
    3 Reflexes are not affected; this is necessary when using magnesium sulfate.
    4 Ritodrine does not affect the client's level of consciousness; it merely relaxes uterine musculature.

40. **4** A positive sign of pregnancy is a urine immunoassay pregnancy test because it is 95% accurate in detecting pregnancy. (b) (OB; AS; PA; PN)

    1 This is a presumptive sign of pregnancy; although nausea can occur during the first trimester because of the secretion of HCG, there are many causes of nausea other than pregnancy.
    2 This is a presumptive sign of pregnancy; there are many other causes of amenorrhea.
    3 This is a presumptive sign of pregnancy; there are other causes of frequency, such as urinary tract infection.

41. **4** Blood sugar level is important because hypoglycemia in early pregnancy can lead to congenital abnormalities; hyperglycemia in late pregnancy may lead to fetal hyperinsulinism and subsequent neonatal hypoglycemia. (b) (OB; PL; ED; HP)

    1 This is too limited a response; assessment without intervention is useless.

2 Appointments should be made by the client; an authoritative approach takes control away from the client and may increase anxiety.
    3 Dietary regulation is usually minimal, with a restriction on excessive carbohydrate ingestion; a limited diet to control weight gain could jeopardize both the fetus and the mother's nutritional status.

42. **4** Fetal heartbeat can be heard with an electronic doppler between 10 and 12 weeks gestation; a fetoscope cannot pick up the fetal heartbeat before the seventeenth week. (a) (OB; IM; ED; PN)

    1 This is too early for the heartbeat to be heard with a fetoscope.
    2 Same as # 1.
    3 This is late; the fetal heart can be first heard with an electronic doppler between 10 to 12 weeks.

43. **1** A negative test implies that placental support is adequate and the fetus is likely to tolerate the stress of labor should it ensue within the week. (b) (OB; AN; PA; PN)

    2 A positive test indicates that the fetus is at increased risk; the fetus has persistent and consistent late decelerations with contractions.
    3 Fetal heart rate accelerations with movement do not require doing an oxytocin challenge test.
    4 Interpretable data does not show signs of hyperstimulation.

44. **2** The lecithin concentration rises abruptly at 35 weeks, reaching a level that is twice the amount of sphingomyelin, which decreases concurrently. (a) (OB; AS; PA; PN)

    1 This ratio is reversed when lung maturity is adequate; it is only early in pregnancy that the sphingomyelin concentration is higher than the lecithin concentration.
    3 At about 30 to 32 weeks' gestation the amounts of lecithin and sphingomyelin are equal; this result indicates lung immaturity.
    4 Although this indicates that the lecithin level is rising, it is not until the L/S ratio is 2:1 that fetal lung maturity is attained.

45. **4** If cord compression is allowed to occur, fetal hypoxia results in central nervous system damage or death; therefore manual elevation of the presenting part is indicated. (b) (OB; IM; TC; IP)

    1 This can be done after elevating the presenting part off the cord; this is necessary because with each contraction the umbilical cord becomes compressed between the maternal pelvis and the presenting part.
    2 This would be unsafe; compression of the cord would continue in this position; the knee-chest or Trendelenburg positions could be used to allow gravity to reduce pressure on the cord.
    3 This is unsafe and too time consuming; immediate intervention is necessary to prevent fetal hypoxia.

46. **4** At birth, circulating maternal glucose is removed; however, the infant still has a high level of insulin and may develop a rebound hypoglycemia. (b) (OB; AS; TC; HN)

    1 The temperature-regulating ability of a neonate born to a mother with diabetes mellitus is similar to that of a normal neonate unless the infant is preterm.

2 Cyanotic episodes, with or without tremors, may be indicative of cardiac problems, not diabetes mellitus.

3 Pathologic jaundice is associated with hemolytic diseases such as Rh and ABO incompatibility, and sepsis, not diabetes mellitus.

47. **3** Often there is a decrease in sexual desire in the first trimester, probably related to nausea and vomiting; if couples are informed about this, they are less likely to become distressed. (b) (OB; IM; ED; PN)

1 Calling the situation a problem may cause further anxiety in the client.

2 The client is asking the nurse for information; the client is unable to answer this question.

4 This does not tell the client why this feeling is occurring; this provides false reassurance.

48. **2** During pregnancy the need for water is increased; it is related to the increased metabolic rate and expanded blood volume; there is no indication of urinary infection. (a) (OB; PL; TC; PN)

1 Fluids must be increased, not decreased.

3 This is unnecessary; there is no indication of urinary infection.

4 The bladder needs to be emptied frequently to prevent urinary stasis and potential ascending infection into the kidneys.

49. **1** Unless a lactose intolerance is present, the client should drink milk; eating dried fruits, high fiber foods, and increasing fluids and activity will aid in lessening constipation. (b) (OB; IM; ED; PN)

2 These are not as beneficial as whole milk and will cause constipation as well.

3 These can cause constipation.

4 Megadoses of vitamins can be harmful; prenatal vitamins are not a substitute for milk.

50. **4** Broccoli is a good source of calcium because it contains approximately 150 mg of calcium per 6 oz cup, compared with a 6 oz cup of milk, which contains 216 mg. (b) (OB; PL; ED; PN)

1 Corn contains about 5 mg calcium per 6 oz cup.

2 Lean meat contains about 20 mg calcium per 6 oz serving.

3 Liver contains about 18 mg calcium per 6 oz serving.

51. **2** The issue of pregnancy is resolved by this time; more awareness of the fetus as a person and the body changes of pregnancy lead to desire to learn about fetal growth, body changes, and nutrition. (b) (OB; IM; ED; PN)

1 This information would be appropriate for the first trimester.

3 This information would be appropriate for the last trimester.

4 Same as # 3.

52. **1** Twins should be suspected with a more rapid increase in fundal height than normal; the nurse should assess for two distinct heartbeats. (c) (OB; AS; PA; PN)

2 Fundal height, not the size of the baby, should lead the nurse to suspect a multiple pregnancy.

3 This cannot be determined until an ultrasound is done.

4 Weight gain will not influence the height of the fundus; a multiple pregnancy is more likely the factor.

53. **4** During the postpartum period a leukocytosis (WBC count of 15,000 to 20,000/mm³) is normal and related to the physical exertion experienced during labor and delivery, not infection. (b) (OB; EV; PA; PP)

1 The leukocytosis is normal and related to physical exertion of labor and delivery, not infection.

2 Same as # 1.

3 This is not a drop in the WBC count because the normal postpartal white blood cell count is between 15,000 and 20,000/mm³.

54. **2** In light of the vaginal bleeding, the priority nursing action is ascertaining if a viable fetus is present. (b) (OB; AS; TC; HP)

1 This is absolutely contraindicated; bright red bleeding is suggestive of placenta previa.

3 Same as # 1.

4 Same as # 1.

55. **2** The Silverman-Anderson Index reflects respiratory status. (c) (OB; EV; PA; HN)

1 The Silverman-Anderson Index does not reflect caloric needs.

3 The Silverman-Anderson Index does not reflect cardiac function.

4 The Silverman-Anderson Index does not reflect neurologic status.

56. **1** Many superficial veins are common in the preterm infant because of the lack of subcutaneous fat deposits. (a) (OB; AS; PA; HN)

2 A positive Babinski reflex is a normal newborn reflex.

3 Absent femoral pulses are indicative of coarctation of the aorta, a congenital heart defect.

4 Flexion of extremities is the posturing of normal term infants; preterm infants usually posture with extremities extended and flaccid.

57. **3** This is a finding consistent with respiratory distress syndrome because of atelectasis and underinflation of alveoli resulting from decreased surfactant in immature lungs. (c) (OB; AS; PA; HN)

1 The rate is much higher in RDS.

2 A lowered pH is more consistent with RDS.

4 Expiratory stridor is present in RDS.

58. **1** Prolonged use of oxygen concentrations above those required to maintain adequate oxygenation have been found to contribute to the occurrence of retrolental fibroplasia (RLF). (a) (OB; PL; TC; HN)

2 Warming and humidifying O₂ will not affect the level in the environment.

3 Retrolental fibroplasia is caused by high blood concentrations of O₂, not by eye exposure to oxygen.

4 Retrolental fibroplasia cannot be prevented by using any preferred route of O₂ administration.

59. **2** Primary manifestations of NEC are feeding intolerance, increased gastric residual of undigested formula, and bile-stained emesis. (c) (OB; AS; PA; HN)

1 This occurs with pyloric stenosis.

3 This occurs with diarrhea; stools in those with NEC are generally reduced in number and contain glucose and blood.

4 This may occur with a cardiac anomaly, not NEC.

60. **1** Prolonged gastric emptying occurs when the baby has NEC; an increase in abdominal girth of

greater than 1 cm in 4 hours is significant and needs immediate intervention. (b) (OB; PL; TC; HN)

2 Formula is stopped and the baby is placed on parenteral fluids.

3 Same as # 2.

4 This will have no therapeutic value for a child with NEC.

61. **3** Touching and holding the infant is the most effective way of promoting mother-infant bonding. (a) (OB; IM; PE; EC)

1 This is an unreal approach; it does not prepare the mother to deal with her ill child.

2 This would prevent the mother from touching and holding the baby; the mother must do this to foster bonding.

4 This provides false reassurance; the nurse does not know if this is true.

62. **2** Apical pulse of 110 = 2; acrocyanois = 1; active motion and flexion = 2; vigorous cry = 2; effective respiratory effort with crying = 2; total Apgar = 9. (b) (OB; AS; PA; NN)

1 This is inaccurate; the infant loses 1 point because of a lack of all-pink color.

3 This is too low; the infant loses only 1 point for not being all pink.

4 Same as # 3.

63. **4** The client's statement, in conjunction with the other findings, suggests urinary retention. (a) (OB; AS; PA; PP)

1 This is unrelated to the other findings; thirst is related to dehydration, whereas the other signs are related to urinary retention.

2 This is an expected postpartal response.

3 This is expected; oxytocin secretion, which is stimulated by infant suckling, causes the uterus to contract.

64. **2** Methergine can cause hypertension and should not be given with an increased blood pressure. (b) (OB; EV; PA; DR)

1 This indicates thrombophlebitis and is not related to Methergine.

3 Methergine does not affect respirations.

4 This is a normal adult finding.

65. **4** Physiologic jaundice is caused by elevated bilirubin levels resulting from breakdown of excessive fetal red blood cells; this occurs on the second or third day of life. (a) (OB; PL; ED; NN)

1 Jaundice is unrelated to breastfeeding.

2 Mottling in the newborn is related to an immature vascular system.

3 This would be evidenced by a decreased urinary output and depressed fontanels.

66. **2** PKU is an inborn error of metabolism involving an inability to properly metabolize phenylalanine, an essential amino acid. (b) (OB; AN; TC; PP)

1 This is metabolized normally in those with PKU.

3 Same as # 1.

4 Same as # 1.

67. **2** This information assists parents to understand the unique features of their newborn and promotes interaction and care during periods of wakefulness. (c) (OB; PL; ED; NN)

1 Most infants are on a demand feeding schedule, not a routine schedule; demand feeding provides for individuality.

3 Printed instructions are inadequate if unaccompanied by a discussion.

4 This is too limited; the parents need a broader discussion of infant behaviors.

68. **1** The priority is to evaluate the progress of labor so that the nurse can plan care. (b) (OB; AS; PA; IP)

2 This question should be asked but is not the first priority.

3 Same as # 2.

4 Same as # 2.

69. **2** The client is in the early part of the first stage of labor, and it is important to help the partner with the role of coach. (b) (OB; IM; ED; IP)

1 It is not necessary to measure the fetal heart rate this often until the second stage of labor; the client may be on an external monitor, which constantly records FHR.

3 Delivery is not imminent at this time.

4 Suggesting that the pain is bad may increase anxiety and produce greater discomfort.

70. **4** Identifying progress and providing encouragement motivates the client and promotes positive feelings about the self. (a) (OB; PL; PE; IP)

1 A client in active labor should not be left alone.

2 Lying flat on her back may induce supine hypotension; side-lying should be encouraged to promote venous return.

3 During this early stage of labor, diversion is therapeutic because the client is not totally involved with herself.

71. **2** This response encourages the client to verbalize concerns; verbalization is an outlet for discharging tension. (a) (OB; IM; PE; EC)

1 This response denies the client's feelings and gives false reassurance.

3 Same as # 1.

4 This response reinforces the client's fears.

72. **3** This fetal heart pattern is known as type III dip or deceleration; it indicates cord compression that may lead to fetal hypoxia. (c) (OB; AN; PA; IP)

1 Beat-to-beat variability indicates a fetus with no nervous system depression.

2 This is a type I dip that results from fetal scalp compression during a contraction and is considered normal.

4 The fetal heart rate does not always drop with a contraction in all labors.

73. **1** Preventing heat loss conserves the infant's oxygen and glycogen reserves, and this is a first priority. (b) (OB; IM; TC; NN)

2 This can be done after provision has been made to prevent heat loss.

3 This is important but not a priority; assessment should be delayed until the infant is warm.

4 Warming the infant will reduce cyanosis if no respiratory obstruction is present.

74. **4** A postpartum chill is a normal occurrence of unknown cause. (a) (OB; EV; PA; PP)

1 This measure is part of the routine postpartum assessment but does not need to be done in relation to the chill.

2 Same as # 1.

3 Same as # 1.

75. **4** The breast buds and genitalia develop at a specified rate and are good indicators of gestational

age. (c) (OB; AS; PA; HN)

1 Weight and length may be influenced both by genetic factors and by prenatal stresses and are not accurate indicators of gestational age.

2 This provides data about the infant's neuromuscular status and is not a specific indicator of gestational age.

3 This is not a good indication of gestational age.

76. **1** The development of bonding between mother and infant is an important psychologic goal and should be facilitated. (b) (OB; PL; PE; EC)

2 It is important for mothers to develop a relationship with ill newborns even if the prognosis is poor.

3 This is a nursing action and does not require a physician's order.

4 Same as # 2.

77. **2** By participating in the infant's care, the client will gain confidence in her own ability to meet the infant's needs. (b) (OB; IM; PE; EC)

1 Watching the provision of care by others would only increase the client's sense of inadequacy.

3 If she is not permitted to care for the infant sooner, the client will have to develop these skills under stress.

4 There is no need for a specialist to care for the infant after discharge.

78. **1** Fatigue will influence the successful use of other coping strategies such as distraction; this may lead to the client's requiring pain medication. (b) (OB; IM; ED; PN)

2 Progesterone is decreased at this time.

3 Energy will enhance the quality of contractions.

4 The client does not push during the first stage of labor; pushing is done during the second stage.

79. **1** A persistent occiput-posterior position causes intense back pain because of fetal compression of the sacral nerves. (a) (OB; IM; ED; PN)

2 This would not cause back pain.

3 Same as # 2.

4 Same as # 2.

80. **3** Low back pain is aggravated when the client is in the supine position because of increased pressure from the fetus as the head rotates. (a) (OB; IM; ED; PN)

1 This position relieves back pain.

2 The knee-chest position is not used in labor except in an emergency situation such as cord prolapse.

4 Same as # 1.

81. **2** Counterpressure alleviates some of the discomfort from the pressure of the fetal head on the sacrum. (a) (OB; IM; ED; IP)

1 Kegel exercises tone the pelvic musculature, not the back.

3 Panting may lead to hyperventilation, which will cause maternal respiratory alkalosis and fetal acidosis.

4 Elevating the legs will increase tension and discomfort.

82. **2** A paper bag helps the client to rebreathe CO_2, which helps correct the respiratory alkalosis. (b) (OB; IM; ED; IP)

1 The client's O_2 level is already elevated; the client needs to elevate the CO_2 level.

3 Anesthesia will further deplete CO_2 and is therefore contraindicated.

4 CO_2 is too dilute in room atmosphere.

83. **2** This is the most difficult part of labor, and the client needs encouragement and support to cope. (b) (OB; AN; TC; IP)

1 Medication at this time will depress the infant and is contraindicated.

3 Fluids should be increased because of the increase in metabolism.

4 Breathing patterns should be complex and should require a high level of concentration to distract the client.

84. **2** Panting and blowing keep the glottis open so that the client cannot hold her breath and bear down. (b) (OB; EV; ED; IP)

1 This pattern interferes with adequate oxygenation of the fetus because it limits the mother's O_2 intake.

3 Although this keeps the pressure of the diaphragm off the contracting uterus, it does not reduce the urge to push.

4 Same as # 3.

85. **2** In the fourteenth week, amniotic fluid is present and small amounts can be withdrawn for testing. (a) (OB; IM; ED; HP)

1 There is no amniotic fluid present at the time of conception.

3 It is more appropriate to do an amniocentesis before quickening is established.

4 This is untrue; an amniocentesis can be performed any time after the fourteenth week; in the last trimester the amount of fluid for testing may be reduced.

86. **1** It is possible that stimulation of the uterus due to the procedure may cause uterine contractions. (a) (OB; AS; TC; HP)

2 This is not necessary because amniocentesis is not done via the vaginal area.

3 This is irrelevant because amniotic fluid is in no way influenced by the intake of fluid.

4 This should not be necessary because the pinprick opening seals up immediately.

87. **2** Once the infant breathes the oxygen in the air, the need for an increased amount of immature erythrocytes decreases. (b) (OB; AN; PA; NN)

1 The infant and mother have independent blood supplies, and Rh− blood does not enter the baby's bloodstream.

3 This is not a common occurrence in newborns; also, symptoms would occur more quickly.

4 Jaundice is not an allergic response.

88. **1** All Rh− mothers with Rh+ infants are candidates for RhoGAM; negative Coombs' indicates absence of Rh antibodies. (c) (OB; AS; TC; HP)

2 When mother and baby both have Rh− blood, RhoGAM is not required.

3 The positive Coombs' indicates the presence of circulating antibodies; therefore RhoGAM is of no use.

4 Same as # 2.

89. **2** Exposure to air dries the nipples by evaporation; exposure also tends to harden the nipples, making them less tender. (b) (OB; IM; TC; PP)

1 If kept from the breast for a prolonged period, the baby may become accustomed to the bottle and not wish to nurse again.

3 This may relieve discomfort but will do nothing to toughen the nipples.

4 Continuous ice packs are used to relieve the discomfort caused by engorged breasts, not sore nipples.

90. **3** The fat pad is present in newborns and infants; the arch develops when the child begins to walk. (b) (OB; AN; PA; NN)
   1 Flat feet are no more common in children than in adults.
   2 The size of the feet is not relevant; arch development is related to walking.
   4 Flat feet are not associated with a deformity such as clubfoot.

91. **2** Coarctation of the aorta results in diminished or absent femoral pulses. (c) (OB; AS; PA; NN)
   1 This has minimal impact on the volume of peripheral circulation (left-to-right shunt).
   3 Same as # 1.
   4 This has no impact on the volume of peripheral circulation (minimal shunting occurs in the newborn period).

92. **1** Right-to-left shunts result in inadequate perfusion of blood; not enough blood flows to the lungs for oxygenation. (c) (OB; AN; PA; NN)
   2 Left-to-right shunts result in too much blood flowing to the lungs; blood is adequately perfused.
   3 Left-sided obstruction to the flow of blood results in decreased peripheral pulses, not cyanosis.
   4 Normally there should be no shunting of blood between the right and left sides of the heart after the ductus arteriosus closes.

93. **2** Because lungs are stressed by increased fluid, increased respirations are the first and best indicators of early congestive heart failure. (c) (OB; AS; PA; HN)
   1 The heart rate would not decrease; it would increase in an attempt to compensate.
   3 This is a normal finding in the newborn.
   4 Cyanosis is not an early sign because there is adequate perfusion of blood.

94. **1** This client will have lower tolerance for pain and greater need for pain relief. (b) (OB; PL; TC; HP)
   2 Larger doses may be needed if this is done.
   3 Delays increase anxiety and discomfort, and larger doses are needed.
   4 Individuals who abuse drugs need more medication than do others because of tolerance.

95. **2** Initially, cold therapy reduces edema and discomfort. (b) (OB; PL; TC; PP)
   1 ASA is contraindicated in the puerperium; there is too great a risk for hemorrhage.
   3 Heat therapy usually begins after 8 to 12 hours of cold therapy; warm, not hot, water would be used.
   4 This provides little or minimal perineal relief.

96. **1** Voiding will be difficult because of peri-urethral edema and discomfort. (b) (OB; EV; PA; PP)
   2 There is nothing to suggest delayed lactation.
   3 There is nothing in the data to suggest that if bonding occurs it would be maladaptive.
   4 This rarely occurs with primigravidas, even when a lot of pushing occurs.

97. **3** The earliest sign of drug withdrawal is CNS overstimulation. (b) (OB; AS; PA; HP)
   1 These have no relation to drug abuse.
   2 These have no relation to drug abuse; most post-

partum women are hungry and thirsty.
   4 Same as # 1.

98. **1** Infection is most commonly transmitted through contaminated hands. (b) (OB; IM; ED; PP)
   2 Tub baths are permitted.
   3 This is contraindicated in the postpartum period until the cervix is completely closed.
   4 Same as # 3.

99. **4** The cytomegalovirus has been recovered from semen, vaginal secretions, urine, feces, and blood (including blood from blood banks); it is commonly found in clients with AIDS. (c) (OB; AN; PA; HN)
   1 This is associated with toxoplasmosis.
   2 Same as # 1.
   3 This is associated with hepatitis B.

100. **4** An infant of less than 37 weeks gestation is considered preterm; a weight of 1000 grams is under the 10th percentile for the gestational age. (b) (OB; AS; PA; HN)
   1 A term infant is gestationally 37 weeks or greater.
   2 The infant is preterm, but the weight is under the 10th percentile for the gestational age.
   3 Same as # 1.

101. **1** A preterm, small for gestational age infant is at risk for problems not seen in the term or average for gestational age infant because of immaturity; this information will help the nurse to anticipate potential problems and aim interventions at prevention. (a) (OB; AN; TC; HN)
   2 The infant will lose weight, but the comparison of weight and gestational age is important for the development of appropriate nursing measures.
   3 The information is documented on the infant's chart, but this is not the overriding reason for obtaining this data.
   4 Same as # 3.

102. **3** Gradually rewarming an infant experiencing cold stress is essential to avoid compromising the infant's cardiopulmonary status. (c) (OB; IM; PA; HN)
   1 An infant experiencing cold stress will become hypoglycemic; the infant uses up glycogen and glucose to maintain the core temperature.
   2 Rapid rewarming of an infant may result in apnea and neonatal stress.
   4 Skin temperatures should be taken at least every 15 minutes until stable.

103. **2** A preterm infant may have a weak suck but usually can be breastfed; the mother may at least attempt it, if the infant is stable. (b) (OB; IM; ED; HN)
   1 The suck may or may not be weak, but a supervised attempt to breastfeed may help the mother get to know the infant and feel competent in providing care.
   3 It does not necessarily take more calories to breastfeed; also, there are immunologic benefits to the preterm infant who receives antibodies through breast milk.
   4 Pumping the breasts may be necessary, but bottle feeding is not needed because this only deters the mother and infant; at 34 weeks if the infant is stable and the mother so desires, breastfeeding should be attempted.

104. **3** This is known as the hormone of pregnancy; to-

gether with estrogen it helps prepare the endometrium for the fertilized ovum, helps maintain pregnancy, and prepares the mammary glands for milk secretion. (a) (OB; AN; PA; PN)
1 This is secreted by the anterior lobe of the pituitary gland; it starts and maintains milk secretion by the mammary glands.
2 It is secreted by the posterior pituitary gland; it stimulates labor contractions and contractile tissue around the nipple during nursing.
4 It is secreted by the adrenal cortex, and it affects carbohydrate metabolism.

105. **1** During pregnancy, a blood volume increase of 30% to 60% and an elevated basal metabolic rate produce an increased need for red blood cells. (b) (OB; AN; PA; PN)
2 There is no data to support the presence of pernicious anemia.
3 There is no indication that the client is allergic to anything.
4 This is related to the Rh factor, not anemia.

106. **2** The male should be treated to prevent the infection from passing back and forth between him and his sexual partner. (a) (OB; EV; ED; PN)
1 A douche is not recommended during pregnancy.
3 This is an ineffective remedy.
4 The organism is most likely present in the partner's urogenital tract; voiding will not prevent recurrence.

107. **3** A continuous trickle is indicative of hemorrhage; immediate medical intervention is required. (b) (OB; IM; TC; IP)
1 Data indicates that the fundus is firm and at the appropriate level.
2 There is no data to indicate a full bladder; the fundus is firm and not dextroverted.
4 This should be done more frequently; however, vital signs do not always change markedly until a large amount of blood is lost.

108. **1** Clients with allergies to penicillin must be evaluated carefully because they may have an allergic response to Velosef as well. (c) (OB; AS; TC; DR)
2 This is unrelated to penicillin hypersensitivity.
3 Same as # 2.
4 Same as # 2.

109. **1** The mother needs to learn the realities of infant behavior and how to cope with them; holding and talking to the baby are consoling measures. (b) (OB; PL; ED; PP)
2 The infant is too young to be given cereal at this time.
3 It is unhealthful to disrupt the baby's sleep pattern.
4 At this age a toy would not be meaningful and would be an inadequate substitute for parental attention.

110. **2** Iron is best utilized when given in an acid medium. (b) (OB; EV; ED; DR)
1 This would decrease the acidity of the stomach; an alkaline medium does not promote absorption of iron.
3 Same as # 1.
4 Same as # 1.

111. **2** Early postoperative ambulation helps prevent many postpartal complications such as thrombophlebitis or constipation. (b) (OB; PL; ED; HP)
1 Discharge commonly occurs around day 5.
3 Clients are permitted to shower after 48 hours.
4 A bowel movement can occur spontaneously if early ambulation and adequate fluids are encouraged.

112. **1** This dilates milk ducts, promotes emptying of the breasts, and stimulates further lactation. (a) (OB; EV; ED; PP)
2 Breast binders may inhibit lactation; they fool the body into thinking that milk secretion is no longer needed.
3 This will contract the milk ducts and interfere with the milk letdown reflex.
4 Large consumption of milk products is not required to stimulate the production of milk.

113. **2** This is the proper attachment and helps compress the milk glands. (a) (OB; EV; PA; NN)
1 This is not a good indication; infant may be sucking on the nipple only.
3 The nipple must be on top of the tongue.
4 This indicates improper attachment.

114. **2** The presence of at least 6 to 8 wet diapers each day indicates sufficient breast milk intake. (b) (OB; EV; ED; NN)
1 This is not a reliable indicator; sleep patterns may vary.
3 This could indicate an inadequate amount of fluid ingestion.
4 This is a poor indicator; not all babies need extra sucking stimulation.

115. **1** This indicates subinvolution and needs further assessment. (a) (OB; EV; TC; PP)
2 This is normal postpartal diuresis.
3 This is the normal milk letdown reflex.
4 This is a normal postpartal concern, especially with a history of infertility.

116. **4** This is the accepted definition of partial placenta previa. (b) (OB; AN; PA; HP)
1 This occurs in abruptio placentae.
2 Same as # 1.
3 This will not lead to placenta previa but will place the fetus in jeopardy.

117. **3** With a low implanted placenta (placenta previa) the presenting part may have difficulty entering the pelvis. (c) (OB; AS; PA; HP)
1 This is difficult with a low-lying placenta.
2 This occurs with abruptio placentae.
4 Placenta previa does not make it difficult to palpate small fetal parts.

118. **2** Blood loss and anemia cause a lowered resistance to infection; the placental site is in the lower uterine segment and is more exposed to the entry of organisms through the vagina in both the antepartal and postpartal periods. (b) (OB; AN; TC; HP)
1 Placenta previa is characterized by painless bleeding.
3 There is a separation from the uterine wall as the uterus expands; there is no tearing of the placenta.
4 Placenta previa is not caused by a genetic factor and would not cause genetic birth defects in the fetus.

119. **4** By counting or weighing pads, an accurate measurement of the amount of blood loss may be obtained. (a) (OB; AS; TC; HP)
1 The vital signs will reflect the effects of the blood loss rather than the amount.
2 Same as # 1.

3 The fundus may be higher than normal because the placenta prevents the descent of the fetus into the pelvis, but the height cannot be used to measure blood loss.

120. **3** Giving the parents true information about what to expect during the procedure will help to allay their fears and encourage their cooperation. (b) (OB; IM; PE; EC)

1 Reassurance is nontherapeutic; amniocentesis is a low-risk procedure, but some complications may occur.

2 If the father is uninformed, viewing the procedure may increase his anxiety even though his presence may be comforting to the mother.

4 The nurse should be able to provide information and interpretation of procedures for clients; delay in answering their questions may increase clients' concerns.

121. **2** A full bladder helps to stabilize the uterus during the ultrasonogram; this allows for better visualization of the fetus; two full glasses of water, drunk about 1 hour before the test, will fill the bladder. (b) (OB; IM; TC; HP)

1 Emptying the bladder is inadvisable because a full bladder supports the uterus and improves visualization of the uterus.

3 Because the procedure is noninvasive, it is unnecessary to cleanse the skin.

4 An enema is contraindicated when bleeding occurs.

122. **3** Vaginal examination may cause separation of the entire placenta with resulting hemorrhage; an immediate cesarean delivery is done to prevent fetal demise. (b) (OB; PL; TC; HP)

1 This would do nothing to save the infant if total placental separation occurs.

2 Delaying labor would not be helpful; immediate cesarean delivery is necessary in this emergency.

4 Same as # 1.

123. **1** A vaginal examination may result in a sudden, severe hemorrhage because of the location of the placenta near the cervical os; whole blood should be ready for administration to prevent shock. (b) (OB; PL; TC; HP)

2 Adults manufacture their own vitamin K, and an injection would not help to prevent bleeding from the placenta.

3 This is an incorrect response; fresh plasma may be used to restore coagulation factors when DIC occurs after severe blood loss.

4 Giving heparin sodium is contraindicated in the presence of hemorrhage.

124. **2** A tuberculin test should not be administered to a client with a known positive tuberculin test because severe reactions can occur at the test site in individuals previously sensitized. (b) (OB; EV; TC; PN)

1 It is more important to know whether the test was positive than if it was done.

3 Unless it was tuberculosis, this would not affect giving the tuberculin test.

4 The priority is a previous positive test.

125. **3** Active immunity occurs when the individual's cells produce antibodies in response to an agent or its products; these antibodies will destroy the agent (antigen) should it enter the body again. (c) (OB; AN; PA; PN)

1 Antigens are foreign substances that enter the body and trigger antibody formation.

2 Antigens do not fight antibodies; they trigger an antibody formation that in turn attacks the antigen.

4 Sensitized lymphocytes do not act as antibodies.

126. **3** A floating fetal head in a primigravida who is in early labor is suggestive of disproportion because engagement usually occurs 2 weeks before term in primigravidas. (c) (OB; AN; TC; IP)

1 This falls within the normal range of 120 to 160 beats per minute.

2 This occurs during early labor when the presenting part bears down on the capillary structure of the cervix.

4 This test confirms the presence of ruptured membranes, which should not cause any problems with delivery.

127. **1** A difficult delivery because of broad fetal shoulders may result in a fractured clavicle, which can be assessed by the findings of a knot or lump, limited arm movement, and a unilateral Moro response. (b) (OB; AS; PA; HN)

2 This reflex involves the feet; it is in no way related to a difficult delivery because of broad shoulders.

3 Same as # 2.

4 This is unrelated to difficult delivery of a baby with wide shoulders.

128. **3** The side-lying position improves the venous return to the heart and increases stroke volume and cardiac output. (a) (OB; PL; TC; HP)

1 This position impairs venous return and may cause supine hypotension syndrome.

2 This position does not promote optimal venous return to the heart.

4 This will cause dyspnea because of increased pressure on the diaphragm from the abdominal organs and fetus.

129. **4** Under normal conditions the heart rate increases with physical activity; the test looks for accelerations of 10 to 15 beats with fetal movements. (b) (OB; AN; PA; HP)

1 This is not a part of the evaluation of the fetus in the nonstress test.

2 Same as # 1.

3 This is used in the stress test (OCT)

130. **4** Nonperiodic accelerations on movement and a baseline variability of 5 to 15 beats indicate fetal well-being. (c) (OB; AS; PA; HP)

1 Early decelerations are associated with fetal head compression.

2 Late decelerations are associated with uteroplacental insufficiency.

3 Variable decelerations are associated with cord compression.

131. **4** The fetus with a borderline cardiac reserve will show hypoxia by a decreased heart rate when there is minimal stress, making the test positive. (b) (OB; AS; PA; HP)

1 The normal baseline measurement would be taken before the test or early in the test to provide a basis of comparison.

2 These decelerations are a response to head compression.

3 There are non-uniform drops in FHR before, during, or after a contraction; they are related to partial, brief cord compression that can be eliminated by changing the mother's position.

132. **2** Preterm infants are at risk for respiratory distress and would be compromised by excessive

use of narcotic analgesics; other supportive measures should be used initially to relieve discomfort. (b) (OB; AN; TC; IP)
1 This is untrue; however, use is limited as much as possible.
3 Although this is taken into consideration, fetal safety is primary, and analgesia is reduced to a minimum.
4 This is untrue; preterm infants are at risk for respiratory distress, and respiratory depression from analgesia may further compromise their immature lungs.
133. **1** The 1-minute Apgar score indicates the need to take resuscitative action, and the 5-minute Apgar indicates whether the action was successful. (b) (OB; AN; TC; HN)
2 Moist oxygen over the face through a funnel to the nose and mouth or stimulation of crying to increase respirations may be sufficient with Apgar scores as low as 5; oxygen under pressure is used when the Apgar is below 4 at 1 minute.
3 The Apgar measurements are for infants of all gestational ages; this infant's response was based on the respiratory effort, heart rate, grimace activity, color, and muscle tone at 1 and 5 minutes after birth.
4 The scores do not indicate a need for this.
134. **4** These are key signs of a pneumothorax, which can occur when an infant is receiving oxygen by positive pressure. (b) (OB; AS; PA; HN)
1 Findings are not normal and need immediate attention.
2 Findings do not indicate this occurrence.
3 Same as # 2.
135. **3** This statement conveys acceptance by the nurse and encourages the mother to verbalize additional concerns; it also explores the mother's understanding of the physician's explanation. (b) (OB; IM; PE; EC)
1 This reply belittles the mother's concern and cuts off further communication.
2 Although this response does acknowledge part of the mother's concerns, it denies her the opportunity of further exploration of her fears that her infant may not respond to therapy.
4 Same as # 1.
136. **4** Research has demonstrated that preterm infants who are allowed to suck on a pacifier during tube feedings take bottle feedings more readily and are discharged sooner. (b) (OB; IM; TC; HN)
1 There is no evidence that non-nutritive sucking is harmful for a preterm infant this size.
2 On the contrary, sucking on a pacifier promotes adaptation to later bottle feedings.
3 Research has identified a benefit of non-nutritive sucking; buck teeth are associated with thumb sucking.
137. **3** Phenergan potentiates the analgesic effect of Demerol; it also acts as an antiemetic if Demerol causes nausea and vomiting. (a) (OB; IM; ED; DR)
1 This is untrue; Phenergan potentiates the analgesic effects of Demerol.
2 Same as # 1.
4 Same as # 1.
138. **3** Methergine, an oxytocic, is used to promote uterine contractions; its vasoconstrictive action can also lead to hypertension, and it should not be used when hypertension is already present. (b)

(OB; EV; TC; DR)
1 In view of the red, edematous episiotomy, this medication is probably being given prophylactically to prevent infection.
2 There is no contraindication to using this medication to relieve the discomfort of the episiotomy.
4 There is no contraindication for use of this drug; it is commonly found as a standing order for postpartum clients to facilitate passage of stool.
139. **4** This is the period when ovulation occurs; the ovum's eruption from the follicle is accompanied by some pain. (a) (OB; AN; ED; FS)
1 The pain is mild, cyclic, and characteristic of mittelschmerz.
2 When menses first begin the client is usually anovulatory and would not experience the pain known as mittelschmerz.
3 The pain will probably occur most frequently when ovulation is well established.
140. **3** A condom covers the penis and contains the semen when it is ejaculated; semen contains a high percentage of HIV in infected individuals. (a) (OB; IM; ED; FS)
1 This is unsafe; although a monogamous relationship is less risky than having multiple sexual partners; if the one partner is HIV positive, the other person is at high risk for acquiring the HIV.
2 This is poor advice; pre-ejaculatory fluid carries the HIV in an infected individual.
4 This is not what the client is asking; most contraceptives do not provide any protection from the HIV.
141. **4** Removing the tube does not bring a halt to menses; endometrial proliferation and shedding will occur as long as the ovaries and uterus are present. (a) (OB; EV; ED; FS)
1 This is true; pregnancy should be delayed 6 to 12 months after a tubal pregnancy.
2 This is true; there is evidence that clients who have one tubal pregnancy are highly susceptible to having another.
3 This is true; pelvic infections can lead to constriction of tubes, and a fertilized ovum may become trapped.
142. **2** This is the only correct definition of dysmenorrhea. (a) (OB; AS; ED; FS)
1 This is known as menometrorrhagia.
3 This is any bleeding that occurs at any time other than during the menstrual period; there may or may not be any pain.
4 This occurs with menopause; menses are also halted during pregnancy.
143. **1** The amniotic fluid is a protective environment; the fetus depends on the placenta, along with the umbilical blood vessels, for obtaining nutrients and oxygen. (b) (OB; EV; ED; PN)
2 This is a true statement and would not require further teaching.
3 Same as # 2.
4 Same as # 2.
144. **1** Because the cervical os is closed, tub bathing cannot cause an ascending infection and may be continued until the onset of labor. (b) (OB; IM; ED; PN)
2 Tub bathing is permitted throughout pregnancy, usually until the onset of labor when the cervical os begins to open.

3 This is untrue; infection may occur only if the cervical os is open and the bathtub is dirty.

4 Same as # 2.

145. 2 Measurement of the fetal structures provides information that is useful in approximating fetal age. (a) (OB; AS; PA; PN)

1 Ultrasound can detect some, but not all, birth defects.

3 This test can detect only physical defects.

4 Ultrasound is done primarily to estimate fetal age, not to approximate linear growth.

146. 1 This is a frequently occurring side effect of this drug, which is a beta$_2$-adrenergic agent that inhibits smooth muscle contractility. (b) (OB; EV; TC; DR)

2 Tachycardia, not bradycardia, frequently occurs.

3 These do not occur with ritodrine.

4 This is not an expected side effect.

147. 1 This block relieves vaginal and perineal pain but does not impair the ability to push. (c) (OB; AN; PA; IP)

2 This relieves uterine pain, not vaginal or perineal pain; the client will not feel contractions.

3 This block relieves pain from the umbilicus to the lower perineum; the client will not feel the urge to push.

4 This relieves pain from the umbilicus to the midthigh; the client will not feel the urge to push.

148. 4 The client becomes very introverted, starts to lose control, and needs assistance and support to help her through this most difficult phase of labor. (a) (OB; PL; TC; IP)

1 This is done throughout labor; it is especially important during the transition phase to help the client maintain control.

2 Same as # 1.

3 Same as # 1.

149. 1 Heat increases milk flow, and because the client is not breastfeeding, this is an undesired outcome; application of cold is recommended to restrict milk flow. (a) (OB; EV; ED; PP)

2 This is a correct statement; a tight, supportive bra will suppress milk production; no further teaching is needed.

3 This is a correct statement; engorgement lasts 48 to 72 hours; no further teaching is needed.

4 This is a correct statement; analgesics will help lessen the discomfort of engorgement; no further teaching is needed.

150. 3 This is due to the arrangement of fatty acids on the glycerol molecule and is related to the natural lipase activity that is present in human milk that has not been heat treated. (b) (OB; AN; ED; PP)

1 The converse is true; lactose content is higher in human milk.

2 It is lower, but protein in human milk is easier for the infant to digest.

4 This is untrue; these factors are found only in human milk.

151. 2 Heart rate below 100 beats per minute = 1; slow and irregular respirations = 1; grimaces in response to suctioning = 1; flaccid muscle tone = 0; and cyanosis = 0; Apgar would total 3. (c) (OB; AN; PA; HN)

1 This score is too low; the infant should receive 1 point for heartbeat, 1 point for respirations, and 1 point for grimacing; thus the assigned score is 3.

3 This is too high; the infant should receive 1 point for heartbeat, 1 point for respirations, and 1 point for grimacing; thus the assigned score is 3.

4 Same as #3.

152. 4 The assessment findings are indicative of a preterm infant; therefore the nurse should closely monitor the infant for signs of respiratory distress syndrome; this occurs frequently in preterm infants because their lungs are immature. (b) (OB; AS; PA; HN)

1 Preterm AGA infants do not develop polycythemia; preterm LGA infants may develop polycythemia, but there is no data to indicate the infant is LGA.

2 Preterm AGA infants may become hypoglycemic.

3 The neonate is preterm, not postterm.

153. 2 If the airway is not patent and gas exchange is inadequate, life cannot be sustained, thus this must be the top priority. (c) (OB; PL; TC; HN)

1 Although body temperature is important because the baby is lacking brown fat and other defense mechanisms needed to maintain temperature, without oxygen, life could not be sustained.

3 Although preventing infection is important because the baby lacks immunity from the mother, without oxygen, life could not be sustained.

4 Although bonding is important to the parent-child relationship, without oxygen, life could not be sustained.

154. 2 Adaptation to the extrauterine environment is largely dependent on the functional capacity of vital organ systems, which is established during intrauterine development; this is measurable in terms of gestational age and weight. (b) (OB; AN; PA; HN)

1 Although these factors may influence health, they are not critical to neonatal survival.

3 Same as # 1.

4 Same as # 1.

155. 2 The nurse applies tactile stimulation after validating that respirations are absent; this action may be sufficient to reestablish respirations in the high-risk neonate with frequent episodes of apnea. (b) (OB; IM; TC; HN)

1 Assessment will not interrupt the period of apnea; respirations must be immediately reestablished.

3 The monitor should be assessed for proper functioning before use.

4 These measures are too invasive and aggressive for initial intervention; gentle stimulation should be attempted first.

156. 3 This is the expected outcome; if output exceeds input, it indicates that the infant is diuresing from the Lasix. (a) (OB; EV; PA; DR)

1 This is not the desired outcome; this would indicate dehydration, which could occur with excessive administration of Lasix.

2 Although important to assess, this is subjective; intake and output would be an objective assessment.

4 Although Lasix can cause hypokalemia, which can precipitate digitalis toxicity, this is not the desired effect of Lasix administration.

157. 1 Confrontation about the active substance abuse

and the mother's diminished ability to safely care for the infant at this time is necessary to help the mother get help and to also protect the baby. (b) (OB; IM; PE; EC)

2 This decision should not be made without input from the mother.

3 This would be unsafe; the mother may not be capable of caring for the infant.

4 Same as # 2.

158. **2** Vitamin C aids in absorption of iron because of its ability to reduce acidity. (b) (OB; PL; ED; PN)

1 This is unrelated to the absorption of iron.

3 Same as # 1.

4 Same as # 1.

159. **2** There is reduced GI motility during pregnancy because of the high level of placental progesterone and displacement of the stomach superiorly and the intestines laterally and posteriorly. (c) (OB; AN; PA; PN)

1 The glomerular filtration rate increases.

3 This is unrelated to the absorption of drugs.

4 HCl secretion decreases.

160. **3** Ultrasound can detect anomalies that can be visualized on the body surface. (a) (OB; AS; PA; HP)

1 This is an internal problem that cannot be identified by ultrasound.

2 Same as # 1.

4 Same as # 1.

161. **3** Probenecid reduces renal tubular excretion of penicillin. (b) (OB; EV; ED; DR)

1 This is unrelated to the concommitant administration of penicillin and probenecid.

2 Same as # 1.

4 Same as # 1.

162. **3** Tetracycline has an affinity for calcium; if used during tooth bud development, it may cause discoloration of teeth. (b) (OB; IM; ED; DR)

1 This is untrue; it causes discoloration of teeth.

2 Same as # 1.

4 Same as # 1.

163. **4** The client is experiencing supine hypotension, which is caused by the gravid uterus compressing the large vessels; side-lying will relieve the pressure, increase venous return, improve cardiac output, and raise blood pressure. (a) (OB; IM; PA; IP)

1 This will not relieve uterine compression of large vessels; the client should be placed on her side.

2 Same as # 1.

3 Same as # 1.

164. **2** The client is hyperventilating; breathing into a paper bag promotes rebreathing of carbon dioxide, relieving respiratory alkalosis. (a) (OB; IM; ED; IP)

1 This will not improve the client's respiratory alkalosis, the problem that is causing the client to hyperventilate.

3 This may cause the client to hyperventilate further.

4 Same as # 1.

165. **3** A full bladder will push the presenting part against the uterus; this can result in irregular, poor-quality contractions. (b) (OB; AS; PA; IP)

1 Before this conclusion is considered, the client's bladder should be emptied to relieve the pressure of the presenting part on the uterus; the client can then be observed to see if regular con-

tractions resume.

2 The client has been dilating and is therefore in true, not false, labor.

4 This would have been established in the admission examination.

166. **4** Pressure on the rectum during contractions would indicate that a multipara is beginning transition. (c) (OB; AS; PA; IP)

1 This occurs when transition is complete; that is, when the client is fully dilated.

2 Same as # 1.

3 This occurs when labor begins, not in the beginning of the transitional phase.

167. **1** This is an incorrect statement; if the client expresses milk from her breasts, she is stimulating milk production and will not relieve engorgement; therefore additional teaching will be necessary. (b) (OB; EV; ED; PP)

2 This is a correct statement; this measure is used to give the body the message that milk production is not needed.

3 This is a correct statement; warm water will promote vasodilation, lead to emptying of breasts, and support further milk production.

4 This is a correct statement; non-breastfeeding mothers do not need extra fluids.

168. **4** The recommended weight gain is 25 to 30 pounds. (a) (OB; AN; PA; PN)

1 This is below the recommended weight gain for pregnancy.

2 Same as # 1.

3 Same as # 1.

169. **2** This amount is recommended by the Food and Nutrition Board of the National Academy of Sciences. (a) (OB; IM; ED; PN)

1 This is too little; a minimum of 30 grams is recommended.

3 This is more than the recommended requirement.

4 Same as # 3.

170. **4** This is the time when the fetus is laying down fat deposits and gaining the most weight. (b) (OB; IM; ED; PN)

1 There is little weight gain during this period of organ development.

2 There is weight gain throughout pregnancy, but it is most marked in the third trimester.

3 Same as # 2.

171. **1** The left breech position indicates that the sacrum is presenting on the left side and the head is in the fundus; fetal heart sounds are best heard in the left upper quadrant. (b) (OB; AS; TC; IP)

2 Fetal heart sounds would be in the upper quadrant, not the lower.

3 Same as # 2.

4 Same as # 2.

172. **2** This is done to prevent pushing, because full dilation has not yet occurred. (a) (OB; EV; TC; IP)

1 This is not done until full dilation; it may tire the mother.

3 This is done in the early part (preliminary phase) of the first stage of labor.

4 This is done in the middle part (accelerated phase) of the first stage of labor.

173. **1** This occurs because pressure on the fetal abdomen from the contractions forces meconium from the bowel. (b) (OB; AS; PA; IP)

2 This is unnecessary; this is a normal occurrence caused by pressure on the fetal abdomen during contractions.

3 Cord prolapse is not an absolute, but it may occur if the presenting part does not fill the pelvic cavity.

4 This is unusual unless there are some accompanying signs of fetal distress, such as prolapsed cord or decelerations.

174. 4 An Apgar rate of 1 will be assigned to the color category; the other four categories have rates of 2, making the Apgar score 9, demonstrating a healthy baby. (b) (OB; AS; PA; NN)

1 This infant would be cyanotic and apneic and would have very diminished muscle tone and reflex responsiveness.

2 Diminished muscle tone and reflexes are characteristic of these infants; they would not be active or crying lustily.

3 This would apply to a healthy infant whose bluish color would be more generalized.

175. 1 RhoGAM will be given only if the infant is Rh positive and the Coombs' test is negative. (c) (OB; PL; ED; HP)

2 RhoGAM is given only to Rh negative mothers to prevent antibody formation and protect future pregnancies; it is never given to the baby.

3 This is useless; antibodies develop after fetal blood enters maternal circulation at the site of placental separation.

4 RhoGAM might be given after twenty-eighth week if the amniocentesis procedure resulted in the escape of some fetal blood into maternal circulation.

176. 2 This avoids the possibility of ingesting infected cysts. (c) (OB; IM; ED; HP)

1 This disease, though more prevalent in foreign countries, is seen in the United States.

3 This is not related to toxoplasmosis.

4 Same as # 3.

177. 1 Bleeding could indicate placenta previa or abruptio placentae, which would be aggravated by oxytocin. (a) (OB; AS; TC; HP)

2 OCT is indicated; sickling may reduce O_2 perfusion to the placenta and compromise the infant during labor.

3 OCT is indicated; blurred vision may indicate PIH; cardiac problems may diminish O_2 perfusion to the placenta and compromise the infant during labor.

4 OCT is indicated; arteriolar spasms may diminish O_2 perfusion to the placenta and compromise the infant during labor.

178. 3 Unless the condom is held, it can be displaced, allowing the sperm to enter the vagina. (b) (OB; IM; ED; FS)

1 This is not true; sperm can be deposited at the beginning of the intercourse without the man's knowledge.

2 When the woman has a rise in temperature, she is most fertile and should avoid intercourse.

4 Spermicidal cream is needed because the diaphragm may be displaced in some positions.

179. 3 There is strong evidence that low protein intake is associated with pregnancy-induced hypertension. (a) (OB; AN; PA; HP)

1 This is too vague; it addresses calories but not the type of calories.

2 This may cause problems, but it is not generally associated with pregnancy-induced hypertension.

4 Lack of minerals may cause other problems but is not generally associated with pregnancy-induced hypertension.

180. 1 Rest is advised to reduce arteriolar spasm, and side-lying promotes more efficient venous return to heart; this improves cardiac output and placental perfusion. (a) (OB; PL; ED; HP)

2 Sodium is necessary to maintain circulatory volume and is not removed from the diet.

3 Because of the increased circulatory volume with pregnancy, the client needs 2000 ml of fluids per day.

4 This may increase general arteriolar spasm; also, venous return is inhibited in the upright position.

181. 4 Blood pressure rises, edema increases, and degenerative changes of the kidney cause increasing proteinuria (3+) as preeclampsia worsens. (b) (OB; AS; PA; HP)

1 This is indicative of a cardiac or respiratory problem; it is not found with worsening hypertension.

2 This may be indicative of placenta previa but is not a common adaptation to worsening of pregnancy-induced hypertension.

3 This is within normal limits.

182. 1 Effective magnesium sulfate therapy reduces edema, thus leading to increased urinary output. (c) (OB; EV; TC; DR)

2 This is a sign of toxicity.

3 Same as # 2.

4 The goal of this therapy is to reduce BP.

183. 1 The gravid uterus no longer compresses major vessels; cardiac output is maintained; glomerular filtration and uterine perfusion rates increase. (b) (OB; IM; TC; HP)

2 Maximizing intraabdominal pressure on the iliac veins will decrease blood flow to the pelvic area.

3 Hemoconcentration occurs in the standing and sitting positions and decreases uterine perfusion.

4 Maximizing aortal compression will decrease uterine blood flow.

184. 1 There is a constant need for evaluation of diabetic status, fetal maturity, and placental functioning. (b) (OB; AN; TC; HP)

2 Insulin requirements vary and are usually increased during the second and third trimesters of pregnancy.

3 Fetal mortality in pregnancies in which diabetes is present is 10% to 15% higher than for pregnancies in which diabetes is not present.

4 Many clients with diabetes deliver vaginally with no problems.

185. 4 In any prenatal situation the goal is an optimally healthy mother and baby, no matter what other factors are involved. (c) (OB; PL; TC; HP)

1 This is false; insulin is given as necessary to maintain acceptable glucose levels.

2 This is an ongoing goal, not a long-term goal.

3 This is important, but delivery of an optimally healthy baby is the priority.

186. 2 An L/S ratio indicates adequacy of pulmonary function, and the baby should be free from major respiratory problems. (a) (OB; AS; ED; HP)

1 There is no indication of fetal distress; immedi-

ate delivery is unnecessary.

3 There is no correlation between L/S ratio and the need for induced labor.

4 The L/S ratio only determines fetal lung maturity; further fetal monitoring will be necessary in the future as with any pregnancy.

187. **4** External pressure is useful for reducing intense sensations caused by a posterior presentation. (a) (OB; IM; TC; IP)

1 Effleurage or breathing techniques may not be enough to reduce the pain associated with back labor.

2 The supine position increases the weight of the uterus and baby on the muscles of the back; it can also cause supine hypotension.

3 Walking aids in increasing labor contractions but does not decrease the pain of back labor.

188. **3** This opens communication and allows the client to verbalize thoughts and feelings. (b) (OB; IM; PE; EC)

1 This ignores the client's needs and cuts off communication.

2 This does not give the client the opportunity to verbalize feelings and needs.

4 This is judgmental; there is not enough data to make this assumption.

189. **4** This is the preferred method for clients with diabetes because it has no physiologic side effects. (a) (OB; IM; ED; FS)

1 Oral contraceptives have a diabetogenic effect; they alter carbohydrate metabolism, and insulin dosage must be adjusted.

2 Because of the possibility of perforation, this method increases the risk of infection for diabetic women.

3 This requires a great deal of self-control and a strong desire to avoid pregnancy, and it is not as effective as a diaphragm.

190. **3** This prevents the cord from drying and the umbilical vessel, which supplies oxygen to the fetus, from collapsing. (b) (OB; IM; TC; IP)

1 Moistening the cord and preserving the oxygen supply to the infant are more critical.

2 This is insufficient monitoring; electronic monitors will be applied; the priority is to keep the cord from drying.

4 This action may lead to further reduction of the fetal oxygen supply because the cord may be compressed.

191. **2** This recognizes the client's feelings, encourages ventilation, and does not encourage alcohol for relaxation. (a) (OB; IM; PE; EC)

1 This gives false reassurance; alcohol should not be encouraged for relaxation.

3 The nurse cannot ensure the physician's response; alcohol should not be encouraged for relaxation.

4 This does not recognize the client's feelings and could put the client on the defensive.

192. **3** This keeps the breast as empty as possible, limiting pressure within the ducts, thereby reducing pain. (a) (OB; IM; ED;PP)

1 This is false; a tight fitting bra will increase pain and suppress milk production; this will impede breastfeeding.

2 Weaning will cause stasis of milk ducts and increase the fullness of the breasts at this time, thereby increasing pain.

4 The causative organism is probably already in the baby's nose and mouth; weaning is not always necessary with mastitis.

193. **4** This is used during the early phase of labor when mild contractions dilate the cervix to 3 cm. (b) (OB; EV; ED; IP)

1 This is used during the transition phase of labor.

2 This is used during the active phase of the first stage of labor.

3 This is used in combination with other breathing patterns; it is a part of the accelerated-decelerated pattern.

194. **4** This is an ROA presentation because the prominence over the symphysis suggests a vertex and the fetal occiput and back are in the right anterior quadrant. (c) (OB; AN; TC; IP)

1 This is ruled out; this fetus is in a vertex, not a breech, presentation.

2 This is ruled out by the presence of irregular lumps on the left side, suggesting that the fetal back is in the mother's right quadrant.

3 The occiput is not located in the left posterior quadrant; the occiput and back are on the mother's right side.

195. **1** Clients should use a panting or blowing pattern to overcome the premature urge to push. (b) (OB; IM; ED; IP)

2 Slow chest breathing is used during the early phase of the first stage of labor.

3 Accelerated-decelerated breathing is used during the first stage of labor.

4 Expulsion breathing should not be used at this time because the cervix is not fully dilated and cervical edema and lacerations can occur.

196. **3** This eases the pressure of the presenting part on the umbilical cord and receives the highest priority. (b) (OB; IM; TC; IP)

1 Oxygen can be given, but this is not the priority.

2 Time should not be wasted trying to locate the fetal heart when the fetus is at risk for hypoxia because of cord compression.

4 A cesarean delivery may be necessary; however, the priority is to ease the pressure on the cord to prevent fetal hypoxia.

197. **2** A client's temperature may be elevated to 100.4° F during the first 24 hours postpartum as a result of dehydration from labor. (b) (OB; AN; PA; PP)

1 Mastitis usually develops after breastfeeding has been established and mature milk is present.

3 This usually begins with a fever of 100.4° F or above on 2 successive days, excluding the first 24 hours postpartum.

4 Urinary tract infections usually become evident later in the postpartum period.

198. **4** Adolescent parents are still involved in the developmental stage of resolving their self-identity; they have not sequentially matured to intimacy and generativity. (a) (OB; AN; ED; EC)

1 Although this may be true, it is not the reason the baby is at risk for neglect or abuse.

2 Same as # 1.

3 Same as # 1.

199. **2** The fetus is at risk for retardation prenatally; proper maternal diet will protect the fetus from buildup of metabolites. (c) (OB; IM; ED; HP)

1 This will not occur if the proper diet is maintained.

3 The fetus is at risk if the maternal diet contains phenylalanine and the infant can inherit phenylketonuria; PKU is transmitted via a recessive gene.

4 The client should remain on a phenylalanine-restricted diet during pregnancy to prevent manifestations of the disease.

200. 3 Screening for the disease results in early diagnosis and treatment, which can prevent mental retardation. (a) (OB; PL; TC; HN)

1 This is not the problem; the major manifestations are mental or neurologic in origin.

2 These children have no problem with physical growth; their problem is mental retardation.

4 The disease is genetic and cannot be acquired other than by inheritance; testing is done for early identification and treatment.

201. 1 The term phenylketonuria is derived from phenylpyruvic acid, which gives urine a mousy, musty odor. (b) (OB; AS; PA; HN)

2 This odor is not present with phenylketonuria.

3 Same as # 2.

4 Same as # 2.

202. 3 Adherence to the diet is necessary for optimal physical growth with no adverse effects on mental development; a diet that is instituted late will not reverse brain damage. (a) (OB; AN; PA; AN)

1 Detection cannot occur until the infant has taken milk or formula that contains phenylalanines for 24 hours and metabolites accumulate in the blood; behaviors indicating mental retardation and CNS involvement usually are evident by about 6 months of age in the untreated infant.

2 There is no phenylalanine at birth; it first becomes measurable after the infant ingests milk or formula.

4 This is untrue; it is related to compliance with the prescribed diet once the diagnosis is made.

203. 1 During periods of active or irregular sleep it is normal for newborns to have some twitching movements and irregular respirations; the vital signs and blood glucose levels are normal. (a) (OB; AS; PA; NN)

2 Hypoglycemia in normal newborns would be characterized by a blood sugar level below 30 mg/100 ml.

3 The normal respiratory rate is 30 to 60; irregular breathing is normal.

4 Twitching is a common finding in normal neonates; it often occurs with crying or stimulation.

204. 3 This statement allows parents an opportunity to obtain additional information and review their options to make an informed decision. (c) (OB; IM; ED; EC)

1 Recent studies do not support any connection between circumcision and penile cancer.

2 This information may have already been discussed with the physician; it may be more helpful for the nurse to review the information at this time.

4 This is a partially true statement; however, the Academy primarily emphasizes that there are no medical indications for this procedure.

205. 3 This is the correct flow rate; 10 units of the drug added to 1000 ml of IV results in a solution where 1 ml = 0.01 mg of the drug; therefore, 1 ml must be administered per minute; multiply the amount to be infused (1 ml) by the drop factor (60) and divide the result by the amount of time in minutes (1). (c) (OB; AN; TC; IP)

1 This is too slow; it should be 60 gtt/min.

2 Same as # 1.

4 This is too fast, it should be 60 gtt/min.

206. 1 Frequent contractions with short relaxation periods may lead to fetal hypoxia. (b) (OB; AN; PA; DR)

2 This is within the normal fetal heart rate range of 120 to 160 during labor.

3 An adverse response to Pitocin is a contraction lasting more than 90 seconds; contractions lasting 30 seconds usually occur in early labor.

4 This intensity is within the normal limits of 50 to 75 mm Hg.

207. 4 After 12 hours, amniotic fluid must be assessed for odor and appearance indicating infection for either mother or infant. (c) (OB; AS; PA; IP)

1 A prolapsed cord usually occurs shortly after membranes rupture; it is very unlikely that it will occur 12 hours later.

2 This is premature separation of a normally implanted placenta; it is totally unrelated to ruptured membranes.

3 This is an abnormally implanted placenta; it is totally unrelated to ruptured membranes.

208. 2 The most common cause of deceleration is compression of great vessels; placing the client on her side relieves compression and enhances venous return. (a) (OB; IM; TC; IP)

1 This can be done after the client is placed on her side; it is important to relieve compression on great vessels first.

3 This will not improve the fetal heart rate; more important is placing the mother in the left lateral position.

4 If deceleration does not improve after the client is placed on her side, then the infusion should be stopped.

209. 3 This is caused by the local anesthetic passing rapidly through the placenta to the fetus and having a quinidine-like effect on the myocardium. (c) (OB; EV; PA; DR)

1 This can occur with general anesthesia.

2 The opposite is true; hypotension may occur.

4 This can occur with epidural or spinal anesthesia when the anesthetic is injected too high.

210. 3 An adequate urinary output, an indicator of good renal function, is necessary to prevent toxicity because $MgSO_4$ is excreted by the kidneys; signs of $MgSO_4$ toxicity are reduced respirations and absent patellar reflexes; therefore baseline assessments should be done. (b) (OB; PL; TC; HP)

1 These are urine tests; they are not significant to $MgSO_4$ toxicity.

2 Deviations in temperature do not indicate $MgSO_4$ toxicity.

4 These are assessments that may indicate worsening preeclampsia, not $MgSO_4$ toxicity.

211. 1 One of the characteristics of SIDS is that subsequent siblings of a SIDS infant have a five times greater risk for SIDS than do infants in the general population. (b) (OB; IM; ED; EC)

2 The opposite is true.

3 This is untrue; they have a greater risk for SIDS.

4 Same as # 3.

212. **2** Because seeing and touching the newborn infant is a species-specific behavior for human attachment, allowing them to hold the infant will promote bonding. (b) (OB; IM; PE; EC)

 1 Although this is a viable action, holding and touching will promote bonding more effectively.

 3 Actual holding and touching promotes bonding more than does just hearing about the baby.

 4 After touching and holding, this action can also contribute to bonding.

213. **1** This has been validated by the literature; also, children thrive as long as their caregivers provide an opportunity for stable relationships to occur. (a) (OB; IM; PE; EC)

 2 This is not validated by current literature.

 3 Same as # 2.

 4 Same as # 2.

214. **1** These animal proteins are complete proteins containing all eight essential amino acids; plant proteins are incomplete. (b) (OB; EV; ED; PN)

 2 These are incomplete proteins; also, comparatively small amounts of protein are contained in these foods.

 3 These are not as good a source of protein as milk, eggs, and cheese.

 4 Same as # 3.

215. **3** Carrots provide the precursor pigment, carotene, which the body converts to vitamin A. (a) (OB; AN; PA; PN)

 1 This contains only about one half the needed vitamin A precursor.

 2 These do not contain any vitamin A precursor.

 4 These contain a very small amount of vitamin A precursor.

216. **3** Massaging the uterus will induce contraction and cause expulsion of clots; frequent massage should be continued to keep the uterus firm and inhibit bleeding. (b) (OB; IM; TC; PP)

 1 This would be done if the client were in shock; the priority intervention now is to massage the uterus and prevent hemorrhage.

 2 Pulse and blood pressure do not change significantly unless large amounts of blood are lost.

 4 This is unnecessary; the client's fundus is boggy and needs to be massaged to help it contract.

217. **2** Compared with the prenatal diet, the diet for lactation requires an increased intake of all food groups, vitamins and minerals, plus increased fluid to replace that lost with milk secretion; calories should be increased by 500 daily and protein by 20 g, raising the protein needed to 70 g daily. (b) (OB; IM; ED; PP)

 1 Breastfeeding mothers need to consume an additional 500 calories and 20 g of protein per day to maintain good milk production.

 3 The client needs a well-balanced diet, not just milk, and she must consume an additional 500 calories a day.

 4 This denies the client's concern; optimal nutrition is necessary to produce an adequate milk supply.

218. **2** Air drying the nipples several times a day hardens the nipples and reduces soreness; changing the position of the neonate while nursing will also relieve sore nipples. (a) (OB; PL; TC; PP)

 1 This would inhibit lactation; the baby must suckle and empty the breasts regularly for milk production to continue.

 3 This may reduce the discomfort, but it will not help the nipples to dry and harden.

 4 This would cause vasoconstriction and lead to milk suppression.

219. **4** Only superficial attention has been directed to hypertension; ongoing health supervision is needed. (a) (OB; AN; TC; FS)

 1 Involving the client is important, but professional supervision is required.

 2 This is untrue; however, limiting sodium intake is too superficial.

 3 Teaching and encouraging the client to engage in self-care is helping the client.

220. **3** The client has the right not to accept the Papanicolaou test today; the nurse must recognize the client's need to talk with the physician first. (b) (OB; IM; PE; EC)

 1 This is inappropriate; this action is not client centered.

 2 This is a subjective conclusion; the client has the right to delay, or even refuse, the test.

 4 The client's need must be recognized first.

221. **2** Because the client's temperature findings reflect that ovulation is occurring, the infertility may be due to a seminal factor; the partner's semen should be examined before more extensive studies or treatments are begun with the woman. (b) (OB; AN; PA; FS)

 1 All other potential problems should be ruled out first; the client does not have a right to receive the drug unless it is appropriate for the problem.

 3 Other potential problems should be ruled out first.

 4 Same as # 3.

222. **1** This recognizes achievement and reinforces the client's positive behavior. (b) (OB; IM; PE; FS)

 2 This focuses on the negative rather than the positive; small gains should be reinforced.

 3 This is inappropriate; the client is reducing her blood pressure and weight with nonpharmacologic strategies.

 4 This implies that the client is not doing enough; the focus should be on the positive, and the gains should be reinforced.

223. **3** Just as after any surgery, pain is a major postoperative problem during the first 24 hours after cesarean delivery. (c) (OB; AN; PA; HP)

 1 Gaseous distention is more likely to occur on day three.

 2 Oral intake is usually limited for the first 24 to 48 hours postoperatively.

 4 Bowels ordinarily do not move for 48 to 72 hours postoperatively.

224. **4** Palpation will indicate if bladder distention is present; the increased intraabdominal space after delivery can result in bladder distention without discomfort. (b) (OB; EV; TC; HP)

 1 Trauma to the area makes surrounding organs atonic; the client may have a full bladder and not feel the urge to void.

 2 A physician's order is needed for catheterization.

 3 Measurement alone is not sufficient for 24 to 48 hours postpartum.

225. **3** Positioning with the head slightly hyperextended and changing the position q 1 to 2 hours helps to drain secretions and can increase O_2 availabe for use by promoting respiratory efforts in a premature infant with immature lung tissue. (b) (OB; AN; TC; HN)

 1 Congenital birth defects are observed for in all

infants, not just those with RDS.

2 This is too low; preterm infants do not shiver.

4 Extensive handling is not desired, but infants do need to be touched.

226. **3** Mothers with Type O blood have anti-A and anti-B antibodies that are transferred across the placenta; this is the most common incompatability because the mother is Type O in 20% of all pregnancies. (b) (OB; IM; PA; HN)

1 This is usually not a problem.

2 Same as # 1.

4 Same as # 1.

227. **4** Multiple pregnancies tend to make the endometrial lining more vulnerable to abnormal implantation. (a) (OB; AN; PA; HP)

1 Primigravidas are the least prone; the endometrium is receptive to normal implantation.

2 Two pregnancies have not compromised the endometrium too much; abnormal implantation is less likely to occur.

3 Age is not known to be a significant factor; also, two pregnancies have not compromised the endometrium too much.

228. **3** The side-lying position decreases pressure on the vena cava from the gravid uterus, assuring more adequate oxygenation of the fetus. (a) (OB; IM; TC; IP)

1 This is not likely to have a significant effect if the client is in active labor.

2 Lying on the back will increase pressure on the vena cava, further compromising the fetus.

4 Without proper positioning, breathing techniques will be less effective.

229. **1** This will indicate whether bleeding may be progressing toward maternal and fetal distress. (b) (OB; AS; TC; IP)

2 This is contraindicated; these examinations may stimulate greater bleeding if the placenta is accidentally dislodged.

3 A fetal monitor would be indicated, because it more accurately records fetal well-being.

4 This is done in the postpartum period, not while the client is in labor.

230. **4** Conservative therapeutic approaches have decreased risks to both mother and infant. (b) (OB; IM; PE; EC)

1 This is not true; conservative approaches are more effective.

2 This is not true; the infant is compromised more than the mother is.

3 Although the prognosis has improved, there is still danger for both mother and infant.

231. **3** When the 5-minute Apgar score is 7 or less, there is a 66% chance that the infant will be neurologically impaired. (c) (OB; AN; PA; HN)

1 The Apgar score does not evaluate hypoglycemia.

2 This may or may not be true; assessment of other factors is necessary.

4 An Apgar score between 0 and 3 necessitates immediate resuscitative measures.

232. **3** This response is nonjudgmental; it permits the client to recognize her own feelings. (b) (OB; IM; PE; EC)

1 This is judgmental; it gives the nurse's opinion on a moral question for the client.

2 This is judgmental; it leaves no room for the client's feelings.

4 This response shifts the burden of decision to the client without offering assistance.

233. **4** A full bladder is required for effective visualization of the uterine contents; the bladder should be empty before an amniocentesis to prevent accidental puncture of the bladder during the procedure. (b) (OB; PL; TC; HP)

1 A full bladder is required for effective sonography.

2 The client voids only after all abdominal tracings are obtained.

3 The bladder may fill within 1 hour; a full bladder is undesirable before an amniocentesis.

234. **1** An invasive procedure such as amniocentesis requires consent. (a) (OB; IM; ED; HP)

2 No vaginal examination is done before amniocentesis.

3 Intravenous therapy is unnecessary.

4 The infection rate is 1%; this is not an appropriate nursing intervention.

235. **2** This provides the opportunity for an evaluation of the client's food intake. (b) (OB; AS; TC; PN)

1 This may prevent further exploration of the diet because the client may answer yes or no.

3 This assumes the client is not eating properly.

4 Same as # 1.

236. **3** Ascorbic acid enhances the absorption of iron. (b) (OB; IM; ED; PN)

1 Iron should be taken in the morning before meals to allow for maximum absorption.

2 Same as # 1.

4 Although milk will decrease stomach irritation, it will not enhance iron absorption.

237. **2** All signs indicate imminent delivery; the perineum should be inspected for appearance of caput. (b) (OB; AS; PA; IP)

1 This is essential but not the initial action.

3 Same as # 1.

4 This is important to know, but inspection is the most important action.

238. **2** An Apgar score of 3 indicates a severely depressed infant with apnea, lowered heart rate, and absent reflexes. (b) (OB; AS; PA; HN)

1 The priority is intubation to obtain a patent airway; the infant is usually apneic and not able to breathe independently.

3 Although this is important, establishing a patent airway and initiating respirations are of greater importance.

4 This would be ineffective; this infant requires resuscitative measures.

239. **2** This metabolic process releases energy and increases heat production in the newborn. (c) (OB; AN; PA; NN)

1 Shivering is the mechanism of heat production for the adult, not for the newborn.

3 This will not be successful unless plentiful brown fat is present.

4 Fatty acids are by-products of the breakdown of brown fat.

240. **1** If suckling or nipple stimulation is discontinued, acini cells degenerate, regressive changes occur, and lactation ends. (b) (OB; IM; ED; PP)

2 Milk secretion starts on the third or fourth day after delivery.

3 High levels of estrogen inhibit anterior pituitary gland secretion of lactogenic hormones.

4 Other than suckling, the stimulant for oxytocin secretion is unknown.

241. **4** Oxytocin (Pitocin) is shown to have an antidi-

uretic effect, acting to reabsorb water from glomerular filtrate. (c) (OB; EV; PA; DR)

1 This may occur in severe PIH, not with prolonged use of Pitocin.

2 Hyperventilation occurs with infection or dehydration, not with prolonged use of Pitocin.

3 This is caused by inappropriate breathing patterns, not by prolonged use of Pitocin.

242. **2** Chances of postpartal hemorrhage are 5 times greater with large infants because uterine contractions may be impaired after delivery. (b) (OB; AN; PA; PP)

1 On the contrary, early breastfeeding will stimulate uterine contractions and lessen the chance of hemorrhage.

3 This does not contribute to postpartum hemorrhage because anesthesia for a pudendal block does not affect uterine contractions.

4 This is a short third stage; a prolonged third stage of labor, 30 minutes or more, may lead to postpartum hemorrhage.

243. **4** BP and pulse may not change significantly until large amounts of blood have been lost; the trickling of blood indicates continuous bleeding. (b) (OB; AS; TC; HP)

1 The pulse becomes very rapid, but not until a significant amount of blood is lost.

2 Blood pressure is normotensive; it usually does not change significantly until a large amount of blood is lost.

3 This is not a sign of impending hemorrhage.

244. **2** From these assessments the nurse can determine unusual weight gain and an increase in blood pressure; both of these are early symptoms of pregnancy-induced hypertension. (c) (OB; IM; TC; HP)

1 The weight gain may not be caused by inappropriate dietary intake but rather by fluid retention.

3 This would be therapeutic for a backache; this answer ignores the possible edema and increased weight gain.

4 The data indicates fluid retention.

245. **3** Sodium is not restricted because restriction decreases blood volume, which in turn reduces placental perfusion. (c) (OB; EV; ED; HP)

1 Losing weight is contraindicated during pregnancy and does not reduce the incidence of pregnancy-induced hypertension.

2 Women at risk for this condition are advised to eat a high-protein diet.

4 Diuretic therapy is dangerous because it decreases blood volume, which in turn reduces placental perfusion.

246. **3** Fluid retention is an undesirable effect of sodium intake. (b) (OB; PL; ED; HP)

1 There is no concern about fluid retention when taking antacids that do not contain sodium.

2 Same as # 1.

4 Same as # 1.

247. **2** Even minimal sensory stimuli can trigger exaggerated cerebral responses such as convulsions; therefore a nonstimulating environment is therapeutic. (b) (OB; AN; TC; HP)

1 A neutral environment has no relation to the length of time antihypertensive drugs must be given.

3 This is an undesired action; intracellular volume should be increased during pregnancy.

4 Neutral environments do not reduce headaches resulting from hypertension.

248. **4** Hypermagnesemia causes extreme muscle depression; calcium gluconate, the $MgSO_4$ antidote, promotes muscle function. (b) (OB; AN; TC; DR)

1 This is used in chelation therapy for lead poisoning.

2 This is used for hyperkalemia.

3 This is an antihypertensive.

249. **1** A copy of the Patient's Bill of Rights is not necessary to give informed consent for treatment. (b) (OB; IM; ED; HP)

2 This information is required to give informed consent.

3 All questions should be answered honestly and in terms that the client can understand.

4 Alternative treatment regimens should be discussed so that the client is able to make an informed choice about which course of treatment to pursue.

250. **2** This is done to determine if any injury has occurred to the fetus or placenta during the procedure. (a) (OB; EV; TC; HP)

1 There is no entry into the vaginal tract with this procedure; bleeding or discharge is not expected.

3 This is a good position to enhance placental perfusion, but it serves no purpose in detecting complications.

4 This is unnecessary; the puncture site seals by itself immediately after removal of the needle.

251. **3** In a normal, regular cycle, ovulation occurs 2 weeks (14 days) before the onset of the next menses. (a) (OB; IM; ED; FS)

1 This would occur in a woman who menstruates every 28 days.

2 This is too early in the cycle; ovulation generally occurs 14 days before the onset of the next menses.

4 This is just the first week of the cycle; ovulation usually occurs 14 days before the onset of the next menses.

252. **1** Heparin can be used before the last trimester of pregnancy because it does not cross the placental barrier and will not cause hemorrhage in the fetus. (c) (OB; IM; TC; DR)

2 This drug can cross the placental barrier and cause hemorrhage in the fetus.

3 Same as #2.

4 Same as #2.

253. **2** Heparin should not be given because 98 seconds is almost three times the normal time it takes a fibrin clot to form (25-36 seconds) and prolonged bleeding may result; the therapeutic range with heparin is 1½ to 2 times normal range. (c) (OB; EV; TC; DR)

1 Heparin must not be increased; the client already has received too much.

3 The medication does not need to be changed; it needs to be stopped.

4 The APTT is not normal but prolonged; it is almost three times the normal rate.

254. **4** As the process of effacement occurs in the latter part of pregnancy, placental separation from the uterus may occur, causing bleeding. (b) (OB; AN; PA; HP)

1 This occurs in separation of a normally implanted placenta (abruptio placentae).

2 This is not usually the first thing to occur; it may

occur after the placenta separates.

3 This is generally not associated with placenta previa at its onset; it may occur later.

255. **3** This response encourages clients to verbalize their feelings. (a) (OB; IM; PE; FS)

1 This is a very insensitive and incorrect statement; there may be nothing wrong with either client.

2 The clients are not interested in the nurse's wishes; the focus should be on them.

4 The clients are not seeking advice about dealing with their parents.

256. **1** This is true; some women find it emotionally unnerving to handle their genitals and discharges. (b) (OB; AN; PE; EC)

2 The data does not support this conclusion.

3 Same as # 2.

4 Same as # 2.

257. **4** This is referred pain from the passage of carbon dioxide through the tubes; this is usually indicative of tubal patency. (b) (OB; IM; ED; FS)

1 The client can resume normal activities as soon as the test is over.

2 The client does not usually experience nausea and/or vomiting.

3 No anesthesic is given; the client's awareness of pain is necessary to evaluate whether carbon dioxide is able to pass through the tubes.

258. **2** This is necessary to keep the sperm viable; if the specimen becomes warm, the sperm will die. (a) (OB; IM; ED; FS)

1 Rubber solvents and preservatives may affect the semen specimen.

3 This may lessen the amount of ejaculate needed for the specimen.

4 The specimen can be collected at any time.

259. **1** Doing this will help the client relax and will lessen discomfort. (b) (OB; IM; PE; EC)

2 This may distract the client but will not produce relaxation.

3 The client may become more anxious if the procedure is hurried.

4 This may make the client more anxious; holding the breath causes tightening of the perineum.

260. **3** There are various foods that can be substituted for meat or animal-related products in planning nutritious meals for the pregnant women who is a vegetarian. (a) (OB; PL; TC; PN)

1 This would be difficult for a client who is a vegetarian.

2 Same as # 1.

4 The client may know good nutrition; this client needs help to adapt the vegetarian diet to meet pregnancy needs.

261. **4** Calcium supplements are available for people who do not consume milk or milk products. (a) (OB; PL; TC; PN)

1 Good dental care and proper mouth hygiene will be more beneficial for maintaining good teeth.

2 Calcium is essential to the pregnant woman's diet for the development of the fetal skeleton; it must be supplemented if the client dislikes milk and milk products.

3 If milk makes the client ill, this would be poor advice and compliance would be suspect.

262. **1** Breast tissue is not palpable in an infant of less than 33 weeks' gestation. (a) (OB; AS; PA; HN)

2 Creases in the palms and on the soles of the feet

are not clearly defined until after the thirty-seventh week of gestation.

3 Ear pinnae spring back in an infant of 36 weeks' gestation.

4 A zero-degree square-window sign is present in an infant of 40 to 42 weeks' gestation.

263. **1** Flaring nares are a compensatory mechanism that attempts to lessen resistance of narrow nasal passages and increase oxygen intake. (a) (OB; AS; PA; HN)

2 Acrocyanosis is not related to respiratory distress but is caused by vasomotor instability; this is a normal occurrence in the newborn.

3 This is a normal finding in the newborn.

4 Same as # 3.

264. **2** Sucking and swallowing reflexes and muscles are immature; this makes oral feeding ineffectual and exhausting. (c) (OB; AN; PA; HN)

1 The metabolic rate is increased because of fatigue and growth needs.

3 Absorption of nutrients is decreased because of immaturity of the intestines.

4 Caloric requirements are increased because of extra growth needs.

265. **4** Weight loss results from the extra sucking effort required to obtain milk flow from the breast. (b) (OB; IM; PE; EC)

1 Time consumption and effort are insufficient reasons to discourage breastfeeding.

2 If the infant is being fed by gavage, the mother's breasts can be pumped and the breast milk can be used for gavage feedings.

3 Breast milk provides good nutrition, protects the infant from necrotizing enterocolitis, and provides antibodies.

266. **1** If the client demonstrates anorexia, crying, and insomnia, the nurse should recognize these as symptoms of depression, not anxiety. (b) (OB; AS; PE; EC)

2 Ambivalence and lethergy can be associated with depression, but they are usually accompanied by anorexia, not increased appetite.

3 Insomnia and ambivalence may be seen with depression, but they are accompanied by anorexia, not increased appetite.

4 Lethargy and anorexia are manifestations of depression, but they are usually accompanied by insomnia rather than prolonged sleep.

267. **2** The head circumference is usually 1 inch larger than the chest; a head circumference 1½ inches smaller than the chest could indicate microcephaly. (c) (OB; AS; PA; HN)

1 According to growth charts, the range of head circumference for boys is just slightly (½ inch) larger than the chest.

3 In anencephaly, the disparity between the head and chest circumference would be much larger than 1½ inches.

4 No molding takes place in cesarean delivery; therefore the head should be about 1 inch larger than the chest at birth.

268. **2** Phototherapy changes unconjugated bilirubin in skin to conjugated bilirubin bound to protein, permitting excretion. (a) (OB; EV; TC; HN)

1 Phototherapy does not affect liver function; the liver does not dispose of bilirubin.

3 Vitamin K has no effect on bilirubin excretion; it is necessary for prothrombin formation.

4 The bilirubin is not excreted via the skin but in the urine and feces.

269. **1** Circumcision is a surgical procedure, and infection can occur; the area should not be exposed to organisms in tub water. (a) (OB; EV; ED; NN)
   2 The diaper should be changed frequently to prevent irritation from the urine.
   3 The petrolatum gauze or A & D ointment prevents the diaper from adhering to the operative site.
   4 There should be only minimal bleeding; excessive bleeding requires immediate attention.

270. **2** If the heart is heard in the upper left quadrant, the baby must be lying in a breech position with the head upright and the heart uppermost. (b) (OB; AS; PA; IP)
   1 Fetal heart tones are heard best in the lower quadrants of the abdomen in cephalic presentations.
   3 Same as # 1.
   4 Same as # 1.

271. **3** The feet or buttocks are not effective in blocking the cervical opening, and the cord may slip through and be compressed. (b) (OB; AS; TC; HP)
   1 Uterine inertia may result from fatigue or cephalopelvic disproportion and is not directly related to fetal position.
   2 Rapid dilation and precipitate labor can occur with infants in cephalic positions as well.
   4 This is a normal occurrence.

272. **4** This is a description of the contractions during the active portion of the first stage of labor. (b) (OB; AS; PA; IP)
   1 This adaptation occurs in the transitional phase

of the first stage of labor.
   2 Same as # 1.
   3 Same as # 1.

273. **2** Transition is the most difficult part of labor, and the client works very hard; beads of perspiration are prominent on the upper lip. (a) (OB; AS; PA; IP)
   1 The bloody show increases during the transitional phase; this occurs from the increased pressure by the presenting part.
   3 This would be seen at the end, not the beginning, of the transitional phase.
   4 This signifies that the client has ruptured the membranes.

274. **4** As the placenta separates and drops down, the cord lengthens in appearance. (b) (OB; AS; PA; IP)
   1 The client may feel a contraction, but it is not nearly as uncomfortable as the painful contractions at the end of the first stage of labor.
   2 Continual seepage occurs when there is hemorrhaging; a large sudden gush of blood heralds placental separation.
   3 The fundus contracts and becomes rounded and firmer.

275. **1** Cold causes vasoconstriction and reduces edema by lessening the accumulation of blood and lymph at the episiotomy site; cold also deadens nerve endings and lessens the pain. (b) (OB; IM; TC; PP)
   2 This may diminish the pain but will not lessen the edema.
   3 This is not used after an episiotomy.
   4 This position will not lessen pain or reduce edema.

Answers and Rationales for Comprehensive Examinations

Comprehensive Examination One
Test 1

1. **2** Studies indicate that a large percentage of children with cerebral palsy had birth weight below 1500 g. (b) (PE; AS; PA; NM)
   1 There is no greater incidence of cerebral palsy in children born by cesarean delivery that is not done for fetal distress.
   3 Studies do not indicate any greater incidence of cerebral palsy in children born to women older than 35 years of age.
   4 The Moro reflex is normally present at birth.

2. **3** Straddling the hip would prevent scissoring by keeping the child's legs abducted. (b) (PE; IM; PA; NM)
   1 Tight wrapping would maintain the child's legs in a scissored position.
   2 An infant seat would not prevent scissoring.
   4 The football hold is used when carrying the child in a supine position with the legs adducted, which promotes scissoring.

3. **4** Cortical control of voluntary muscles occurs between 2 and 4 months. (c) (PE; IM; ED; NM)
   1 Cerebral palsy is not diagnosed by the presence of joint deformities; these may develop later because of spastic muscle imbalance.
   2 Parents have a right to be informed of their child's diagnosis as soon as possible.
   3 The neurologic lesions are fixed and will neither progress nor regress.

4. **1** The therapy program in use in the home should be incorporated into the nursing care plan to maintain continuity. (a) (PE; PL; TC; NM)
   2 The child should have a regular diet appropriate for his developmental age.
   3 The child has social needs, and interaction should be promoted; there is no need for a private room.
   4 The parents should be encouraged to stay with the child and actively participate in his care.

5. **1** Bile salts are used to aid digestion of fats and absorption of the fat-soluble vitamins A, D, and K. (b) (ME; IM; ED; DR)
   2 Bile salts play no role in prothrombin production.
   3 Bile salts are not necessary to stimulate the secretion of bilirubin.
   4 Bile salts do not initiate the contraction of the common bile ducts.

6. **3** Aldosterone, a corticosteroid, causes sodium and water retention and potassium excretion by the kidneys. (b) (ME; AS; PA; FE)
   1 Hypovolemia would not occur with increased aldosterone levels because sodium and water are retained.
   2 Potassium is excreted in the presence of aldoster-

one and therefore would not accumulate and cause arrythmias.
   4 Calcium is unaffected by aldosterone.

7. **4** Aldactone is a potassium-sparing diuretic often used in conjunction with thiazide diuretics. (a) (ME; AN; PA; DR)
   1 Both diuretics do this, so it is not a particular advantage of Aldactone.
   2 Same as # 1.
   3 Same as # 1.

8. **4** Malnutrition and liver damage lead to reduced serum albumin level, failure of capillary fluid shift mechanism, and resulting ascites. (b) (ME; AN; PA; FE)
   1 Sodium level is usually excessive with cirrhosis.
   2 Vitamins are unrelated to ascites.
   3 Iron promotes hemoglobin synthesis; this is unrelated to cirrhosis.

9. **3** This increases oncotic pressure, which pulls interstitial fluid into the blood vessels, restoring blood volume. (c) (ME; AN; PA; FE)
   1 Salt-poor albumin is not given to increase protein stores.
   2 This is provided by total parenteral nutrition, not salt-poor albumin.
   4 This has no effect on diverting blood flow away from the liver.

10. **3** The damaged liver causes rising ammonia levels resulting in CNS irritation, producing behavioral changes. (c) (ME; PL; ED; GI)
    1 The liver cannot metabolize protein, and a low-protein diet is indicated.
    2 Chlorpromazine is detoxified by the liver and is therefore contraindicated in severe hepatic disease.
    4 Kidney function is usually not affected.

11. **2** Reducing the blood pressure is done to prevent seizures. (a) (OB; PL; TC; HP)
    1 Bleeding is not generally a problem with pregnancy-induced hypertension unless abruptio placentae occurs.
    3 Anxiety may be present, but the elevated pressure is the priority problem.
    4 Unless the client is in a very salt-poor state that contributes to hypovolemia, the compensatory state of vasospasm will not occur.

12. **2** Vasospasms of placental vessels occur because of elevated blood pressure; the placenta may separate prematurely (abruptio placentae). (b) (OB; PL; TC; HP)
    1 Placenta previa occurs because of abnormal implantation and is not related to vasospasm.
    3 This is scant amniotic fluid and is usually not associated with hypertensive disorders of pregnancy.
    4 Isoimmunization in pregnancy is associated with Rh disease, not hypertension.

13. **3** Rising blood pressure with a widening pulse pressure indicates cerebral edema, which can cause convulsions. (a) (OB; EV; TC; HP)
    1 This generally does not occur unless the sedated client is not carefully observed; premature delivery is not indicated by blood pressure changes.
    2 Bleeding is not associated with pregnancy-induced hypertension unless abruptio placentae occurs.
    4 Cessation of fetal heartbeat would indicate fetal death rather than a change of maternal blood pressure.

14. **2** Monitoring of weight and intake and output is an indicator of an edematous state; the high-protein diet is essential for fetal growth. (b) (OB; PL; PA; HP)
    1 Diuretics and low-salt diets will gradually decrease circulating fluid, creating hypovolemia, which decreases placental circulation.
    3 Diuretics are contraindicated in pregnancy because they decrease circulating fluids and may impair fluid supply to the placenta.
    4 Fractional urines serve no purpose with clients who have pregnancy-induced hypertension.

15. **2** An output of 25 ml/hr would not permit proper excretion of the magnesium sulfate; excess magnesium levels can cause respiratory and cardiac depression. (b) (OB; EV; TC; DR)
    1 Respirations at this rate are normal; a rate of at least 16 breaths per minute should be present before each dose of magnesium sulfate.
    3 Loss of patellar reflex is indicative of magnesium sulfate toxicity; the next dose should not be given.
    4 This is the expected response to magnesium sulfate.

16. **1** Calcium gluconate is the antidote for magnesium sulfate toxicity. (a) (OB; PL; TC; DR)
    2 Adrenalin is a vasoconstrictor and is not used as an antidote for magnesium sulfate toxicity.
    3 Neo-Cortef is a steroid and is not used to counteract magnesium sulfate toxicity.
    4 Calcium gluconate, not calcium chloride, is the antidote.

17. **3** This helps the client to feel important enough for the nurse to remember their meeting and be on time. (b) (PS; IM; PE; TR)
    1 This would not only be unsafe but may make the client feel that the nurse does not care enough to stay.
    2 Feelings should never be ignored but should be accepted as important to the client.
    4 The client is mistrustful of others and will probably not believe the nurse; caring is best demonstrated through behavior.

18. **3** This gives direction to the relationship and provides a blueprint for future evaluation of progress. (b) (PS; AN; TC; TR)
    1 This is an aspect of the therapeutic relationship but is not the most important; what the client wants to achieve takes priority.
    2 Same as # 1.
    4 Same as # 1.

19. **2** The nurse is making an observation; bringing it to the attention of the client is an initial step in understanding that behavior. (a) (PS; IM; PE; TR)
    1 This is premature because the client may not even be aware of the anxiety.

3 This is premature and does not allow for self-recognition of feelings.
    4 This is requesting an explanation from the client that the client probably is incapable of making.

20. **1** A first step in any therapeutic relationship should include setting parameters such as time and frequency. (c) (PS; PL; PE; TR)
    2 There is no need to carry this out during the termination phase because it is part of the initial ground rules.
    3 This is part of the working phase of a therapeutic relationship and therefore not an initial intervention.
    4 The nurse should not deviate from the original contract.

21. **3** Closeness increases anxiety, which cannot be tolerated; hostility is used to keep people away. (b) (PS; EV; PE; TR)
    1 This is true, but the expression of hostility is not really a flare-up in this situation.
    2 Regressive behavior is the resumption of behavior that is characteristic of an earlier stage of development; hostility does not fit this definition.
    4 Hostility is more extreme than assertiveness and is not an indication of improvement.

22. **3** An additional meeting is important to deal with the problem of termination with the client. (b) (PS; IM; PE; TR)
    1 The client is avoiding the nurse, and the nurse must reach out to help the client with the termination process.
    2 This would not be a therapeutic termination because the issues would not be resolved for the client.
    4 The nurse may want to do this; however, the focus should be on the needs of the client.

23. **1** Axillary lymph nodes are an early site of metastasis and thus are removed. (a) (SU; EV; ED; RG)
    2 Pectoral muscles are not removed in a modified radical mastectomy.
    3 This is not removed in this type surgery; leaving the skin intact improves healing.
    4 The entire breast is removed in this type surgery.

24. **4** Drainage will flow with the force of gravity; therefore the dependent point should be checked for bleeding. (b) (SU; EV; TC; RG)
    1 Turning the client on the affected side is usually painful and should be avoided; the client should turn to the unaffected side.
    2 The drainage is assessed for amount and characteristics; it is not emptied hourly, only once per shift or when necessary.
    3 Pressure dressings are rarely used today when a portable suction device is employed; if the drainage on the dressing is excessive, the physician should be notified.

25. **4** As drainage collects and occupies space, the original level of negative pressure decreases; the less negative pressure, the less effective the drainage. (a) (SU; AN; TC; RG)
    1 It is easy and safe to empty regardless of the amount of drainage in the unit.
    2 A one-way valve between the tubing and the collection chamber prevents drainage from entering the tubing and causing trauma to the wound.
    3 Drainage can be accurately measured by the cal-

ibrations on the unit or in a graduated container after emptying.

26. **2** Compressing the device expels air in the unit, and closing the plug while it is compressed reestablishes the closed system. (a) (SU; IM; TC; RG)
1 A portable suction device is never attached to a mechanical suction machine.
3 This facilitates drainage by gravity, not negative pressure.
4 Milking the tubing promotes patency but will not create negative pressure.

27. **2** These movements require muscle contraction, putting pressure on blood vessels, increasing tissue oxygen, and thus promoting circulation. (c) (SU; AN; PA; RG)
1 Lymphedema is assessed by measuring the circumference of the extremity, not by doing exercises.
3 Contractures are a rare complication following a mastectomy.
4 Muscle atrophy is not a common complication following a mastectomy.

28. **4** These would be signs of infection and should be reported to the physician. (a) (SU; EV; ED; IT)
1 There is little subcutaneous fat in the thoracic area, and the skin may be taut at the operative site, appearing irregular.
2 This is a sign of healing that is expected and normal.
3 This results from severance of nerves and formation of scar tissue, which are expected and normal.

29. **2** This is important in determining whether the baby has maternally transmitted antibodies against measles. (b) (PE; AS; PA; BI)
1 This baby has no vaccination against measles because this is not done until the baby is older than 1 year of age.
3 This has no relationship to present exposure.
4 Same as # 3.

30. **4** This is the optimum age for measles vaccination because antibodies are no longer present to block formation of new infant antibodies. (a) (PE; IM; PA; BI)
1 This is too early; the baby would still have antibodies from the present vaccination.
2 Same as # 1.
3 Same as # 1.

31. **2** Using Nägele's rule to calculate, the estimated date of delivery (EDD) is the date of LMP plus 7 days minus 3 months; spotting is fairly common at time of expected menstrual period. (a) (OB; AN; PA; PN)
1 This is an incorrect calculation; this is too early.
3 This is an incorrect calculation; this is too late.
4 Same as # 3.

32. **3** Right occiput anterior is a vertex presentation; the fundus has a soft rounded mass, which is the buttock; therefore this is cephalic presentation; the irregular curvature on the right indicates the fetal spine, and the bumpy projections on the left indicate the extremities. (b) (OB; AS; PA; IP)
1 This is a transverse lie with right scapula (shoulder) presenting anteriorly.
2 Left sacrum posterior is a breech presentation; the fetal part in the fundus would be firm.
4 The fetal spine would be on the left side in the left occiput posterior position.

33. **2** Examining for a prolapsed cord is the first prior-

ity after the membranes rupture. (b) (OB; AS; TC; IP)
1 The fetal heart rate should be assessed after it has been determined that the cord has not prolapsed.
3 The client probably does not have to void; the priority action is checking for prolapsed cord.
4 This can be done after checking for a prolapsed cord and assessing the fetal heart rate.

34. **3** Counterpressure against the sacrum during contractions affords some relief from the discomfort of back pain. (a) (OB; IM; PA; IP)
1 It is difficult to predict the length of labor for any client.
2 This does not respond to the situation; the husband should be included in providing comfort to the client.
4 Same as # 2.

35. **2** Various waveforms can indicate damage to different areas of the heart. (a) (ME; IM; ED; CV)
1 Auscultation can detect various heart sounds.
3 Cardioversion, not an ECG, is used to change heart rhythm.
4 An ECG taken during a stress test determines the endurance of the heart.

36. **3** Xylocaine usually reduces the irritability of the heart. (c) (ME; IM; TC; DR)
1 At present, manually stimulating the heart is not needed.
2 Stimulating the cough reflex will not affect an irritable heart muscle.
4 Treating the PVCs is the first priority.

37. **4** Vertigo may be a symptom of hypotension. (b) (ME; EV; TC; DR)
1 Dizziness is not a normal sensation after morphine.
2 Hypotension is a side effect, not an allergic response to morphine.
3 Raising the client's head may aggravate symptoms.

38. **3** The physician must be consulted because the decision depends on the amount of damage and extent of healing. (c) (ME; IM; PE; EC)
1 This is a medical decision that depends on amount of damage, not how client feels.
2 It would be false reassurance to determine an exact time and date.
4 Same as # 1.

39. **3** This statement leaves communication lines open. (c) (PS; IM; PE; SD)
1 This response discounts the client's thoughts and may increase agitation.
2 This provides false reassurance; it does not provide security because the client may believe the nurse is one of those trying to kill her.
4 This supports client's delusional system.

40. **1** Rephrasing allows for further communication, expresses understanding, and does not belittle the client's feelings. (c) (PS; IM; PE; SD)
2 "Why" questions make a client defensive, and the wording implies the client's delusion could be true.
3 Presenting reality to the client at this time only raises anxiety and leads the client to defend the delusion.
4 This is false reassurance; in any event, a suspicious client would not believe the nurse.

41. **2** The brief, frequent contacts are less threatening and help to build trust. (b) (PS; PL; TC; SD)

1 This supports the client's delusional system, thus increasing suspiciousness.

3 The client needs to be observed to prevent self-harm as a result of delusional thinking.

4 This would increase suspiciousness; the client needs consistent caregivers to help increase her trust level.

42. **2** Delusions are a way the unconscious defends the individual from real or imagined threats. (b) (PS; AN; PE; SD)

1 This is logical thinking that is formulated from an illogical base; delusions do not have a logical base.

3 Illusions are false interpretations of actual external stimuli.

4 Delusions are precipitated by feelings of anxiety, not by anger.

43. **1** This simply states reality without attempting to argue the client out of her delusion; it is best to avoid physical contact at this time. (c) (PS; IM; PE; SD)

2 This denies the client's feelings and directly attacks the delusional system, forcing the client to defend it.

3 Touching the client's arm can be frightening and overwhelming at this time.

4 This is false reassurance; the client does not feel safe, and the nurse's saying it does not make it so.

44. **2** Periorbital edema is indicative of excess fluid; kidneys are inflamed and the output of urine is lessened. (b) (PE; EV; PA; RG)

1 The symptoms do not indicate excess fluid.

3 Diarrhea and polyuria would lead to fluid deficit.

4 Same as # 1.

45. **2** Glomerulonephritis is associated with a history of a prior streptococcal infection of the throat. (a) (PE; AS; PA; RG)

1 A streptococcus infection, not the measles virus, is associated with glomerulonephritis.

3 Glomerulonephritis is not an inherited disease; it usually follows a streptococcal infection.

4 There are no immunizations that would cause glomerulonephritis.

46. **2** The child's health improves, the appetite increases, and the blood pressure normalizes with the reduction of edema. (b) (PE; PL; TC; RG)

1 Ambulation does not have an adverse effect on the disease; most children voluntarily restrict their activities during the acute phase.

3 Fluids should not be forced, because the kidneys are inflamed and cannot tolerate large amounts.

4 Sodium is lowered, not eliminated; sodium restriction is not tolerated well by children and may further restrict their appetite.

47. **3** 7200 ml ÷ 24 hours = 300 ml/hour. (a) (SU; AN; PA; FE)

1 This is an inadequate hourly rate; the rate should be 300 ml/hr.

2 Same as # 1.

4 This is an excessive hourly rate; the rate should be 300 ml/hr.

48. **1** Deep breathing provides an active role in controlling pain; this is a positive coping skill. (c) (SU; PL; ED; NM)

2 This could increase pain.

3 Distraction techniques are usually ineffectual in the presence of severe pain; contraction may add additional pain.

4 Understanding the importance of care will not reduce severe pain; health teaching should be initiated before, not during, a procedure.

49. **1** High-protein drinks have twice the calories per volume of other fluids and provide protein for wound healing. (b) (SU; PL; PA; IT)

2 Fruit juices are comparably low in calories; potassium need not be restricted at this time; potassium is restricted during the hypovolemic stage (first 48 to 72 hours after burn injury).

3 Low-sodium milk does not contain adequate calories to help meet the high metabolic rate associated with burns.

4 More fats are not indicated; increased calories in the form of protein and carbohydrates are needed.

50. **2** Client participation provides for a sense of control, and a consistent approach provides a routine with no surprises; these approaches may limit pain and promote compliance with the regimen. (b) (SU; PL; TC; IT)

1 Preparation of the equipment and explanation of the procedure should be performed before the procedure; when performed during the procedure it wastes time, which can prolong pain.

3 Changing staff disrupts the client's routine and sense of trust.

4 This is too hot; the water should be approximately 100°F.

51. **3** An autograft is a permanent graft that should not be rejected; the nurse needs to assess the site immediately. (a) (SU; EV; TC; IT)

1 An autograft is a permanent graft that should not need to be replaced.

2 This could raise the anxiety of the client and draws a conclusion before assessment of the site; infection is usually associated with purulent drainage.

4 The nurse needs to assess the site; the responsibility of assessment should not be left up to the client.

52. **3** Insulin needs may decrease in early pregnancy because of increased fetal needs and the possibility of nausea and vomiting; insulin needs increase in the second and third trimesters as a resistance to insulin develops; the blood sugar is monitored to prevent ketoacidosis and ensuing harm to the fetus. (a) (OB; IM; ED; HP)

1 This is untrue; even the nondiabetic woman makes a dietary adjustment to keep pace with the increased demands of pregnancy; in addition, insulin needs increase in the second and third trimesters.

2 Most nutrient requirements, not just protein, increase in pregnancy.

4 This is untrue; pregnancy causes a resistance to insulin, and more insulin is required in the second and third trimesters.

53. **1** This is giving correct information in a nonthreatening manner; fetal-placental status may deteriorate because of falling estriol levels, which occur in a diabetic mother. (c) (OB; IM; ED; HP)

2 Fetal viability—as determined by lung maturity, not size—would influence the time of delivery; the route would be determined by fetal and maternal status, not just size.

3 This client does not show any signs of toxemia; in addition, delivering early does not prevent development of toxemia; however, the client with

severe preeclampsia may be delivered early to prevent eclampsia.

4 Neonates generally develop hypoglycemia shortly after birth; however, early delivery has no effect on this development.

54. 1 Because the newborn's GI tract is sterile, the infant does not have the bacteria that are necessary to synthesize vitamin K; it is vitamin K that functions to stimulate the liver's production of clotting factors. (a) (OB; AN; PA; DR)

2 The vitamin K does not replace the necessary bacteria; the bacteria will develop once oral feedings are established.

3 A prolonged prothrombin time indicates potential clotting problems for the newborn and would not be deliberately produced.

4 Vitamin K has no relation to the absorption of biliary salts.

55. 2 The properly fitted diaphragm, when used correctly with spermicidal gel, is 98% to 99% effective and has low risk for complications. (b) (OB; EV; ED; FS)

1 Oral contraceptives are not recommended for women with diabetes because of their effect on carbohydrate metabolism and the risk of major cardiovascular complications.

3 The intrauterine device carries a high risk of infection, which is already increased in diabetic women.

4 Sterilization is recommended only if there is severe renal disease or proliferative retinopathy associated with diabetes.

56. 2 This position allows the lungs more room to expand, thus affording more comfort; this enables the child to breathe better. (a) (PE; IM; PA; RE)

1 This position would increase difficulty in breathing; it does not allow for chest expansion.

3 Same as # 1.

4 Same as # 1.

57. 2 Epinephrine produces sympathetic nervous system side effects such as tachycardia and hypertension. (b) (PE; EV; TC; DR)

1 Hypertension, not hypotension, is a common side effect.

3 Pallor, not flushing, is a common side effect.

4 This is not a common side effect; this medication is given to decrease respiratory difficulty.

58. 1 This drug is a local irritant to the GI tract. (c) (PE; EV; ED; DR)

2 This is not a side effect; theophylline is given to ease respirations.

3 This is not a side effect; frequent urination is expected because the drug often produces diuresis.

4 This is not a side effect.

59. 1 Moderate exercise, including baseball and skiing, that involves starting and stopping does not overtax the respiratory mechanism; endurance exercises such as basketball, soccer, and wrestling are not well tolerated. (c) (PE; PL; ED; RE)

2 Endurance exercise overtaxes the respiratory mechanism.

3 Same as # 2.

4 Same as # 2.

60. 2 Anxiety, shakiness, and insomnia occur early; within 24 hours convulsions, delirium, tachycardia, and death can occur. (b) (PS; AN; PA; SA)

1 Withdrawal is rarely life threatening but does cause severe discomfort such as abdominal cramping and diarrhea.

3 Withdrawal does not cause life-threatening symptoms but does result in severe exhaustion and depression.

4 Same as # 1.

61. 3 The addict is unable to adequately deal with reality; drugs help blur reality and reduce frustrations. (c) (PS; PL; PE; SA)

1 Drug users are concerned with reality; drug use is often an attempt to blur the pains of reality.

2 It is possible, although not easy, but it does require a change in attitude and a deconditioning process.

4 Education of the public has been extensive, but the new user of drugs does not believe addiction will develop.

62. 4 This moves the emphasis from facts to feelings; it focuses on the client without setting the direction for communication. (c) (PS; IM; PE; PR)

1 This is a rhetorical question because the client has already brought up the topic.

2 This asks a direct question that the client will probably be unable to answer.

3 This denies the client's feelings and cuts off further communication.

63. 2 There is usually a history of interpersonal difficulties; clients are unable to engage in the give and take a relationship requires. (b) (PS; AN; PE; PR)

1 The parents of these individuals rarely impose any discipline or limits at all.

3 There is no direct relationship between antisocial personality disorders and sexual aberrations.

4 There is no diminished contact with reality; these clients are in contact with reality; they just do not care about it.

64. 1 This client does not need to be on the surgical unit; his problem is emotional; it is unfair to upset the other clients; he should be removed from this unit. (c) (PS; EV; PE; PR)

2 An individual cannot be accused of stealing unless actual proof is obtained.

3 This action supports the client's feelings that any means can be used to justify a desired goal.

4 This would accomplish little because the client would deny he took them.

65. 2 Anxiety about the behavior is absent, as is motivation for change; these persons are unwilling to accept help. (b) (PS; AN; PE; PR)

1 These individuals do not experience feelings of guilt about their behavior.

3 More than life-style needs to change; the client's entire view of life and interpersonal response is involved.

4 It is not a resistance to demonstrating feelings but a total lack of feeling for others.

66. 3 Change is always accompanied by some anxiety and pain; without motivation, change will not occur. (b) (PS; EV; PE; PR)

1 These usually do not work unless the individual is motivated to change.

2 The life-style of these individuals is rarely limited because they tend to be rather gregarious and outgoing; in reality, they attempt to live by their guile.

4 His parents' reactions would be of little influence at this age.

67. 3 Type I diabetes is classified as insulin-dependent diabetes mellitus (IDDM) because the person

needs exogenous insulin to maintain carbohydrate, fat, and protein metabolism. (b) (ME; AN; PA; EN)

1 Gestational diabetes (GDM) occurs only during pregnancy; this client is not pregnant.

2 Impaired glucose tolerance diabetes (IGT) describes glucose levels higher than normal but lower than those diagnostic for diabetes mellitus.

4 Type II diabetes is classified as non-insulin–dependent diabetes mellitus (NIDDM) because the condition can be controlled with diet, exercise, and oral hypoglycemics, not insulin.

68. **3** Obesity is a known predisposing factor to diabetes mellitus; the exact relationship is unknown. (b) (ME; AS; PA; EN)

1 Alcohol intake is not known to predispose to diabetes mellitus, and alcohol lowers the blood sugar.

2 High-cholesterol diets and atherosclerotic heart disease are associated with diabetes mellitus.

4 Diabetes insipidus is a disease caused by too little ADH and has no relation to diabetes mellitus.

69. **4** 160 mg/100 ml is above the normal fasting blood glucose level, which is between 60 and 110 mg/100 ml; this is indicative of diabetes mellitus. (b) (ME; AS; PA; EN)

1 This would indicate hypoglycemia, not hyperglycemia.

2 Same as # 1.

3 This is an expected blood glucose level in the nondiabetic individual.

70. **2** Regular insulin is short acting, and it peaks in 2 to 4 hours, which is just at or before lunch. (a) (ME; PL; TC; DR)

1 This is too soon; regular insulin peaks in 2 to 4 hours.

3 This is too late; regular insulin peaks in 2 to 4 hours.

4 Same as # 3.

71. **4** These are early signs of hypoglycemia or too much insulin; the client should be taught to take additional food. (c) (ME; EV; ED; EN)

1 These are symptoms of hyperglycemia.

2 Same as # 1.

3 Same as # 1.

72. **3** Insulin in tablet form would be inactivated by gastric juices; insulin given by injection bypasses the destructive gastric juices. (b) (ME; IM; ED; EN)

1 Oral agents do not contain insulin because it would be inactivated in the stomach; they contain substances, such as sulfonylurea, that stimulate beta cells to produce insulin.

2 This does not answer the client's question; inadequate understanding of the treatment regimen will result in client noncompliance.

4 This is incorrect information for a client who is currently insulin-dependent; this provides false reassurance.

73. **2** This is an accurate statement; each gram of carbohydrate contains 4 calories per gram. (a) (ME; PL; ED; EN)

1 This is too few calories; carbohydrates contain 4 calories per gram.

3 This provides too many calories; fats contain 9 calories per gram.

4 This provides too many calories; no nutrient contains this many calories per gram.

74. **3** Ketoacidosis occurs when insulin is lacking and carbohydrates cannot be used for energy; this increases the breakdown of protein and fat, causing Kussmaul respirations, decreased alertness, decreased circulatory volume, metabolic acidosis, and acetone breath. (a) (ME; EV; PA; EN)

1 Hyperosmolar non-ketotic coma usually occurs in non-insulin dependent diabetes because available insulin prevents breakdown of fat.

2 The Somogyi effect is a rebound hyperglycemia induced by severe hypoglycemia; there is not enough data to determine if this occurred.

4 Hypoglycemia is manifested by cool moist skin, not hot dry skin or Kussmaul respirations.

75. **4** A lung is a highly vascular area that accommodates a large portion of intravascular volume; once a portion is removed, the remaining lung tissue is at risk for pulmonary congestion. (c) (SU; AN; PA; RE)

1 When an intravenous solution is administed correctly, this should not occur.

2 Same as # 1.

3 Same as # 1.

76. **2** The first chamber collects drainage; the second chamber provides for the underwater seal; the third chamber controls the amount of suction by the depth of the tube under the water. (c) (SU; AN; TC; RE)

1 The first chamber, not the third chamber, collects drainage.

3 The second chamber, not the third chamber, provides an underwater seal.

4 Although this occurs in a three-chamber system, the main purpose of the third chamber is to control suction.

77. **4** All amino acids are needed for the synthesis of various proteins, but the term *essential* refers to those amino acids the body cannot make, which are thus essential in the diet. (b) (SU; IM; ED; GI)

1 All amino acids, not just essential amino acids, contain nitrogen.

2 All amino acids, not just essential amino acids, are necessary for rebuilding body tissue.

3 All amino acids in a protein contribute the same number of calories for energy.

78. **3** This is a normal cardiopulmonary symptom in pregnancy; it is caused by an increased ventricular rate and an elevated diaphragm. (b) (OB; AS; PA; HP)

1 This is pathologic, a sign of impending cardiac decompensation.

2 Same as # 1.

4 Same as # 1.

79. **3** Forceps reduce the mother's need to push, thereby conserving energy; regional anesthesia does not compromise cardiovascular function. (b) (OB; PL; TC; HP)

1 Induced labor is often more stressful and painful than natural labor.

2 Major abdominal surgery is performed on clients with cardiac problems only when absolutely necessary.

4 Same as # 1.

80. **2** In this position the gravid uterus impedes venous return; this causes reduced cardiac output and results in reduced placental circulation.

(a) (OB; AN; TC; IP)

1 This may be partially true, but more significantly, it is the least comfortable position and may cause hypotension and reduced placental perfusion.

3 Even if true, this is not significant as a factor of labor.

4 This is false; it can lead to supine hypotension.

81. **1** In the first 48 hours there is a rapid fluid shift, which causes an increase in cardiac output and blood volume; this taxes an already compromised heart. (b) (OB; PL; PA; HP)

2 This is false; the first 48 hours are crucial because of the rapid fluid shift and the stress of increased cardiac output on a compromised heart.

3 Progressive ambulation starting 48 hours after delivery is recommended.

4 This is not recommended because this will further increase circulating blood volume and necessitate an increase in cardiac workload.

82. **3** This provides for collection of more data. (a) (OB; AS; ED; PP)

1 This implies that things are not well, and the mother may be to blame.

2 This could make the mother guilty about not meeting her baby's needs.

4 This is a negative comment that closes communication.

83. **3** Positive and negative experiences connected with previous illness or hospitalization will influence the child's response and adaptation to this and subsequent hospitalization. (c) (PE; AS; PE; GD)

1 This will not be too meaningful because a 5-year-old may not have too great an understanding of the illness.

2 The priority care at this time should be directed to the child's coping abilities.

4 This is not a priority; the child's present acute illness must be attended to first.

84. **2** Vague symptoms frequently prolong the accurate diagnosis of the leukemic process; all of these are early signs related to the leukocyte alteration. (a) (PE; AS; PA; BI)

1 Mouth lesions and an enlarged liver are not common symptoms of early leukemia; the early symptoms are usually vague and nonspecific.

3 Alopecia is not a common sign of early leukemia; the early symptoms are usually vague and nonspecific.

4 Splenomegaly is not a common sign of early leukemia; the symptoms are usually vague and nonspecific.

85. **3** The child needs to know that he will remain awake, and he should be prepared to experience the pressure of the aspiration or the biopsy needle entry, and he should know that he will not be incapacitated following the test. (b) (PE; IM; ED; BI)

1 This is a false statement; false statements must be avoided or the child will not trust what is said in the future.

2 The child will be permitted to ambulate freely.

4 A bone marrow specimen is obtained through a puncture wound; sutures are not necessary.

86. **3** Although this is a somewhat rapid rate of flow for a 5-year-old, the response is accurate based on the given facts. (b) (PE; AN; TC; FE)

1 This rate would deliver less than the prescribed rate in the prescribed time.

2 Same as # 1.

4 This rate would deliver more than the prescribed rate in the prescribed time.

87. **2** Constipation and paralytic ileus are frequent problems because of decreased nerve innervation of the GI tract; they are symptomatic of neurotoxicity. (b) (PE; EV; TC; DR)

1 Vincristine causes leukopenia, which increases susceptibility to infection; it does not cause these reactions.

3 This is not a toxic effect; it is not necessary to check bowel sounds if diarrhea is present.

4 This is not a factor in development of constipation; fluid can be given intravenously if nausea is present.

88. **4** Today, 5-year survival for children with acute lymphocytic leukemia exceeds 60% in most treatment centers. (c) (PE; AN; PA; BI)

1 This projected prognosis is too favorable; 5-year survival occurs in about 60% of children treated.

2 This projected prognosis is too fatalistic; 5-year survival occurs in about 60% of children treated.

3 Same as # 2.

89. **3** This helps to decrease the gag reflex, therefore easing the passage of the tube. (b) (SU; IM; TC; GI)

1 This is false reassurance; the procedure is not painful but is uncomfortable.

2 This does not take advantage of gravity; the side-lying position makes naso-oral cavities less accessible to the individual passing the tube.

4 This will make it more comfortable but will interfere with swallowing, which is necessary during the procedure.

90. **4** An acid pH means the tube is still in the stomach; a pH greater than 7 indicates the tube has reached the small intestine. (c) (SU; IM; TC; GI)

1 This tube must advance to the intestine; securing it would inhibit this movement.

2 The client does not need to remain in bed.

3 A client with a nasogastric or intestinal tube is kept npo.

91. **4** Infection is the most common complication; sterile technique at the catheter insertion site must be maintained. (b) (SU; PL; TC; GI)

1 This is not necessary; the catheter is sutured in place, and reasonable movement is permitted.

2 Excessive weight gain or loss is not a complication of total parenteral nutrition.

3 The client should be taught to leave the infusion pump as set and to call the nurse if the alarm rings.

92. **2** Drainage from the small intestine contains residual digestive enzymes that cause the skin to break down. (a) (SU; PL; PA; GI)

1 An ileostomy will continually drain liquid stool; regular bowel habits are impossible.

3 An ileostomy will continually drain liquid stool; this is unrelated to diet; the stool is excreted before fluid can be reabsorbed in the large intestine.

4 An ileostomy cannot be controlled because stool is too liquid in quality.

93. **4** The stoma secretes mucus immediately following surgery and continues to secrete mucus mixed with serum and blood because of surgical

trauma; fecal drainage begins in about 72 hours. (b) (SU; EV; PA; GI)

1 Drainage will not be clear; it will be serosanguinous because of the trauma of surgery.
2 Drainage that is bloody with clots would indi-

cate hemorrhage; the expected drainage is mucoid and serosanguinous.
3 This would not occur until about 72 hours after surgery.

How to Use Worksheet 1: Errors in Processing Information

Common errors in processing information are listed in the left-hand column of this worksheet. At the top of the worksheet is a row of blank spaces for inserting the number of the question missed. Directly below each number, check any errors you made in answering that question. You may have made more than one type of error in an answer.

Worksheet 1: Errors in processing information

Question number																					
Did not read situation/question carefully																					
Missed important details																					
Confused major and minor points																					
Defined problem incorrectly																					
Could not remember terms/ facts/concepts/principles																					
Defined terms incorrectly																					
Focused on incomplete/incorrect data in assessing situation																					
Interpreted data incorrectly																					
Applied wrong concepts/principles in situation																					
Drew incorrect conclusions																					
Identified wrong goals																					
Identified priorities incorrectly																					
Carried out plan incorrectly/incompletely																					
Was unclear about criteria for evaluating success in achieving goals																					

How to Use Worksheet 2: Knowledge Gaps

Types of common knowledge gaps are listed along the top of this worksheet. Write a brief description of topics you want to review in the spaces provided. For example, if you missed a question on administration of a particular drug, write the drug name and problem (e.g., dosage) in the appropriate space under the column labeled *Pharmacology*.

Worksheet 2: Knowledge gaps

Basic science	Skills/ procedures	Basic human needs	Growth & develop-ment	Normal nutrition	Psycho-social factors	Clinical area/ topic	Stressors/ coping mechanisms	Patho-physiology	Pharma-cology	Therapeutic nutrition	Legal implications	Other

Test 2

94. **1** These clients can better work through their underlying problems when the environment is controlled, demands are reduced, and the routine is simple. (b) (PS; AN; PE; PR)
   2 Preventing these clients from carrying out rituals can precipitate panic reactions.
   3 Because anxiety stems from unconscious conflicts, the environment alone is not enough to effect resolution.
   4 The intent of therapy should be to help the client gain control, not to enable others to do the controlling.

95. **4** This sets an unrealistic limit that would increase anxiety by removing a defense the client needs at this time; rituals cannot be this controlled until other defenses are developed to replace them. (b) (PS; EV; PE; PR)
   1 This is done in therapy as the client's condition improves; insight must be developed slowly to minimize anxiety.
   2 This would increase self-esteem and self-control, not increase anxiety.
   3 This would reduce, not increase, anxiety because the client would feel free to express feelings.

96. **4** It is important to set limits on behavior, but it is also important to involve the client in decision making. (b) (PS; IM; PE; PR)
   1 This would increase anxiety, because the client uses the ritual as a defense against anxiety.
   2 This is a nontherapeutic approach; some limits must be set by the client and the nurse together.
   3 This is a nontherapeutic approach; rarely can a client be distracted from a ritual.

97. **3** These symptoms are a defense against anxiety resulting from decision making, which triggers old fears; the client needs support. (b) (PS; EV; PE; PR)
   1 This is judgmental; the client should be encouraged to work through the symptoms, not to avoid risk.
   2 This is judgmental; an increase in anxiety does not necessarily mean the client does not want to attain the goal.
   4 This denies the client's overwhelming anxiety and lacks realistic support.

98. **1** A resting tremor is typically present when the hand is not involved in a purposeful activity; also known as nonintention tremor; the tremor is caused by decreased neurotransmitter substance. (a) (ME; AS; PA; NM)
   2 An intention tremor is exhibited or intensified when purposeful movements are attempted.
   3 This implies the tremor is under the client's control; the tremor with Parkinson's disease is not voluntary.
   4 Parkinson's may be idiopathic, but the cause of the tremor is known.

99. **3** Levodopa can cross the blood-brain barrier and be converted to dopamine, a substance depleted in Parkinson's. (b) (ME; PL; TC; DR)
   1 Dopamine is not given because it does not cross the blood-brain barrier.
   2 Vitamin B$_6$ can reverse the effects of some anti-Parkinson's disease medications and is contraindicated.
   4 Isocarboxazid is an MAO inhibitor used for treatment of severe depression.

100. **1** Because of the serious side effects of Levodopa, a thorough daily nursing assessment is a priority. (c) (ME; PL; TC; DR)
   2 This is an incomplete assessment; isolating this as a priority would be indicated if there was a fluid imbalance.
   3 This is an incomplete assessment; vital signs would be a priority if there was an additional abnormality or indication beyond the drug therapy.
   4 This is incomplete; it is only one part of a thorough nursing assessment.

101. **2** Elastic stockings help decrease venous pooling of blood and help maintain systemic blood pressure when the client stands up. (b) (ME; IM; PA; CV)
   1 Orthostatic hypotension occurs on rising to an upright position; gait training will not affect this.
   3 An alteration in dosage may be ordered by the physician, but sudden withdrawal is dangerous and unwarranted.
   4 This may increase intravascular fluid volume temporarily but will not affect reflexes involved in orthostatic hypotension.

102. **2** The need for the basic four continues throughout life, although the quantities needed may be less. (a) (ME; PL; ED; GD)
   1 The priority is to educate the client, although home-delivered meals may be one way to provide adequate nutrition.
   3 Aging per se has no effect on nutritional needs; however, it may influence digestion and/or absorption of food.
   4 Protein is needed every day, but it need not be in the form of meat.

103. **4** This response recognizes the concern and provides accurate information that may reduce anxiety. (b) (SU; IM; ED; EC)
   1 This does not recognize feelings and provides inaccurate information; impotence rarely if ever occurs with this operation.
   2 This is inaccurate information; impotence usually does not result; it is possible after perineal prostatectomy.
   3 This reply closes off communication and transfers responsibility to the physician.

104. **2** Spasms result from irritation of the bladder during surgery; they decrease in intensity and frequency as healing occurs. (c) (SU; IM; ED; RG)
   1 Fluids should be increased to help flush the urinary tract and prevent stasis.
   3 This is too long; it would indicate hemorrhage; after the first few hours, drainage should be dark red and then gradually turn pink.
   4 The Valsalva maneuver should be avoided because it may initiate prostatic bleeding.

105. **3** Clients may develop cerebral edema caused by excessive absorption of irrigating solution by the venous sinusoids during surgery. (c) (SU; EV; TC; RG)
   1 The surgery is performed through the urinary meatus and urethra; there is no suprapubic incision.
   2 The procedure is usually performed under spinal anesthesia; the supine position is maintained for 8 to 12 hours.
   4 The client is initially npo and then advanced to a

regular diet as tolerated; continuous irrigation supplies fluid to flush the bladder.

106. **3** This is the correct flow rate; multiply the amount of fluid to be infused (175 ml) by the drop factor (15) and divide this result by the amount of time in minutes (1 hr × 60 min). (b) (SU; AN; PA; FE)

1 This rate would deliver less than the prescribed amount of fluid.

2 Same as # 1.

4 This rate would deliver more than prescribed amount of fluid.

107. **3** Straining at stool should be avoided for 4 to 6 weeks after surgery to permit healing and avoid initiating bleeding. (a) (SU; EV; ED; RG)

1 The client has carcinoma and needs continued medical supervision.

2 Sexual intercourse should be avoided for 3 to 4 weeks after surgery.

4 This is insufficient fluid; at least 2500 ml/day should be consumed.

108. **3** This is most common as the disbelief of actually being pregnant is experienced. (b) (OB; IM; PE; EC)

1 Depression is more commonly seen in the third trimester and postpartum.

2 Rejection is more commonly seen in the third trimester.

4 Narcissism is more commonly seen in second and third trimesters.

109. **4** Fasting results in hypoglycemia, which can cause nausea. (b) (OB; PL; ED; PN)

1 Fluids need not be increased but should be consumed between meals.

2 Calcium intake will not change the nausea.

3 This intake would not be sufficient to meet the normal nutritional needs of the mother and fetus.

110. **1** Total blood volume increases 50%, which necessitates the heart pumping harder and working more to accommodate this increase. (b) (OB; AN; PA; PN)

2 Although the renal threshold is lowered, the major changes occur in the cardiovascular system.

3 Changes in hormonal levels occur but are not as profound as changes in the cardiovascular system.

4 There are no changes in the system itself, but pressure from the growing uterus can result in altered patterns of elimination.

111. **1** The influence of progesterone and the pressure of the gravid uterus slows GI motility. (a) (OB; AN; PA; PN)

2 There is a decrease in ovarian activity.

3 There is an increase in the glomerulofiltration rate because of the increased fluid volume.

4 The pulmonary capacity stays relatively stable as the thoracic cage widens to accommodate lung volume.

112. **3** Forcing fluids fills the bladder, which is necessary to push the uterus up for good ultrasound viewing. (b) (OB; IM; TC; PN)

1 This has no relation to ultrasound preparation; fasting places the fetus in jeopardy.

2 The bladder must be full, not empty, for better visualization of the uterus.

4 The gastrointestinal tract is not involved.

113. **2** This relieves some of the pain because it pro-

vides support to the incised abdominal wall. (a) (OB; IM; TC; PP)

1 The symptoms do not indicate a need for this action.

3 Same as # 1.

4 Analgesics will not relieve the discomfort associated with coughing unless stress placed on the incision by coughing is relieved.

114. **2** This is a correct description of talipes equinovarus. (b) (PE; AS; PA; SK)

1 This describes talipes calcaneovarus.

3 Same as # 1.

4 This describes talipes equinovalgus, also known as rocker-bottom foot.

115. **1** Casts are changed weekly to accommodate the rapid growth in early infancy. (b) (PE; PL; TC; SK)

2 This is not frequent enough in early infancy; the cast could become too tight because of rapid growth.

3 Soiling is not usually a problem because casts for clubfoot do not extend to the perineal area.

4 This is too frequent; muscles and tendons would not be stretched and relaxed enough between cast changes to affect foot position.

116. **4** Exercising should be done often; association with a specific activity makes it easier to incorporate into the life-style, leading to increased compliance. (b) (PE; EV; ED; SK)

1 This is not frequent enough.

2 Same as # 1.

3 Although this is frequent enough, such a rigid schedule is difficult to follow with an infant, and compliance becomes more difficult.

117. **2** Exploration allows the nurse to assess the client's knowledge and fears. (b) (PE; IM; ED; EC)

1 This is false reassurance; it may occur again.

3 This is not true; this would imply a dominant mode of transmission.

4 This is not true; this would imply an autosomal recessive mode of transmission.

118. **4** Subcostal incisional pain causes the client to splint and avoid deep breathing, which impedes air exchange in the alveoli. (c) (SU; AN; PA; GI)

1 The location of the incision does not increase the risk of hemorrhage.

2 The site is not specifically a vulnerable location for infection.

3 This can be a postoperative problem, but it is unrelated to the incision site.

119. **2** The incision is just below the diaphragm; deep breathing causes tension and pain. (b) (SU; EV; PA; GI)

1 Clients with nasogastric tubes mouth breathe, limiting nasal irritation.

3 Dressings do not encircle the abdomen; they should not be tight enough to restrict respirations.

4 It would not move because it is sutured in place; it is unlikely to cause cramps because it is not in the intestines.

120. **3** Bile drainage for the first 24 hours is usually 300 to 500 ml; kinks in the tubing hinder the flow. (c) (SU; IM; TC; GI)

1 Drainage of 150 ml is less than expected in the first 24 hours.

2 Further intervention is necessary because this amount of bile is less than normal.

4 Clamping the tube is contraindicated in the first 24 hours.

121. **1** This reduces the risk of introducing irrigant into the lungs. (a) (SU; AS; TC; GI)
  2 This is irrelevant to nasogastric tube irrigation.
  3 Same as # 2.
  4 This increases the risk of introducing irrigant into the lungs if tube placement is not checked first.

122. **2** Lactated Ringer's is an alkaline solution that replaces bicarbonate ions lost from T-tube bile drainage, thus preventing or treating acidosis. (c) (SU; EV; TC; FE)
  1 This is unrelated to the effectiveness of this IV solution.
  3 Same as # 1.
  4 Same as # 1.

123. **2** Clients should be allowed to maintain some control, depending on their ability to perform a given task. (b) (SU; AS; TC; FE)
  1 Able clients should be supported to perform self-care.
  3 This is immaterial.
  4 The client has indicated willingness by the request.

124. **1** Being overweight is a predisposing factor to wound dehiscence because of decreased vascularity and fragility of adipose tissue. (b) (SU; AS; PA; GI)
  2 This does not contribute to dehiscence; a T-tube helps remove bile from the common bile duct.
  3 Age does not really contribute to dehiscence.
  4 This causes discomfort, not dehiscence.

125. **4** The decreased respiratory drive resulting from excessive O_2 administration indicates CO_2 narcosis. (c) (ME; IM; TC; RE)
  1 There are no indications that secretions have increased.
  2 This is inappropriate; a confused client cannot answer questions about the confusion.
  3 Increasing O_2 administration will further diminish respiratory drive until respiratory arrest occurs.

126. **1** More data is needed about activities of daily living to evaluate noncompliance before revising the care plan. (b) (ME; AS; TC; RE)
  2 This is nonproductive because it places blame for the illness on the client.
  3 Same as # 2.
  4 Same as # 2.

127. **2** The client has indicated engagement in activities contrary to the medical regimen and to his own best interests. (b) (ME; AN; PE; RE)
  1 No knowledge deficit exists; the client demonstrates knowledge about cessation of smoking and doing breathing exercises.
  3 Thought processes were not altered until noncompliance affected the Po_2 and Pco_2; the client's behavior does not indicate altered thought processes.
  4 The behavior does not indicate self-care deficit.

128. **2** Aminophylline acts as a vasodilator, and hypotension results when vessels are dilated. (c) (ME; EV; TC; DR)
  1 Increased diuresis, not oliguria, is a common side effect.
  3 Tachycardia, not bradycardia, is a common side effect.

4 Tachypnea, not hypoventilation, is a common side effect.

129. **4** This technique promotes nasal breathing, which negates the effects of aerosol medication; a loose seal around the mouthpiece allows for inhalation through the mouth. (c) (ME; EV; ED; RE)
  1 This is a correct technique; the nebulizer tip must be past the lips to deliver medication.
  2 This is a correct technique; it promotes contact of medication with the bronchial mucosa.
  3 This is a correct technique; it prolongs and improves delivery of the medication to the respiratory mucosa.

130. **1** Clients need to understand the cycle as a physiologic event that can be dealt with, not as a life-threatening crisis. (b) (ME; PL; ED; RE)
  2 Though helpful, this is not primary in helping to break the cycle of fear, dyspnea, and inactivity.
  3 This is insufficient to break the cycle.
  4 Same as # 3.

131. **2** This is a fragmented, pressured, nonsequential pattern of speech typically used during a manic episode. (a) (PS; AS; PE; MO)
  1 These are fixed false beliefs that others are plotting to do harm; they are typically found in clients with paranoid schizophrenia.
  3 This is the pattern of speech found in clients with schizophrenia; usual connections between words and phrases are lost to the listener and meaningful only to the speaker.
  4 These are repetitive, purposeful, and intentional behaviors that are carried out in a stereotyped fashion; they are typically found in clients with obsessive-compulsive disorders.

132. **1** This shows acceptance and protects the client and others from possible aggressive behavior. (b) (PS; PL; PE; MO)
  2 This is a threatening approach that increases feelings of inadequacy.
  3 Explanations are not helpful because the client's easy distractibility interferes with understanding.
  4 Both clients would be very responsive to external stimuli; therefore this action could lead to loss of control for both.

133. **4** Antipsychotics are usually prescribed to calm the agitated client during the period of waiting for lithium to become effective. (c) (PS; AN; TC; DR)
  1 Chlorpromazine is a major tranquilizer that has a different, not a potentiating, mechanism of action.
  2 Chlorpromazine is a major tranquilizer that has no effect on lithium toxicity.
  3 The drugs are used to control symptoms of mania; most clients do not progress to depression from the manic phase.

134. **3** This will help decrease irritability and impulsiveness caused by the client's increased responsiveness to changing stimuli. (b) (PS; PL; PE; MO)
  1 This is not helpful because of the client's easy distractibility and minimal attention span.
  2 A strange environment and new staff tend to increase anxiety level, not reduce manipulation.
  4 At this time, the client may misidentify this approach as threatening and may retaliate by aggression.

135. **2** This involves no element of competition and still

allows for channeling of excessive energy. (b) (PS; PL; TC; MO)

1 The sense of competition and increased stimulation may raise the client's anxiety.

3 This requires fine motor skill from a client who is hyperactive and whose attention span is limited.

4 The client is too hyperactive to complete this task and may respond with distractibility or aggressiveness toward others.

136. **4** The client will be able to attend to grooming because lithium effectively controls and reduces grandiosity, poor judgment, and psychomotor hyperactivity. (b) (PS; EV; TC; DR)

1 This would not reflect an effective response to lithium.

2 Same as # 1.

3 Same as # 1.

137. **2** The exact reason is unknown, but three factors appear related: lead in the environment; toxins in the environment; and characteristics of the child and the parents. (c) (PE; IM; ED; NM)

1 This is only one of the three etiologic factors.

3 Same as # 1.

4 Same as # 1.

138. **4** Bone marrow is most susceptible to lead toxicity; interference with hemoglobin biosynthesis leads to early signs of anemia. (c) (PE; AS; PA; BI)

1 This is a late response indicating central nervous system involvement.

2 This is a serious, life-threatening, late response.

3 This is a late response indicating kidney shutdown; loss of protein and other substances occurs first.

139. **3** Damaged nerve cells do not regenerate; once mental retardation has occurred, it is not reversible. (a) (PE; AN; PA; NM)

1 Changes in this system are reversible with treatment.

2 Same as # 1.

4 Same as # 1.

140. **1** The desired outcome is the increased excretion of lead in the urine. (b) (PE; EV; TC; DR)

2 This is expected when lead initially equilibrates to the blood; until the lead is excreted in the urine, the treatment is not considered a success.

3 Fecal elimination of lead is not as satisfactory as urinary elimination and is not as successful in ridding the soft tissues of lead.

4 This is a desirable effect, but it does not determine the success of therapy; also, the amount is difficult to determine.

141. **1** The child should be given an outlet for tension, and playing with a syringe and doll is the most appropriate in this situation. (a) (PE; PL; PE; EC)

2 This is part of the preparation, but not the most important; the child must be allowed to express his feelings; the child is too young to comprehend too much.

3 This may ease some of the discomfort, but an outlet for feelings should be provided.

4 The child's fear is not caused by unfamiliar adults but by the painful treatments.

142. **2** Applying moist or dry heat relieves muscle pain through vasodilation, increases circulation to the area, and facilitates drug absorption. (b) (PE; PL; TC; NM)

1 Movement most likely will be difficult and cause more discomfort.

3 This will cause more discomfort because the injection site is tender.

4 This will prolong the discomfort by slowing the rate of absorption of the drug by vasoconstriction.

143. **4** Lead toxicity and Ca EDTA both damage the proximal renal tubules, resulting in the abnormal excretion of protein and other substances. (c) (PE; EV; TC; RG)

1 This does not occur with lead toxicity, nor is it likely to occur with the Ca EDTA preparation, which replaces calcium.

2 Bone marrow damage is caused by lead toxicity only.

3 Lead encephalopathy causes serious elevation of intracranial pressure; this is not related to Ca EDTA.

144. **1** The mother should see her infant as soon as possible so that she can acknowledge the reality of the delivery and begin bonding. (b) (OB; PL; PE; EC)

2 A delay retards maternal-infant bonding.

3 This is an independent nursing action.

4 Same as # 2.

145. **4** By not acknowledging baby's sex, the client indicates that she has not released her fantasy baby and accepted the real one. (a) (OB; AN; PE; EC)

1 The mother has acknowledged the infant's sex by using "he," and her question denotes a relationship.

2 Same as # 1.

3 The mother incorporated the infant into the family by this statement.

146. **1** Focusing on the client's feelings permits her to work through her fears. (b) (OB; IM; PE; EC)

2 This statement does not encourage the client to focus on her feelings.

3 Same as # 2.

4 This closes off communication and does not allow the client to verbalize her feelings.

147. **4** Retractions are a prominent feature of respiratory problems in premature infants because of their compliant chest walls. (b) (OB; AS; PA; HN)

1 This rate is still within the normal range of 120 to 160 per minute.

2 A rapid respiratory rate of 40 to 60 is normal in neonates.

3 This is more indicative of low body temperature, not respiratory distress.

148. **4** Immature neurologic and chemical respiratory mechanisms cause apnea in premature infants; tactile stimulation will start breathing. (b) (OB; IM; PA; HN)

1 This is not done unless the infant is cyanotic or blood Po_2 is low.

2 This is not done unless the infant shows signs of obstructed airway.

3 This is done only if the infant does not respond to tactile stimulation.

149. **3** Insensible and intestinal fluid losses are increased during phototherapy; extra fluid prevents dehydration. (c) (OB; PL; TC; HN)

1 This is unnecessary unless changes from baseline occur.

2 The total body needs to be exposed to light.

4 A Guthrie test is done for PKU screening.

150. **1** This is necessary to provide for some normal psychosocial contact. (b) (OB; PL; PE; HN)

2 All parts of the body may contain bilirubin deposits and should be exposed to the light.

3 This may block light rays from acting on bilirubin deposits; frequent cleansing after voiding and defecation will prevent skin excoriation.

4 Radiant heaters are not used; only fluorescent bulbs are used.

151. **4** Increased levels of steroids and aldosterone cause sodium and water retention. (c) (ME; AS; PA; EN)

1 Hypertension would be expected.

2 The extremities would be thin; subcutaneous fat deposits occur in the upper trunk, especially the back between the scapula.

3 Hyperglycemia, not hypoglycemia, occurs because of increased secretion of glucocorticoids; hyperglycemia is sustained and not restricted to the morning hours.

152. **3** High levels of steroids result in emotional changes; the actual cause is unknown, but knowing the response may help the client to better cope with her son's behavior. (b) (ME; IM; ED; EN)

1 The changes are not permanent with adequate therapy.

2 This is unnecessary; the problem has been excessive production of steroids.

4 Weight loss, not weight gain, would indicate an improving condition.

153. **1** This decreases pressure on the sella turcica, as well as promoting venous return, thus limiting cerebral edema. (b) (SU; PL; TC; NM)

2 Gentle oral hygiene is performed, excluding brushing of teeth to prevent trauma to the surgical site.

3 Although deep breathing is encouraged, initially coughing is discouraged to prevent increasing intracranial pressure.

4 There is no need to limit oral fluids because of the presence of nasal packing.

154. **4** The pulse pressure is obtained by subtracting the diastolic from the systolic blood pressure reading; pulse pressure widens as intracranial pressure increases. (a) (SU; AN; PA; NM)

1 This is the pulse deficit.

2 This is measured with systolic and diastolic blood pressure readings.

3 This is determined by various diagnostic techniques used in cardiology; this is the role of the physician, not the nurse.

155. **2** Corticosteroids inhibit the inflammatory response and increase an individual's susceptibility to infection. (c) (SU; AN; TC; EN)

1 Urinary stasis is unrelated to Decadron; Decadron will promote diuresis.

3 The client will be hypertensive, not hypotensive, until stabilized.

4 With therapy, the client should lose weight.

156. **1** This will help to decrease the client's anxiety, provide a safe environment, and compensate for impaired cognition. (b) (PS; PL; PE; OR)

2 Restraints may increase confusion and agitation; they should be used only when absolutely unavoidable.

3 Reality orientation should be employed when

necessary.

4 Focusing on coping skills would increase the client's feelings of inadequacy; coping skills are on the unconscious level.

157. **2** A change in environment and introduction of unfamiliar stimuli precipitate confusion in the elderly client with organic brain syndrome; with appropriate intervention, including frequent reorientation, confusion can be reduced. (b) (PS; AN; PA; OR)

1 This is untrue; this is a stereotype.

3 This is untrue; reality orientation can reduce confusion.

4 Same as # 3.

158. **3** A small light in the room may prevent misinterpretation of shadows, which can heighten fear and alter the perception of the environment. (b) (PS; IM; TC; OR)

1 This is unnecessary; sedatives should be used sparingly in the aged because they may further confuse and agitate the aged client.

2 This is unsafe; a disoriented and confused client should not be isolated but closely observed.

4 Less restrictive intervention should be used first; restraints may not be necessary.

159. **2** This provides for turning in bed; putting siderails up and down will not interfere with the restraint, which can be easily removed in an emergency. (a) (PS; IM; TC; OR)

1 This is contraindicated; it would restrict shoulder, elbow, wrist, and upper trunk movement.

3 This is unsafe; it would restrict leg movement and turning; the client could injure himself by partially falling from the bed.

4 Same as # 1.

160. **2** The client will need reassurance and support after this frightening experience. (a) (PS; IM; PE; OR)

1 This provides false reassurance.

3 This is inappropriate; the client has an organic brain disorder and will have limited recall of recent teaching.

4 This is inappropriate; the priority is to allay anxiety; also, there is no need to stand the client up to take the pulse.

161. **3** Respiratory isolation is necessary because meningitis is most commonly spread by droplet infection, which is carried by airborne microorganisms. (c) (PE; IM; TC; NM)

1 This is unnecessary; meningitis is not a blood-borne disease.

2 This is unnecessary; meningitis is not transmitted via the feces.

4 This would be unnecessary; the client's immune system is not affected; others must be protected from the client's infection.

162. **3** This private room will provide isolation; also, being close to nurses' station will facilitate frequent neurologic monitoring. (b) (PE; PL; TC; NM)

1 This is unsafe; it would permit cross-infection; a private room is necessary to prevent transmission of airborne droplets.

2 This is unsafe; it interferes with frequent monitoring of the client.

4 Same as # 1.

163. **2** This action would encourage the mother to leave and reassure her that someone will be with and

will comfort the child. (b) (PE; IM; PE; EC)

1 The mother has said she must leave; convincing her to stay will make her feel guilty about having to leave.

3 Same as # 1.

4 The mother has indicated she is upset when the child is upset; the mother knows the way to the elevator; this intervention meets no one's needs.

164. 1 The position of maximal safety and comfort is side-lying because the client's neck is arched backwards and the spine is an inverted "C". (b) (PE; IM; TC; NM)

2 This is contraindicated; this would increase intracranial pressure.

3 This would be impossible because the child is in a rigid opisthotonic position; this could be injurious to the child.

4 Same as # 3.

165. 2 If the IV infused at the prescribed rate of 45 ml/hr × 5 hrs, 225 ml would have infused, leaving 275 ml in the bottle. (b) (PE; EV; TC; FE)

1 This is incorrect; an excessive amount of fluid has been infused.

3 Same as # 1.

4 This is untrue; the IV should be delivered at 45 ml/hr and should be monitored continually.

166. 3 With a microdrip set up, the nurse should know that the number of ml/hr equals the number of micro gtts/min; thus 55 ml/hr = 55 micro gtts/min. (b) (PE; AN; TC; FE)

1 This is too low; this rate would not deliver the required amount of solution.

2 Same as # 1.

4 This rate is too high; it would deliver more than the required amount of solution.

167. 4 A serious side effect of chloramphenicol (Chloromycetin) is aplastic anemia, a common reaction to the drug; blood studies would monitor RBCs. (c) (PE; EV; TC; DR)

1 This is unrelated to chloramphenicol.

2 A decrease, not an increase, in RBCs occurs.

3 Same as # 1.

168. 4 Baseline pulse and respiratory rates will aid in monitoring treatment efficacy and identifying concurrent problems such as CHF and bradydysrhythmias. (a) (ME; IM; PA; CV)

1 This could precipitate respiratory distress; semi- to high-Fowler's position should be maintained.

2 This is not the priority at this time; this may be done later.

3 This is unnecessary; it is unrelated to hypertension.

169. 1 Furosemide (Lasix) is a diuretic with a rapid onset of action, particularly when given intravenously. (a) (ME; IM; ED; FE)

2 This is contraindicated; at this time, the client has a fluid volume excess; potassium needs will be addressed later.

3 Hearing loss is associated only with high doses; 20 mg is a small dose.

4 Burning is not associated with IV administration of furosemide.

170. 4 This helps to prevent aspiration and opens the airway. (a) (ME; IM; TC; RE)

1 This is contraindicated; it could injure the client and does nothing to establish an airway.

2 Same as # 1.

3 This is unsafe; a client having a seizure should

not be left unattended; an airway must be established.

171. 2 Sodium absorbs water in the kidney's renal tubules; when dietary intake is decreased, water is not reabsorbed and edema is reduced. (b) (ME; AN; PA; FE)

1 This will not be caused by a low-sodium diet; this will cause fluid to enter the intravascular compartment.

3 This is untrue; a decrease in sodium will prevent the reabsorption of water; furosemide stimulates the Loop of Henle.

4 Adequate hydration is the major factor that diminishes the thirst response.

172. 3 Lemon juice adds flavor and is low in sodium. (a) (ME; IM; ED; FE)

1 Carbonated beverages generally contain sodium; coffee, whether it is decaffeinated or not, does not contain sodium.

2 This is unnecessary.

4 This is unnecessary; canned vegetables generally contain sodium.

173. 2 The solution with the greatest number of particles is hyperosmolar and exerts an osmotic force, pulling fluid in its direction. (b) (ME; AN; ED; FE)

1 On the contrary; water moves to the side with the greater number of particles.

3 This is untrue; the opposite occurs.

4 Same as # 3.

174. 4 Thrombophlebitis is a common complication of immobility in situations related to the application of traction. (b) (SU; AS; TC; SK)

1 This is contraindicated during use of Buck's traction; positioning with a pillow to relieve back pressure is permitted for short periods.

2 This is contraindicated; this could cause further soft tissue injury and pain for the client.

3 This interferes with the pull of traction; it would cause further soft tissue injury and pain for the client.

175. 3 Lying on the affected side causes adduction, which may result in dislocation of the femoral head. (c) (SU; PL; PA; SK)

1 This is too long a period; partial weight bearing will be permitted sooner, depending on the extent of surgery and the progression of healing.

2 Partial weight bearing on the affected leg is contraindicated for at least 2 to 3 weeks.

4 This is contraindicated; it would put too much pressure on the operative site; the leg on operative side should be kept in abduction.

176. 4 Heparin interferes with activation of prothrombin to thrombin and inhibits aggregation of platelets. (b) (SU; AN; PA; DR)

1 This is not the action of Heparin.

2 Same as # 1.

3 Same as # 1.

177. 2 Active ROM increases venous return from the unaffected leg, preventing complications of immobility, including thrombophlebitis (b) (SU; AN; PA; CV)

1 Although isotonic exercises do promote muscle strength, that is not the purpose at this time; the priority is to prevent further thrombi from developing.

3 These isotonic exercises are being performed on the unaffected extremity; there should be no dis-

comfort.

4 These activities will prevent, not limit, venous inflammation.

178. **2** Alcohol frequently reduces inhibitions and is one of the leading causes of violent behavior. (a) (PS; AS; PA; SA)

1 This factor alone rarely precipitates abusive behavior.

3 Same as # 1.

4 Same as # 1.

179. **3** Encouraging conversation allows the abused individual an opportunity to verbalize feelings and may ultimately lead to development of possible coping strategies. (b) (PS; IM; PE; CS)

1 This focuses on a topic that may not be the client's concern; the client should be permitted to direct the topic of conversation.

2 This is not the legal responsibility of the nurse at this time.

4 Same as # 1.

180. **2** Parental role support and contact with other adults is very important in parenting. (b) (PS; AS; PE; CS)

1 This is untrue; the client is in a state of crisis, which would indicate present defenses are ineffective.

3 No personality type is specifically associated with abusive behavior.

4 Although lack of knowledge may lead to unrealistic expectations of the child, this factor alone does not significantly contribute to abusive behavior.

181. **2** Identifying potential health problems and planning and implementing programs aimed at these problems is primary prevention. (b) (PS; AN; TC; CS)

1 There is no such term; legal intervention would be a form of secondary prevention.

3 These are interventions such as legal orders of protection or temporary removal of the child from the situation.

4 These are interventions such as long-term or permanent removal of the child from the home.

182. **1** The first action should be to dry the infant and place him under a warmer to prevent chilling, thereby decreasing the possibility of development of metabolic acidosis. (b) (OB; IM; PA; NN)

2 This is not the priority at this time; conserving body heat takes precedence.

3 This would not be done until after the baby is warmed.

4 This is useless without an adequate airway.

183. **3** The desquamation occurs from prolonged exposure to amniotic fluid, causing cracking, peeling, and drying of skin in the post-term baby. (b) (OB; AS; PA; HN)

1 This indicates a preterm infant.

2 Same as # 1.

4 Creases would cover the entire sole of each foot.

184. **1** After laboring all night the client is tired. (c) (OB; PL; PA; PP)

2 This would be premature; the client is not ready to learn.

3 This assessment would be too frequent and would interfere with the client's rest.

4 This is necessary only the first time the client ambulates; otherwise the client can ambulate ad lib.

185. **2** Nipple soreness often occurs when there is incorrect positioning of the newborn's mouth on the breast; also, nipples still need to toughen in response to sucking. (b) (OB; AS; PA; PP)

1 This is premature; the cause of soreness must be determined first and will dictate what type of intervention is necessary.

3 Same as # 1.

4 Same as # 1.

186. **3** The fundus tends to stay at or slightly above the umbilicus for about 24 hours, then decreases in size about one finger-breadth per day. (a) (OB; AS; PA; PP)

1 This would be the position in the first 24 hours postpartum.

2 Same as # 1.

4 This would be the position on the fourth or fifth day.

187. **4** Lochia serosa is similar in appearance to serosanguinous drainage and generally appears on third or fourth postpartum day. (a) (OB; AS; PA; PP)

1 There is no such term.

2 Lochia alba consists of leukocytes, decidua, epithelial cells, mucus, and serum; this appears 10 days postpartum and lasts 2 to 6 weeks.

3 Lochia rubra is initially bright red, changing to dark red or reddish brown; it consists mainly of blood, decidua, and trophoblastic debris; it occurs immediately after delivery, lasting for 2 to 3 days.

How to Use Worksheet 1: Errors in Processing Information

Common errors in processing information are listed in the left-hand column of this worksheet. At the top of the worksheet is a row of blank spaces for inserting the number of the question missed. Directly below each number, check any errors you made in answering that question. You may have made more than one type of error in an answer.

Worksheet 1: Errors in processing information

Question number																					
Did not read situation/question carefully																					
Missed important details																					
Confused major and minor points																					
Defined problem incorrectly																					
Could not remember terms/ facts/concepts/principles																					
Defined terms incorrectly																					
Focused on incomplete/incorrect data in assessing situation																					
Interpreted data incorrectly																					
Applied wrong concepts/principles in situation																					
Drew incorrect conclusions																					
Identified wrong goals																					
Identified priorities incorrectly																					
Carried out plan incorrectly/incompletely																					
Was unclear about criteria for evaluating success in achieving goals																					

How to Use Worksheet 2: Knowledge Gaps

Types of common knowledge gaps are listed along the top of this worksheet. Write a brief description of topics you want to review in the spaces provided. For example, if you missed a question on administration of a particular drug, write the drug name and problem (e.g., dosage) in the appropriate space under the column labeled *Pharmacology*.

Worksheet 2: Knowledge gaps

Basic science	Skills/ procedures	Basic human needs	Growth & develop- ment	Normal nutrition	Psycho- social factors	Clinical area/ topic	Stressors/ coping mechanisms	Patho- physiology	Pharma- cology	Therapeutic nutrition	Legal Implications	Other

Test 3

188. **3** Nitroglycerin causes vasodilation, increasing the flow of blood and oxygen to the myocardium and reducing anginal pain. (a) (ME; EV; TC; DR)
   1 The tingling indicates that the medication is fresh; relief of pain is the only indicator of effectiveness.
   2 The pulse rate should decrease because of vasodilation.
   4 Nitroglycerin does not promote the formation of new blood vessels.
189. **1** Breaking up the tablet increases the surface area of the tablet, which permits it to dissolve faster. (b) (ME; IM; ED; DR)
   2 If taken with water, the tablet is held away from the site of absorption or may even be swallowed.
   3 This would slow absorption because saliva helps to dissolve the tablet.
   4 This does not hasten absorption and may even impair its ability to dissolve.
190. **2** This response recognizes the client's and family's concerns and encourages further verbalization of feelings. (b) (ME; IM; PE; EC)
   1 This response does not focus on the client's and family's underlying concerns and keeps the discussion on a physiologic level.
   3 This provides false reassurance and cuts off further verbalization of feelings.
   4 Same as # 3.
191. **3** Myocardial necrosis causes a rise in body temperature within the first 24 to 48 hours, which gradually returns to normal within a week. (b) (ME; PL; PA; CV)
   1 This is unnecessary; this is an expected response and not an emergency.
   2 Coughing necessitates the use of the Valsalva maneuver, which is contraindicated because it can precipitate arrhythmias.
   4 This temperature did not result from a respiratory complication.
192. **1** These foods are low in sodium and calories. (a) (ME; EV; ED; CV)
   2 Stir-fried Chinese vegetables are made with soy sauce, which is very high in sodium, and cornstarch, which is high in calories.
   3 Canned tuna fish and celery are high in sodium.
   4 Beef is high in calories, and carrots are high in sodium.
193. **4** The ability to endure progressive activity indicates that collateral circulation has improved cardiopulmonary functioning. (c) (ME; IM; ED; CV)
   1 Perspiration is an expected and desired adaptation to promote heat loss through evaporation.
   2 Intermittent claudication is related to peripheral arterial occlusive disease, not cardiopulmonary function.
   3 Breathing when jogging should be regular and deep to meet the oxygen demands of the body during exercise.
194. **4** Normal eating patterns are not lost when a laryngectomy is performed. (c) (SU; IM; ED; RE)
   1 Air goes directly to the trachea, bypassing the nose and olfactory organs.
   2 There is no passage of air from the lungs to the mouth, and the ability to sip through a straw is lost.

3 There is no passage of air from the lungs to the nose, and the ability to blow the nose is lost.
195. **2** Semi-Fowler's position helps to maintain the head in proper body alignment and facilitates respiration. (b) (SU; PL; PA; RE)
   1 The side-lying position inhibits respiratory excursion.
   3 This position may cause flexion of the neck, which would inhibit respiration and place pressure on the suture line.
   4 Same as # 3.
196. **3** A patent airway is always a priority concern; therefore removal of secretions is imperative. (a) (SU; AN; PA; RE)
   1 This is an important postoperative concern but does not occur immediately.
   2 This is an important postoperative intervention but is not the priority immediately after surgery.
   4 Same as # 2.
197. **3** Initial attempts at oral feeding may cause a choking feeling that may produce severe coughing and raise secretions. (c) (SU; IM; PA; RE)
   1 The pain medication may cause a decrease in the client's respiratory effort and may also depress the cough reflex.
   2 A progressive diet is started with liquids, not pureed foods.
   4 Swallowing does not have an adverse effect on the suture line; a nasogastric tube would not be used because it could traumatize the suture line.
198. **3** This frustration reveals readiness to deal with the problem of speech that may be best demonstrated by a person with a laryngectomy. (c) (SU; PL; PE; EC)
   1 This type of answer leaves the client in limbo and offers no plans for goal setting.
   2 The healing of the incision in no way affects learning a new way of speaking.
   4 This closes off communication, but the client's frustration reveals a need for positive action.
199. **1** It is important to determine if the client is thinking about suicide; the direct approach is most appropriate. (a) (PS; AS; PE; MD)
   2 This approach denies the client's feelings and may be false reassurance.
   3 This approach not only denies the client's feelings but also tells her she has no right to feel the way she does.
   4 This approach tells the client that her feelings do not have top priority.
200. **4** A formal plan demonstrates determination, concentration, and effort, with conclusions already thought out. (b) (PS; AS; PE; MD)
   1 Many clients verbalize their suicidal thoughts as they are working on their decision and plan of action; suicide is not always attempted for the attention it achieves.
   2 Talking about suicide does not give clients the idea; verbalizing feelings may help reduce clients' need to act out.
   3 Failure to successfully complete the suicidal act can add to feelings of worthlessness and stimulate further acts.
201. **4** A rapid mood upswing and psychomotor change frequently signals that the client has made a decision and has developed a plan for suicide. (b) (PS; EV; PE; MD)

1 This statement is typical in the depressed client and does not really signal a change in mood.

2 Same as # 1.

3 Same as # 1.

202. **2** This is a true statement that assures the client that it is effective. (b) (PS; IM; PE; MD)

1 This response does not answer the client's question.

3 This response puts off answering the client's question by referring it to the physician.

4 ECT does not change usual patterns of behavior although it does interrupt disturbed or disturbing acting-out behavior.

203. **3** Anectine produces respiratory depression because it inhibits contractions of respiratory muscles. (a) (PS; EV; TC; DR)

1 Because the client is not permitted anything by mouth for 8 to 10 hours before the treatment, this is not a major problem.

2 As a muscle relaxant, Anectine prevents convulsions.

4 The loss of memory results from the ECT treatment, not from Anectine.

204. **1** This is a true statement that addresses the client's concern. (b) (PS; IM; PE; MD)

2 This approach denies the client's fears and feelings and could be frightening and upsetting.

3 This approach denies the client's fears and feelings and may not be the most important thing to the client at this time.

4 This approach denies the client's fears and feelings and really does not address her current concern.

205. **1** With a cleft in the lip the baby will be unable to suck like other newborns. (a) (PE; PL; PA; GI)

2 This is not necessary because intake and output will be normal once a feeding method is established.

3 This is common for all newborns, not just a baby with a cleft lip.

4 This is contraindicated in a newborn because the normal alignment of the spine will be interfered with if the head is elevated at all times.

206. **3** After surgery the baby will be lying on the back, a position different from the prone position most newborns prefer. (b) (PE; IM; ED; GI)

1 The baby is too young and will miss out on some oral gratification with this method.

2 Constant restraint of the arms would be injurious to arm growth, as well as to the infant's need to move about.

4 Babies with a cleft lip need increased burping time because they tend to swallow large amounts of air during feeding.

207. **2** Cleansing after feeding keeps the suture line from becoming infected. (b) (PE; EV; ED; IT)

1 The baby should be held and cuddled during feeding.

3 This exerts pressure on the suture line and may cause wound separation.

4 Same as # 3.

208. **4** This would minimize the sucking and yet not be irritating to the suture line. (b) (PE; PL; TC; GI)

1 Intravenous infusions do not supply the necessary caloric intake.

2 This is not used since it would be irritating to the nostrils.

3 No nipple should be used because the baby should not suck.

209. **2** An explanation of how the restraints work and why may reassure the mother. (b) (PE; AN; TC; GI)

1 Using things routinely does not explain why they are being used now; this is an unsatisfactory response.

3 This implies strict adherence to the physician's wishes without any thinking or understanding by the nurse.

4 This is most unreassuring because it gives the mother the feeling that the baby is not being watched at all times.

210. **1** Intrauterine devices should be inserted during menses because the cervical os is slightly dilated and the chance of pregnancy is slim. (c) (OB; IM; ED; FS)

2 An IUD should not be inserted at this time; this is the proliferative phase of the menstrual cycle.

3 An IUD should not be inserted at this time; this is the secretory phase of the menstrual cycle.

4 Same as # 3.

211. **4** The cervical mucus is clear and stretchable (spinnbarkeit) at ovulation because of maximum estrogen stimulation. (c) (OB; IM; PA; FS)

1 These characteristics do not normally occur at any point during the cycle.

2 Same as # 1.

3 Same as # 1.

212. **2** The diaphragm is used in conjunction with spermicidal jelly or cream, which remains active for only 6 to 8 hours. (a) (OB; EV; ED; FS)

1 Removal this soon would allow motile sperm to pass through the cervical os.

3 The diaphragm may be left in place as a mechanical barrier but the spermicidal jelly or cream becomes inactive after 6 to 8 hours.

4 The diaphragm may be left in place for this period of time but may cause an unpleasant odor.

213. **3** The ovum is fertilizable for 12 to 24 hours, and sperm remain motile for about 72 hours. (a) (OB; PL; PA; FS)

1 The fertility period is longer than this.

2 This time period is too long before ovulation and too short after ovulation.

4 The fertility period is shorter than this.

214. **2** At this time the tube is unable to expand to the size of the growing pregnancy. (a) (OB; AS; PA; HP)

1 The size of the fertilized egg at this time is miniscule and will cause no problem.

3 Tubal pregnancies cannot advance to this stage because of the tube's inability to expand with the growing pregnancy.

4 Same as # 3.

215. **3** The ruptured tube will be removed; repair of the tube may result in scarring, predisposing to another tubal pregnancy. (a) (OB; PL; TC; HP)

1 The D and C would be effective only in cleaning out the uterine cavity; no pregnancy contents are in the uterus with a tubal pregnancy.

2 The uterus is usually uninvolved in a tubal pregnancy, and this would make the woman incapable of future pregnancy.

4 This is a procedure for removing myomas (fibroids) from the uterus.

216. **2** Shock ensues rapidly in a ruptured ectopic pregnancy, and internal loss of blood may indicate

profound hemorrhage. (c) (OB; EV; PA; HP)

1 The nurse can observe hyperventilation by watching the client's breathing patterns; rapid respirations, rather than a rapid pulse, would be expected.

3 Extreme anxiety is not usually associated with lightheadedness unless there is hyperventilation.

4 The symptoms are not inclusive enough to indicate infection; there is no indication of fever or rising white blood count.

217. **3** Removing a tube does not impair the ovarian ability to release an egg, which may be fertilized in the remaining tube. (a) (OB; PL; PE; EC)

1 There is no absolute way of knowing whether or not another tubal pregnancy will ensue.

2 There is no information given that states the client is Rh negative.

4 This is unrelated to tubal pregnancy, as well as incorrect information, because douching cannot reach a fertilized egg.

218. **3** This helps allay guilt, reduces anxiety, and assists with coping. (c) (PS; IM; PE; CS)

1 It is too soon for this intervention.

2 The client should be considered before a clergyman is called.

4 This is a last resort because this delays the grieving process.

219. **1** Because of the shock and trauma it is expected that the client will have an alteration in normal coping mechanisms. (b) (PS; AN; PE; CS)

2 The client does not project falsely positive opinions about himself to enhance his self-regard; it is more likely that his problem is an alteration in meeting life's demands and handling stress.

3 The diagnosis is for the client; no family is mentioned in the situation.

4 No information is presented to indicate that the client cannot distinguish between the self and nonself.

220. **2** The client's grieving process is severe and extended, indicating dysfunction. (b) (PS; AN; PE; CS)

1 The data does not support this; the client is communicating effectively with the nurse.

3 This is not as specific as identifying grieving; also, low motivation is not the reason for the client's inability to cope.

4 There is not enough data to support this conclusion.

221. **1** Guilt feelings can prolong the grieving process because the individual is overwhelmed by both the guilt and grief, and consequently the energy to cope with either is absent. (c) (PS; AN; PE; CS)

2 Ambivalent feelings about the deceased, not the death itself, can prolong grief.

3 There is no data to support this.

4 Usually the opposite is true; the support provided would hasten resolution of grief.

222. **2** During this stage the nurse comes to a conclusion about the collected data and makes a diagnosis. (c) (PS; AN; TC; CS)

1 The nurse gathers and clusters data during this stage of the nursing process.

3 During this stage, the nurse sets priorities, establishes goals, identifies outcome criteria, and develops a nursing care plan.

4 The client's response to nursing care is assessed in relation to the stated outcome criteria to determine if goals have been met.

223. **2** The nursing diagnosis consists of two parts: the statement of the client's health status (health problem) and the related factors (probable causes). (c) (PS; AN; TC; CS)

1 The nursing diagnosis includes a statement of the problem; the client's needs are addressed in the plan of care.

3 Although the client's responses may reflect health status, this is only one part of the diagnosis.

4 A medical diagnosis describes a disease process; a nursing diagnosis describes a person's response to a disease process, condition, or situation.

224. **4** This is realistic, specific, and measurable; it relates to the client's stated nursing diagnosis. (a) (PS; PL; PE; CS)

1 This may be unrealistic and cannot be made without involvement of the family.

2 This is an unrealistic goal.

3 There is no data to indicate he is thinking negatively about himself or others.

225. **3** Hyperthyroidism raises the metabolic rate and need for oxygen; this results in increased heart rate and myocardial irritability. (b) (ME; AS; PA; EN)

1 These are signs associated with myxedema and hypothyroidism.

2 Same as # 1.

4 Same as # 1.

226. **2** Additional studies such as T_3 and T_4 will be necessary to confirm hyperthyroidism; it is not reliable to base the diagnosis on RAI alone. (c) (ME; IM; ED; EN)

1 This test uses ^{131}I, which emits radioactive particles for at least 24 hours; these are excreted in the urine.

3 Test results are affected by many medications, especially those containing iodine.

4 This test measures uptake of ^{131}I by the thyroid gland; it does not measure levels of thyroid hormone.

227. **2** Propylthiouracil can cause a depression of leukocytes and platelets. (c) (ME; EV; TC; DR)

1 Therapy will be continued for at least 6 to 8 weeks, even if the client's temperature and pulse return to normal.

3 They are given with milk, juice, or food to prevent gastric irritation.

4 Drug therapy decreases the risk of postoperative hemorrhage because it decreases the size and vascularity of the thyroid gland.

228. **2** These are signs of congestive heart failure, which may develop with the persistent tachycardia that is present with hyperthyroidism. (c) (ME; AS; PA; EN)

1 These are expected to occur with hyperthyroidism and need not be reported immediately.

3 Same as # 1.

4 Same as # 1.

229. **1** Immediate treatment in this emergency focuses on reduction of oxygen demands and thus cardiac workload to prevent cardiac decompensation. (b) (ME; AN; TC; EN)

2 The need is for an increase in fluid intake to compensate for that lost because of the very high metabolic rate.

3 This is not likely because drugs are metabolized more rapidly in this condition; there is a danger of exaggerated effects with hypothyroidism.

4 Clients with thyrotoxicosis are more apt to develop hypoglycemia from the high metabolic rate.

230. **4** This permits air to enter through the mouth along with the medication from the nebulizer; slow deep breaths deliver medication deep into the lung. (a) (ME; IM; ED; RE)

1 It is impossible to breathe through the mouth with the lips sealed around the mouthpiece; shallow breaths are ineffective in delivering medication into the lung.

2 This is a nasal spray that does not deliver medication to the lung.

3 This would not deliver the medication to the lungs but would deposit it in the oral cavity.

231. **4** Because the affected lung will not expand, aeration of the lung will not be complete and breath sounds will be diminished. (a) (SU; AS; PA; RE)

1 This occurs with asthma, not with a pneumothorax.

2 This occurs with congestive heart failure, not with a pneumothorax; with a pneumothorax there is no air in the alveoli to produce rales.

3 This is a broad term that includes all abnormal breath sounds; it is not specific to pneumothorax.

232. **4** Negative pressure is exerted by gravity drainage or by suction through the closed system. (a) (SU; AN; PA; RE)

1 In a pneumothorax associated with COPD there is an accumulation of air, not fluid.

2 Though the discomfort may be lessened, this is not the primary purpose.

3 Subcutaneous emphysema in the chest wall is most frequently associated with clients receiving air under pressure, as in ventilator treatment.

233. **1** All these interventions promote aeration of the expanding lung and maintenance of function in the arm and shoulder on the affected side. (c) (SU; PL; PA; RE)

2 Cough suppressants would not be indicated, because coughing and deep breathing are to be encouraged.

3 Drainage is marked with time tapes on the side of the device; the system is not broken for emptying; when full, the entire device is replaced.

4 Clamps are not necessary and should be avoided in almost all instances because of the danger of tension pneumothorax.

234. **3** The collection device must be kept below the level of the chest to prevent backflow of fluid into the pleural space. (a) (SU; IM; TC; RE)

1 The chest tube should almost never be clamped; this may precipitate a tension pneumothorax.

2 There is no reason to disconnect the chest tube from the water seal system; this could allow atmospheric air to enter the pleural space.

4 For transport, suction should be turned off and the tubing disconnected distal to the water seal connection.

235. **4** Palpation is the most invasive technique of the assessment skills; infants do not tolerate invasive procedures as well as they do less threatening maneuvers. (b) (PE; AS; TC; GD)

1 Auscultation is less invasive than palpation; the accuracy of auscultation may be affected if it is done after a more invasive technique that produces crying, thus making auscultation more difficult.

2 Inspection is the least invasive procedure and should be done first.

3 Percussion of the lung fields can be frightening to an infant but is generally tolerated better than palpation; it should be done toward the end of the assessment but before palpation.

236. **4** This is the most appropriate family nursing diagnosis because it is the alteration in parenting that forms the basis for the other problems experienced by the child and family. (c) (PE; AN; ED; GD)

1 Altered nutrition is a problem for the child but only indirectly for the family; the history does not support child abuse.

2 Sensory-perceptual alteration is a diagnosis that is related most specifically to the infant; the problem can be resolved by addressing the parenting problems.

3 Potential for injury is not an actual problem at this time because there is no history or evidence of physical abuse.

237. **4** This is appropriate for a 4-month-old; the child enjoys squeezing and hearing the sound of the squeaker. (a) (PE; PL; ED; GD)

1 This is appropriate for a child 12 to 24 months of age.

2 This is appropriate for a child 16 months of age.

3 This is appropriate for a child 10 to 12 months of age.

238. **2** This is normal developmental behavior for 18-month-olds; however, they may have trouble coming down the stairs. (b) (PE; EV; PA; GD)

1 This is above the level of an 18-month-old child.

3 Same as # 1.

4 Same as # 1.

239. **2** White spots (Koplik's spots) and the rash with coryza are very indicative of measles (rubeola). (c) (PE; EV; PA; IT)

1 Varicella (chickenpox) has skin lesions rather than a rash and lesions in the mouth.

3 Rubella (german measles) does not cause Koplik's spots.

4 Scarlet fever does not cause Koplik's spots but a strawberry-red tongue.

240. **2** The diagnosis is based on the presence of five out of six specific symptoms including fever, trunk rash, enlarged cervical lymph nodes, bilateral congestion of the conjunctiva, edema, and redness of the extremities. (c) (PE; AS; PA; NM)

1 An elevated ASO titer may be seen with a streptococcal infection.

3 This is non-specific to Kawasaki disease; the sedimentation rate is elevated in the presence of inflammation with many disorders.

4 This is not present in Kawasaki disease.

241. **4** When children are allowed to have some control in their care, their cooperation and willingness to tolerate procedures and medications are enhanced. (b) (PE; PL; PE; EC)

1 A child's favorite food should never be used to disguise medication because it will likely cause an aversion to that food and can affect the child

nutritionally.

2 Bribing sets up a nontherapeutic relationship between the child and the nurse and should not be used.

3 The nurse should be truthful about the taste of medication so that the child can have an opportunity to suggest ways to deal with the taste.

242. **1** This is a form of doxorubicin, which is cardiotoxic and causes arrhythmias. (b) (ME; EV; TC; DR)

2 Toxicity causes severe, not minor, dermatitis.

3 This is a side effect of doxorubicin, not a toxic effect.

4 Same as # 3.

243. **3** Respiratory tract infection may be the first clinical sign of bone marrow suppression. (b) (ME; EV; TC; DR)

1 This is an expected, non–life-threatening side effect.

2 Same as # 1.

4 This is not a side effect of doxorubicin.

244. **1** Rewording of the client's statement is paraphrasing that promotes further verbalization. (b) (ME; IM; PE; EC)

2 This is not an interviewing technique; immediate movement to intervention cuts off communication.

3 This is not paraphrasing; this merely repeats the client's exact words.

4 This is a therapeutic technique, but it is not paraphrasing.

245. **1** At the very minimum, the role of a witness is to attest to the validity of the signature. (a) (SU; AN; TC; EC)

2 This is the responsibility of the physician.

3 Clients also need to know about the outcomes and risks of surgery.

4 A consent is valid for the length of the hospital stay.

246. **1** This is a gram-negative antibiotic given to decrease bacteria in the colon, which should limit postoperative infection. (c) (SU; PL; TC; GI)

2 This would be used for a client with ruptured esophageal varices, not for one having a hemicolectomy.

3 These are used for constipation; oil retention enemas would not be ordered before surgery; tap water enemas until clear might be ordered.

4 This is contraindicated; a diet to decrease bulk and empty the colon would be ordered.

247. **1** This procedure removes fluids and gas from the GI tract, which permits better healing of the surgical area and minimizes nausea. (a) (SU; AN; TC; GI)

2 Tube feeding would be contraindicated after gastrointestinal surgery.

3 This is not the purpose in this situation; the tube is used to decompress the stomach.

4 The tube decompresses the stomach, not the large bowel.

248. **3** Baked fish is a low-residue, low-fat, high-protein, and non–gas-producing food that is usually well tolerated. (b) (SU; EV; PA; GI)

1 This irritates the gastrointestinal tract and stimulates mucus production.

2 This has fiber and irritates the gastrointestinal tract.

4 Same as # 2.

249. **2** Goodell's sign, or softening of the cervix, occurs at 8 to 9 weeks gestation. (c) (OB; AS; PA; PN)

1 Lightening or settling of the fetal presenting part into the pelvis usually occurs 2 weeks before the onset of labor in nulliparas.

3 Braxton-Hicks are intermittent, cramplike contractions that usually occur toward the end of pregnancy and may be mistaken by the mother for the onset of labor.

4 This refers to the fetal movements usually perceived by the mother between the sixteenth and twentieth weeks of gestation.

250. **1** At about the twentieth to twenty-second week of gestation, the top of the fundus is at the level of the umbilicus. (c) (OB; AS; PA; PN)

2 In a normal pregnancy this would be too low for a pregnancy between the fifth and sixth month.

3 In a normal pregnancy, this would be too high for 20 to 22 weeks of gestation.

4 Same as # 2.

251. **3** The client should be assessed further for signs of abruptio placentae by looking for cessation of uterine activity, fetal heart deceleration, and falling blood pressure. (b) (OB; IM; TC; IP)

1 This is unsafe; the status of the fetus and mother must be assessed immediately.

2 This is not the priority; the status of fetus is paramount.

4 This is unsafe; the status of fetus is primary; in a partial abruptio placentae, placing the client in a supine position would further compromise blood flow to the fetus.

252. **4** These are characteristics associated with children who have Down's syndrome; a mongoloid slant of the eyes is also present. (a) (OB; AS; PA; HN)

1 Although low-set ears occur with Down's syndrome, microencephaly and a high-pitched cry may indicate a variety of neurologic problems; the last two symptoms are part of a syndrome known as cri-du-chat.

2 Only low-set ears occur with Down's syndrome; all of these symptoms occur with Trisomy 18.

3 Webbed neck and widely spaced nipples are associated with Turner's syndrome.

253. **2** This is a pictorial analysis of chromosomes usually done on peripheral blood, which will show chromosomal abnormalities such as the translocation found in Down's syndrome. (b) (OB; PL; PA; HN)

1 This is a test that is done before delivery.

3 Karyotyping, not a buccal smear, is done on peripheral blood.

4 This test does not assess chromosomal aberrations.

254. **2** This is an accurate and nonjudgmental response. (b) (OB; IM; PE; EC)

1 This is a judgmental response that questions the mother's decision making and deals only with the present.

3 Same as # 1.

4 This response recognizes the client's feelings but cuts off communication because it ends the discussion.

255. **1** Unwavering adherence to the same principles and regulations promotes safe, firm limits. (a)

(PE; PL; PA; GD)

2 This stifles the child's natural development in learning to explore.

3 Injuries are promoted when there is lack of care.

4 This hinders the child's freedom to explore and enjoy the surroundings.

256. **2** The child is developing autonomy, is curious, and learns from experience. (a) (PE; AN; PA; GD)

1 The toddler is still attempting to distinguish himself as separate from his parents.

3 The toddler is still learning from his own experience; he is at the level of parallel, not interactive, play.

4 Older siblings often are not good role models because they tend to be careless.

257. **4** This will give the child adequate time to adjust and prepare for the surgery without presenting it too far in advance. (b) (PE; PL; ED; GD)

1 This is appropriate for a toddler.

2 This is too far in advance; the child will forget or build up a great deal of fear.

3 Same as # 2.

258. **4** Palpation would create a risk of rupturing the tumor mass. (b) (PE; IM; TC; RG)

1 There is no related contraindication for IV medication.

2 Diapers can be worn as long as there is no palpation.

3 This is unnecessary; no calculi are present.

259. **1** Because the tumor is of renal origin, the renin-angiotensin mechanism can be involved and blood pressure monitoring is very important. (c) (PE; PL; TC; RG)

2 This could put pressure on the involved area, causing rupture of the tumor and seeding of cancer cells.

3 Same as # 2.

4 This is unnecessary; no infection is present.

260. **2** Between the ages of 3 and 5 years, death is viewed as a departure or sleep, which is reversible. (c) (PE; AN; PE; GD)

1 This occurs at 9 or 10 years of age; death is viewed as reversible by the preschooler.

3 Children of all ages have some concept of death.

4 The early school-age child of 6 or 7 years personifies death and sees it as horrible and frightening; this is consistent with the concrete thinking present at this age.

261. **3** This moves from clean to dirty and keeps microorganisms away from the urinary meatus to prevent an ascending infection. (b) (PE; EV; ED; RG)

1 Fluid should be encouraged to maintain urinary function and prevent urinary stasis.

2 Contact sports should be avoided to prevent trauma to the remaining kidney.

4 This is not necessary; the child's immune system is not depressed.

262. **2** The opportunity must be provided for the client to practice language skills; family participation must be accepted and recognized. (a) (ME; IM; PA; NM)

1 This demeans the spouse and cuts off communication.

3 Same as # 1.

4 This is contraindicated; the spouse should be involved in the client's care.

263. **1** Clients with left-sided hemianopsia ignore whatever is in the left field of vision. (c) (ME; EV; PA; NM)

2 This would occur if the client had right hemianopsia and wished to see what he was eating.

3 This would occur with right hemiparesis, not with hemianopsia.

4 Indicates hemiparesis, not hemianopsia.

264. **1** Placing the walker flat on the floor provides stability; putting weight on the walker equalizes weight bearing on upper and lower extremities. (b) (ME; IM; ED; SK)

2 It is not possible to move the walker and have it bear weight at the same time; walker should be flat on the ground when stepping forward.

3 This is unsafe; this places the walker too far in front of the client for safe transfer of body weight.

4 All four points of the walker should be flat on ground when the client is stepping forward.

265. **3** Safety becomes a priority when the client has hemiparesis and hemianopsia. (b) (ME; PL; ED; NM)

1 Although a balance between activity and rest is important, the client does not have to maintain bedrest.

2 All the basic four nutrients should be included in the diet; there is no need to reduce protein intake.

4 Oxygen is generally unnecessary.

266. **3** A 6-year-old should have resolved the developmental task of initiative vs guilt. (a) (PS; AN; ED; BA)

1 Resolution of identity vs role diffusion occurs at adolescence.

2 Resolution of intimacy vs isolation occurs at adulthood.

4 This is part of Maslow's hierarchy of needs; the need for love and belonging arises once physical and safety needs are met.

267. **2** Excessive motor activity with intermittent head banging is self-destructive behavior that can result in injury. (a) (PS; AN; TC; BA)

1 This is not the most important nursing diagnosis according to the data presented; prevention of self-injury is primary.

3 Same as # 1.

4 Same as # 1.

268. **1** All nursing care is directed toward preventing injury, particularly with a self-destructive client. (b) (PS; PL; TC; BA)

2 Although this is important, prevention of injury is the priority.

3 Same as # 2.

4 Same as # 2.

269. **2** An increased attention span in school indicates that the child has improved. (b) (PS; EV; PE; BA)

1 A child of age six is not usually enuretic at night even without hyperactivity; there is no data to indicate enuresis in this situation.

3 This would indicate that the child has not made sufficient progress to be ready for discharge.

4 This would indicate that the child has not made progress because children should enjoy playing with peers at this age.

270. **2** Phobias are specific fears that serve as a means of coping with generalized anxiety. (b) (PS; AN;

PE; AX)

1 Anxiety, not depression, is related to phobias; finding a direct connection to life events is often difficult.

3 Anxiety, not obsession, is related to phobias.

4 A direct connection to life events is often difficult to find.

271. **3** This is a realistic essential first step; the problem and related feelings must be thoroughly explored before solutions can be developed. (a) (PS; AN; PE; AX)

1 This would be a long-term goal.

2 Same as # 1.

4 This is an inappropriate goal; a direct connection to life events is often difficult to find.

272. **4** This is not uncommon in breech presentation because the contracting uterus exerts pressure on the lower colon, forcing out the meconium. (c) (OB; AS; PA; IP)

1 This would not only be unusual with a breech position but also ominous, because it may be an indication of fetal distress.

2 This is not observable during usual external monitoring; the fetus would have to be attached to a special ECG apparatus.

3 Mild vaginal show is expected; heavy flow might indicate abruptio placentae or placenta previa.

273. **2** Because of increased blood loss associated with cesarean delivery, the client should be well hydrated before surgery to maintain adequate blood volume. (c) (OB; PL; PA; IP)

1 Only routine monitoring of vital signs is necessary unless there has been some indication of infection or PIH.

3 Unless the fetus is extremely premature or in distress, there is no reason for admission to the neonatal ICU.

4 This is not relevant; just before surgery is done, the skin will be cleansed.

274. **2** Abdominal surgery, especially pelvic surgery, predisposes the client to the risk of hemorrhage. (b) (OB; AN; TC; PP)

1 An impaired gas exchange would be an appropriate diagnosis for a client who is immobilized.

3 The position of the fetus is unrelated to tissue perfusion.

4 Regional anesthesia is related to impaired physical mobility and sensory-perceptual alterations, not altered tissue perfusion.

275. **2** By dealing with his or her own emotions first, the nurse can be more sensitive to the needs of the client. (c) (OB; AS; PE; EC)

1 Complete control is not, and should not, be the goal of the nurse.

3 The focus should be on the client's feelings, not the nurse's.

4 A time of crisis is not the time to teach; the client is not ready to learn.

276. **4** This response encourages the client to discuss her fears and anxieties. (a) (OB; IM; PE; EC)

1 This response does not focus on the client's feelings; it cuts off communication between the nurse and the client.

2 This is false reassurance; it denies the client's feelings and cuts off communication.

3 This gives inaccurate information; this conclusion has not been documented, and this response adds to the guilt felt by the client.

277. **4** The cerebellum is involved in synergistic control of the skeletal muscles and the coordination of voluntary movement. (a) (SU; AN; PA; NM)

1 Basal ganglia are concerned with large subconscious movements and muscle tone; damage here may cause paralysis as in stroke, or involuntary movements and uncontrollable shaking as in Parkinson's disease.

2 The parietal lobe is concerned with localization and two-point discrimination; tumors here cause motor seizures and sensory function loss.

3 The occipital lobe is concerned with special sense perception; tumors here cause visual disturbances, visual agnosia, or hallucinations.

278. **4** Tomography provides a three-dimensional view of cranial contents and defines outlines of masses and other abnormalities. (a) (SU; AS; TC; NM)

1 Myelography is an x-ray examination of the spinal cord and vertebral canal, not the cranium.

2 Electromyography measures electrical currents produced by skeletal muscles, not the cranium.

3 This is not done; removal of CSF in the presence of increased intracranial pressure may cause compression of the brain stem.

279. **1** Shampooing is done carefully to avoid scratching the scalp, which would provide a portal of entry for microorganisms. (b) (SU; PL; TC; IT)

2 Narcotics are not used because of possible central nervous system depression.

3 Fluids are withheld preoperatively; they may also be restricted because of cerebral edema.

4 Enemas are contraindicated; the client should avoid straining because it increases intracranial pressure.

280. **2** Decadron is a corticosteroid with antiinflammatory effects. (a) (SU; EV; TC; DR)

1 Decadron will not keep the tumor from growing; it will only reduce fluid content and therefore cell size, not number.

3 Decadron does not promote fluid reabsorption, which is undesirable because it increases fluid retention and therefore cerebral edema.

4 Decadron does not promote sedation; sedation is not desired because it could mask symptoms.

281. **1** Euthanasia is a crime and is against the law in every state. (a) (SU; AN; PE; EC)

2 Euthanasia is against the law in all states.

3 Neither physicians nor nurses have the legal authority to perform acts of euthanasia; it is a crime.

4 This is not negligence; it is a crime.

How to Use Worksheet 1: Errors in Processing Information

Common errors in processing information are listed in the left-hand column of this worksheet. At the top of the worksheet is a row of blank spaces for inserting the number of the question missed. Directly below each number, check any errors you made in answering that question. You may have made more than one type of error in an answer.

Worksheet 1: Errors in processing information

Question number																				
Did not read situation/question carefully																				
Missed important details																				
Confused major and minor points																				
Defined problem incorrectly																				
Could not remember terms/facts/concepts/principles																				
Defined terms incorrectly																				
Focused on incomplete/incorrect data in assessing situation																				
Interpreted data incorrectly																				
Applied wrong concepts/principles in situation																				
Drew incorrect conclusions																				
Identified wrong goals																				
Identified priorities incorrectly																				
Carried out plan incorrectly/incompletely																				
Was unclear about criteria for evaluating success in achieving goals																				

How to Use Worksheet 2: Knowledge Gaps

Types of common knowledge gaps are listed along the top of this worksheet. Write a brief description of topics you want to review in the spaces provided. For example, if you missed a question on administration of a particular drug, write the drug name and problem (e.g., dosage) in the appropriate space under the column labeled *Pharmacology*.

Worksheet 2: Knowledge gaps

Basic science	Skills/ procedures	Basic human needs	Growth & develop- ment	Normal nutrition	Psycho- social factors	Clinical area/ topic	Stressors/ coping mechanisms	Patho- physiology	Pharma- cology	Therapeutic nutrition	Legal Implications	Other

Test 4

282. **3** Because the vagina has no sphincter, holding the labia permits the solution to enter, fill, and irrigate the vaginal vault. (b) (OB; IM; ED; PN)
    1 A bulb syringe should never be used because it may cause an air embolism.
    2 This is a possible position to empty the vaginal vault after the fluid has been instilled.
    4 The douche tip should never be inserted more than 3 inches during pregnancy.

283. **3** If carbohydrate intake is reduced, protein is utilized for energy, thereby lowering the recommended elevated protein requirements for pregnancy. (b) (OB; AN; PA; PN)
    1 Additional calories are needed to spare protein.
    2 This is not the reason for avoiding dieting during pregnancy.
    4 This is untrue.

284. **2** The placenta begins to age after term, and the fetus may be deprived of oxygen and nutrients. (c) (OB; AN; PA; HP)
    1 Usually these infants lose weight because of placental deprivation.
    3 Infection may be caused by premature rupture of membranes or a lack of sterile technique, not postmaturity.
    4 This is unrelated; maternal diabetes usually results in early delivery.

285. **4** These babies have been nutritionally deprived by placental insufficiency and put their fists in their mouths to try to satisfy their hunger. (a) (OB; AS; PA; HN)
    1 This is not present in the postmature infant but in the preterm infant.
    2 Postmature infants lose weight because of insufficient nutrition from the aging placenta.
    3 The postmature infant is alert and awake immediately after birth and tends to stay awake for long periods.

286. **3** Necrotic tissue and blood in an area that is moist, warm, and dark make an excellent culture media. (b) (OB; AN; ED; NN)
    1 The diaper is kept below the level of the umbilicus; although the site may be touched by clothing, the clothing should be 100% cotton to allow for drying of the cord.
    2 This is untrue; Wharton's jelly is present and provides a protective barrier.
    4 This is untrue; newborns carry antibodies from the mother.

287. **4** The newborn's intake of milk is gradual and small; at the same time he is emptying the bowel of meconium, thus a weight loss occurs. (b) (OB; AN; PA; NN)
    1 This is untrue; slight weight loss after delivery is a normal physiologic response.
    2 Same as # 1.
    3 Same as # 1.

288. **4** This is breast engorgement, which immediately precedes milk production on the second to fourth day postpartum. (b) (OB; AN; PA; PP)
    1 This is impossible because the breasts have not filled with milk yet; engorgement is occurring.
    2 Milk production has not yet begun; this is engorgement, which precedes milk production.
    3 Acini cells do not become overdistended because of the supply-and-demand nature of milk pro-duction; in addition, milk production is not yet established; the client is engorged.

289. **4** Rest is required during active inflammation of the joints to prevent injury; once active inflamation has receded, an activity and exercise regimen can begin. (a) (ME; AN; TC; SK)
    1 The extent of the arthritis is not the determinant; whether the process is in exacerbation or remission is the deciding factor.
    2 Although this is true, physical therapy is not performed during acute exacerbation of the arthritis.
    3 This is untrue; physical therapy would not be prescribed during a period of exacerbation.

290. **2** ASA is irritating to the stomach lining and can cause ulceration; the presence of food, fluid, or antacids decreases this response. (a) (ME; IM; ED; DR)
    1 Tylenol does not contain the antiinflammatory properties present in aspirin; tinnitus should be reported to the physician.
    3 This should be reported to the physician, not the dentist.
    4 This is unnecessary as long as aspirin is taken with food.

291. **1** The need for acceptance of life as fulfilling and meaningful is the major task of the elderly. (b) (ME; AN; ED; GD)
    2 This is the task of adulthood (21 to 45 years); it involves establishment of a family and guiding of next generation.
    3 The task of the adolescent (12 to 20 years) is establishing identity through work and development of relationships and occupation.
    4 This is the task of young adulthood (18 to 25 years); it involves establishment of an intimate relationship and occupation.

292. **1** Flexion and extension prevents tightening of muscles and tendons. (b) (ME; PL; ED; SK)
    2 This is the result of cerebellar changes; it is not related to immobility.
    3 This is an abnormal sensation and is related to neurologic, not musculoskeletal, alterations.
    4 Weightbearing, not exercise, would promote the development of osteoblasts.

293. **2** Aging causes reduction in skin lubrication that results in dry skin. (a) (ME; PL; PA; IT)
    1 This influences how much assistance is necessary, not the frequency of bathing.
    3 This influences safety factors applicable during the bath, not the frequency of bathing.
    4 This influences what bath products may be used, not the frequency of bathing.

294. **1** This encourages tissue regeneration and prevents creation of a moist area conducive to infection. (a) (ME; PL; TC; IT)
    2 A high-caloric diet is appropriate to provide energy for tissue repair.
    3 This creates a warm, moist, protein-containing medium that is ideal for growing pathogens.
    4 Placing the client in one position will promote development of additional decubitus ulcers.

295. **4** Preadolescents and young adolescents are most at risk and can be most successfully treated. (a) (PE; PL; TC; SK)
    1 Scoliosis would not be identifiable in children of this age.

2 Some students with scoliosis might be identified, but it may be too late for adequate treatment.

3 80% of clients with idiopathic scoliosis are pre-adolescents and young adolescents, not pre-schoolers.

296. **4** This is the correct definition. (a) (PE; AN; PA; SK)

1 There are no pathologic changes in the vertebrae.

2 This is a description of lordosis.

3 This is a description of kyphosis.

297. **2** An exercise program and the Milwaukee brace are the treatments of choice for mild structural scoliosis. (b) (PE; IM; ED; SK)

1 Exercises alone are used only with scoliosis that is related to posture, not structure.

3 Exercises are to be encouraged regardless of the type of scoliosis.

4 Although compliance will affect the ultimate outcome of treatment, exercises alone are not helpful in this type of scoliosis.

298. **2** Properly chosen clothes can minimize the appearance of the brace, especially if an effort is made to keep up with the current styles. (a) (PE; IM; PE; EC)

1 There is no data to indicate that the child will not adjust to the treatment regimen.

3 This has a negative connotation that emphasizes the client's problem.

4 This may be misinterpreted as false praise, and a trusting nurse-client relationship may not develop.

299. **3** Reapplication destroys any surviving ova (nits). (a) (PE; IM; ED; IT)

1 Personal items can be soaked in pediculicidal solution; clothing and linen should be laundered in hot water and dried in a hot drier.

2 Once the hair has been shampooed, there is no reason to isolate the child.

4 This is untrue; excessive use can cause an eczematous rash and central nervous system disturbances.

300. **1** Transmission occurs through direct contact with infected individuals and indirect contact with contaminated articles; crowded conditions aid transmission. (a) (PE; IM; ED; IT)

2 Pediculosis can also be transmitted by contact with infested clothing, personal articles, or bedding.

3 All socioeconomic groups are equally affected.

4 Lice are not carried or transmitted by household pets.

301. **4** This statement focuses on the client's perceptions and promotes further communication. (c) (PE; IM; PE; EC)

1 This statement is valid but accusatory; it discourages further communication.

2 This reads too much into the client's statement and may be too emotionally charged.

3 This is untrue; there is a higher incidence of lice in people with poor personal hygiene.

302. **4** The nurse provides support in a nonjudgmental way by sharing information and observations about the child. (c) (PS; IM; PE; BA)

1 This is false reassurance that does not provide support; the mother recognizes something is wrong.

2 This indirectly indicates that the parent may be

at fault; it negates the mother's need for support and increases her sense of guilt.

3 Same as # 2.

303. **4** Autistic children relate best with objects, which can be used as a bridge in interpersonal relationships; this begins at the child's level. (b) (PS; IM; PE; BA)

1 Autistic children will not initiate contact or interactions.

2 Autistic children usually have difficulty tolerating being touched.

3 Autistic children often become agitated when movement is restricted and personal space is invaded.

304. **3** The autistic child needs protection from self-injury. (b) (PS; IM; TC; BA)

1 The autistic child has difficulty following directions, especially when out of control.

2 The autistic child cannot separate herself from her behavior; a punitive approach will decrease the child's self-esteem.

4 This can only be permitted if it does not place the child in jeopardy.

305. **1** This is the most complete definition of bulimia. (b) (PS; AN; PE; BA)

2 This may occur with bulimia, but it is not the definition.

3 Same as # 2.

4 Although clients with bulimia do consume large amounts of food in private, they do eat in public.

306. **1** Individuals with bulimia have many unmet dependency needs that they attempt to meet by the use of food. (c) (PS; AS; PE; BA)

2 Individuals with bulimia talk freely about their problems, though the discussion is usually on a superficial level.

3 Individuals with bulimia tend to be unable to make decisions; though they may appear obstinate at times, there is no rigidity of character.

4 Individuals with bulimia tend to be extroverted rather than demonstrating a flattened affect.

307. **3** Bulimia is characterized by the binge-purge cycle; most clients withdraw from others and vomit after an eating binge. (b) (PS; AS; TC; BA)

1 Although individuals with bulimia may hoard food, this behavior frequently occurs later, when limits are put on their intake.

2 Although some individuals with bulimia may perform excessive exercises, this is a more common finding with the diagnosis of anorexia nervosa.

4 Most individuals with bulimia do not seek support or socialization after a binge, though they may socialize at other times.

308. **2** The nurse should be alert for dehydration caused by fluid loss through vomiting in the binge-purge cycle. (b) (PS; AS; TC; BA)

1 Hyperglycemia would not be expected because of the vomiting that follows a binge.

3 Hyperactivity would not be expected because most individuals with bulimia withdraw and vomit after a binge.

4 Weight gain would not be expected because of the purging that usually follows a binge.

309. **3** This is the only way the nurse can be certain of the amount of food and fluid vomited. (c) (PS; PL; TC; BA)

1 An accurate intake and output is difficult to

maintain unless the individual is closely observed.

2 Weighing daily would not help to assess the individual's electrolyte or nutritional status.

4 Searching for hoarded food establishes a negative relationship and documents lack of trust.

310. **2** Bed rest with the leg extended prevents trauma caused by hip flexion and provides time for the insertion site to heal. (b) (SU; PL; ED; CV)

1 Mild sedation and local infiltration are used for adults; the client is conscious.

3 With the femoral approach, bed rest is maintained for several hours.

4 The physician will thoroughly review test results and may consult other physicians before answering.

311. **1** When neither rest nor nitroglycerin relieves the pain, there may be acute myocardial infarction. (a) (SU; IM: ED; CV)

2 This is expected; anginal pain can, and often does, radiate.

3 This is expected; acute myocardial infarction causes profuse, not mild, diaphoresis, which should be reported.

4 This is expected; activity increases cardiac output, causing angina.

312. **2** Informed consent means the client must comprehend the surgery, the alternatives, and the consequences. (b) (SU; IM; TC; CV)

1 This explanation is not within nursing's domain.

3 The nurse's signature documents the client has given informed consent; however, this follows after the nurse determines the client's comprehension.

4 This is true, but it does not determine the client's ability to give informed consent.

313. **4** More than 80% of those who have this surgery have marked relief of their symptoms. (c) (SU; AN; ED; CV)

1 So far, studies have failed to show that bypass surgery affects life span.

2 The surgery itself does not affect the disease process; clients must also reduce risk factors (obesity, smoking, and poor diet).

3 This depends on the client's presurgical condition and occupation, not the surgery itself.

314. **1** Clients should be familiar with these people and hear from them what will be experienced. (b) (SU; PL; ED; CV)

2 Most clients do not want or need a minutely detailed description.

3 Although discharge plans should be mentioned, they are not the primary focus at this time.

4 The client's whole body, not just the specific area, will be prepped and shaved.

315. **3** These arrhythmias may result from postoperative inflammation around the SA node area. (c) (SU; EV; TC; CV)

1 This syndrome occurs later, not immediately.

2 Same as # 1.

4 Hemoglobin and hematocrit levels usually fall; anemia can be a problem.

316. **2** Because the client is up more at home, edema usually increases. (c) (SU; IM; ED; CV)

1 Serosanguinous drainage will persist after discharge.

3 These symptoms will persist longer, because it takes 6 to 12 weeks for the sternum to heal.

4 These should not be expected and are in fact signs of postpericardotomy syndrome.

317. **3** Abrupt discontinuation of Inderal may cause an acute myocardial infarction. (b) (SU; IM; ED; DR)

1 Alcohol is contraindicated for clients taking Inderal.

2 The pulse rate can go much lower as long as the client feels well and is not dizzy.

4 Clients should never increase medications without a physician's direction.

318. **2** Delivery is imminent; contamination will be minimized by catching the infant on a clean surface. (b) (OB; AN; TC; IP)

1 Panting will hold back the infant and exhaust the mother.

3 This is not the priority; delivery is imminent.

4 It is too late; the nurse is capable of assisting the mother and should remain with her.

319. **3** This prevents too rapid expulsion of the head, which can lead to increased intracranial pressure in the infant and a perineal laceration in the mother. (c) (OB; IM; TC; IP)

1 This is unnecessary; precipitate delivery is caused by forceful uterine contractions that expel uterine contents.

2 At this time the urge to push is uncontrollable and she will be unable to take prolonged deep breaths.

4 Vigorous pushing will cause too rapid expulsion, leading to increased intracranial pressure in the infant and laceration in the mother.

320. **1** The sudden change of pressure tends to tear away the dural linings. (c) (OB; AN; PA; HN)

2 This occurs before delivery and is unrelated to precipitate labor; this may occur in placenta previa or abruptio placentae.

3 This occurs normally during labor as the baby's head descends into the birth canal.

4 Although this could occur, the placenta usually is expelled shortly after the fetus.

321. **4** Immature thermoregulation necessitates keeping the infant warm to prevent acidosis. (c) (OB; IM; TC; NN)

1 It is too soon to evaluate hemorrhagic condition of the mother; the placenta has not yet been delivered.

2 There is no hurry; as soon as the infant breathes, the umbilical cord no longer functions.

3 There is no hurry; the placenta may not separate for 30 minutes without danger.

322. **2** Suckling will induce neural stimulation of the posterior pituitary gland, which in turn will release pitocin and cause uterine contractions. (b) (OB; IM; PA; IP)

1 This will not help if the uterus is not contracting.

3 If the placenta is still attached to the uterine wall, this may disconnect the cord from the placenta.

4 This could cause a uterine prolapse.

323. **4** This is the most frequent route of transmission. (b) (OB; AN; PA; HN)

1 There is no evidence of toxoplasmosis being transmitted via this route.

2 Same as # 1.

3 The genital tract is not locally affected.

324. **3** Growth retardation is evident and common in

infants with toxoplasmosis. (c) (OB; AS; PA; HN)

1 This is a normal assessment in a healthy neonate.

2 Same as # 1.

4 This is a normal characteristic in the dark-pigmented neonate.

325. **3** Fever, malaise, and headache may accompany local reactions. (b) (ME; AS; ED; RG)

1 This is of viral origin; there is no cure, and antibiotics are ineffective.

2 Vesicles on genitalia rupture, causing very painful ulcerations.

4 This is uncommon, but a virus can survive for short periods of time on fomites.

326. **1** The initial attack is both local and systemic; recurrent attacks are milder and localized. (a) (ME; IM; ED; RG)

2 Although good health habits may limit recurrence, they will not totally prevent it.

3 There is recurrence in 50% of clients.

4 Recurrent attacks are precipitated by physical and emotional stress, not by sexual activity.

327. **2** Liberal fluid intake will prevent crystal formation. (a) (ME; EV; ED; DR)

1 Phenazopyridine is expected to give the urine a red-orange color.

3 Antacids will interfere with the absorption of sulfisoxazole.

4 Although the urine should be observed for crystals, straining is not necessary.

328. **2** These are measurable responses to therapy and are the desired outcomes. (b) (ME; EV; TC; RG)

1 This is too much; it is approximately double the amount that is necessary.

3 No dietary restrictions are necessary.

4 There is no need to limit activities.

329. **1** An acid ash diet, including cranberries, lowers the pH of the urine and discourages pathogenic growth. (a) (ME; AN; ED; RG)

2 The glomerular filtration rate is not affected.

3 An acid medium will discourage further growth but will not kill existing organisms.

4 Acid urine does not soothe bladder walls.

330. **2** Voiding flushes the lower portion of the urinary tract of microorganisms introduced during intercourse. (c) (ME; PL; ED; RG)

1 Most citric juices will increase the alkalinity of the urine, promoting bacterial growth.

3 This promotes the transfer of microorganisms to the urethra, where they could ascend to the bladder.

4 When used correctly, tampons do not increase the risk of cystitis.

331. **2** This answers the client's question and provides an accurate description of a cystoscopy. (a) (SU; AN; ED; RG)

1 No dye is used.

3 This is not a computerized examination.

4 This procedure does not involve x-ray films or dye.

332. **3** Withdrawn clients can tolerate personal contact only for short periods of time. (b) (PS; PL; PE; SD)

1 The client could not function in this type of group.

2 The client has a problem with interpersonal relations, therefore this would not work.

4 Allowing the client to be alone would not relieve

anxiety; it would foster withdrawal.

333. **4** Neologisms are newly coined words with personal meanings to the client with schizophrenia. (b) (PS; AN; PE; SD)

1 Clanging is the association of words by sound rather than meaning.

2 Echolalia is parrot-like echoing of spoken words or sounds.

3 Echophrasia (echolalia) is parrot-like echoing of spoken words or sounds.

334. **1** The nursing goal is to keep the client oriented by involving her in activities with other people; even though the client probably could not follow any game rules, the activity provides involvement with the nurse. (c) (PS; IM; TC; SD)

2 This would have no effect on the client's behavior.

3 This is not therapeutic and implies that the client is actually talking to someone.

4 This is not therapeutic and allows the client to withdraw further rather than orienting her to reality.

335. **4** The tranquilizer helps control anxiety and acting-out behavior, making the client more approachable. (c) (PS; AN; TC; DR)

1 Although the medication may produce this effect, it is not the primary purpose of administration.

2 Same as # 1.

3 Same as # 1.

336. **1** This statement attempts to understand the symbolism, reflects and acknowledges the client's feelings, and helps to preserve ego integrity. (c) (PS; IM; PE; SD)

2 This validates the client's delusion and does not test reality.

3 This is false reassurance; the nurse cannot fully understand the symbolism and therefore cannot make this promise.

4 This rejects the client's feelings; it does not address the client's fears of being harmed.

337. **3** The intestine is obstructed by thick, tenacious, pasty meconium. (b) (PE; AS; PA; EN)

1 This is common in most newborns because of destruction of immature erythrocytes; it may be physiologic or pathologic.

2 A rapid respiratory rate is normal in infants; respirations accelerate with movement and crying.

4 Imperforate anus is a congenital malformation in which the anal opening is obliterated; it is not associated with cystic fibrosis

338. **1** Nutrients such as protein, carbohydrates, and fats are not digested and are not properly absorbed by the intestinal mucosa. (b) (PE; AN; PA; EN)

2 It is not the retention of carbon dioxide, but the deprivation of nutrients and oxygen to all body cells that retards physical growth.

3 There is no evidence that the child has an atrial ventricular defect.

4 These children lose high concentrations of sodium and chloride in perspiration.

339. **1** Treatment is done several hours after meals to avoid regurgitation and several hours before meals so that unpleasant odor and taste do not affect eating. (b) (PE; PL; PA; RE)

2 Postural drainage should not be done before meals because the unpleasant odor and taste will

interfere with eating.
3 Treatment is done more frequently than this.
4 Same as # 3.

340. **3** Impaired fat absorption necessitates lowering dietary fat; more calories are needed because of poor absorption of nutrients. (c) (PE; PL; PA; EN)
1 A high-carbohydrate diet is correct, but because salt depletion via sweating is a hazard, children are encouraged to use salt generously.
2 A high-protein diet is recommended, but fat must be avoided because fat absorption is impaired.
4 A low-fat diet is recommended, but these children need high-salt diets to replace the large amount of salt lost by sweating.

341. **3** A 2½-year-old is capable of fitting large wooden pieces into the puzzle; this activity challenges the child's ability to recognize shapes. (b) (PE; PL; ED; GD)
1 This is a toy suitable for the young infant.
2 Same as # 1.
4 This is more appropriate for the child of 12 months who is becoming adept at motor skills.

342. **4** Hot climates are contraindicated for children with cystic fibrosis because sweating brings about excessive loss of sodium chloride. (c) (PE; EV; ED; EN)
1 This is advisable because it will keep the child from sweating.
2 Pancreatic enzymes are essential to help digest the nutrients so that they can be absorbed by the intestinal mucosa.
3 After passage of the feces associated with this disorder, the rectum may become inflamed if not properly cleaned.

343. **3** The client's measured output is about 400 ml in 24 hours based on the available history; insensible losses are 400 to 500 ml in 24 hours. (c) (ME; AN; PA; FE)
1 Based on the history, the client's expected urinary output should be about 400 ml in the next 24 hours; this is far less than 900 ml.
2 This is insufficient fluid to help prevent hypostatic pneumonia; fluid intake is only one of many factors involved.
4 Hyperkalemia in acute renal failure is caused by inadequate glomerular filtration and is not related to fluid intake.

344. **3** Vital signs monitor cardiorespiratory status; hyperkalemia can cause serious cardiac arrhythmias that must be treated. (c) (ME; EV; TC; FE)
1 The cardiac arrest team is always on alert and will respond when called for a cardiac arrest.
2 The priority is medical attention, and the physician should be notified immediately.
4 A repeat laboratory test would take time and probably reaffirm the original results.

345. **4** Insulin causes an increased rate of flow of potassium into the cells, which will then reduce the circulating blood levels of potassium. (c) (ME; AN; PA; FE)
1 Insulin will not lower the metabolic rate.
2 This response halts communication and is nonsupportive.
3 Blood sugar levels are usually not elevated in clients with acute renal failure.

346. **1** Dialysis removes chemicals, wastes, and fluids usually removed from the body by the kidneys. (a) (SU; IM; PA; RG)
2 This is a threatening response and can cause an increase in client's level of anxiety.
3 The mention of heart problems is a threatening response and may cause increased fear or anxiety.
4 Dialysis does not speed recovery; it helps maintain fluid and electrolyte balance.

347. **3** Turning from side to side will change the position of the catheter, thereby freeing its drainage holes, which may be obstructed. (b) (SU; IM; TC; RG)
1 Taking fluids into the gastrointestinal tract does not influence the drainage of dialysate from the peritoneal cavity.
2 This improves pulmonary ventilation and helps in maintaining comfort but does not improve the flow of dialysate from the catheter.
4 The position of the catheter should be changed only by the physician.

348. **1** Heat promotes vasodilation, which aids shift of urea, a large molecular substance, from blood vessels into the dialyzing solution. (c) (SU; AN; PA; RG)
2 Heat does not affect the shift of potassium into the cells.
3 The removal of metabolic wastes is affected in renal failure; this does not affect the metabolic processes themselves.
4 Excess serum potassium is removed by dialyzing with a potassium-free solution, not by heat.

349. **3** In the diuretic phase, fluid retained during the oliguric phase is excreted and hypovolemia may occur. (c) (ME; AS; PA; RG)
1 This develops in the oliguric phase when glomerulofiltration is poor.
2 Same as # 1.
4 Diuresing is an indication of improved renal functioning, not progression into failure.

350. **3** This is a noninvasive, relatively harmless way to visualize the location of the placenta. (b) (OB; AN; PA; HP)
1 This is used for removing amniotic fluid for diagnosis and fetal evaluation, not for placenta previa.
2 This is an invasive surgical procedure used for diagnostic purposes other than the location of the placenta.
4 This is a visualization of the amniotic fluid via vaginal examination; it is contraindicated because it may detach the placenta.

351. **3** Because normal implantation occurs in the upper third of the uterus, a low-lying placenta would be an abnormal implantation. (b) (OB; EV; PA; HP)
1 Abruptio placentae is the premature separation of a normally implanted placenta.
2 Placenta previa usually occurs with a fully developed, normal placenta that is abnormally located.
4 Infarctions may appear on a placenta because of some interference with the blood supply; this is not related to position.

352. **2** This response presents facts that help to reduce guilt. (b) (OB; IM; PE; EC)
1 This is an inadequate explanation and gives the client no idea of what is happening.

3 This is untrue, and labor may not be beginning at this time.

4 This is very unreassuring, as well as incorrect, because placenta previa can occur in a woman with a normal uterus.

353. **4** Rhythmic uterine contractions are positive signs of beginning labor. (b) (OB; AS; PA; HP)

1 This has no relation to the onset of labor; it is more likely a sign of further placental separation.

2 This is not a sign of labor but a sign of fetal distress that demands medical attention.

3 This is not a sign of labor; it may indicate that placental separation has ceased.

354. **4** Lack of remorse indicates weak superego, the aspect of personality concerned with prohibitions. (b) (PS; AN; PE; PR)

1 This aspect of personality is not underdeveloped.

2 The ego is not related to acting-out behavior.

3 Same as # 1.

355. **3** Limit setting must be consistent with a client who is using manipulative behavior; a unified approach is vital because the client will play the staff against each other. (a) (PS; IM; PE; PR)

1 This must be a group decision, not the responsibility of one staff member alone; the client is unable to set limits on herself.

2 Limit setting is required to control inappropriate behavior.

4 The most important concept is unity of approach, not degree of manipulation.

356. **2** When action on either side of a conflict creates anxiety, a physical reason for not acting at all may unconsciously be used. (c) (PS; AN; PE; AX)

1 These individuals do not enjoy their illness; their anxiety is relieved by it.

3 These individuals are in contact with reality.

4 These disorders are disabling; the client truly believes the symptoms are real.

357. **4** The symptoms prevent the individual from being forced to move in either direction on the conflict; symptoms thus reduce anxiety and remove the conflict. (b) (PS; AS; PE; AX)

1 The individual is not frightened or upset because the symptoms relieve the anxiety.

2 The individual is not happy and cheerful but is relieved by the reduction in anxiety.

3 The individual is not sad and depressed but is relieved by the reduction in anxiety.

358. **1** Discussion should not be initiated by the nurse; symptoms should be accepted but should not be the focus of discussion. (c) (PS; PL; TC; AX)

2 This response would increase anxiety because it focuses on unconscious feelings about the paralysis.

3 This response would increase anxiety and deny the client's symptoms; in reality this client cannot make herself walk.

4 This response would increase anxiety and take away the client's unconscious defense.

359. **3** Individuals who have somatoform disorders are really ill; they need care and a nonthreatening environment. (c) (PS; PL; TC; AX)

1 The client requires physiologic and emotional care; without movement, venous stasis and atrophy of the "paralyzed" limbs can occur.

2 Same as # 1.

4 The client is ill and requires good physical and emotional care.

360. **2** The complications of diabetes, along with those of aging, account for a higher incidence of chronic complications. (b) (ME; AN; PA; EN)

1 The incidence of chronic complications is higher in those with adult-onset diabetes.

3 The onset of adult diabetes is usually slow, whereas in juveniles it is sudden and dramatic.

4 Adults with NIDDM do secrete endogenous insulin, but secretion is slow and subnormal.

361. **2** Diabetic retinopathy is characterized by neovascularization. (b) (ME; AS; PA; EN)

1 Arthritic changes of the hand are not a usual complication associated with diabetes mellitus.

3 Peripheral vascular disease is indicated by dependent rubor and pallor on elevation.

4 Clients who are diabetic have peripheral neuropathy, which is characterized by hypoactive reflexes.

362. **2** With diabetic ketoacidosis, serum lipid levels can go so high that the serum appears opalescent and creamy. (c) (ME; AS; PA; EN)

1 With diabetic ketoacidosis the BUN is generally elevated because of dehydration.

3 This is unrelated to diabetic ketoacidosis.

4 With diabetic ketoacidosis the hematocrit is generally elevated because of dehydration.

363. **2** An open wound needs sterile technique, and these supplies are not sterile. (b) (SU; IM; TC; IT)

1 This is unsafe, a clean basin and washcloth are not sterile.

3 This is irrelevant; client safety is a priority.

4 This is unnecessary; the physician has already indicated the type of soak desired.

364. **4** Elevation in the first 24 hours helps prevent edema; continued elevation may lead to hip contractures. (a) (SU; PL; PA; SK)

1 The stump dressing is usually changed at least twice a day; this can be done by the nurse.

2 The client is usually taken out of bed on the second postoperative day.

3 Hemorrhage and infection are the two most common complications.

365. **2** There is better control with short-acting (regular) insulin, and emergencies can be handled more quickly. (c) (SU; AN; PA; EN)

1 This is untrue; the level of glucose must be maintained as close to normal as possible.

3 This is untrue; the occurrence is greater when the client is receiving exogenous insulin.

4 This is not the reason for using regular insulin; both oral hypoglycemics and insulin are available.

366. **4** This response acknowledges and reflects the client's feelings and encourages further communication. (b) (SU; IM; PE; EC)

1 This is true, but telling the client this serves no therapeutic purpose at this time.

2 The nurse does not know how the client's family feels; this response takes the focus off the client.

3 This response negates the client's feelings.

367. **4** A nasogastric tube is used postoperatively to decompress the stomach and limit tension on the suture line. (b) (PE; IM; TC; GI)

1 Vomiting indicates obstruction of the nasogastric tube; the initial action should be to check the patency of the nasogastric tube.

2 To limit pressure on the suture line, oral feedings should not be used in the immediate postoperative period when the gastric tube is in place.

3 This is too soon for signs of infection to occur.

368. **3** Previous experiences with projectile vomiting are frightening; an explanation that surgery has eliminated this, as well as support and encouragement of the parents as they resume care of their infant, are necessary. (a) (PE; EV; PE; EC)

1 Not used initially, oral feedings are reinstituted with clear liquids and electrolytes and progressing to formula as tolerated.

2 No special nipple is required; these are used for infants with cleft lip and/or palate.

4 This is untrue; the data indicates the mother is eager to assist with other aspects of care.

369. **4** This is an autosomal-recessive disorder; each parent contributes one affected gene. (b) (PE; AN; PA; BI)

1 There is only a 50% chance that a child will have the sickle cell trait, not sickle cell anemia.

2 Same as # 1.

3 All of the children from these parents will have the sickle cell trait but not sickle cell anemia.

370. **2** Oxygen limits further sickling and compensates for compromised oxygen transportation capacity of hemoglobin. (a) (PE; IM; TC; BI)

1 There is too much swelling and pain in the joints during a crisis for this intervention.

3 Increased hydration is necessary to promote hemodilution, improve circulation, and reverse sickling.

4 Cold will constrict blood vessels, further depleting oxygenation to affected parts; warmth is preferable.

371. **2** Strenuous exercise leads to increased cellular metabolism, causing tissue hypoxia, which can precipitate sickling. (b) (PE; EV; ED; BI)

1 This is detrimental to the developmental needs of a 6-year-old and may result in social isolation.

3 Fluid should never be restricted; keeping the child well hydrated helps to prevent sickling.

4 This is unnecessary unless the other children have an infectious disease; peer relationships should be encouraged.

372. **1** Discussion with parents who have children with similar problems helps to reduce some of their discomfort and guilt. (b) (PE; PL; PE; EC)

2 Some parents do not choose to avoid future pregnancies and should not be forced to do so.

3 When not in crisis, the child should be allowed to attend school and should not be developmentally damaged by social isolation.

4 There is no recommended therapeutic climate for these children, and moving may not be beneficial to the child or the family.

373. **3** Semi-Fowler's position will localize the spilled stomach contents in the lower part of the abdominal cavity. (b) (SU; IM; TC; GI)

1 This position will exert pressure on the abdomen, which may be uncomfortable for the client.

2 This position exerts pressure against the diaphragm, inhibits breathing, and intensifies discomfort.

4 Same as # 2.

374. **4** The nurse should auscultate the abdomen and listen for bowel sounds, which signify the passage of flatus. (a) (SU; IM; PA; GI)

1 The first bowel movement occurs after peristalsis returns and after food is eaten.

2 Peristalsis should return before the tenderness of the abdomen subsides.

3 Nausea may be present even though peristalsis has begun.

375. **1** Drainage is bright red initially and gradually becomes darker red during the first 24 hours. (b) (SU; EV; PA; GI)

2 If the nasogastric tube is functioning correctly, gastric distention will not occur.

3 If the nasogastric tube is functioning correctly, secretions will be removed and vomiting will not occur.

4 Because the bowel was emptied before surgery and the client is now npo, there would be no expected intestinal activity.

How to Use Worksheet 1: Errors in Processing Information

Common errors in processing information are listed in the left-hand column of this worksheet. At the top of the worksheet is a row of blank spaces for inserting the number of the question missed. Directly below each number, check any errors you made in answering that question. You may have made more than one type of error in an answer.

Worksheet 1: Errors in processing information

Question number																			
Did not read situation/question carefully																			
Missed important details																			
Confused major and minor points																			
Defined problem incorrectly																			
Could not remember terms/facts/concepts/principles																			
Defined terms incorrectly																			
Focused on incomplete/incorrect data in assessing situation																			
Interpreted data incorrectly																			
Applied wrong concepts/principles in situation																			
Drew incorrect conclusions																			
Identified wrong goals																			
Identified priorities incorrectly																			
Carried out plan incorrectly/incompletely																			
Was unclear about criteria for evaluating success in achieving goals																			

How to Use Worksheet 2: Knowledge Gaps

Types of common knowledge gaps are listed along the top of this worksheet. Write a brief description of topics you want to review in the spaces provided. For example, if you missed a question on administration of a particular drug, write the drug name and problem (e.g., dosage) in the appropriate space under the column labeled *Pharmacology*.

Worksheet 2: Knowledge gaps

Basic science	Skills/ procedures	Basic human needs	Growth & develop-ment	Normal nutrition	Psycho-social factors	Clinical area/ topic	Stressors/ coping mechanisms	Patho-physiology	Pharma-cology	Therapeutic nutrition	Legal implications	Other

Comprehensive Examination Two
Test 1

1. **2** In pregnancies in which the fetus has a neural tube defect, alpha fetoprotein leaks into the amniotic fluid, causing abnormally high levels; at 14 to 16 weeks there is a sufficient amount of amniotic fluid present. (c) (OB; AS; PA; PN)
   1 This is too early to safely obtain amniotic fluid.
   3 This is not the optimal time for diagnostic testing for birth defects; the optimal time for an amniocentesis is when the uterus enters the abdominal cavity: there is sufficient amniotic fluid available, and the fetus is still small.
   4 Same as # 3.

2. **3** Preventing infection and trauma are the priorities; rupture of the sac may lead to meningitis. (a) (OB; IM; TC; HN)
   1 This can be done before the infant leaves the delivery room; the priority is care of the sac.
   2 The Apgar reveals 9/10; there is no respiratory complication.
   4 The sac must be protected before this is done.

3. **2** This provides an accurate statement of why scalp veins are used in infants; other veins are not well developed for IV therapy. (b) (PE; IM; ED; CV)
   1 The absorption rate through a peripheral vein is the same regardless of placement.
   3 The infant will still need to be restrained to prevent her pulling out the IV or rolling over on it.
   4 Placement of the needle is not related to whether the solution is irritating; D5/E48 is not irritating to veins.

4. **2** Normal head circumference is 13 to 14 inches (33 to 35.5 cm) and about 1 inch greater than the chest circumference. (b) (PE; AS; PA; NM)
   1 The head is too large.
   3 Same as # 1.
   4 The chest circumference is within normal limits.

5. **3** Prevention of infection continues as a priority both before and after the repair of the sac. (b) (PE; PL; TC; NM)
   1 This is unrealistic; newborns lose weight in the first few days of life.
   2 This is not the priority at this time.
   4 A neurologically impaired infant would not be given sedatives because it would interfere with accurate assessment.

6. **4** Gastric returns would indicate correct placement. (a) (PE; IM; TC; GI)
   1 This could cause undue trauma regardless of where the tube is.
   2 Further assessment is necessary.
   3 This is unsafe until correct placement is verified; feeding could enter the lung if the tube is not in the stomach.

7. **3** The presenting clinical symptoms must be evaluated in light of a complete and detailed history of present and past episodes, life-style practices, and family history. (b) (ME; AS; PA; CV)
   1 This is insufficient by itself for diagnosis.
   2 A stress test would be dangerous at this point.
   4 Same as # 1.

8. **2** Changes in an ECG will reflect the area of the heart that has been damaged because of hypoxia. (a) (ME; AN; ED; CV)
   1 A stethoscope is used to detect heart sounds.
   3 Medical intervention such as cardioversion or cardiac medications, not an ECG, can alter heart rhythm; an ECG will reflect heart rhythm, not change it.
   4 This is accomplished through a stress test; this uses an ECG in conjunction with physical exercise.

9. **3** Multiple premature ventricular contractions can eventually fall on a T wave, causing ventricular fibrillation; this rhythm must be immediately interrupted with a drug that reduces cardiac irritability. (c) (ME; IM; TC; DR)
   1 This is unnecessary; a cardiac arrest has not occurred.
   2 This will not interrupt the arrhythmia.
   4 This is unsafe; the arrhythmia must immediately be interrupted.

10. **3** Both Lanoxin and Pronestyl decrease cardiac conduction, with resultant depression of the myocardium. (b) (ME; EV; TC; DR)
    1 These drugs do not influence respirations.
    2 These drugs do not influence the CNS.
    4 These drugs do not influence the body's reflexes.

11. **2** Peripheral muscular hypoxia precipitates carpopedal spasm in the presence of hypocalcemia. (b) (ME; AS; PA; FE)
    1 Although this sign indicates hypocalcemia, it is elicited by tapping over the facial nerve.
    3 This indicates thrombophlebitis when pain results from dorsiflexing the foot.
    4 This indicates the loss of position sense; swaying results when the client stands still with the feet close together and the eyes closed.

12. **4** Toxicity can result because the action of calcium ions is similar to that of digitalis. (c) (ME; AN; TC; DR)
    1 Calcium can be added to this solution.
    2 If calcium infiltrates, sloughing of tissue will result.
    3 Calcium cannot be added to solution containing carbonate or phosphate because a dangerous precipitation will occur.

13. **3** Cholesterol is an essential precursor of body substances such as vitamin D and steroid hormones; although some is synthesized by the body, a small amount is needed in the diet. (c) (ME; IM; ED; CV)
    1 Polyunsaturated fats come from vegetable sources; saturated fats come from animal sources, coconut oil, and palm oil.
    2 Same as # 1.
    4 The diet must contain some cholesterol, and this should come from plant sources.

14. **1** The caloric distribution of the "Prudent Diet" proposed by the American Heart Association is 30% fat (less than 10% saturated fat), 50% carbohydrates (35% complex carbohydrates), and 20% protein. (a) (ME; IM; ED; EC)
    2 This is untrue; this would be discouraging and encourages noncompliance.
    3 Fried foods are not advocated on the "Prudent Diet"; peanut oil is a mono-unsaturated fatty acid; these acids should not exceed 15% of the kilocalories of the diet.
    4 Same as # 2.

15. **1** Clients who have lost contact with reality can be assisted to reestablish contact by being provided structured activities. (b) (PS; PL; PE; MO)

2 This client is responding to voices, not reality; limit setting is reality oriented and is usually ineffective unless it involves directing the client to dismiss the voices.

3 Although this may decrease the hallucinations, it takes a long time to establish such a relationship and the client needs help now.

4 The client represents no immediate threat to herself or others; isolating the client would decrease her contact with reality and would most likely increase the hallucinations.

16. **4** This response provides feedback, which helps communication stay on track and demonstrates the nurse's interest in the client as a person. (b) (PS; IM; PE; MO)

1 This response would only increase the client's anxiety and anger; it may precipitate acting-out behavior.

2 Ignoring a client does not help the situation, nor does it demonstrate the nurse's interest or concern.

3 This response would not set limits but would create feelings of rejection.

17. **1** Quickness is used for safety; an attitude of concern may help to reduce client anxiety. (b) (PS; IM; TC; MO)

2 The client must be told why sedation is being used.

3 Same as # 2.

4 A client this upset would never agree; the client may harm herself or others and must be sedated.

18. **3** This drug suppresses activity in key regions of the subcortical area of the CNS; it also has antihistaminic and anticholinergic effects. (a) (PS; EV; TC; DR)

1 These symptoms are not associated with Vistaril.

2 Same as # 1.

4 Same as # 1.

19. **2** Decreased sodium intake can accelerate lithium retention, with subsequent toxicity. (c) (PS; IM; ED; DR)

1 This is unrelated to the administration of lithium.

3 Same as # 1.

4 Same as # 1.

20. **4** Weight gain may be indicative of fluid retention; renal problems have been reported with lithium therapy. (c) (PS; EV; TC; DR)

1 This has no relationship to the administration of lithium.

2 Same as # 1.

3 Same as # 1.

21. **4** Levels close to 2 mEq/liter are dangerously close to the toxic level; immediate action must be taken. (c) (PS; EV; TC; DR)

1 The level is dangerously high, and the priority is the immediate notification of the physician rather than continued monitoring.

2 The therapeutic range for lithium is 0.6 to 1.2 mEq/liter.

3 Same as # 2.

22. **1** Anemia may result because of the possible bone marrow depressant effect of this drug. (a) (ME; IM; TC; EN)

2 This would be unsafe; a physical examination and blood studies are necessary to determine the cause of the the client's symptoms.

3 An increase may result in toxic effects if the client is taking the maximum dose.

4 This is unsafe; this is not the role of the nurse.

23. **4** This limits edema in the operative area and promotes respirations. (b) (SU; IM; PA; EN)

1 This would promote edema in the operative area, and the edema could compromise respirations.

2 Same as # 1.

3 Same as # 1.

24. **3** Drainage flows by gravity. (c) (SU; EV; TC; EN)

1 Although this might be done, it does not take into consideration that drainage flows by gravity.

2 This is unsafe; this would interfere with the healing process.

4 This is unsafe; lifting and replacing dressing would contaminate the surgical site.

25. **4** Because of the anatomic position of the parathyroids, they may be accidentally removed during surgery. (c) (SU; EV; TC; EN)

1 This is unlikely; the thyroid is nearer to the trachea.

2 This is unlikely; the thoracic cavity is not entered.

3 This is unlikely; this usually results from a blunt blow.

26. **4** Hyperextension of the neck places tension on the suture line. (b) (SU; AN; PA; EN)

1 The cervical vertebrae are designed to flex and hyperextend; there should be no ill effects.

2 Hyperextension would not cause this.

3 Same as # 2.

27. **3** Pelvic examination would reveal dilation and effacement. (c) (OB; AS; PA; IP)

1 This indicates only the presence of estrogen in cervical mucus; determines ovulation, not true labor.

2 Contractions are also present with Braxton-Hicks contractions, which are not true labor.

4 This only differentiates between amniotic fluid and urine; rupture of the membranes can occur with or without the onset of true labor.

28. **2** According to Erikson, identity vs role confusion is the developmental conflict of the adolescent. (a) (OB; AN; ED; EC)

1 Ego integrity vs despair is the developmental conflict of the older adult.

3 Industry vs inferiority is the developmental conflict of the school-age child.

4 Intimacy vs isolation is the developmental conflict of the young adult.

29. **4** The iron needs of the adolescent are high because of growth requirements and often poor nutrition; needs are increased by the demands of pregnancy. (b) (OB; AS; PA; PN)

1 This is not common in pregnant adolescents.

2 Same as # 1.

3 Same as # 1.

30. **4** This reduces pressure on the cord, increasing oxygen to the fetus. (a) (OB; IM; TC; IP)

1 Although this may eventually be done, the priority is to relieve pressure on the cord.

2 Same as # 1.

3 This promotes placental perfusion but would not relieve pressure on the cord.

31. **2** Immediate delivery is necessary to prevent fetal

hypoxia and death. (a) (OB; PL; TC; HP)

1 This is unsafe; contractions would increase pressure on the cord, causing fetal hypoxia.

3 This is unsafe; the fetus is in distress, and immediate delivery is necessary.

4 This is unsafe; this would increase pressure on the cord.

32. **3** Newborn does not have intestinal flora to synthesize; vitamin K (Aquamephyton) increases prothrombin that is necessary for clotting. (b) (OB; AN; PA; NN)

1 This is not affected by vitamin K.

2 Same as # 1.

4 Same as # 1.

33. **2** Application of cold relieves discomfort, and the binder provides support and aids in pressure atrophy of acini cells so that no more milk will be produced. (c) (OB; IM; TC; PP)

1 Severe restriction of fluid will not prevent engorgement and might cause dehydration.

3 This is suitable for the engorged breastfeeding mother because it promotes comfort and stimulates milk production.

4 Same as # 3.

34. **3** The cusps of the valves may be fused or the infundibulum below may be hypertrophied, thus restricting blood flow to the lungs. (c) (PE; AN; PA; CV)

1 This is untrue; pulmonic stenosis is a congenital condition that results from the failure of tissues to develop normally in utero.

2 The mitral valve is not involved in pulmonic stenosis.

4 The tricuspid valve is not involved in pulmonic stenosis.

35. **2** Pulmonic stenosis increases resistance to blood flow, causing right ventricular hypertrophy; with right-sided heart failure there is an increase in pressure on the right side of the heart. (c) (PE; AN; PA; CV)

1 The pressure would be decreased in pulmonic stenosis.

3 Same as # 1.

4 Same as # 1.

36. **3** Intravenous analgesics will be used because numerous infusions are in place, as well as monitors with which to observe physiologic responses. (c) (PE; PL; TC; NM)

1 IM analgesics are not necessary because circulatory access is available.

2 Oral analgesics are not as effective as IV analgesics.

4 This is false reassurance; it is rarely possible to relieve all pain immediately postoperatively.

37. **4** Iron is excreted in the feces, and the change in color is due to the insoluble iron compound in the stool. (a) (PE; AS; ED; DR)

1 This is not associated with iron; it occurs with pyridium administration.

2 This is associated with GI bleeding, not iron administration.

3 This should not occur with proper administration of the iron; iron elixir should be diluted in fluid and administered with a straw; the teeth should immediately be brushed after administration.

38. **3** This prevents seepage of Imferon up through the

needle track, thereby limiting staining of the skin. (a) (PE; IM; TC; DR)

1 This length needle is too short to get into a muscle; a 1½ to 2 inch needle is required; the gauge of the needle is too small for the viscosity of Imferon; a 19- to 22-gauge needle is required.

2 Aspiration would still be performed with the Z-track method.

4 This is unsafe; massage would force Imferon into the subcutaneous tissue, causing irritation and staining.

39. **2** During acute cholecystitis, low-fat liquids are permitted; skim milk is low in fat and contains protein, which will eventually promote healing. (c) (SU; PL; ED; GI)

1 Egg yolks contain fat and should be avoided.

3 Beef, even if it is lean, contains fat and should be avoided.

4 Gas-forming vegetables should be avoided.

40. **1** All tubes should immediately be attached to appropriate collection devices to permit drainage; T-tube and nasogastric tube drainage lessens tension on the operative site. (b) (SU; IM; TC; GI)

2 A T-tube should not be fastened to the bed sheets; a T-tube is surgically positioned in the common bile duct, and tension on the tube must be avoided to prevent accidental removal.

3 A T-tube drains by gravity and is never irrigated by the nurse.

4 This is not the priority at this time; this would be done later at the change of shift or when the collection devices get too full.

41. **4** This expands collapsed alveoli and enhances surfactant activity, thereby preventing atelectasis. (c) (SU; PL; PA; RE)

1 This promotes exhalation, not inhalation.

2 This clears accumulated secretions from the pulmonary tree; it does not directly promote alveolar expansion.

3 This promotes collapse of, not expansion of, alveoli.

42. **3** A T-tube drains by gravity into a small collection bag; gravity drainage is enhanced by the right side-lying or semi-Fowler's position. (b) (SU; PL; TC; GI)

1 The right side-lying position facilitates drainage and should be encouraged.

2 A T-tube drains by gravity, not intermittent suction.

4 A T-tube is never irrigated by the nurse; it drains by gravity.

43. **3** The return of brown color to the stool indicates that bile is entering the duodenum and being converted to urobilinogen by bacteria. (b) (SU; AN; PA; GI)

1 The serum bilirubin is not affected.

2 The liver is not tender; the incisional site and the operative area, under and below the liver, is tender.

4 This is unrelated to the flow of bile after cholecystectomy.

44. **3** Bile, which aids in fat digestion, is not as concentrated as before surgery; once the body adapts to the absence of the gall bladder, the client should be able to tolerate a regular diet that contains fat. (b) (SU; IM; ED; GI)

1 This is an inappropriate priority at this time; a

temporary avoidance of fatty foods with the gradual resumption of a regular diet is the priority.

2 Initially the client should still avoid fatty foods unless the physician indicates otherwise.

4 Same as #1.

45. **3** This identifies the client's feelings. (a) (PS; IM; PE; AX)

1 This is an unrealistic question; the cause of anxiety is on an unconscious level.

2 This response moves the focus away from the client.

4 This disregards the client's comment and avoids feelings.

46. **4** This portrays a nonjudgmental attitude that recognizes the client's needs. (b) (PS; IM; PE; AX)

1 This is untrue; it implies that crying will make it all better.

2 The client is upset that she cannot control her crying.

3 This is unrealistic; the cause of the anxiety, and hence the crying, is on an unconscious level.

47. **1** The lack of a social support system can precipitate feelings of isolation. (a) (PS; AN; PE; AX)

2 The data does not support this nursing diagnosis.

3 Same as # 2.

4 Same as # 2.

48. **2** The loss of a job can bruise the ego, particularly when there is a lack of a social support system. (a) (PS; PL; PE; AX)

1 Feelings should be expressed, not limited; attempting to decrease crying frequently increases it.

3 The focus should be on the client's self-acceptance.

4 The client does not know the cause of the crying; it is not necessarily an expression of sadness.

49. **2** Pressure of the uterus against major blood vessels reduces circulation; decreased perfusion of the placenta can result. (a) (OB; AN; PA; IP)

1 This could possibly prolong labor, but this is not the most essential reason; it is known that women who stand and walk during labor have shorter labors.

3 This does not interfere with the movement of symphysis pubis.

4 This is false; it can lead to supine hypotension.

50. **2** The longest and strongest contractions occur at the end of the first stage; a backache is common. (a) (OB; AS; PA; IP)

1 In this stage contractions are well spaced, with time to relax in between.

3 The fetal head begins to crown and would be seen at the perineum.

4 This is the period between the birth of the baby and the delivery of the placenta.

51. **3** Lochia can accumulate under the buttocks; it cannot be accurately observed with the client in a supine position. (b) (OB; IM; TC; IP)

1 Overstimulation can cause uterine atony.

2 Vital signs should be taken q 15 minutes during the fourth stage of labor, which continues for 1 hour after delivery.

4 This is too soon for ambulation.

52. **2** Bladder distention causes uterine displacement, which interferes with uterine contractions and may lead to postpartum hemorrhage. (a) (OB; AS; PA; PP)

1 Retained placental fragments often cause bright red bleeding and boggy uterus; there is no data to support this.

3 During normal involution the uterus is not deviated to the right.

4 There is no such thing as second-degree uterine atony.

53. **4** This offers the mother the opportunity to identify what is bothering her about caring for her baby. (c) (OB; IM; PE; PP)

1 This minimizes the client's feelings and offers false reassurance.

2 Same as #1.

3 This response could put the client on the defensive.

54. **2** This frequently begins with what parents describe as clumsiness that becomes progressively worse; the cerebellum controls coordination. (b) (PE; AS; PA; NM)

1 At this age, sutures are completely closed and the tumor would be contained in the cranium.

3 Seizures usually occur with cerebral or supratentorial tumors.

4 This is a very late sign of tumor involvement.

55. **1** The cerebellum is the most common area; symptoms of increased intracranial pressure result from obstruction of cerebrospinal fluid flow. (b) (PE; AN; PA; NM)

2 This is an uncommon site in children.

3 Same as # 2.

4 Same as # 2.

56. **3** This indicates the child's level of understanding to the nurse, and explanation can then proceed at this level. (c) (PE; PL; ED; GD)

1 Although the school-age child appreciates some detail, extensive detail is inappropriate.

2 Doll play is more appropriate for younger children; it is inappropriate in this instance.

4 Role playing is inappropriate and nontherapeutic at this time.

57. **2** If the drainage progresses beyond the markings, it would enable the nurse to determine whether an abnormal amount of drainage was occurring. (a) (PE; IM; TC; NM)

1 This is not an emergency; some drainage is expected.

3 In the immediate postoperative period, the dressing is to be removed only by the neurosurgeon.

4 This would not enable the nurse to monitor progression of the drainage.

58. **3** Cerebellar astrocytomas, unlike those in the cerebrum, are slow growing and benign, with a cure rate of 80% to 90% after surgery. (b) (PE; IM; PE; EC)

1 Other infratentorial tumors, such as medulloblastomas, are more rapid growing and highly malignant.

2 This is not true of a cerebellar astrocytoma.

4 Same as # 2.

59. **2** This is an emergency situation that demonstrates sudden pressure on the third cranial nerve on the affected side from displacement of the tentorium or uncus. (c) (PE; AN; PA; NM)

1 Response to severe pain is generally equal in both eyes.

3 This is inaccurate; reduced pressure would not

cause one pupil to dilate; more likely, increasing pressure would cause this response.

4 An autonomic response to fear would affect both pupils equally.

60. **3** The disease is most common in this age-group; it has a slight predilection for men. (b) (ME; AN; ED; EC)

1 Incidence is not limited to any age-group.

2 The opposite is true.

4 This is not completely accurate; sometimes it is possible; this response depersonalizes the wife's concern.

61. **1** This is the definitive diagnostic test for Hodgkin's disease. (a) (SU; IM; ED; BI)

2 This is a diagnostic device to assess bony metastasis of cancers other than Hodgkin's disease.

3 These are not indicated for Hodgkin's disease; they are usually used for radiotherapy or diagnosis of thyroid diseases.

4 This is not used to diagnose Hodgkin's disease; it can identify the extent of the disease by locating abdominal or chest lesions.

62. **3** Cells are vulnerable to specific drugs through the stages of mitosis, and a combination bombards the malignant cells at various stages. (a) (ME; IM; ED; DR)

1 This is true, but it is not the reason for using a combination of drugs.

2 This is not true; the side effects of a drug are not ameliorated by combination with others.

4 There is more than one stage of Hodgkin's, but this is not the reason for using a combination of drugs.

63. **2** This is a plant alkaloid that is cell cycle specific; it affects cell division during metaphase by interfering with spindle formation and causing cell death. (c) (ME; IM; ED; DR)

1 This is typical of antimetabolites such as Fluorouracil.

3 Antibiotics such as Dactinomycin act in this way.

4 Alkylating agents such as nitrogen mustard act in this way.

64. **1** This is responsible for the effectiveness of alkylating agents, of which nitrogen mustard is one. (c) (ME; AN; TC; DR)

2 Some drugs are believed to act in this way, but nitrogen mustard is not.

3 This is the mechanism of action of antimetabolites.

4 Antibiotics used in cancer chemotherapy are believed to act in this way.

65. **2** This is a common and expected side effect of vincristine. (c) (ME; EV; TC; DR)

1 Tingling is associated with hypocalcemia, which is not induced by nausea and vomiting.

3 Burning and tingling are not related to vasoconstriction, but rather to neurotoxicity.

4 Prednisone is not known to cause neurotoxicity.

66. **1** This occurs with the administration of Adriamycin and may alarm the client. (c) (ME; EV; ED; DR)

2 This is true for mithramycin, not the drugs in this protocol.

3 This is not true for drugs in this protocol.

4 Adriamycin is not given orally, only via the IV route.

67. **1** This assesses the client's level of alcohol abuse

by direct questioning. (b) (PS; AS; TC; SA)

2 The client probably would not bring up the subject, because denial is often used to cope with alcohol abuse.

3 This is a judgmental approach that uses manipulation and decreases the client's self-esteem.

4 This is not straightforward and will decrease trust.

68. **4** This provides reality-based feedback for the client withdrawing from alcohol. (b) (PS; IM; PE; SA)

1 Shadows will increase the chance of distortions and illusions.

2 This focuses on hallucinations and delusions rather than on reality.

3 Physical restraints will increase agitation and should be applied only as a last resort.

69. **3** This points out reality and does not support the client's hallucinations. (b) (PS; IM; PE; SA)

1 This feeds into the client's hallucination and provides false reassurance.

2 The client has hallucinations, not illusions.

4 Same as # 1.

70. **4** During detoxification this provides safety and prevents suicide, which is a real threat. (b) (PS; PL; TC; SA)

1 Restraints tend to upset the client further; if at all possible, they should not be used.

2 This type of client does not usually lose his hearing, so there is no need to shout.

3 Bright light is preferable to dim light, which creates shadows and increases illusions and misinterpretations.

71. **3** This helps the client recognize and adhere to established limits and goals. (b) (PS; IM; PE; SA)

1 This reinforces the client's pattern of manipulation.

2 Same as # 1.

4 This response can be degrading and reinforces the client's manipulative behavior.

72. **3** Most injuries to abused children are not life threatening; protection takes priority over immediate treatment. (c) (PS; PL; TC; CS)

1 Treatment of medical injuries is the physician's primary responsibility.

2 The nurse is often the first individual to see the abused child and must establish protection even before the physician arrives.

4 An accurate diagnosis of child abuse may take time and must be fully investigated.

73. **1** Self-awareness is an essential element in providing support, understanding, and empathy to others. (a) (PS; AS; PE; CS)

2 Although important, this data does not take priority at this time.

3 Although essential, this may in reality be a deterrent to the interpersonal relationship.

4 Meeting emotional needs cannot be accomplished until an interpersonal relationship is established.

74. **3** Most child abusers have been abused themselves; they do not know how to deal with the rage they feel. (b) (PS; PL; PE; CS)

1 Therapy should focus on and encourage the sharing of feelings, not personal parenting information.

2 Parents in abusing parent groups have already admitted and begun to seek help for their prob-

lem.

4 This type of presentation usually alienates individuals who are struggling with their own difficulties.

75. **2** This is a very common manifestation caused by vascular disease, particularly renal vascular disease (renin/angiotensin mechanism). (c) (ME; AS; PA; CV)

1 Weight loss is common.

3 Lymphadenopathy does not generally occur.

4 Peripheral nerves, not cranial nerves, can be involved.

76. **4** This acknowledges the client's apprehension and encourages further communication. (a) (SU; IM; PE; EC)

1 This is perhaps true, but it does not foster communication; the client may focus on the word pain.

2 This does not address the client's feelings and may cause more anxiety.

3 This negates the client's feelings and promotes false reassurance.

77. **3** As long as the client has no nausea or vomiting, there are no diet restrictions. (b) (SU; IM; ED; GI)

1 The biopsy site will be sutured and should not get wet.

2 The client should not disturb the dressing; it should be changed by the physician on a follow-up visit.

4 Temperature elevation is not a usual response and may indicate infection.

78. **4** Autoimmune response plays a role in the development of polyarteritis, although drugs and infections may precipitate it. (c) (ME; IM; ED; CV)

1 Men are affected three times more frequently than women.

2 Arteriolar pathology can affect any organ or system.

3 The disease is often fatal, usually as a result of congestive heart failure or renal failure.

79. **4** Mood changes can occur as a side effect of steroid therapy. (c) (ME; EV; TC; DR)

1 This denies the value of the client's statement and provides false reassurance.

2 The client has already stated he does not know why this is happening.

3 This is difficult to do, because the direction a situation will take cannot always be anticipated.

80. **2** The client has signs of diabetes, which may result from steroid therapy; testing the blood glucose level is a method of screening for diabetes mellitus, thus gathering more data. (b) (ME; AS; PA; EN)

1 The symptoms presented are not those of fluid retention, but of diabetes mellitus.

3 The symptoms are not those of benign prostatic hypertrophy.

4 This would not be as accurate as a blood glucose level.

81. **2** Buck's traction is an example of traction applied directly to the skin by moleskin and ace bandages. (b) (SU; AN; PA; SK)

1 Skeletal traction is applied directly to the bony skeleton.

3 Balanced suspension traction keeps the affected extremity elevated off the bed.

4 There is no such traction.

82. **1** The client's major concern at this time is pain caused by inappropriate handling. (b) (SU; IM; PE; SK)

2 This is not the major concern, and false reassurance should not be given.

3 The number of personnel will not necessarily ensure careful handling; this does not address the client's primary concern.

4 Diversion at this time would not be an appropriate response to the client's primary concern.

83. **4** Because more people are living longer, this problem of the elderly, especially elderly women, is increasing. (c) (SU; AN; PA; GD)

1 This is unrelated to osteoporosis; fat does not contain calcium.

2 This is unrelated to osteoporosis.

3 Early retirement does not necessarily imply inactivity or immobility.

84. **1** Yogurt, which contains calcium, is easily digested because it contains the enzyme lactase, which breaks down milk sugar. (a) (SU; AN; PA; GI)

2 These are deficient in calcium.

3 Same as # 2.

4 Same as # 2.

85. **2** The data indicates impending shock; the dressing should be assessed for signs of hemorrhage. (c) (SU; EV; TC; CV)

1 Although this may eventually be done, it is not the priority.

3 There are no signs of respiratory distress; if the hemorrhage is confirmed, the supine position is preferable.

4 This is unsafe; the client may be hemorrhaging and needs immediate assessment.

86. **3** The client needs to know details of transfer to assist appropriately and avoid injury. (a) (SU; IM; ED; SK)

1 More commonly, no weight bearing is permitted on operative leg at first.

2 This is not advisable because this could disrupt the repair of the affected hip.

4 This is unnecessary; the client may touch the floor with the foot but may not bear weight on this extremity.

87. **4** Stimulation of the autonomic nervous system is a normal response to cord compression during uterine contraction. (c) (OB; EV; PA; IP)

1 This is unnecessary; this is a normal response to cord compression during a contraction.

2 Same as # 1.

3 Same as # 1.

88. **2** Bradycardia (baseline FHR below 120 beats per minute) may indicate fetal distress and may require medical intervention. (b) (OB; IM; TC; IP)

1 The normal fetal heart rate is 120 to 160 beats per minute.

3 There is no indication of maternal distress; the fetus may be in distress.

4 This is dangerous; the fetus may be in distress, and time should not be spent on monitoring.

89. **2** Heat causes vasodilation and an increased blood supply to the area. (b) (OB; PL; PA; PP)

1 This is not the purpose of the sitz baths.

3 Cleansing is done immediately after voiding and defecating with a perineal bottle filled with cleansing solution.

4 Relaxation of the rectal sphincter is promoted by

the sitz bath; this will provide comfort but will not increase healing.

90. **4** Prevention of infection is the priority. (b) (OB; EV; ED; PP)
  1 This provides comfort but is not the priority.
  2 Stair climbing may cause some discomfort but is not detrimental to healing.
  3 It is not necessary to stop sitz baths as long as they provide comfort.

91. **3** Because intussusception creates intestinal obstruction where the intestine "telescopes" and becomes trapped, passage of intestinal contents is lessened; stools are red and currant jelly-like from the mixing of stool with blood and mucus. (a) (PE; AS; PA; GI)
  1 This is not as important to assessment as is observable behavior associated with crying.
  2 Accurate fluid intake and output records are im-

portant, but they are not essential to confirming this diagnosis.
  4 Bowel sounds would not be significantly affected.

92. **1** Atropine is a vagolytic and drying agent used preoperatively. (a) (PE; AN; TC; DR)
  2 This is a narcotic analgesic.
  3 This is a tranquilizer.
  4 This is a sedative.

93. **1** This is a behavior seen in 9- to 12-month-olds; this is the most advanced behavior listed, and thus the most unusual for this age. (b) (PE; AS; ED; GD)
  2 This is a behavior seen in 6- to 8-month-olds.
  3 This is a coordination ability seen in 5- to 7-month-olds.
  4 This is a coordination ability seen in 3- to 5-month-olds.

How to Use Worksheet 1: Errors in Processing Information

Common errors in processing information are listed in the left-hand column of this worksheet. At the top of the worksheet is a row of blank spaces for inserting the number of the question missed. Directly below each number, check any errors you made in answering that question. You may have made more than one type of error in an answer.

Worksheet 1: Errors in processing information

Question number																				
Did not read situation/question carefully																				
Missed important details																				
Confused major and minor points																				
Defined problem incorrectly																				
Could not remember terms/ facts/concepts/principles																				
Defined terms incorrectly																				
Focused on incomplete/incorrect data in assessing situation																				
Interpreted data incorrectly																				
Applied wrong concepts/principles in situation																				
Drew incorrect conclusions																				
Identified wrong goals																				
Identified priorities incorrectly																				
Carried out plan incorrectly/incompletely																				
Was unclear about criteria for evaluating success in achieving goals																				

How to Use Worksheet 2: Knowledge Gaps

Types of common knowledge gaps are listed along the top of this worksheet. Write a brief description of topics you want to review in the spaces provided. For example, if you missed a question on administration of a particular drug, write the drug name and problem (e.g., dosage) in the appropriate space under the column labeled *Pharmacology*.

Worksheet 2: Knowledge gaps

Basic science	Skills/ procedures	Basic human needs	Growth & develop- ment	Normal nutrition	Psycho- social factors	Clinical area/ topic	Stressors/ coping mechanisms	Patho- physiology	Pharma- cology	Therapeutic nutrition	Legal Implications	Other

Test 2

94. **3** Class A diabetes is gestational diabetes, and the woman will demonstrate symptoms only when pregnant; this is the client's first pregnancy and her first sign of diabetes; it is too early for secondary complications. (a) (OB; AS; PA; HP)
   1 This is class C diabetes, which is more severe.
   2 Retinopathy is usually present in class D diabetes or higher.
   4 Same as # 2.

95. **3** The likelihood of pregnancy-induced hypertension increases fourfold, probably because of a preexisting vascular condition. (a) (OB; AN; PA; HP)
   1 Most pregnant women have increased appetites; excessive weight gain may be caused by a macrosomic infant and hydramnios.
   2 Clients with diabetes have increased, rather than decreased, amniotic fluid.
   4 Abnormal implantation may occur because of scarring or uterine abnormalities, not because of diabetes.

96. **3** L/S ratios, which indicate fetal lung maturity, are performed on amniotic fluid. (a) (OB; AS; PA; HP)
   1 This is irrelevant; this is not the primary purpose for examining amniotic fluid.
   2 This is determined by the less invasive procedure of ultrasonography.
   4 Amniocentesis would be done between the sixteenth and twentieth weeks to determine genetic disorders.

97. **2** This is done to reduce the possibility of bladder puncture. (a) (OB; IM; TC; HP)
   1 Medications are not given because of their effect on the fetus.
   3 This procedure is not done via the colon, so fecal material does not have to be expelled.
   4 The mother may eat and drink before the test; a hungry mother may cause a restless fetus.

98. **4** Hypoglycemia may be present because of sudden withdrawal of maternal glucose and increased insulin production by the infant. (c) (OB; AN; TC; HN)
   1 This is not the priority until the blood glucose level is determined.
   2 The umbilical vein may be used for starting an IV; it should not be obliterated.
   3 This can be delayed for 2 hours; determination of the blood glucose level is the priority.

99. **1** A patent airway is the first priority, and the necessary equipment must be immediately available. (a) (PE; PL; TC; RE)
   2 Although helpful, this is not the priority.
   3 Same as # 2.
   4 This would be appropriate for convulsions, which are not associated with croup; respiratory promotion is the priority.

100. **2** Laryngeal spasms can occur abruptly; patency of the airway is determined by constant assessment for symptoms of respiratory distress. (a) (PE; AS; TC; RE)
   1 This is important, but maintenance of respiration has priority.
   3 The fever should be treated, but it is not critical at 103° F; maintenance of respiration has priority.

   4 Same as # 1.

101. **4** These are signs of increasing hypoxia; a tracheotomy may be necessary to maintain an open airway. (b) (PE; IM; TC; RE)
   1 Increased O_2 therapy can induce carbon dioxide narcosis.
   2 The symptoms are not indicative of increased secretions; suctioning can precipitate sudden laryngospasm.
   3 This is ineffective for laryngeal spasms.

102. **1** These are some of the first signs of hypoxia; the airway must be kept patent to promote oxygenation. (b) (PE; AS; PA; RE)
   2 The client will not be able to communicate verbally after a tracheotomy.
   3 These are late signs of hypoxia; suctioning should have been done well before this time.
   4 These are late signs of respiratory difficulty; suctioning and other measures should have been done well before this time.

103. **3** Erosion of blood vessels may lead to hemorrhage, a life-threatening situation further complicated by decreased prothrombin production. (c) (ME; AS; PA; GI)
   1 Increased intraabdominal pressure may cause this; there is no immediate threat to life; assessment for bleeding takes priority.
   2 Same as # 1.
   4 Although this may cause gastritis, there is no immediate threat to life; assessment for bleeding takes priority.

104. **4** The enlarged liver impairs venous return, leading to increased portal vein hydrostatic pressure and fluid shift into the abdominal cavity. (c) (ME; AN; PA; GI)
   1 Ascites is not related to the interstitial fluid compartment.
   2 Increased serum albumin causes hypervolemia, not ascites.
   3 Bile plays an important role in digestion of fats, but it is not a major factor in fluid balance.

105. **1** The bladder should be empty to avoid injury during insertion of the abdominal trocar. (b) (SU; IM; TC; GI)
   2 This is unrelated to the procedure; however, it would be preferable to offer fluids after the procedure if allowed.
   3 The upright position is assumed to allow accumulation of fluid in the lower abdomen by gravity.
   4 Although regular monitoring of girth is important, it is not necessary immediately before this test.

106. **1** Fluid may shift from the intravascular space to the abdomen as fluid is removed, leading to hypovolemia and compensatory tachycardia. (c) (SU; EV; PA; GI)
   2 A paracentesis should decrease the degree of distention.
   3 The fluid shift can cause hypovolemia with resulting hypotension, not hypertension.
   4 This sign of dehydration may occur, but it is not as vital or immediate as signs of shock.

107. **2** This ensures that the liver does not move as it does with normal respiratory excursions. (b) (SU; IM; TC; GI)
   1 Movement or breathing increases the danger of

damage to the liver.

3 There is no rationale for this, and it is difficult to carry out.

4 Lying on the right side, not the left side, after the procedure applies pressure at the insertion site, preventing hemorrhage.

108. **2** This therapy permits relative isolation of the tumor area and saturation with the drug(s) selected. (b) (SU; AN; TC; GI)

1 These effects cannot be confined completely to the treated area; some migration still occurs.

3 This is not true; this procedure requires medical and nursing supervision.

4 Combinations of drugs can also be administered via IV or oral routes.

109. **3** Regression to a more immature, helpless developmental level is normal and should be supported at this point. (b) (SU; PL; PE; EC)

1 The client's behavior does not indicate anger.

2 Denial is not the response described.

4 The client's behavior is inconsistent with the need for more control.

110. **4** A continual level of the drug is maintained to keep the terminally ill client comfortable. (a) (ME; PL; PA; NM)

1 The client should not have to request this medication; it should be given routinely.

2 This medication contains morphine and cocaine; the potential for addiction is no less than with other narcotics; addiction is not a major concern for the terminally ill client.

3 This medication is in liquid form and is taken orally.

111. **1** Percussing over fluid produces a dull sound, not the normal tympanic sound. (c) (ME; AS; PA; GI)

2 Bowel sounds do not indicate much about ascites.

3 This would assess for dependent edema, not ascites.

4 Respiratory distress is evident with ascites but is not an early sign.

112. **1** Delusions are false, fixed beliefs that have a minimal reality base. (a) (PS; AN; PE; SD)

2 Tactile hallucinations are false sensory perceptions of touch without external stimuli.

3 Loose associations are verbalizations that sound disjointed to the listener.

4 Ideas of reference are false beliefs that every statement or action of others relates to the individual.

113. **3** The client's low self-esteem makes her doubt her boyfriend loves her; her statements reflect her feelings. (c) (PS; AS; PE; SD)

1 The client's statements do not represent hallucinations because they are not false sensory perceptions.

2 The client's statements do not reflect confusion or disorientation, but false beliefs.

4 Setting limits after the fact would not be effective in any situation; limits must be set when the situation occurs.

114. **4** This presents the reality of the situation and helps support the client during a threatening hallucination. (b) (PS; IM; PE; SD)

1 Clients cannot be distracted from hallucinations without competing stimuli.

2 This would encourage withdrawal and isolation and would not stop the hallucinations.

3 This would have little effect on the client's behavior and would not stop the hallucinations.

115. **2** This reflects the client's feelings and opens channels of communication. (c) (PS; IM; PE; SD)

1 This provides false reassurance; it is really not the same food, because it is on the client's plate.

3 This response denies the client's feelings; this will not foster development of trust.

4 This is false reassurance; the delusional client would believe the nurse knows what part to taste.

116. **2** A sharing of views helps to support the client's trust in herself and others; participation increases self-esteem. (c) (PS; EV; PE; SD)

1 Asking clients to defend their point of view is threatening.

3 Suspicious clients are sensitive to others' feelings; this may be viewed as a lack of trust.

4 Pressuring the client to explain behavioral changes increases anxiety and the need to use defenses.

117. **1** Because suspicious clients lack trust and have difficulty sharing feelings, this healthy behavior should be recognized. (b) (PS; EV; PE; SD)

2 Focusing on the staff's concerns ignores the client's needs; the staff's attitude could decrease self-esteem.

3 The client's feelings are rejected when blanket statements are given; this only responds to part of the client's concerns.

4 A detailed description at this time may increase the client's fears.

118. **4** As the lower uterine segment stretches and thins, tearing and bleeding occurs at the lower implantation site. (b) (OB; AS; PA; HP)

1 This is usually associated with abortion or an ectopic pregnancy.

2 This is associated with abortions, but cramping and backache are usually present.

3 This is usually associated with abruptio placentae rather than placenta previa.

119. **1** This would give the client a familiar gauge in estimating the amount of bleeding she is experiencing. (a) (OB; AS; PA; HP)

2 Weakness is a subjective system and may not truly reflect blood loss.

3 The presence of clots does not indicate the amount of bleeding.

4 This may indicate a problem but does not relate to the amount of bleeding.

120. **4** The nurse palpates the abdomen to locate the head, back, and small parts of the fetus; the location of these parts reveals the position of the fetus. (a) (OB; AS; PA; IP)

1 This can be done by lightly placing the hand on the fundus during a contraction; no other maneuver is necessary.

2 Uterine involution is measured in the postpartum period.

3 The station can be ascertained only on vaginal examination, which is not part of the Leopold maneuvers, and would not be done with placenta previa.

121. **3** If the bleeding continues, both mother and fetus are at risk and a cesarean delivery would be indicated. (a) (OB; PL; TC; HP)

1 This is desired in all situations, not just in placenta previa.

2 This may be a medical decision and would be difficult for the nurse to control.

4 It is best to deal with reality; diversion at this time is unrealistic.

122. **3** In grand multiparas observation for failure of the uterus to contract after delivery is a priority. (c) (OB; PL; TC; HP)

1 This can be done only after the mother is in stable condition.

2 This is an important goal, but it is not primary or life-threatening.

4 This is not a priority goal immediately after delivery; it also is not common after abdominal delivery.

123. **3** Pelvic rocking on the first postoperative day would be very painful and could traumatize the wound site. (a) (OB; EV; ED; HP)

1 Foot circles promote circulation in the lower extremities.

2 Leg bends promote circulation in the lower extremities and help to alleviate gas pains.

4 Shoulder circles relieve neck stiffness associated with bed rest.

124. **2** A specimen must be obtained and analyzed before the physician can prescribe treatment. (a) (PE; PL; TC; GI)

1 The organism can be identified only by laboratory analysis of a specimen.

3 The priority is identifying the organism, then handwashing techniques can be taught.

4 This is not a reportable communicable disease.

125. **4** The pinworm emerges when the client is asleep to lay its eggs; these can be collected from the perianal area by applying tape upon awakening. (a) (PE; PL; ED; GI)

1 Any larvae on the perianal area would have been removed by the bath.

2 The larvae would not have been deposited yet because the adult pinworm would still be in the bowel; it emerges when the client is asleep.

3 Any larvae that were present in the morning would probably have been wiped away.

126. **3** This infestation is transferred by the the oral-anal route, and handwashing is the most effective method to prevent transmission. (a) (PE; EV; ED; GI)

1 Pinworms are found in the rectum or colon and travel to the perianal area only when the person sleeps.

2 This is not the usual mode of transmission.

4 Cats do not transmit this disease.

127. **3** This would indicate a lack of understanding of the necessity of taking antibiotics for a full 10 to 14 days or until a follow-up urine culture is negative. (a) (PE; EV; ED; RG)

1 Bubble bath can be a source of irritation to the meatus, which can predispose to a urinary tract infection and thus should be avoided.

2 Wiping from front to back prevents contamination of the meatus with fecal contents.

4 Stasis is the primary predisposing factor to a urinary tract infection, thus voiding when feeling the urge is important; the bladder should be emptied every 3 to 4 hours.

128. **2** The basement membrane of the glomerulus becomes permeable to protein that is lost in the urine; decreased serum protein reduces the oncotic pressure in the capillaries, which normally helps to hold fluid within the vascular system. (c) (PE; AN; PA; FE)

1 The basement membrane becomes permeable to protein, not impermeable to water.

3 Nephrosis is characterized by hypoproteinemia; increased oncotic pressure pulls fluid from interstitial space into the intravascular compartment.

4 Hypoproteinemia causes decreased oncotic pressure, which results in hypovolemia; sodium and water are retained to counter the hypovolemia.

129. **4** Severe edema is usually present, and change of position is necessary to prevent breakdown of tissue. (c) (PE; PL; TC; IT)

1 Play periods would be permitted during remission but not during the edema phase to limit energy expenditure.

2 Fluids are not forced and may even be restricted during periods of edema.

3 A high-protein diet minimizes negative nitrogen balance; a low-protein diet is used in renal failure with azotemia.

130. **3** The shift of fluid predisposes to hypovolemia; increased thready pulse and hypotension are signs of shock. (c) (PE; AS; PA; RG)

1 This does not usually occur as an early complication of this disease; it is a major complication of glomerulonephritis.

2 This is not a complication of nephrotic syndrome, although pulmonary effusion may occur.

4 Tubular reabsorption of sodium is increased to replenish vascular volume; therefore potassium would be excreted.

131. **3** School-age children enjoy competition, have manipulative skills, and are creative. (a) (PE; IM; ED; GD)

1 These are appropriate for the toddler who is developing fine motor skills.

2 This activity is inappropriate during the acute phase of nephrotic syndrome because it requires too much energy.

4 Magazines would interest an older child who would be more proficient in reading.

132. **1** Poor appetite and decreased energy are associated with an accumulation of toxic waste; associated anemia accounts for the pallor. (c) (PE; AN; PA; RG)

2 An elevated temperature would be present; an infection would not cause muddy pallor.

3 Discontinuing the corticosteroids and diuretics if prescribed might result in recurrence of edema in steroid-dependent children; pallor would not occur.

4 Once remission has occurred, usual activities can be resumed with discretion.

133. **2** Low concentrations of oxygen do not reduce the stimulus to breathe and prevent carbon dioxide narcosis. (a) (ME; IM; PA; RE)

1 Sedatives would further depress respirations and increase the carbon dioxide level.

3 Chronic hypercapnia is present; additional carbon dioxide only adds to the problem and results in carbon dioxide narcosis.

4 Respiratory obstruction causes difficulty on expiration; deep breathing will aggravate this situation.

134. **2** Hypoxia stimulates production of large quantities of erythrocytes in an attempt to compensate for lack of oxygen. (b) (ME; AN; PA; BI)

1 Hypercapnia is an increase in Pco_2 in extracellular fluid; there is no direct effect on blood cell counts.

3 White blood cell production increases, but hemoglobin and hematocrit are not measures of white blood cell counts.

4 There is a loss of extracellular fluid in acute infections with fever, but in a chronic condition this fluid is replenished.

135. **4** Decreased normal breath sounds result from reduced air flow, pleural effusion, and destruction of lung tissue. (c) (ME; AS; PA; RE)

1 There is an increased A-P diameter (barrel chest) because of air trapping and enlargement of lungs with loss of recoil ability.

2 There is enlargement of accessory muscles, which are used during the expiratory phase to help force air out.

3 There is an increased expiratory phase because of entrapment of air and collapse of airways.

136. **2** Improving ventilation provides comfort, maintains existing lung function, and prevents further lung damage. (a) (ME; AN; PA; RE)

1 Maintaining hydration thins secretions so that there is less interference in achieving the goal of improved ventilation.

3 Some decrease in hypoxia will promote comfort, but the primary problem is too much carbon dioxide rather than too little oxygen; oxygen should not exceed 2L.

4 Correcting the bicarbonate deficit will not help ventilation but will correct the accompanying respiratory acidosis.

137. **2** The aim of therapy is to eliminate the causative agent, which can be determined from culture and sensitivity tests of sputum. (a) (ME; EV; TC; RE)

1 Pulmonary function studies indicate air volume that may fall within the normal range despite the presence of bronchopneumonia.

3 Bronchoscopy shows the appearance of the bronchi but does not indicate the presence or absence of microorganisms.

4 A lung scan permits visualization of lung vasculature but does not provide data on the condition of the lung tissue itself.

138. **3** Forcing fluids helps to liquefy secretions, enabling the client to clear the respiratory tract by coughing. (b) (SU; PL; PA; RE)

1 The use of cotton balls around a tracheostomy introduces the risk of aspiration of one of the cotton fibers.

2 Excessive suctioning will irritate the mucosal lining of the respiratory tract and can actually result in more secretions.

4 An occlusive dressing would totally block air exchange.

139. **4** Cor pulmonale is right-sided heart failure caused by pulmonary congestion; edema results from increasing venous pressure. (c) (ME; AS; PA; CV)

1 This is caused by alterations in oxygen and hydrogen ion levels and their effects on the central nervous system.

2 Same as # 1.

3 A productive cough is symptomatic of the original condition—COPD.

140. **2** Initial rapid assessment will determine priorities of care and subsequent actions. (c) (ME; PL; TC; CV)

1 Although important, obtaining a history and x-ray films can be postponed until bleeding is controlled and injuries are assessed.

3 A thorough physical assessment is too time consuming initially; open wounds can be covered at a later time.

4 Intravenous therapy and transfusions will be ordered, but baseline data is needed to assess the client's response.

141. **3** Limitation of increased intracranial pressure and resultant brain damage depends on frequent systematic observation. (c) (ME; AS; PA; NM)

1 There is no indication that hyperactivity is present.

2 This is unrealistic; the state of consciousness should be observed, but otherwise rest is not contraindicated.

4 Mannitol is administered to reduce cerebral edema; there is no indication as yet that this will be needed.

142. **1** Mediastinal structures move toward the uninjured lung, reducing oxygenation and venous return. (c) (SU; AS; PA; RE)

2 This is a result of cardiac contusion and usually occurs from sternal, not lateral, compression.

3 Flail chest is a closed chest injury; open pneumothorax results from penetrating injury to the chest wall.

4 This is unusual with a crushing chest injury.

143. **3** The chamber closest to the client collects drainage, and the second chamber acts as the water seal. (c) (SU; AN; TC; RE)

1 The water seal in a two-chamber system is provided by the second chamber.

2 Suction requires the addition of a third chamber or a modified system.

4 In a one-chamber system the seal and drainage are combined and there is no suction chamber.

144. **4** Lying on the affected side increases drainage and allows the unaffected lung to expand to the fullest extent. (c) (SU; IM; PA; RE)

1 This will not facilitate drainage and leads to pooling of drainage in the operative site.

2 Same as # 1.

3 This is undesirable because this may not allow the unaffected lung to fully expand and provide maximum oxygenation.

145. **2** Nerve and vascular injury and significant blood loss may be present. (b) (SU; AS; PA; SK)

1 False reassurance is never appropriate.

3 Closed fractures generally do not require operative reduction; they are usually reduced by manipulation.

4 This is a medical decision that has not yet been made; closed fractures generally are reduced by manipulation.

146. **4** Stable vital signs are the major indicators that transfer will not jeopardize the client's condition. (b) (SU; AS; TC; CV)

1 Restlessness may be a sign of shock; the client needs further assessment.

2 The vital signs are not stabilized, and transfer at this time is contraindicated.

3 These are signs of increased intracranial pressure, and the client should not be transferred at this time.

147. **2** Furniture and loose rugs can interfere with crutch walking and should be removed to prevent further injury. (a) (SU; PL; ED; SK)

1 The client may shower if the cast is protected from becoming wet.

3 There is no documentation that vitamin C enhances healing; it prevents capillary fragility.

4 This is a medical decision.

148. **1** Initially the nurse should not discuss the client's appearance since this focuses on a symptom rather than the feelings. (b) (PS; IM; PE; BA)

2 This focuses on a symptom rather than the feelings; in addition, the client does not believe she looks bad.

3 The client's objective is not suicide; the client has an unconscious desire to remain childlike.

4 Stating the rules would not accomplish anything and will not convince the client to eat.

149. **2** The client expects the nurse to focus on her eating, and the emphasis should be placed on feelings rather than actions. (b) (PS; IM; PE; BA)

1 Threats will not convince the client to eat; this response sets up a challenge that the nurse will not win.

3 This is a threat that will not convince the client to eat; privileges are associated with a contracted weight gain.

4 This is a threat that will not convince the client to eat; the client believes she is fat and is not concerned about malnutrition.

150. **4** These individuals need peer group relations to validate their feelings and to experience peer group pressures. (c) (PS; PL; PE; BA)

1 These individuals totally relate their attractiveness to thinness; they have amenorrhea and diminished libido.

2 These individuals rarely have trouble making decisions, so they do not have to be forced into the role.

3 These individuals have a remarkable store of energy that does not reflect their malnourished state.

151. **3** This action still permits the client to deal with feelings of anxiety in an acceptable way. (b) (PS; AN; TC; PR)

1 This action does not allow the client any outlet for dealing with extreme anxiety, which is a priority need at this time.

2 The anxiety is too great for the client to understand why handwashing is necessary.

4 Recognition must precede the development of insight; neither can be done until the level of anxiety is reduced.

152. **1** A therapeutic relationship is easier to establish when anxiety is lowered; the use of paper towels may ultimately facilitate communication. (b) (PS; IM; PE; PR)

2 This may increase anxiety further, thus hindering the development of a therapeutic relationship.

3 This is untrue and only reinforces the use of dirt as a defense against real feelings and increases anxiety.

4 This will cause further anxiety and hinder the development of a therapeutic relationship.

153. **4** The nurse shows an understanding of the client's needs by not totally restricting the handwashing. (c) (PS; IM; PE; PR)

1 Continued handwashing does not reveal an understanding of the problem or a sign of progress.

2 This denies the client's feelings, is untrue, and will close off any communication.

3 At this time, the client is still too anxious and is incapable of dealing with the reasons for handwashing.

154. **3** Reducing anxiety limits the need for these obsessive-compulsive actions. (c) (PS; PL; TC; PR)

1 This is a temporary action that does not deal with the feelings that cause anxiety.

2 Menial tasks may decrease feelings of self-worth; these individuals do not have a need to expiate guilt.

4 Simple repetitive activities are not therapeutic for this client and could increase anxiety.

155. **1** This prevents the spread of infection to others; isolation is a priority that should be immediately implemented. (a) (PE; IM; TC; NM)

2 There is no indication that the child is dehydrated; fluid maintenance is a continuing goal.

3 This would not be given because these children are sensitive to stimuli and movement causes increased discomfort.

4 There is no indication that the child needs oxygen, and it would not be given routinely.

156. **4** This measure assesses for increasing intracranial pressure, which may occur if drainage channels are obstructed by the bacterial infection. (b) (PE; PL; TC; NM)

1 This is insufficient monitoring; many changes could occur in this time span.

2 Antibiotics are administered intravenously throughout the course of treatment.

3 Parents can visit if they are taught how to carry out the isolation procedures.

157. **3** The formula is drop factor (60) ÷ time in minutes (60) × desired hourly volume (800 ÷ 24) = drops per minute; the correct answer is 33 drops per minute. (b) (PE; AN; TC; FE)

1 This is too slow; a rate of 3 drops/min would deliver 72 ml in 24 hours.

2 This is too slow; a rate of 6 drops/min would deliver 144 ml in 24 hours.

4 This is too fast; a rate of 60 drops/min would deliver 1440 ml in 24 hours.

158. **4** Tetanus immunoglobulin (TIG) contains ready-made antibodies and only confers short-term passive immunity. (b) (PE; AN; TC; BI)

1 Immune globulins confer passive artificial immunity.

2 Passive immunity is temporary.

3 Immune globulins are antibodies and do not stimulate the formation of antibodies.

159. **2** Tetanus immune globulin should not cause anaphylaxis because it is derived from human serum. (b) (PE; AN; TC; BI)

1 It is necessary to perform skin tests for both types of medications to determine the presence of sensitivity.

3 Tetanus immune globulin is not as effective as the antitoxin, but it is not derived from horse serum and should not cause anaphylaxis.

4 These medications always carry the risk of hypersensitivity; it cannot be assumed they can be safely given to everyone.

160. **1** Toxoids are modified toxins that stimulate the body to form antibodies, lasting up to 10 years, against the specific disease. (c) (PE; AN; TC; BI)

2 Toxoids give artificial active immunity.

3 Passive immunity is temporary; even the natural type derived from the mother does not last longer than the first year of life.

4 Only by having the disease can lifelong natural immunity become possible; toxoids confer active artificial immunity.

161. **1** Edema associated with the inflammatory reaction after surgery limits the conduction of sound. (c) (SU; AN; PA; NM)

2 This should not happen because the inner ear is not involved in this surgery.

3 This is extremely unlikely.

4 If the graft slips out, the hearing loss would be worse than before surgery.

162. **4** The motor fibers of the facial nerve innervate the superficial muscles of the face and scalp. (b) (SU; AS; PA; NM)

1 This is a sensory response that may be manifested when the injury is to the sensory branch of the facial nerve.

2 Same as # 1.

3 This response is usually not related to damage to the facial nerve but may indicate infection.

163. **4** Urinary retention and distention are common problems after a cystoscopy because of urethral edema. (b) (SU; EV; TC; RG)

1 Although not usual, inability to void deserves further investigation because infection can follow retention of urine.

2 Fluids dilute the urine and reduce the chance of infection after cystoscopy.

3 More conservative methods such as running water or a sitz bath should be attempted; catheterization carries a risk of infection.

164. **1** A continuous flushing of the bladder dilutes the bloody urine and empties the bladder, preventing clots. (a) (SU; AN; TC; RG)

2 Only the kidneys form urine; fluid instilled into the bladder does not affect kidney function.

3 Urinary output can be easily measured regardless of the amount of fluid instilled.

4 This system does not exert any additional pressure within the bladder; it may also prevent obstruction.

165. **1** This action monitors the tube for patency; retained fluid raises intravesicular pressure, causing discomfort similar to the urge to void. (b) (SU; IM; TC; RG)

2 Total intake and output have no relationship to the client's present feeling that there is a need to void.

3 This is true; however, the integrity of the gravity system should be ascertained before this reason can be assumed.

4 The need to take vital signs is not indicated by the client's complaint; the physician is not called unless the blocked tube cannot be corrected.

166. **2** This action causes the bladder muscle to contract, initiating painful bladder spasms. (a) (SU; IM; ED; RG)

1 Narcotics may dull the pain, but they will not necessarily limit muscle spasms.

3 Instillation of fluid will not decrease bladder spasms and may be irritating and precipitate additional spasms.

4 Manipulating the catheter may precipitate additional spasms.

167. **4** This suggests metastasis to the bone, which results in pain and risk of pathologic fractures. (b) (SU; PL; TC; SK)

1 Measuring intake and output is necessary for any

client with prostatic cancer because of the high risk of obstruction, not just because of these results.

2 Seizure precautions are not necessary; a serum alkaline phosphatase elevation indicates bone, not brain, involvement.

3 An elevated serum alkaline phosphatase does not significantly affect the pH.

168. **4** This acknowledges the impact of this diagnosis on the client and should explore what is really known. (a) (ME; IM; PE; EC)

1 This statement is untrue and gives false reassurance.

2 Same as # 1.

3 There is no evidence of ineffective coping, especially since the client has returned to work.

169. **1** Optic nerve inflammation is an early effect of multiple sclerosis caused by lesions in the optic nerves or their connections. (a) (ME; IM; ED; NM)

2 Tumors of the brain cause increased intracranial pressure because the skull cannot expand.

3 This causes blindness as a result of increased intraocular pressure, not inflammation of the optic nerve.

4 At present there is no evidence of viral infection of any kind in multiple sclerosis.

170. **3** Emotional outbursts are common and fleeting in these clients; it is best not to emphasize them. (b) (ME; IM; PA; NM)

1 The client may be unaware of the reason; inappropriate responses and emotional outbursts are common.

2 The client is unable to control this emotion, and focusing on it may exaggerate the outburst.

4 The client is probably unaware of the cause of the crying, and saying it is normal is not reassuring.

171. **2** Steroids decrease the inflammatory process around the optic nerve, thus improving vision. (a) (ME; EV; PA; DR)

1 Pain in the extremities is not common unless spasms are present; steroids do not relieve spasms.

3 Steroids are not effective in easing muscle contractions.

4 Steroids are usually associated with increased emotional lability.

172. **3** Muscle contraction causes neuronal stimulation; multiple foci of demyelination cause interruption or distortion of the impulse, resulting in intention tremors. (b) (ME; AN; PA; NM)

1 There are no tremors when the client is inactive; this is a resting tremor that is usually associated with parkinsonism.

2 There are no tremors when the person is asleep.

3 Intention tremors are associated with muscle contraction, not feelings; stress can exacerbate the symptoms of MS.

173. **4** A home-care program would be more efficient and cost effective; this couple can manage with proper assistance. (b) (ME; PL; TC; GD)

1 There is nothing in the history to demonstrate that a skilled nursing facility is necessary.

2 Because the couple appear able to function with assistance at home, it is not necessary to move them at this time.

3 Same as # 2.

174. **4** It is too costly and a poor delegation of manpower to use a professional nurse indefinitely in the home. (a) (ME; PL; TC; GD)
    1 Clients prefer to stay in a familiar environment and will achieve their maximal potential regardless of the area.
    2 Multidisciplinary services on a part-time basis in the home would be more therapeutic and cost effective than placement in a nursing home.
    3 Part-time personal care assistance in the home would be more therapeutic and cost effective than placement in a nursing home.

175. **4** Familiarity with the environment and orientation to staff may help promote security and feelings of trust. (b) (PS; IM; PE; OR)
    1 A person under stress cannot assimilate much information; verbiage can only lead to more confusion and anger.
    2 This denies the client's feelings, is disrespectful, and provides false reassurance.
    3 This statement denies feelings and is false reassurance because all personnel are not involved with the client.

176. **3** Destruction of brain cells decreases cognitive abilities, and learning and thinking are compromised. (b) (PS; AS; PA; OR)
    1 Psychologic stress and changes caused by aging result in a decreased capability to adapt to the environment; familiar routines provide security.
    2 The attention span would be decreased.
    4 This is not specific to organic mental syndrome or aging; it depends on the individual.

177. **2** This lessens anxiety, promotes verbalization, reduces guilt, and helps the family feel useful. (b) (PS; IM; PE; TR)
    1 The "why" creates defensiveness; the information is incorrect, and crying helps to relieve tension.
    3 This is false reassurance.
    4 This is a generalized personal opinion; the nurse at this time does not know about family relationships.

178. **1** Familiarity with situations and continuity add to the client's sense of security and foster trust in the relationship. (b) (PS; PL; PE; OR)
    2 Although this helps individualize care, continuity is the priority.
    3 Some degree of flexibility by the nurse would help to individualize care.
    4 Detailed explanations are apt to be forgotten; instructions should be simple and to the point and given when needed.

179. **1** This is a therapeutic approach that indicates awareness of the client's feelings and encourages verbalizations. (a) (PS; IM; PE; OR)
    2 Moralizing is a roadblock to effective communication.
    3 This is diverting the client's attention to something else and ignoring the client's attempt to verbalize.
    4 This conveys a judgmental or critical attitude toward the client's actions.

180. **3** Extravasation of blood at the separation site into the myometrium causes a tetanic, board-like uterus. (b) (OB; AS; PA; HP)
    1 This is associated with placenta previa; pain and possible minimal external bleeding occur in abruptio placentae.

2 The uterus is rigid because of filling with blood and clots.
    4 This occurs with placenta previa; there is little external bleeding with abruptio placentae; if any does occur, it is dark red.

181. **2** In abruptio placentae there is uterine bleeding that results in massive internal hemorrhage, causing hypovolemic shock. (b) (OB; AS; PA; HP)
    1 Jaundice occurs only when there is seepage of bilirubin into subcutaneous tissues and skin; this is not associated with abruptio placentae.
    3 Convulsions are associated with pregnancy-induced hypertension; there is no information indicating the presence of this condition.
    4 It is more likely that with internal bleeding, blood pressure will fall rather than increase.

182. **3** This indicates afibrinogenemia; massive clotting in the area of the separation has resulted in a lowered circulating fibrinogen level. (b) (OB; AS; PA; HP)
    1 This is found in the postpartum period; a boggy uterus indicates a relaxed uterus with either placental membranes or clots present.
    2 Blood clots indicate normal fibrinogen levels; however, clots may indicate poor uterine contraction and should be explored further.
    4 This is not indicative of shock, which would be a likely occurrence with the uncontrolled bleeding of DIC.

183. **2** Gravid means pregnant, so gravida III indicates a third pregnancy. (a) (OB; AN; PA; IP)
    1 Neither para nor gravida indicates whether there are living children.
    3 Para and gravida do not refer to the gestational age of babies at birth.
    4 Gravida does not identify either induced or spontaneously aborted pregnancies.

184. **2** The cervix is 50% effaced and 6 cm dilated. (b) (OB; AS; PA; IP)
    1 When the cervix is 6 cm dilated the individual is beyond the early stage of labor.
    3 The transitional phase of labor begins when the cervix is 8 cm dilated.
    4 In the second stage of labor the cervix is fully dilated and 100% effaced.

185. **4** Greenish fluid is indicative of meconium, which is released by the fetus; it is considered an indicator of fetal distress unless the fetus is in breech position. (a) (OB; PL; TC; IP)
    1 This is normal; it is not indicative of any problem.
    2 A bloody show is normally present and may increase at the end of the first stage of labor; this is not indicative of any problem.
    3 This is a normal occurrence as labor progresses; it is not indicative of any problem.

186. **3** Bulging of the perineum is caused by the presence of the fetal head and usually signifies imminent delivery. (b) (OB; IM; PA; IP)
    1 Catheterization is indicated earlier in labor so that uterine contractions are not impeded; voiding will occur spontaneously with pushing.
    2 During the second stage of labor, the client is encouraged to push, not pant, with each contraction.
    4 Pain medication at this time is harmful to the fetus; it crosses the placental barrier and causes respiratory distress.

187. **4** Pitocin will cause the uterus to contract, which will assist in separating the placenta from the uterine wall. (b) (OB; EV; TC; DR)

    1 Prolactin, not pitocin, stimulates milk production.

    2 Relaxation of the uterus is undesirable and would not result in separation of the placenta.

    3 Pitocin has no analgesic effect.

How to Use Worksheet 1: Errors in Processing Information

Common errors in processing information are listed in the left-hand column of this worksheet. At the top of the worksheet is a row of blank spaces for inserting the number of the question missed. Directly below each number, check any errors you made in answering that question. You may have made more than one type of error in an answer.

Worksheet 1: Errors in processing information

Question number																			
Did not read situation/question carefully																			
Missed important details																			
Confused major and minor points																			
Defined problem incorrectly																			
Could not remember terms/facts/concepts/principles																			
Defined terms incorrectly																			
Focused on incomplete/incorrect data in assessing situation																			
Interpreted data incorrectly																			
Applied wrong concepts/principles in situation																			
Drew incorrect conclusions																			
Identified wrong goals																			
Identified priorities incorrectly																			
Carried out plan incorrectly/incompletely																			
Was unclear about criteria for evaluating success in achieving goals																			

How to Use Worksheet 2: Knowledge Gaps

Types of common knowledge gaps are listed along the top of this worksheet. Write a brief description of topics you want to review in the spaces provided. For example, if you missed a question on administration of a particular drug, write the drug name and problem (e.g., dosage) in the appropriate space under the column labeled *Pharmacology*.

Worksheet 2: Knowledge gaps

Basic science	Skills/ procedures	Basic human needs	Growth & develop- ment	Normal nutrition	Psycho- social factors	Clinical area/ topic	Stressors/ coping mechanisms	Patho- physiology	Pharma- cology	Therapeutic nutrition	Legal Implications	Other

Test 3

188. **1** Steroids cause gluconeogenesis and glycogenolysis, both of which raise blood glucose levels. (c) (ME; AN; PA; EN)

    2 This event is in the future and would not cause sufficient stress to elevate the serum glucose level to this degree at this time; retirement may be welcomed and may not cause stress.

    3 There is no data to indicate that this is a stressful event for the clinet.

    4 This is a chronic condition that has probably been incorporated into the client's coping patterns; it would not cause sufficient stress to elevate the serum glucose level to this degree.

189. **4** These are classic symptoms of ketoacidosis due to the respiratory system's attempt to compensate by blowing off excess carbon dioxide, a component of carbonic acid. (b) (ME; AS; PA; EN)

    1 This is indicative of insulin shock.

    2 This is a hypersensitivity reaction; it is unrelated to diabetes mellitus.

    3 Diaphoresis is associated with insulin shock, not diabetic ketoacidosis.

190. **1** This is the correct flow rate; 500 units of insulin added to 500 ml of IV results in a solution wherein 1 ml contains 1 unit of the drug; therefore 60 ml must be administered in 30 minutes; to determine flow rate multiply the amount to be infused (60) by the drop factor (10) and divide this result by the amount of time in minutes (30). (b) (ME; AN; TC; DR)

    2 This would deliver an excessive amount of insulin.

    3 Same as # 2.

    4 Same as # 2.

191. **2** Hypoglycemia affects the central nervous system causing headache and nervousness, and the sympathetic nervous system causing diaphoresis. (b) (ME; EV; TC; DR)

    1 These are not signs of insulin shock; excessive thirst and malaise are clinical symptoms of diabetes; hunger, not anorexia, is related to insulin shock.

    3 Dry skin and drowsiness are associated with ketoacidosis.

    4 These signs are all associated with ketoacidosis.

192. **2** Hypoglycemia stimulates the production of ACTH, glucagon, glucocorticoids, growth hormone, and catecholamines; this produces glycogenolysis and gluconeogenesis and results in hyperglycemia. (b) (ME; AN; PA; EN)

    1 This would result in hyperglycemia, not hypoglycemia.

    3 Same as # 1.

    4 Excessive glucose intake causes hyperglycemia, not gluconeogenesis.

193. **3** Exercise causes muscle contractions, which require an increase in arterial circulation to supply oxygen and nutrients for energy being expended. (a) (ME; PL; ED; CV)

    1 This would reduce arterial blood flow; the legs should be kept dependent.

    2 Hot water is contraindicated because it can burn the skin and/or cause drying; also, individuals with diabetes have neuropathies, which alter the perception of temperature.

    4 This is important for the person with diabetes, but it does not improve arterial blood flow.

194. **3** Covering exposed burned surfaces limits contamination by microorganisms and prevents exposure to air, which increases pain. (b) (SU; IM; TC; IT)

    1 This is unsafe; this would traumatize the skin.

    2 Same as # 1.

    4 Same as # 1.

195. **4** No bowel sounds are present; therefore the client must remain npo. (b) (SU; IM; PA; IT)

    1 This is unsafe; the client must be kept npo until bowel sounds are present, and then only fluids with electrolytes are indicated.

    2 Urinary output is adequate; there is no need to increase IV fluids.

    3 Same as # 1.

196. **2** Maintaining a patent airway is the priority; inhalation burns may have occurred. (a) (SU; AN; PA; RE)

    1 This is extremely important but not the first priority.

    3 Same as # 1.

    4 Same as # 1.

197. **2** This indicates infection and should immediately be reported. (a) (SU; EV; PA; IT)

    1 Serosanguinous oozing is to be expected.

    3 This is not a problem.

    4 This indicates healing and is desirable.

198. **4** Of the selections offered this is the highest in calories and protein, which are needed for the increased basal metabolic rate and for tissue repair. (c) (SU; PL; TC; IT)

    1 These foods do not provide as high an amount of calories and protein as the correct choice.

    2 Same as # 1.

    3 Same as # 1.

199. **2** Shortening of the affected leg occurs because of the overriding of bone fragments. (a) (SU; AS; PA; SK)

    1 The affected leg should not be moved because it can cause further damage to nerves and blood vessels.

    3 Same as # 1.

    4 Although bruising may be present with a fracture, it also may be present from soft tissue injury.

200. **3** Arterial perfusion and the presence of hemorrhage must be assessed hourly to prevent complications or identify problems early. (a) (SU; EV; TC; SK)

    1 This is unsafe; this will interfere with the pull of traction.

    2 Same as # 1.

    4 Same as # 1.

201. **4** Drug dose and frequency are adjusted according to these readings to enhance efficacy; therapeutic levels are maintained. (a) (SU; EV; TC; DR)

    1 Peak and trough levels reveal nothing about allergic reactions.

    2 Renal clearance would affect the readings, but adequate renal function must be determined before therapy to avoid toxicity.

    3 A sustained drop in fever is the desired outcome, not reduction just at peak serum levels of the drug.

202. **4** This is the correct flow rate; the amount to be in-

fused (50) is multiplied by the drop factor (10) and the result is divided by the amount of time in minutes (30). (b) (SU; AN; TC; DR)

1 This rate is too slow; this would not deliver the desired dosage in 30 minutes.

2 Same as # 1.

3 Same as # 1.

203. **4** This is a prime time for symptoms of a pulmonary embolus to appear. (b) (SU; EV; TC; SK)

1 This would not require nursing intervention; a productive cough would indicate a respiratory infection.

2 This could result from the inflammatory process; the temperature-regulating mechanisms in the aged may be slightly compromised, and they may show a slight elevation in body temperature for a longer period of time after surgery.

3 All weight bearing is being done by the unoperative leg at this time, and fatigue may be expected.

204. **2** Absence of peptidase results in inability to metabolize the gliadin fraction of grains; this results in excessive glutamine that is toxic to the mucosal cells. (a) (PE; AN; PA; GI)

1 This is unrelated; meconium is present in the first bowel movements before the introduction of food.

3 This does not occur.

4 Fluid balance is not the basic problem with celiac disease; however, dehydration can occur in celiac crisis.

205. **4** Frankfurter has grain filler; parents should read labels and unless they are sure of ingredients, should not feed the food to the child. (b) (PE; EV; ED; GI)

1 This does not contain gluten.

2 This does not contain gluten; this is a substitute for grain foods.

3 Same as #2.

206. **1** The diet must be followed forever because there will always be an absence of peptidase; some variations to this diet may be allowed, but this should not be promised. (b) (PE; IM; ED; GI)

2 This is untrue; each phase of child development may have problems related to dietary management; follow-up care is needed to prevent crises.

3 This is untrue; gluten must be avoided for a prolonged period of time and usually indefinitely.

4 This is untrue; a restricted diet is never easy to follow, especially for a growing child.

207. **1** Favorable personality change within 1 to 2 days attests to the effectiveness of the diet; other improvements take longer. (c) (PE; EV; PA; GI)

2 Usually anorexia is not a problem; if it does occur, it does so during bouts of diarrhea.

3 This occurs after the personality change.

4 Same as # 3.

208. **3** Autonomy leads to exploring and self-feeding; child may eat food not on the diet. (b) (PE; AS; ED; GD)

1 Although this is a common characteristic of a toddler, it would not lead to the child eating restricted foods.

2 Same as # 1.

4 Same as # 1.

209. **3** Skin-to-skin contact between mother and infant is most effective in maintaining the infant's body temperature; heat is transferred by conduction. (a) (OB; IM; PA; NN)

1 This is not very effective and leaves much of the baby exposed; a blanket and warmer would also be necessary.

2 Bathing the infant should be delayed until the body temperature is stabilized.

4 Oxygen is not administered unless the infant is experiencing respiratory and cardiac difficulties; oxygen has a cooling effect.

210. **2** A strong cry indicates good respiratory function and is assigned a value of 2. (a) (OB; AS; PA; NN)

1 The heart rate should be over 100 per min and therefore is assigned a value of 1.

3 If the flexion of the arms and legs is only slight and movement is diminished, the value assigned is 1.

4 A value of 1 is assigned when the body is pink and the extremities are blue.

211. **1** The liver is usually palpable in the newborn at 2 cm below the costal margin. (a) (OB; AS; PA; NN)

2 The stomach is never palpable, and the borders are not detectable.

3 The pancreas is never palpable because it is located in the posterior portion of the abdominal cavity.

4 The gall bladder is not palpable because it is a posterior structure.

212. **2** Dislocation of the hip limits abduction to less than 90 degrees. (b) (OB; AS; PA; NN)

1 This is a normal finding in the newborn; maternal hormones cause loosening of ligaments, which allows abduction to 90 degrees.

3 It is normal for the legs to be of equal length.

4 Fixation of the hips is not affected by dislocation.

213. **2** The fontanels, anterior and posterior, are both open at birth. (b) (OB; AS; PA; NN)

1 Closed sutures are abnormal and may prevent normal brain growth during the first year.

3 This is cephalohematoma, an abnormal but common finding, indicating injury to the head during the labor process.

4 This would indicate dehydration.

214. **3** Central cyanosis (blue lips and face) indicates lowered oxygen of the blood caused by either decreased lung expansion or right-to-left shunting of blood. (b) (OB; AS; PA; HN)

1 This is normal in the newborn.

2 Same as # 1.

4 This is not an abnormal finding because peripheral circulation of the infant is poor; blueness disappears when the baby is warm.

215. **4** The greatest danger associated with depression is self-inflicted injury when feelings, especially anger, are internalized. (b) (PS; PL; PE; MO)

1 This is false reassurance; this is not supportive of the client's feelings at this time.

2 The client is unable to control or regulate her own behavior at this time.

3 A low-calorie diet would be more appropriate because of the client's decreased physical activity.

216. **1** This is direct quotation of the client's statement with no added value judgments. (b) (PS; AS; PE; MO)

2 This is subjective judgment and interpretation of what the client actually said.

3 Same as # 2.

4 Same as # 2.

217. **3** It is necessary to assess behavior changes that clue the nurse to impending suicidal acting out. (b) (PS; IM; TC; MO)
    1 Because there has been no overt acting out, continuous observation may threaten the client's ability to maintain self-control.
    2 Detailed explanations are inappropriate and overwhelming for a client with psychomotor retardation.
    4 The depressed client cannot follow involved interesting activities because of psychomotor retardation.

218. **1** The effects of the tricyclic antidepressants are cumulative; it may be some time before improvement is noted. (b) (PS; IM; ED; DR)
    2 It is not a nursing function to determine drugs for the client.
    3 Antidepressant drugs are effective in the treatment regardless of the length of the depression.
    4 This is false; antidepressants help relieve the physical and mental discomforts of the depressed client.

219. **2** This response recognizes capability without adding stress or increasing dependency. (c) (PS; IM; PE; MO)
    1 This increases dependency, which is not therapeutic.
    3 This does not address the client's needs and is punitive.
    4 This attempts to manipulate compliance; the client cannot accept responsibility for the future.

220. **4** A change in behavior may indicate the client has worked out a plan for suicide; the potential for acting out on suicide increases when physical energy returns. (b) (PS; IM; TC; MO)
    1 This is not indicated at this time.
    2 This may increase the client's feelings of inadequacy, because it implies the client did not look well before.
    3 The client should not be considered for discharge simply because of a change in behavior.

221. **3** A large percentage of HIV-positive individuals eventually develop AIDS. (b) (PE; AS; PA; BI)
    1 Although blood transfusions can place someone at risk, a positive serologic status places a person at highest risk for AIDS.
    2 An immature reticuloendothelial system does not indicate the potential development of AIDS.
    4 The presence of an opportunistic infection alone is not an indication of AIDS.

222. **3** This statement acknowledges the mother's feelings. (c) (PE; IM; PE; EC)
    1 This statement gives false hope.
    2 This statement does not address the mother's feelings.
    4 Same as # 2.

223. **1** This statement is not true because the virus could still be transmitted if the result was a false negative. (c) (PE; EV; ED; BI)
    2 Blood screening has improved and has reduced the incidence of transmission, but it is still not perfect.
    3 Blood that tests negatively can seroconvert at a later time.
    4 This is a true statement; members of high-risk groups are more apt to be HIV positive.

224. **3** The Centers for Disease Control have determined that health professionals should use gloves when coming into direct contact with body fluids and blood of HIV-infected individuals because these fluids contain the virus. (a) (PE; PL; TC; BI)
    1 Approaching the bedside does not expose the health care worker to the virus.
    2 Contact should not be limited; this does not allow for optimal care of the client.
    4 Gloves, mask, and gown are not needed when the health worker is not in contact with body fluids and blood.

225. **1** The estrogen and progesterone in birth control pills increase the amount of renin, which in turn increases production of angiotensin, a potent pressor substance. (a) (OB; EV; TC; FS)
    2 This is untrue.
    3 This is not usually serious; it often indicates a low hormone level; it is corrected by changes in the type of medication prescribed.
    4 Anovulation is the desired effect of oral contraceptives.

226. **2** The objective is to stimulate ovulation near the fourteenth day of the menstrual cycle, which is achieved by taking the drug on the fifth through the ninth days; there is an increase in the pituitary gonadotrophins LH and FSH, with subsequent ovarian stimulation. (b) (OB; EV; ED; DR)
    1 There is insufficient estrogen at this time for Clomid to be effective this early in the cycle.
    3 This is too late in the cycle.
    4 There are insufficient hormones to be effective.

227. **1** This shows understanding and offers reassurance that this is a normal side effect; this response also offers a possible solution. (a) (OB; EV; ED; DR)
    2 This indicates a problem where one probably does not exist.
    3 This side effect continues as long as the drug is continued.
    4 This side effect has nothing to do with ovulation.

228. **4** An objective examiner confirms the fetal movements; this eliminates subjectivity by the client. (b) (OB; AS; PA; PN)
    1 This is a softening of the lower uterine segment, a presumptive sign of pregnancy.
    2 This could be caused by a variety of situations other than pregnancy; it is a probable sign of pregnancy.
    3 Only a probable sign of pregnancy because of possible false negative readings.

229. **3** The term *atherosclerosis* means a thickening of the arterial lining by lipid plaques, which become atheromas. (a) (ME; AN; PA; CV)
    1 Atheromas develop within the lining of the artery, not within the muscle tissue.
    2 Mobilization of free fatty acids will produce an acid-base imbalance.
    4 Arterial pressure is increased as a result of renin.

230. **1** Lunch meat is processed and has high sodium levels to help in preservation. (a) (ME; PL; ED; CV)
    2 Canned salmon is high in sodium, but fresh salmon is not.
    3 Broccoli does not have significant sodium levels.
    4 Beef is lower in sodium than are preserved meats; however, beef is high in saturated fat.

231. **4** The taste for salt is learned from habitual use and can be unlearned or reduced with health-improvement motivation and creative salt-free food preparation. (c) (ME; IM; ED; FE)
    1 The taste for salt is learned.

2 This is untrue; substitutes often have a metallic taste.

3 This is unsafe; abnormally high potassium levels can result.

232. **2** Research has shown that decreasing stress will decrease the rate of atherosclerosis development. (a) (ME; PL; ED; CV)

1 Saturated fats in the diet increase atherosclerosis.

3 Exercise is thought to decrease atherosclerosis and the formation of lipid plaques.

4 Same as # 3.

233. **4** Client safety always has the highest priority over any other client needs. (a) (PS; PL; TC; SD)

1 This is a later priority.

2 Same as # 1.

3 Same as # 1.

234. **1** This is an accurate and concise explanation of Haldol's effects; it blocks postsynaptic dopamine receptors in the brain. (a) (PS; IM; ED; DR)

2 This is not true; it is a tranquilizer, and it does not alter mood.

3 Same as # 2.

4 This drug lowers the seizure threshold.

235. **2** Photosensitivity is a side effect of many antipsychotic medications. (c) (PS; EV; TC; DR)

1 This is a precaution associated with lithium, not with Haldol.

3 Avoiding tyramine-containing foods is a precaution associated with MAO inhibitors, not with Haldol.

4 These symptoms are side effects of lithium, not of Haldol.

236. **1** Talking with others in similar circumstances provides support and allows for sharing of experiences. (a) (PS; IM; TC; TR)

2 This is not therapeutic; it offers false reassurance.

3 The feeling of guilt has not been expressed.

4 This avoids the client's concerns and cuts off communication.

237. **3** These are the classic symptoms of neuroleptic malignant syndrome, which is caused by neuroleptic-induced blockage of dopamine receptors. (c) (PS; EV; TC; DR)

1 These are side effects of Haldol, but they are not signs of neuroleptic malignant syndrome.

2 Same as # 1.

4 Same as # 1.

238. **4** Grief reactions to the impending loss and security present in the one-to-one relationship need to be anticipated. (c) (PS; EV; PE; TR)

1 There should not be a disintegration of the personality.

2 This phase occurs early in the one-to-one relationship, not at termination.

3 This behavior may occur in the early phase of a working relationship.

239. **3** The client's systolic reading is 32mm Hg above the baseline reading and the diastolic reading is 15mm Hg above the baseline; a marked increase indicating a hypertensive disorder of pregnancy would be 30mm Hg for the systolic reading and 15mm Hg for the diastolic reading. (c) (OB; AS; TC; HP)

1 This is an insufficient rise to indicate a hypertensive disorder of pregnancy.

2 Same as # 1.

4 Although this would indicate hypertension, it would be too far advanced for a person who normally exhibits a low blood pressure.

240. **1** The increased circulating plasma volume during pregnancy requires more protein to sustain the plasma protein level essential for normal capillary fluid shift mechanism and correction of hypovolemia. (c) (OB; PL; TC; HP)

2 It is impossible to eliminate all salt; salt is usually not restricted in hypertensive disorders of pregnancy; only excessive salt intake is discouraged.

3 Caloric intake should not be restricted during pregnancy because of the associated increased BMR and the needs of the developing fetus.

4 The person is hypervolemic, not hypovolemic; iron promotes RBC production, not an increased circulating blood volume.

241. **2** Inadequate protein decreases colloidal osmotic pressure within the vascular space, allowing fluid to shift into the interstitial spaces. (b) (OB; EV; PA; HP)

1 Protein does not affect heart rate.

3 Bleeding gums are due to a deficiency in vitamin C or platelets, not protein.

4 Petechiae result from an abnormality in the clotting mechanism such as thrombocytopenia.

242. **1** This indicates failure to resolve conflicting feelings about pregnancy that commonly occur in the first trimester. (c) (OB; PL; PE; EC)

2 This is a normal feeling in the third trimester.

3 Same as # 2.

4 Same as # 2.

243. **3** Respiratory distress or arrest may occur when the serum level of magnesium sulfate reaches 12 to 15 mg/dl; deep tendon reflexes disappear when the serum level is 10 to 12 mg/dl; the drug is withheld in the absence of deep tendon reflexes. (c) (OB; EV; TC; DR)

1 This is an inappropriate assessment to determine client response to magnesium sulfate; deep tendon reflexes need to be assessed.

2 Same as # 1.

4 Same as # 1.

244. **2** Respiratory depression occurs in magnesium sulfate toxicity because of CNS depression. (c) (OB; EV; TC; HN)

1 This is not a sign of magnesium sulfate toxicity.

3 Same as # 1.

4 Same as # 1.

245. **2** Mottling of the skin results from hypothermia in the newborn. (a) (OB; IM; PA; NN)

1 Feeding will not increase temperature.

3 This is not necessary; the baby requires warming.

4 This is not necessary; this is a normal phenomenon that usually indicates falling temperature; the baby requires warming.

246. **4** SGA infants have little subcutaneous fat or glycogen stores. (b) (OB; AS; PA; HN)

1 Increased intracranial pressure is not characteristic of SGA infants.

2 This would provide no therapeutic value for this SGA infant.

3 Intestinal bleeding is not common in SGA infants.

247. **4** A rising reticulocyte count indicates accelerated erythropoietic activity that may reflect increased

RBC destruction; increased RBC destruction raises the bilirubin level, causing jaundice. (c) (OB; AN; PA; HN)

  1 This test does not reflect respiratory functioning; however, ultimately with hemorrhage the respiratory rate will be elevated.

  2 Although the reticulocyte count may be elevated with chronic blood loss, there is no data to indicate the baby is bleeding.

  3 In this instance the sedimentation rate or WBCs, not the reticulocytes, would be elevated.

248. **1** Talking about what actually happened helps the client sort out the truth from confused thoughts and begins to help the client accept what happened as a part of the history. (b) (PS; IM; PE; CS)

  2 Most rapes are planned in advance and are violent acts of the perpetrators, who are responsible for their behavior; nevertheless, the victim often feels unjustifed guilt related to the incident.

  3 The victim should be told of the legal services available; legal counsel should come from a legal authority.

  4 If the client does not want to discuss intimate details, this should be respected.

249. **3** The client needs to feel in control to prevent ego deterioration. (c) (PS; PL; PE; CS)

  1 It is too soon after the rape to discuss this.

  2 Same as # 1.

  4 Although the nurse should always be available and supportive; feelings of anger are usually not the initial response.

250. **3** When the rape victim chooses to prosecute the rapist, the victim must prove that rape occurred; the accused is innocent until proven guilty. (a) (PS; AN; TC; CS)

  1 The perpetrator tries to establish innocence in a rape case; the victim must prove that the rapist is guilty.

  2 The medical team may be asked to provide evidence at the trial, but the victim must prove that the rapist is guilty.

  4 Guilt or innocence will be established by a jury, with the burden of proof placed on the victim.

251. **2** This eliminates the nurse's subjectivity from the report. (a) (PS; IM; TC; CS)

  1 This would allow for subjectivity.

  3 This is unrelated to the rape itself; this would allow for subjectivity.

  4 This is not part of the responsibility of the medical team.

252. **3** Systemic antibiotics are necessary to eradicate the streptococcal organism, which caused the primary infection, impetigo. (b) (PE; PL; TC; RG)

  1 This would not prevent glomerulonephritis; this is part of the local therapy for impetigo.

  2 Same as # 1.

  4 This would not prevent glomerulonephritis.

253. **2** Weight monitoring is the most useful means of assessing fluid balance and changes in the edematous state; 1 L of fluid weighs about 2.2 pounds. (b) (PE; PL; TC; FE)

  1 This is not as accurate as daily weights; fluid can be trapped in the third compartment with no alteration in intake and output.

  3 This would be subjective and inaccurate.

  4 This is unreliable; these may or may not be altered with fluid shifts.

254. **2** Preschoolers are active, sociable individuals who enjoy the company of peers and become bored when isolated. (c) (PE; IM; PA; GD)

  1 Five-year-olds have a limited ability to understand complex explanations of cause and effect; they employ concrete thinking.

  3 This will increase agitation and be punitive.

  4 Although this would provide some distraction, it is better to permit peer contacts.

255. **4** Bed rest promotes decreased cardiac output; it also decreases tissue catabolism, which lowers the workload of the kidneys, eventually increasing filtration by the renal glomeruli; limiting activity also helps lower the blood pressure. (b) (PE; PL; ED; RG)

  1 The activity level depends on the response to therapy.

  2 Bed rest is necessary during the acute phase of illness.

  3 Same as # 1.

256. **3** Hoarseness is caused by the inability of the vocal cords to come close during speech when a tumor exists. (b) (SU; AS; PA; RE)

  1 Aphasia refers to an expressive or receptive communication deficit as a result of cerebral disease; it is not related to laryngeal cancer.

  2 Dysphagia is a late sign, occurring when the tumor is large enough to compress the esophagus.

  4 Dyspnea is a late sign, occurring when the tumor is large enough to obstruct air flow.

257. **2** This is the correct amount;
0.3mg : 0.4mg = Xml : 0.5ml;
X = 0.4ml or 6 minims. (b) (SU; AN; TC; DR)

  1 This would be an overdose.

  3 This would be an inappropriately low dose.

  4 Same as # 3.

258. **4** The client will be unable to speak because a tracheostomy tube is in place to prevent edema from blocking the airway; writing provides an alternate form of communication. (a) (SU; IM; PE; RE)

  1 This has no effect; the client's ability to hear or understand is not affected.

  2 The client cannot speak with a tracheostomy tube in place.

  3 Same as # 1.

259. **1** The amount of solution (1000) is divided by the hourly amount to be infused (150) which equals 6.66; the decimal portion of the result must be converted to minutes (0.66 x 60 min), which equals 40 minutes plus the 6 hours. (b) (SU; AN; TC; FE)

  2 The solution should be infused before this time.

  3 Same as # 2.

  4 Same as # 2.

260. **1** Subcutaneous emphysema refers to the presence of air in the tissue that surrounds an opening in the normally closed respiratory tract; the tissue appears puffy, and a crackling sensation is detected under the fingertips as trapped air is compressed between the tissue. (b) (SU; AS; TC; RE)

  2 The lungs are not affected.

  3 Gas exchange, and thus blood gases, are not affected.

  4 Same as # 2.

261. **3** The client is nervous and afraid of leaving home; the priority is provision for safety and security needs. (c) (PS; PL; PE; AX)

1 Unless the client is provided with a sense of security, adjustment is likely to be unsatisfactory because the anxiety will most likely escalate.

2 The client is experiencing memory loss and may not be able to remember what precipitated admission to the hospital; some memory loss may be due to high anxiety and thought blocking.

4 This cannot be done until anxiety is reduced.

262. **3** Without trust, the nurse-client relationship will achieve nothing. (a) (PS; AN; PE; TR)

1 Trust comes first.

2 Although rapport is important, trust must be developed first.

4 Same as # 2.

263. **4** The person transfers anxieties to objects, usually inanimate objects, which are then avoided to decrease anxiety. (a) (PS; AN; PA; AX)

1 Projection, the attributing of undesirable traits or unacceptable feelings or motivations to others, is not the main defense mechanism used by someone with a phobia.

2 Regression, the return to an earlier more comfortable level of adjustment, is not the main defense mechanism used by someone with a phobia.

3 Repression, the pushing of unacceptable impulses or ideas into the unconscious, is not the main defense mechanism used by someone with a phobia.

264. **4** No specific diet is recommended; the client is encouraged to avoid meals that overdistend the stomach and foods that cause GI distress. (c) (ME; PL; PA; GI)

1 High-fat dairy products increase GI secretion and should be avoided.

2 There is no need for a mechanical soft diet, which would be appropriate for those who have difficulty with chewing and swallowing.

3 The client does not have to be restricted to a liquid diet.

265. **1** Ranitidine inhibits histamine at H$_2$ receptor sites in parietal cells, which inhibits gastric secretion. (c) (ME; AN; PA; DR)

2 This drug does not regenerate the gastric mucosa; the drug prevents its erosion by gastric secretions.

3 This is not the direct action of this drug; this is the action of antacids.

4 This would be undesirable; gastric hormones increase gastric acid secretion.

266. **2** Antacids are most effective when taken after digestion has started but before the stomach begins to empty. (b) (ME; EV; ED; DR)

1 The antacids would interfere with the absorption of nutrients.

3 Same as # 1.

4 Antacids should be taken before the onset of pain; pain indicates that gastric irritation has begun, and the aim of treatment is to protect the GI mucosa.

267. **2** Eating in a semirecumbent position slows gastric emptying, thereby preventing premature gastric dumping of contents. (c) (SU; PL; ED; GI)

1 This would speed gastric emptying and should be avoided.

3 Same as # 1.

4 Same as # 1.

268. **3** Gastric secretions, which are electrolyte rich, are lost through the NG tube; the imbalances that result could prove life threatening. (a) (SU; EV; TC; FE)

1 This is unsafe; if respiratory intubation has occurred, aspiration will result.

2 This is unsafe; this could result in suture line disruption.

4 This is unnecessary and could damage the suture line.

269. **2** This objective includes observable client behavior, which is specified by amount and time and therefore is measurable. (b) (SU; AN; TC; RE)

1 This objective is not stated in measurable terms.

3 This is a statement, not an objective.

4 Same as # 1.

270. **4** This technique is required when a wound is infected to prevent the spread of infection to others. (b) (SU; IM; TC; IT)

1 This may be used with clients who are immunosuppressed and at risk for infection.

2 This technique is used when changing dressings to protect the client from infection.

3 Wound or peritoneal infections are transmitted through incisional drainage, not feces.

271. **4** School-age children are most concerned about school, if not for the academics, for the social aspects. (b) (PE; AS; ED; GD)

1 School-age children are generally not this future oriented.

2 This may be of some concern, but not as much as is school.

3 School-age children generally look at physicians as authority figures and do not doubt their competence.

272. **4** Children, because of the demands of growth and their dietary indiscretions, have a more fragile glucose balance. (a) (PE; IM; ED; EN)

1 The fragility of glucose balance is not due to resistance to treatment, but rather to the changing requirements associated with growth.

2 This is untrue; it is more often associated with non–insulin-dependent diabetes mellitus.

3 This is untrue; hypersensitivity is unrelated to either type of diabetes mellitus.

273. **1** An infection will increase the metabolic rate, which eventually results in hyperglycemia. (c) (PE; EV; ED; EN)

2 This would cause hypoglycemia.

3 Same as # 2.

4 Same as # 2.

274. **1** Insulin, a hormone and protein, when taken orally is destroyed by digestive enzymes, particularly pepsin. (b) (PE; IM; ED; DR)

2 It is not neutralized; it is inactivated by digestive enzymes.

3 This is untrue.

4 The potency of insulin is not just reduced, it is totally inactivated.

275. **1** Specialized insulin receptors on insulin-sensitive cells transport glucose through cell membranes, making it available for use. (a) (PE; AN; ED; EN)

2 This is not the action of insulin.

3 Same as # 2.

4 Same as # 2.

276. **1** Saccharin is an non-nutritive substitute; aspartame is made of two amino acids, phenylalanine

and aspartic acid, and is metabolized as such. (b) (PE; IM; ED; EN)

2 Honey, a fructose, provides 1.3 times as many Kcal as does table sugar and must be calculated into the diet.

3 Simple sugars may be used in controlled amounts and must be calculated into the diet.

4 Foods do not have to taste sweet to contain sugar.

277. **2** Baseline vital signs are extremely important; physical assessment precedes diagnostic measures and intervention. (b) (ME; AS; PA; RE)

1 A sputum specimen should be obtained after vital signs and before administration of antibiotics.

3 This would be done after the physician makes a medical diagnosis; this is not an independent function of the nurse.

4 This might be done after it is determined if a specimen for blood gases is needed; this is not usually an independent function of the nurse; oxygen is only administered independently by the nurse in an emergency situation.

278. **2** The data presented indicates an infectious process within the lung. (a) (ME; AN; PA; RE)

1 The cardinal signs would be pain in the lower lobe at the height of inspiration and a pleural friction rub.

3 The cardinal signs would be barrel chest, resonance on percussion, and thick tenacious sputum.

4 Although fever and chills can occur later in the disease, the cardinal signs are irritating cough, chest pain, and shortness of breath.

279. **3** This recognizes the client's feelings and encourages communication. (b) (ME; IM; PE; EC)

1 Although this may be true, it does not encourage further communication.

2 This question sounds accusatory; it ignores the client's feelings and discourages communication.

4 This statement negates the client's feelings and discourages communication.

280. **2** The client may become injured in many ways during a seizure, and trauma prevention is a priority. (b) (ME; PL; ED; NM)

1 Especially early in therapy, many anticonvulsants can cause GI disturbances; they should be taken with food.

3 Others should be aware of the condition and taught how to help in case of a seizure.

4 This is untrue; symptoms and treatment of seizure disorders vary greatly.

281. **1** Ataxia is a side effect of phenytoin, and drug continuation may cause cerebellar damage. (c) (ME; EV; ED; DR)

2 Massaging the gums should be done regularly to prevent gingival hyperplasia, which can result from phenytoin therapy.

3 The client should report the rash but keep taking the drug; withdrawal may precipitate a seizure.

4 This sign of toxicity should be reported.

How to Use Worksheet 1: Errors in Processing Information

Common errors in processing information are listed in the left-hand column of this worksheet. At the top of the worksheet is a row of blank spaces for inserting the number of the question missed. Directly below each number, check any errors you made in answering that question. You may have made more than one type of error in an answer.

Worksheet 1: Errors in processing information

Question number																				
Did not read situation/question carefully																				
Missed important details																				
Confused major and minor points																				
Defined problem incorrectly																				
Could not remember terms/ facts/concepts/principles																				
Defined terms incorrectly																				
Focused on incomplete/incorrect data in assessing situation																				
Interpreted data incorrectly																				
Applied wrong concepts/principles in situation																				
Drew incorrect conclusions																				
Identified wrong goals																				
Identified priorities incorrectly																				
Carried out plan incorrectly/incompletely																				
Was unclear about criteria for evaluating success in achieving goals																				

How to Use Worksheet 2: Knowledge Gaps

Types of common knowledge gaps are listed along the top of this worksheet. Write a brief description of topics you want to review in the spaces provided. For example, if you missed a question on administration of a particular drug, write the drug name and problem (e.g., dosage) in the appropriate space under the column labeled *Pharmacology.*

Worksheet 2: Knowledge gaps

Basic science	Skills/procedures	Basic human needs	Growth & development	Normal nutrition	Psychosocial factors	Clinical area/topic	Stressors/coping mechanisms	Patho-physiology	Pharma-cology	Therapeutic nutrition	Legal implications	Other

Test 4

282. **1** This will help to elicit any fantasy the child may have; it helps the child understand that treatment is not a punishment. (c) (PE; IM; PE; EC)

2 This is not currently supported as a cause; this is inappropriate discussion for a 4-year-old.

3 This is inappropriate for a 4-year-old and does not elicit feelings.

4 This is inappropriate; it may be frightening.

283. **2** The symptoms are caused by unrestricted white blood cell proliferation and resultant decreased platelet production. (a) (PE; AS; PA; BI)

1 These are not the presenting symptoms; this occurs through infiltration of the vascular organs of the reticuloendothelial system by immature WBCs.

3 Pain is not an early symptom; the skin will be pale.

4 Papilledema is not a common presenting symptom because the blood-brain barrier is an initial deterrent.

284. **4** This accurately responds to the parents' question, reinforcing what the physician explained. (b) (PE; IM; ED; BI)

1 This would abdicate teaching responsibilities.

2 This is an insensitive response that places the parents in a defensive position.

3 This statement reinforces parental insecurity about the information they have recently received from the physician; this may increase anxiety.

285. **3** Platelets are rapidly administered to avoid destruction after hanging the IV. (b) (PE; IM; TC; BI)

1 Dextrose solution is not appropriate for flushing a blood derivative line because it may clog the IV line.

2 Platelets should not hang for a long time because of their fragility.

4 This is too long an interval; during infusion of blood derivatives, vital signs are more closely monitored.

286. **2** Anxiety and stress tend to close communication; this in turn intensifies the reaction to illness and death. (c) (PS; PL; PE; CS)

1 This is true, but the focus should be on mutual understanding by all members.

3 The family system could not solve all its problems at this time because of the emotional turmoil of its members.

4 This is false; the family must begin to deal with feelings before death occurs.

287. **2** How people handled grief in the past provides clues to their coping patterns when dealing with current grieving. (b) (PS; AN; PA; CS)

1 Although these are important, past experiences with grief are paramount.

3 Same as # 1.

4 Same as # 1.

288. **1** This is the intentional touching of one person by another without permission of the person touched. (b) (PS; EV; TC; CS)

2 This is an intentional act, without touching, that makes a person fearful or produces reasonable apprehension of bodily harm.

3 This refers to the right of clients to have their private affairs protected.

4 This applies to written permission for procedures and treatments to be performed.

289. **3** Because the client is feeling a loss of control, it would be important to include the client in revision of the plan. (b) (PS; PL; TC; CS)

1 This is very authoritarian and places total control with the nurse.

2 This does not consider changes in the client or the client's feelings.

4 This is unnecessary; these are the nurse's functions and judgments, not the physician's.

290. **1** This demonstrates the client's diminished anger and is a realistic assessment and acceptance of present capabilities and limitations. (b) (PS; EV; PE; CS)

2 This shows dependency; either the client has given up or is being sarcastic.

3 This shows dependency and suggests the client has given up.

4 Anger is still apparent at loss of decision making; there is no real evidence of sharing.

291. **3** This provides the family member with an opportunity to express his feelings. (a) (PS; IM; PE; CS)

1 This shuts off communication and abdicates nursing responsibility toward the client.

2 This is false reassurance and cuts off communication.

4 Although true, this statement really does not address the family's concerns.

292. **2** Breast palpation should be done in the supine position with a small towel roll under the shoulder of the palpated side. (a) (ME; EV; ED; IT)

1 This is a correct procedure for breast self-examination.

3 Same as # 1.

4 Same as # 1.

293. **4** Lack of symmetry and palpation of a thickening are signs of a possible breast mass. (a) (ME; EV; TC; IT)

1 This is a common deviation, that is within normal limits.

2 Engorgement is an expected response to menstrual hormones.

3 Premenstrual engorgement may cause the breast to feel lumpy.

294. **3** Reflecting these feelings gives the client the opportunity to express fears and provides a chance to explore family history. (b) (SU; IM; PE; EC)

1 Although true, this provides false reassurance.

2 This supports the client's fears of cancer and blocks communication.

4 This statement is probing and does not address the client's fears.

295. **4** When clients in obvious crisis appear depressed, anxious, and desperate, the nurse should question them regarding the presence of suicidal thoughts, because immediate hospitalization may be required. (b) (SU; IM; PE; EC)

1 Further assessment and exploration is needed before encouraging clients to admit themselves to a psychiatric facility.

2 Running away from problems does not help solve them, nor will escaping bring lasting relief.

3 When the client is overwhelmed with problems, it is difficult to think positively and to focus on the good things in life.

296. **3** At this time breast engorgement is minimal, and this provides a regular examination cycle. (a) (ME; EV; ED; IT)
    1 Premenstrual breast engorgement may cause the breast to feel lumpy.
    2 Breast consistency is altered by the menstrual cycle; the same date each month would fall in a different stage of the cycle.
    4 Ovulation is occurring, and hormones may influence breast consistency.

297. **1** Itching associated with jaundice is believed to be caused by an accumulation of bile salts in the skin. (a) (ME; AS; PA; GI)
    2 This symptom may occur but is not related to jaundice.
    3 Same as # 2.
    4 This symptom is not related to jaundice.

298. **2** This response provides needed information and establishes the opportunity for further discussion of surgery. (b) (SU; IM; PE; EC)
    1 This implies the other approaches are as effective as surgery; this places doubt in the client's mind that surgery is the most effective option.
    3 This is an inappropriate response; the competence of the physician was not questioned, but there exists a need for a further discussion of the treatment; making this type of referral is not the nurse's role.
    4 This is false reassurance; it cuts off communication and does not address the need for further discussion.

299. **4** The common bile duct passes through the head of the pancreas; it is often constricted or obstructed by the neoplasm. (c) (ME; AN; PA; GI)
    1 This is the prehepatic cause of jaundice; it is not applicable in this situation.
    2 This is a hepatic cause of jaundice; it is not applicable in this situation.
    3 This would not cause jaundice.

300. **2** This behavior indicates that the client is comfortable; therefore the medication regimen is effective. (b) (SU; EV; TC; NM)
    1 The efficacy of Demerol decreases when the drug is given orally; this is too soon after surgery to alter the route.
    3 This is the accepted dose; no data exists to indicate it is excessive for this client.
    4 This is not necessary; the medication regimen is effective.

301. **3** This individualized information would be the best basis for predicting the outcome of therapy. (b) (SU; PL; TC; EC)
    1 This would be useful, but it is not specific for this client.
    2 This knowledge would not be helpful in understanding the likelihood of additional problems associated with the current cancer.
    4 Same as # 2.

302. **3** Protein deficiency causes a low serum albumin, which permits fluid shifts from the intravascular to the interstitial compartment, causing edema; decreased protein also causes anemia; protein intake must be increased. (b) (ME; AN; PA; GI)
    1 Although a deficiency of iron would result in anemia, it would not cause the other symptoms.
    2 Hypokalemia would not cause these symptoms; it causes cramps and weakness.
    4 This is unrelated to these symptoms; it is an es-

sential fatty acid.

303. **4** In a client with perforated viscera, barium could leak out of the intestinal tract and cause inflammation and/or abscess. (b) (ME; AN; TC; GI)
    1 Serum potassium would be unaffected; barium is insoluble and would not affect blood content.
    2 Barium studies are not contraindicated and could be useful in diagnosing ulcerative colitis and Crohn's disease.
    3 Although it may be irritating, this does not contraindicate barium studies.

304. **2** Taking the drug in the early morning mimics normal adrenal secretions; food and/or antacid helps reduce gastric irritation. (a) (ME; EV; ED; DR)
    1 The food helps decrease gastric irritation; however, normal diurnal rhythms could be altered.
    3 Steroids cause gastric irritation and should be taken with food.
    4 Diurnal rhythms may be altered, and steroids are ulcerogenic; they should be taken with more than just a snack.

305. **4** Impulse conduction of skeletal muscles is impaired with decreased K^+ levels; muscular weakness and cramps may occur. (b) (ME; EV; ED; FE)
    1 Hyperactive reflexes indicate hyperkalemia, not hypokalemia.
    2 The pulse would be weak and irregular with hypokalemia because of an impaired conduction system in the cardiac muscles.
    3 Diarrhea is caused by hyperkalemia, not hypokalemia.

306. **2** This fat-binding agent would also bind and eliminate the fat-soluble vitamins such as vitamins A, D, and K. (c) (ME; EV; TC; GI)
    1 This is not a fat-soluble vitamin and would be unaffected.
    3 Same as # 1.
    4 Same as # 1.

307. **3** To avoid symptoms, these clients often refuse to eat and become malnourished; a high-calorie, high-protein diet is advised. (a) (ME; PL; ED; GI)
    1 This is not a problem in Crohn's disease.
    2 Same as # 1.
    4 This is a secondary problem that results from malnutrition; correcting the malnutrition will increase strength.

308. **2** Diabetic mothers have a tendency toward placental insufficiency, which can threaten fetal well-being during labor; an OCT can determine this. (c) (OB; AN; TC; HP)
    1 This would be an assumption; the situation gives no reason to deduce this because the mother had a living child the first time.
    3 OCT does not measure any plasma levels.
    4 This is true, but it is not the reason for doing the test.

309. **1** A semi-Fowler's position will avoid hypotension and is recommended for safety and comfort. (a) (OB; PL; TC; HP)
    2 This position is used for shock or a prolapsed cord, not OCT.
    3 Sims' position would make monitoring very difficult.
    4 Usually no vaginal examination is necessary, and the lithotomy position is very uncomfortable for long periods.

310. **2** This is the definition of a positive OCT result. (c) (OB; AN; TC; HP)
  1 There is no correlation between OCT and a cesarean delivery.
  3 A normal fetal heart rate is 120 to 160.
  4 Other fetal assessment methods should be used before labor is induced.
311. **3** Statistics show that 40% to 60% of the infants develop herpes. (b) (OB; AN; PA; HN)
  1 This is too low; 40% to 60% of the infants develop herpes.
  2 Same as # 1.
  4 This is too high; 40% to 60% of the infants develop herpes.
312. **2** A gown and gloves must be worn to prevent contamination of the nurse from blood or body secretions. (a) (OB; IM; TC; HP)
  1 This is not sufficient protection for the nurse.
  3 A mask is not needed because the virus is not airborne.
  4 Same as # 1.
313. **1** Wound and skin precautions include wearing a gown and gloves; this protects the nurse from the virus. (a) (OB; PL; TC; HP)
  2 This is used for fecal contamination.
  3 This is done for the client's protection, not the nurse's; in caring for a client with herpes the nurse needs to be protected.
  4 A mask is not needed because the virus is not airborne.
314. **4** The virus disintegrates rapidly on contact with soap. (b) (OB; EV; ED; HP)
  1 This is unnecessary; only meticulous hand washing is required.
  2 The lesion is in the genital area, not on the lips; kissing will not affect the infant.
  3 This is not necessary, because soap effectively disintegrates the virus.
315. **4** Vomiting frequently accompanies a head injury because of increased intracranial pressure and stimulation of the vomiting reflex. (a) (PE; AS; PA; NM)
  1 A positive Babinski reflex is normal and expected in a 10-month-old child.
  2 This would be within the normal range for a child this age.
  3 A 10-month-old child would not complain of a headache; persistent vomiting is an objective sign.
316. **2** The buttocks should be elevated just enough to slip a hand underneath; this permits the weight of the body to act as a countertraction. (a) (PE; PL; TC; SK)
  1 This is counterproductive because it eliminates the pull of the traction.
  3 This indicates too much weight is being applied.
  4 Same as # 1.
317. **3** This prevents the pelvis and hips from rotating and places equal stress on the growing extremities. (b) (PE; IM; ED; SK)
  1 This is a description of Russell traction.
  2 This is a description of Buck's extension.
  4 This is a balanced suspension traction that is used for a fractured femur in adults.
318. **1** This is an iron-rich food appropriate for slight anemia, which has probably occurred from blood loss into the tissues at the site of the injury. (b) (PE; IM; TC; BI)

2 This is not necessary unless there is a marked decrease.
  3 If internal bleeding occurred there would have been earlier signs other than a reduction in hemoglobin and hematocrit.
  4 Same as # 2.
319. **3** Calcium promotes osteoblastic activity, and calories support the growth and energy needs of the 2-year-old. (a) (PE; PL; ED; SK)
  1 Extra calories are converted to adipose tissue; if calcium needs are met, sufficient phosphorus will be ingested.
  2 The level of purine does not affect bone repair; a decrease in calories would not support growth and development.
  4 Bone tissue responds to sufficient calcium in the diet; if injury had occurred to the soft tissues, a high-protein diet would be necessary.
320. **2** Clients should know why they are there, what to expect, and what is to be accomplished. (a) (PS; PL; PE; TR)
  1 This would come after the explanation of the purpose of the group.
  3 Same as # 1.
  4 This is not necessary to define; this is a long-term goal.
321. **3** This rejects the behavior, not the client; it helps separate the client from the behavior. (c) (PS; IM; PE; SD)
  1 This does not help the client learn self-control; it rejects both the client and the behavior.
  2 Part of recovery is learning acceptable behavior; ignoring inappropriate behavior does not help.
  4 Isolating clients keeps them from learning more acceptable responses.
322. **4** Sexual anxiety and conflict occur with this disorder; uncertainty is projected onto others to defend the ego. (b) (PS; IM; PE; SD)
  1 The anxious client may not be able to handle being confronted with feelings; this may precipitate a panic reaction.
  2 This avoids the issue and is a threatening response; this could increase anxiety.
  3 This validates ideas of reference and is an inappropriate response.
323. **1** A person who can handle the activities of daily living and function in society is considered mentally healthy. (b) (PS; EV; PE; SD)
  2 Insight into one's problems is of no use if one is unable to function in society.
  3 Everyone uses defense mechanisms; the degree to which they are used determines mental health.
  4 Some anxiety is necessary; anxiety causes problems when it is overwhelming for an extended time.
324. **4** This is characteristic of tardive dyskinesia, an irreversible phenothiazine-induced neurologic disorder. (b) (PS; EV; PE; MO)
  1 This drug would cause sedation, not insomnia.
  2 This is a reversible side effect.
  3 This is unrelated to phenothiazine.
325. **2** Hard candy may produce salivation, which helps alleviate the anticholinergic-like side effect of dry mouth that is experienced with phenothiazine. (b) (PS; EV; ED; MO)
  1 This is unnecessary.
  3 Fluids should be encouraged, not discouraged;

fluids may alleviate the dry mouth.

4 This is unnecessary; although these drugs can cause leukopenia and agranulocytosis, they do not cause thrombocytopenia.

326. **4** Sitting quietly with a severely withdrawn client can provide an opportunity for nonthreatening interaction. (b) (PS; PL; PE; MO)

1 Entering a withdrawn client's body space is intrusive and stressful; it often precipitates a need for further withdrawal.

2 Placing demands on the withdrawn client causes a sense of threat, increased anxiety, and a need for additional withdrawal.

3 The client is unable to deal with even a one-to-one relationship at this time.

327. **3** The nurse offers support and uses clear, simple terms to allay the client's anxiety. (a) (PS; IM; ED; MO)

1 This may be too frightening or confusing to the client.

2 When anxiety is high, the client cannot retain details, and details may lead to added fears.

4 The client generally is kept npo before ECT to prevent aspiration during treatment.

328. **2** This provides for release of tension with no element of competition; success in a simple project increases the sense of accomplishment and worth. (b) (PS; PL; TC; MO)

1 This allows the client to withdraw further.

3 This is too cheerful; this could result in excessive stimuli and increase the client's irritation.

4 The client has psychomotor retardation and may not be able to cope with fine details at this time.

329. **2** Initiating interactions demonstrates that the depressed person is attempting to change behavior patterns. (b) (PS; EV; PE; MO)

1 Clients who attempt to modify behavior to please others make only superficial changes.

3 Avoiding people is a reinforcement of the depressed life-style.

4 Solitary activities are nonthreatening but do not deal with the problem of impaired relationships.

330. **1** Intestinal antibiotics and a complete cleansing of the bowel with enemas until returns are clear are necessary to reduce the possibility of fecal contamination when the bowel is resected. (a) (SU; PL; TC; GI)

2 The bladder will be removed, so there is no need for a Foley catheter.

3 A clear liquid diet is usually prescribed for several days with npo for at least 8 hours before surgery.

4 This is not necessary; there is no evidence of urinary infection.

331. **4** By narrowing the tube, flow rate is reduced and cramping due to distension is lessened. (a) (SU; IM; TC; GI)

1 This is unsafe; this would increase the discomfort.

2 There is no need to discontinue the enema; flow should be slowed or temporarily interrupted until discomfort subsides; an effective enema must be administered before surgery.

3 This would result in the administration of a Harris flush; the purpose of the preoperative enema is to evacuate the bowel of feces, not flatus.

332. **2** Urine should drain continually from the conduit because there is no sphincter control unless a continent conduit is created. (b) (SU; EV; TC; RG)

1 This is expected; the stoma may be swollen and red for several weeks after surgery.

3 This is expected; bowel sounds should be diminished because of anesthesia and intestinal manipulation and surgery.

4 Vomiting is a common occurrence after anesthesia.

333. **3** Nasogastric suction is maintained to prevent pressure on the intestinal anastamosis; no oral fluids are permitted until peristalsis resumes and suction is stopped; giving fluids with suction causes loss of electrolytes. (c) (SU; IM; TC; GI)

1 This has no bearing; the return of peristalsis and removal of the nasogastric tube are determinants.

2 This drains immediately unless it is a continent conduit; this has no bearing on when oral fluids can be started.

4 This would be too long to wait; sips of water are permitted when peristalsis returns and suction is removed; this usually takes 2 to 3 days.

334. **4** The nurse should determine the location, intensity, and other characteristics of the pain before initiating intervention. (a) (SU; EV; TC; NM)

1 Assessment should occur before nursing intervention.

2 This is not specific to pain assessment.

3 Same as # 1.

335. **2** Bed rest weakens the perineal and abdominal muscles used in defecating; ambulation promotes peristalsis and improves muscle tone, thereby facilitating expulsion of flatus and promoting defecation. (a) (SU; PL; PA; RG)

1 Early ambulation will not prevent this complication.

3 Same as # 1.

4 There will be no retention because the surgery involved removal of the bladder and the creation of a permanent urinary diversion.

336. **1** This common response to local anesthesia occurs for a short period because of a fall in the blood pressure. (b) (OB; EV; TC; IP)

2 This could be a response to a developing infection or dehydration, but rarely relates to local anesthesia.

3 This is associated with an allergic response, which is not a common adaptation to a local anesthetic.

4 Same as # 3.

337. **2** This value indicates a highly concentrated urine and requires additional hydration of the client. (a) (OB; IM; PA; IP)

1 This reading is meaningless unless a comparison with other readings indicates a decrease and the possibility of shock.

3 Tinges of blood in the urine may indicate bladder injury and are not related to the client's fluid status.

4 Increasing the IV rate in the presence of urinary suppression would be unsafe because it could cause hypervolemia.

338. **2** The muscular action during ambulation facilitates the return of venous blood to the heart. (a) (OB; IM; PA; PP)

1 This is unrelated; the baby is usually given to the mother in the delivery room to begin the

bonding process.

3 Early ambulation would not prevent this complication.

4 Same as # 3.

339. **3** This is a symptom of separation of the incision; further evaluation should be made because dehiscence is always a possibility. (c) (OB; EV; TC; PP)

1 A sharp, severe pain may result from other causes, and a continuation of the activity even with splinting is unsafe.

2 This would not be done without further evaluation of the source of the pain experienced by the client.

4 This is only part of the assessment; an analgesic would alleviate the pain but would do nothing about the underlying problem.

340. **3** This would indicate that the kidneys are secreting adequate urine and the urinary sphincter tone has not been affected by the catheter. (b) (OB; EV; TC; PP)

1 This indicates retention with overflow; the client urinates small amounts but does not completely empty the bladder.

2 The absence of bacteria indicates the absence of infection but does not portend the return of urinary function.

4 Although the total amount of urine indicates adequacy of kidney function, it does not reflect sphincter control or the possibility of retention.

341. **4** The Harris drip or flush removes accumulated gas in the intestine, which reduces distention of the abdomen. (b) (OB; EV; PA; PP)

1 Stimulating evacuation is not the purpose of a Harris drip; a bowel movement would indicate the procedure was done improperly.

2 The returns of a Harris drip usually contain small amounts of fecal material; it is not for cleansing the bowel.

3 The fluid is not retained; small amounts are instilled slowly and then permitted to return, taking gas with them.

342. **2** Cold causes vasoconstriction and reduces edema; it may also help to reduce fever. (b) (PE; AN; PA; RE)

1 Cold mist is less comfortable, because the environment is cold and damp.

3 Heat dries secretions.

4 Absorption via the mucosa is insignificant and cannot be considered fluid intake.

343. **2** This reduces energy requirements, allows for rest, and lessens the demand for oxygen. (b) (PE; IM; PA; RE)

1 This is not done unless respiratory distress is extremely severe; it increases restlessness and energy demands.

3 Although this loosens secretions in the lungs, it should not be used when the infant is in distress.

4 This positional change will not reduce energy and oxygen demands.

344. **3** The function of sucking requires more oxygen and therefore tires the child. (b) (PE; PL; PA; RE)

1 Parenteral fluids do not provide complete calorie needs.

2 IVs have no effect on vagal stimulation.

4 Laryngospasm, or spasmodic closing of the glottis, which results from edema, is not related to oral feedings.

345. **4** Redness and pain are signs of phlebitis; the site should be changed to avoid further inflammation and possible thrombus formation. (c) (PE; IM; TC; CV)

1 Continuing administration can lead to further irritation and even permanent damage to the vein.

2 Same as # 1.

3 Although this is generally true, there is no indication that this is what is occurring in this situation.

346. **1** Care for an infant after croup should be directed toward good personal care, proper nutrition, and stimulation. (a) (PE; PL; ED; GD)

2 Three-month-old infants need environmental stimuli.

3 The infant does not require additional fluids if all feedings are consumed.

4 Croup is not directly related to antigen-antibody responses.

347. **3** By the standards of normal growth and development the anterior fontanel is known to close between 13 and 18 months of age. (c) (PE; IM; ED; GD)

1 This is too early; early closure may impede the growth of the infant's brain, impairing mental development.

2 Same as # 1.

4 The closure should have occurred by 18 months; delayed closure may indicate neurologic difficulties.

348. **4** This is a reflective statement that conveys acceptance and encourages further communication. (b) (SU; IM; PE; EC)

1 This is false reassurance that does not lessen anxiety.

2 The reliance on a pill to help the client in this instance evades the problem and cuts off further communication.

3 This is too direct; this statement does not encourage the client to discuss his feelings.

349. **4** Inadequate oxygenation can cause premature ventricular contractions. (c) (SU; AN; PA; CV)

1 The reverse is true; postoperative pain can increase the respiratory rate.

2 Hypoxia can precipitate respiratory acidosis; hyperventilation causes respiratory alkalosis.

3 Although this may be true, it does not explain why adequate oxygenation is important.

350. **2** During open heart surgery the conductive system of the heart can be damaged because of the trauma of surgery. (c) (SU; EV; PA; CV)

1 Hypoxia causes tachycardia, not bradycardia.

3 Shock results in a weak rapid pulse, not bradycardia.

4 Congestive heart failure causes a rapid pulse rate, not bradycardia.

351. **3** Sleep deprivation alone can cause these disturbances. (b) (SU; IM; PA; NM)

1 The constant lights of an intensive care unit limit sleep.

2 Pain limits or interrupts periods of sleep and rest.

4 Lack of contact with significant others increases anxiety and feelings of isolation and can lead to disturbances in rest.

352. **1** A cancerous mass can grow into the lumen of the intestines, altering the shape of the stool; stools may be ribbonlike or pencil thin. (a) (ME; AS;

PA; GI)

2 This is not specific to intestinal cancer.

3 Same as # 2.

4 Same as # 2.

353. **4** The intestinal lumen is narrowed by the large mass, and contraction of the proliferate fibrous tissue causes an obstruction. (b) (ME; AS; PA; GI)

1 Diarrhea may occur but usually alternates with constipation.

2 This usually results from a perforation of the bowel that is caused by a buildup of pressure behind the obstruction.

3 Dehydration usually does not occur unless there is severe vomiting and/or diarrhea.

354. **4** This diet is low in fiber, and after digestion and absorption, there is very little substance to be eliminated. (b) (SU; AN; TC; GI)

1 This diet does not affect the bacterial milieu of the intestine.

2 This diet does not promote peristalsis, the products of digestion remain in the intestine longer, and flatus is increased.

3 Although a low-residue diet is less irritating, this is not the primary reason for its use before surgery.

355. **1** This is caused by manipulation of abdominal contents and the depressant effects of anesthesia and analgesics. (a) (SU; AN; PA; GI)

2 An absence of fiber, not fluids, decreases peristalsis.

3 A nasogastric tube decompresses the stomach; it does not cause cessation of peristalsis, with which there is no output.

4 Edema would not totally interfere with peristalsis; edema may cause peristalsis to be less effective but some output would still result.

356. **3** The client's feelings, knowledge, and skills concerning the colostomy must be assessed before discharge. (b) (SU; AN; ED; EC)

1 After a colostomy the client is usually placed on a regular diet and told only to eliminate gas-producing foods.

2 Frequently the client no longer needs a dressing on the incision at this time.

4 Individuals should not be coaxed into doing something they are not ready to do, particularly on a long-term basis.

357. **2** This is an open-ended question that should elicit the desired information. (b) (PE; AS; PE; EC)

1 This is not an open-ended question because it can be answered yes or no.

3 This question can be answered with a yes or no and does not elicit what the child feels about the situation.

4 This may establish that the child knows where she is but does not elicit if she knows why she is there.

358. **3** If there is a trickle of blood from the operative site, the child will swallow frequently; this is usually the first sign of hemorrhage. (b) (PE; EV PA; RE)

1 The child with a sore throat tries very hard not to swallow too much.

2 Swallowing frequently is not a specific reaction to general anesthesia.

4 The child may need suctioning, but the presenting symptoms for this intervention would be restlessness or a color change, such as cyanosis.

359. **4** This would numb the nerve endings and reduce pain; cold also produces vasoconstriction, limits edema, and prevents hemorrhage. (a) (PE; PL; ED; NM)

1 This could dislodge a clot and cause bleeding.

2 Aspirin has anticoagulant properties that could increase the risk of bleeding and should therefore be avoided.

3 Hard candies can scratch the operative site and dislodge the clot and should therefore be avoided.

360. **2** Adenoids can obstruct nasal breathing, interfering with the senses of taste and smell. (b) (PE; EV; PA; RE)

1 Speech should not be affected because the vocal cords are not within the operative area.

3 The vocal cords are outside the operative area; the site should be healed and not cause discomfort when swallowing.

4 The operative site should be healed and not cause discomfort when swallowing.

361. **4** History demonstrates that the client has had a difficult time controlling impulsive behavior and has consistently exhibited poor judgment; this indicates ineffective coping. (a) (PS; AN; PE; PR)

1 This is not an accepted nursing diagnosis.

2 Same as # 1.

3 This is a psychiatric diagnosis, not a nursing diagnosis.

362. **3** The client needs positive relationships with other adults, but clear, consistent limits must be presented to minimize attempts at manipulation. (a) (PS; PL; PE; PR)

1 This is not a therapeutic approach.

2 This is not a therapeutic approach; clear, consistent limits are necessary to prevent manipulation.

4 This is a judgmental attitude that should be avoided.

363. **4** The client is incapable of accepting responsibility for his problems and blames society for his behavior. (b) (PS; AS; PE; PR)

1 This response demonstrates insight, and these individuals rarely develop insight into their problems.

2 Same as # 1.

3 Same as # 1.

364. **3** Ovulation usually occurs 14 days before menses; in a 35-day cycle, ovulation may occur as late as the twenty-first day. (b) (OB; EV; ED; FS)

1 This is the proliferative phase of the cycle; ovulation has not yet occurred.

2 If the woman has a 28-day cycle, ovulation could be expected at this time.

4 The ovum has already passed out of the fallopian tube and can no longer be fertilized.

365. **2** Pelvic rocking exercises, in which the lower back can be pressed onto the floor by contracting the abdominal muscles, reduce back pain. (c) (OB; EV; PA; PN)

1 Leg lifts help to strengthen the abdominal muscles and promote circulation in the lower extremities.

3 Kegel exercises are used to tone pelvic floor muscles.

4 Tailor sitting stretches the muscles of the inner thigh and tones the muscles of the outer thigh.

366. **2** Pain caused by deep penetration by the male partner is common in late pregnancy and can be reduced by using alternative positions such as rear entry. (a) (OB; PL; ED; PN)
    1 This should not be suggested until other alternatives have been tried.
    3 This is unnecessary because this is common during the third trimester.
    4 Douching is not recommended and does not lubricate the vagina; a water-soluble lubricant is more effective.

367. **4** Kegel exercises tone the pelvic floor muscles and prepare the area for the second stage of labor. (c) (OB; IM; ED; PN)
    1 This alleviates backache and strengthens the abdominal muscles.
    2 This helps the abdominal musculature.
    3 Same as # 1.

368. **4** Leakage of fluid could be caused by ruptured membranes, predisposing to an ascending infection and infection of the fetus. (a) (OB; EV; ED; PN)
    1 This is a common discomfort of pregnancy caused by the shift in the center of gravity because of the enlarged uterus.
    2 Leukorrhea is common during pregnancy because of increased vascularity of the cervix and increased production of mucus.
    3 Braxton-Hicks contractions are painless contractions of the uterus occurring at irregular intervals throughout pregnancy.

369. **3** Panting or blowing breathing patterns make it impossible to push. (a) (OB; IM; ED; IP)
    1 This causes respiratory alkalosis and fetal acidosis, which would be undesirable.
    2 Pelvic rocking exercises are used to alleviate backache.
    4 Deep-breathing exercises between contractions increase oxygenation and help maintain relaxation; this is unrelated to pushing.

370. **3** These symptoms, in addition to a history of rheumatic fever, would require an assessment for other cardiopulmonary symptoms. (b) (ME; AS; PA; CV)
    1 Loss of appetite in conjunction with shortness of breath and the history of rheumatic fever make gastrointestinal symptoms secondary in importance.
    2 Anorexia and weight gain do not indicate a nutritional problem but a fluid balance problem.
    4 There is no reason to investigate the gynecologic and sexual history in relation to the current problem.

371. **1** The heart muscle begins to fail, and the muscle does not contract with enough strength to pump sufficient blood to meet the body's metabolic needs. (c) (ME; AN; PA; CV)
    2 Hypervolemia can precipitate congestive heart failure in individuals with a diseased heart, but it is not specific to rheumatic heart disease.
    3 Hypertension and arteriosclerosis can add stress to this situation, but they are not the reason for this client's congestive heart failure.
    4 Heart valves can become stenotic or regurgitant as a result of rheumatic fever; however, congestive heart failure will occur only when the heart can no longer pump an adequate amount of blood to maintain cardiac output.

372. **1** Digoxin slows the heart rate, which is reflected in a slowing of the pulse; it also increases kidney perfusion, which promotes urine formation, resulting in diuresis and decreased edema. (b) (ME; EV; TC; DR)
    2 Digoxin does not increase pulse rate or blood pressure.
    3 Digoxin lowers the pulse rate and produces diuresis as a result of improved cardiac output.
    4 Digoxin will not affect a defective valve or reduce a heart murmur.

373. **4** The major cause of skin cancer is exposure to the sun's ultraviolet light, a form of radiation. (a) (ME; AN; PA; IT)
    1 Although environmental pollutants may have some bearing, they are not considered the major cause of skin cancer.
    2 This is not a causative factor.
    3 Same as # 2.

374. **3** This provides factual information and addresses the client's concern. (b) (ME; IM; PE; EC)
    1 This reinforces the client's fears instead of pointing out reality.
    2 This does not speak to the client's concern and may increase anxiety.
    4 This may provide reassurance but does not permit further exploration of concern.

375. **2** Steroids are used for their antiinflammatory, vasoconstrictive, and antipruritic effects. (b) (ME; EV; ED; DR)
    1 Steroids increase fluid retention.
    3 Steroids increase the incidence of secondary infections by masking symptoms.
    4 Although steroids have an antipruritic effect, their major purpose after surgery is the antiinflammatory effect.

How to Use Worksheet 1: Errors in Processing Information

Common errors in processing information are listed in the left-hand column of this worksheet. At the top of the worksheet is a row of blank spaces for inserting the number of the question missed. Directly below each number, check any errors you made in answering that question. You may have made more than one type of error in an answer.

Worksheet 1: Errors in processing information

Question number																				
Did not read situation/question carefully																				
Missed important details																				
Confused major and minor points																				
Defined problem incorrectly																				
Could not remember terms/ facts/concepts/principles																				
Defined terms incorrectly																				
Focused on incomplete/incorrect data in assessing situation																				
Interpreted data incorrectly																				
Applied wrong concepts/principles in situation																				
Drew incorrect conclusions																				
Identified wrong goals																				
Identified priorities incorrectly																				
Carried out plan incorrectly/incompletely																				
Was unclear about criteria for evaluating success in achieving goals																				

How to Use Worksheet 2: Knowledge Gaps

Types of common knowledge gaps are listed along the top of this worksheet. Write a brief description of topics you want to review in the spaces provided. For example, if you missed a question on administration of a particular drug, write the drug name and problem (e.g., dosage) in the appropriate space under the column labeled *Pharmacology*.

Worksheet 2: Knowledge gaps

Basic science	Skills/ procedures	Basic human needs	Growth & develop-ment	Normal nutrition	Psycho-social factors	Clinical area/ topic	Stressors/ coping mechanisms	Patho-physiology	Pharma-cology	Therapeutic nutrition	Legal implications	Other